# The Clinical Practice of
# Drug Information

*Edited by*

## Michael Gabay, PharmD, JD, BCPS

Director, Drug Information Group
Clinical Associate Professor
University of Illinois at Chicago
Chicago, Illinois

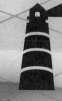

JONES & BARTLETT
LEARNING

*World Headquarters*
Jones & Bartlett Learning
5 Wall Street
Burlington, MA 01803
978-443-5000
info@jblearning.com
www.jblearning.com

Jones & Bartlett Learning books and products are available through most bookstores and online booksellers. To contact Jones & Bartlett Learning directly, call 800-832-0034, fax 978-443-8000, or visit our website, www.jblearning.com.

Substantial discounts on bulk quantities of Jones & Bartlett Learning publications are available to corporations, professional associations, and other qualified organizations. For details and specific discount information, contact the special sales department at Jones & Bartlett Learning via the above contact information or send an email to specialsales@jblearning.com.

05788-1

**Production Credits**
VP, Executive Publisher: David D. Cella
Publisher: Cathy L. Esperti
Associate Editor: Sean Fabery
Associate Director of Production: Julie C. Bolduc
Associate Production Editor: Kristen Rogers
Director of Marketing: Alisha Weisman
Marketing Manager: Grace Richards
Production Services Manager: Colleen Lamy
Rights and Media Manager: Joanna Lundeen
Art Development Assistant: Shannon Sheehan

VP, Manufacturing and Inventory Control:
  Therese Connell
Composition: Cenveo Publisher Services
Cover Design: Kristin E. Parker
Rights and Photo Research Coordinator:
  Ashley Dos Santos
Cover Image: Grid: © immrchris/ShutterStock, Inc.; Swirls:
  © Bocos Benedict/Shutterstock
Printing and Binding: Edwards Brothers Malloy
Cover Printing: Edwards Brothers Malloy

**Library of Congress Cataloging-in-Publication Data**
The clinical practice of drug information / edited by Michael Gabay.
    p. ; cm.
  Includes bibliographical references and index.
  ISBN 978-1-284-02623-8
  I. Gabay, Michael, editor.
  [DNLM: 1. Drug Information Services. 2. Pharmaceutical Services. QV 737.1]
  RA975.5.P5
  362.17'82--dc23
                                        2014049075

6048

Printed in the United States of America
19 18 17 16 15   10 9 8 7 6 5 4 3 2 1

# CONTENTS

**Chapter 5**    **Primary Sources of Information**              **71**

*Joshua L. Conrad, PharmD*

**Chapter 6**    **Introduction to Clinical Study Design**       **87**

*Joshua L. Conrad, PharmD, and Heather A. Pace, PharmD*

**Chapter 7**  **Research Study Design**  **125**

*Lara K. Ellinger, PharmD, BCPS*

**Chapter 14**    **Evidence-Based Medicine**   **253**
*Miki Goldwire, PharmD, MSc, BS, BCPS, and*
*Jason Babby, PharmD, BCPS*

**Chapter 20**   **Medical Writing and Peer Review**   **425**

*Heather J. Ipema, PharmD, BCPS, and Maria G. Tanzi, PharmD*

**Chapter 21**   **Informatics and Clinical Decision Support**   **445**

*Christine D. Sommer, PharmD, MA*

# PREFACE

*The Clinical Practice of Drug Information* was conceived as a core educational resource for faculty, students, and pharmacists with an interest in the key concepts of drug information. These concepts include drug information resources, clinical trial design, biostatistics, and literature evaluation, among others. Drug information as a clinical practice has evolved significantly over the years with the advent of evidence-based medicine and the expanding role of residency-trained drug information specialists into diverse practice settings, such as medication use policy, medication safety, and clinical informatics. This resource was developed to not only educate individuals on traditional drug information topics, but to provide an extensive background on more recent practice areas.

*The Clinical Practice of Drug Information* was developed with the aid of seasoned academics and practitioners from a variety of universities, hospitals and health systems, and companies. Each of the individuals involved in the preparation of this resource has either significant involvement in educating students and/or real-world experience in drug information practice.

## ORGANIZATION OF THE TEXT

*The Clinical Practice of Drug Information* is organized in a manner in which drug information concepts are introduced in a comprehensible fashion and built upon logically throughout the resource. Initial chapters provide an overview and examples of the varying types of drug information resources and the systematic approach to answering drug information requests. These are followed by multiple chapters on clinical study design, biostatistics, and errors in clinical research. Finally, chapters on evidence-based medicine, medication safety, medication use policy, formulary management, medical writing, and informatics provide individuals with an all-encompassing review of these drug information–related topics.

## FEATURES AND BENEFITS

Each chapter includes the following features:

- *Chapter Objectives* present the chapter's desired outcomes to the reader.
- *Chapter Outlines* indicate the topics to be covered in the chapter.
- *Key Terms* help the reader quickly identify critical new terms.

Where appropriate, *Case Studies* have been incorporated; the goal here is to explain the information in a logical manner through case studies that are clear and comprehensible to the student or educator. Other helpful features within the resource include medication use evaluation and formulary templates, an in-depth glossary of terms, a comprehensive index, and an example grading rubric for journal club presentations.

Unique topics within this resource include academic detailing and industry relationships, informatics, and more in-depth coverage of statistical concepts, including noninferiority, correlation and regression, epidemiology and measures of associated risk, and errors in clinical research.

## INSTRUCTOR RESOURCES

Online ancillary materials, including a Test Bank containing potential examination questions, Slides in PowerPoint format presenting the material within the chapters, and an Instructor's Manual, provide added value to educators. These materials should assist individuals responsible for teaching drug information principles in developing and executing their courses.

The provision of drug information remains a key component of pharmacy practice; therefore, practitioners and students require a strong background in drug information concepts. This resource, *The Clinical Practice of Drug Information*, will assist educators, students, and pharmacists with identifying drug information resources, evaluating the biomedical literature, practicing evidence-based medicine, and understanding the growing role of drug information specialists in various areas of pharmacy practice. We hope that this resource is a useful tool for drug information educators, students, and practitioners alike!

Michael Gabay

# ABOUT THE EDITOR

**Michael Gabay, PharmD, JD, BCPS,** is currently a Clinical Associate Professor and Director of the Drug Information Group at the University of Illinois at Chicago (UIC) College of Pharmacy. He received his bachelor of science in pharmacy and doctor of pharmacy degrees from the University of Minnesota. Dr. Gabay completed a pharmacy practice residency at Fairview University Medical Center in Minnesota in 1998 and a specialty residency in drug information at UIC in 1999. Dr. Gabay also completed his doctor of jurisprudence at Loyola University of Chicago College of Law in 2007. He teaches pharmacy students in a drug information and biostatistics course at UIC and is the UIC PGY2 Drug Information Residency Program Director.

# CONTRIBUTORS

Keri C. Anderson, PharmD, BCPS
Assistant Professor
School of Pharmacy
South University
Savannah, Georgia

Jason Babby, PharmD, BCPS
Drug Information Clinical Pharmacy Coordinator
Department of Pharmacy
The Mount Sinai Hospital
New York City, New York

Allison Bernknopf, PharmD, BCPS
Associate Professor
College of Pharmacy
Ferris State University
Kalamazoo, Michigan

Catherine Brown, PharmD, MSM, BCPS
Pharmacist Specialist, Drug Information
MultiCare Health System
Clinical Assistant Professor
School of Pharmacy
University of Washington
Tacoma, Washington

Jamie N. Brown, PharmD, BCPS, BCACP
Drug Information Specialist
Pharmacy Service
Durham VA Medical Center
Durham, North Carolina

Luigi Brunetti, PharmD, MPH, BCPS
Clinical Associate Professor
Ernest Mario School of Pharmacy
Rutgers, The State University of New Jersey
Piscataway, New Jersey
Clinical Pharmacy Specialist in Internal Medicine
Robert Wood Johnson University Hospital Somerset
Somerville, New Jersey

Jacquelyn Bryant, PharmD
Critical Care Pharmacy Specialist
Department of Pharmacy
Georgia Regents Medical Center
College of Pharmacy
University of Georgia
Augusta, Georgia

Christine K. Choy, PharmD, BCPS
Assistant Professor
School of Pharmacy
University of Maryland
Baltimore, Maryland

Sabrina W. Cole, PharmD, BCPS
Medication Policy and Outcomes Director
Intermountain Healthcare
Salt Lake City, Utah

Joshua L. Conrad, PharmD
Director of Patient Safety and Clinical Utility
Epocrates
San Francisco, California

Vern Duba, MA
Clinical Assistant Professor
College of Pharmacy
The University of Iowa
Iowa City, Iowa

Lara K. Ellinger, PharmD, BCPS
Clinical Assistant Professor
College of Pharmacy
University of Illinois at Chicago
Chicago, Illinois

McKenzie C. Ferguson, PharmD, BCPS
Director, Drug Information and Wellness Center
Assistant Professor
Southern Illinois University–Edwardsville
Edwardsville, Illinois

Kelli Garrison, PharmD, BCPS
Manager, Medication Use Policy and Informatics
Adjunct Assistant Professor
South Carolina College of Pharmacy
Medical University of South Carolina
Charleston, South Carolina

Miki Goldwire, PharmD, MSc, BS, BCPS
Associate Professor
Faculty, Drug Information Service
School of Pharmacy
Regis University
Denver, Colorado

Yvette Grando Holman, RPh, PharmD, BCPS
Pharmacy Clinical Supervisor
St. Charles Medical Center
Bend, Oregon
Clinical Affiliate Faculty and Adjunct Faculty
School of Pharmacy
Pacific University–Oregon
Hillsboro, Oregon

Conor Hanrahan, PharmD, BCPS
Drug Information Specialist
Intermountain Healthcare
Salt Lake City, Utah

Evelyn R. Hermes DeSantis, PharmD, BCPS
Clinical Professor
Ernest Mario School of Pharmacy
Rutgers, The State University of New Jersey
Piscataway, New Jersey
Director of Drug Information Services
Robert Wood Johnson University Hospital
Somerville, New Jersey

Heather J. Ipema, PharmD, BCPS
Clinical Assistant Professor
Drug Information Group
College of Pharmacy
University of Illinois at Chicago
Chicago, Illinois

Yash J. Jalundhwala, MS
Research Assistant
Center for Pharmacoepidemiology and Pharmacoeconomic Research
College of Pharmacy
University of Illinois at Chicago
Chicago, Illinois

Vicki R. Kee, PharmD, BCPS
Drug Information Pharmacist
Adjunct Assistant Professor
Iowa Drug Information Service
College of Pharmacy
The University of Iowa
Iowa City, Iowa

Dianne May, PharmD, BCPS
Clinical Associate Professor, Drug Information
Campus Director for Pharmacy Practice Experiences–Augusta
College of Pharmacy
University of Georgia
Augusta, Georgia

Andrea L. McKeever, PharmD, BCPS
Director, Drug Information Center and Residency Program
Associate Professor
School of Pharmacy
South University
Savannah, Georgia

Heather A. Pace, PharmD
Assistant Director, Drug Information Center
Clinical Associate Professor
School of Pharmacy
University of Missouri–Kansas City
Kansas City, Missouri

Alexandra Perez, PharmD, MS
Assistant Professor
College of Pharmacy
Nova Southeastern University
Fort Lauderdale, Florida

Jennifer Phillips, PharmD, BCPS
Assistant Professor
College of Pharmacy
Midwestern University–Chicago
Downers Grove, Illinois

Simon Pickard, PhD
Assistant Director, Center for Pharmacoepidemiology and
    Pharmacoeconomic Research
Associate Professor
College of Pharmacy
University of Illinois at Chicago
Chicago, Illinois

Ryan Rodriguez, PharmD, BCPS
Clinical Assistant Professor
Drug Information Group
College of Pharmacy
University of Illinois at Chicago
Chicago, Illinois

Jennifer C. Samp, PharmD, MS
Senior Manager, Health Economics and Outcomes Research
Abbvie
North Chicago, Illinois

Christine D. Sommer, PharmD, MA
Supervisor, Drug Interactions
Editor, Evaluations of Drug Interactions
FDB (First Databank, Inc.)
St. Louis, Missouri

Joan Stachnik, MEd, PharmD, BCPS
Clinical Associate Professor
College of Pharmacy
University of Illinois at Chicago
Chicago, Illinois

Maria G. Tanzi, PharmD
Clinical Assistant Professor
Drug Information Group
College of Pharmacy
University of Illinois at Chicago
Chicago, Illinois

Erin M. Timpe Behnen, PharmD, BCPS
Director, Drug Information and Wellness Center
Associate Professor
Southern Illinois University–Edwardsville
Edwardsville, Illinois

Sherilyn VanOsdol, PharmD, BCPS
Assistant Professor
Medication Outcomes Center
School of Pharmacy
University of California, San Francisco
San Francisco, California

Kristina E. Ward, PharmD, BCPS
Director, Drug Information Services
Clinical Associate Professor
College of Pharmacy
University of Rhode Island
Kingston, Rhode Island

# REVIEWERS

Leona Blustein, PharmD
Assistant Professor of Clinical Pharmacy
Department of Pharmacy Practice and Pharmacy Administration
University of the Sciences
Philadelphia, Pennsylvania

Mary L. Chavez, PharmD, FAACP
Professor and Chair of Pharmacy Practice
Rangel College of Pharmacy
Texas A&M Health Science Center
Kingsville, Texas

Cathy H. Ficzere, PharmD, BCPS
Associate Professor and Chair of Pharmacy Practice
College of Pharmacy
Belmont University
Nashville, Tennessee

Jennifer Kirwin, PharmD, BCPS
Associate Clinical Professor
School of Pharmacy
Northeastern University
Boston, Massachusetts

Tina Christi Lopez, PharmD, MSc
Associate Professor and Director of the Drug Information Center
Feik School of Pharmacy
University of the Incarnate Word
San Antonio, Texas

# INTRODUCTION TO DRUG INFORMATION PRACTICE

Michael Gabay, PharmD, JD, BCPS
Andrea L. McKeever, PharmD, BCPS

## CHAPTER OBJECTIVES

- ▸ Describe the history of drug information practice.
- ▸ Identify the various practice settings for drug information specialists.
- ▸ Summarize the American College of Clinical Pharmacy (ACCP) Drug Information Practice and Research Network (DI PRN) recommendations for the practice of drug information.
- ▸ Review the core drug information competencies taught as part of pharmacy education.
- ▸ Describe advanced drug information skill sets obtained as part of postgraduate year 1 (PGY1) pharmacy practice and postgraduate year 2 (PGY2) drug information residency training.
- ▸ Discuss future directions and challenges for the clinical practice of drug information.

1

# CHAPTER OUTLINE

# KEY TERMS

Academia                              Drug information residency
Drug information                      Drug information specialist

# INTRODUCTION

The clinical practice of **drug information** involves the efficient retrieval, evaluation, and communication of medication information in order to assist in care decisions, develop evidence-based recommendations, and improve patient outcomes.[1,2] For the majority of pharmacists, the provision of drug information is a routine component of daily practice. For pharmacists with advanced training and/or work experience, drug information is a specialized area of clinical pharmacy practice—a practice area that has been documented to be associated with decreased drug costs and a reduction in hospital mortality rates.[3] The goal of this chapter is to provide a brief overview of the history and evolution of drug information practice and education.

# HISTORY

Drug information as a specific area of pharmacy practice was initially described in the early 1960s. In August 1962, the University of Kentucky opened the doors of the first formal drug information center (DIC) in the United States.[4] The center was conceived as having multiple purposes (**Table 1-1**) and one overarching goal—to "support, assist, and promote a rational drug therapy program" at the University of Kentucky. The center aimed to achieve this goal through educating and influencing current and future healthcare providers with regard to appropriate patient-specific drug selection. The creation of the University of Kentucky DIC marked one of the initial steps in the metamorphosis of the pharmacist from drug distributor to medication therapy expert and integral member of the patient care team.

With the success of the University of Kentucky experience, additional DICs were established throughout the 1960s to the 1980s.[5] According to the results of a survey by Rosenberg and colleagues, the number of pharmacist-operated DICs in the United States reached an apex in 1986 ($n = 127$).[6] However, other survey data reported continued growth in the number of formalized DICs until the early 1990s.[7] The number of operational DICs, particularly long-established university-based centers, has been on the decline over the past few decades. In the last DIC status survey, published by Rosenberg and colleagues in 2009, only 75 formal DICs were still operational.[8] This significant decrease is more than likely due to a confluence of factors, including widespread availability of electronic medication information resources, changes in pharmacy practice and education, and alterations in funding sources.

**TABLE 1-1** Purposes of the University of Kentucky Drug Information Center, Established in 1962

- To be a source of comprehensive drug information for the evaluation and comparison of medications
- To serve as a teaching aid for the various healthcare-related colleges (i.e., medicine, dentistry, nursing, and pharmacy)
- To influence medical students and physicians with regard to selection of appropriate, patient-specific medications
- To influence nurses to collect more information about the medications administered to patients
- To influence pharmacy students with regard to their new role as "drug consultants"
- To become a possible source of drug information for healthcare practitioners throughout Kentucky
- To serve as a potential center for adverse drug event reporting
- To serve as a stimulus for the establishment of other DICs and potentially serve as a training center for the staff within these newly established centers

Data from Parker PF. The University of Kentucky drug information center. *Am J Hosp Pharm*. 1965;22:42-47.

Not only has the number of existing DICs decreased, but the types of services provided have also undergone a transformation. Provision of drug information services on a nonprofit basis and education of healthcare professionals remain key components of the mission statement of most DICs; however, an increasing number of DICs have expanded, or plan to expand, into a variety of fee–for–service activities (**Table 1-2**).[9] Fee-for-service clients may include individual hospitals and health systems, pharmacy benefit management companies, pharmaceutical manufacturers, medical education companies, law firms, community pharmacies, major healthcare corporations, pharmacy schools, and state or federal agencies. Furthermore, drug information specialists themselves have "broken free" from employment specifically within a formal DIC and now practice in a multitude of settings.

**TABLE 1-2** Potential Fee-for-Service Activities Offered by Drug Information Centers

- Responses to individual drug information requests
- Single drug, drug class, and disease state formulary reviews
- Consultative services for pharmacy and therapeutics (P&T) committees
- Disease-specific treatment algorithms and step-care documents
- Continuing education programs for healthcare professionals in various formats (e.g., written, live, webinar)
- Slide kits
- Database development and validation
- Writing projects, including dossiers, standard response letters, manuscripts, newsletters, and posters
- Documents in patient-specific language
- Training programs for sales representatives and medical science liaisons
- Advisory board and consensus conference development
- Drug information and literature evaluation courses

Data from Gabay M. Generate revenue with drug information services. *Pharmacy Purchasing & Products*. 2013;10(5):50, 52.

# PRACTICE SETTINGS

**Drug information specialists** can now be found engaging in the clinical practice of drug information in a variety of settings, including **academia**, institutional health systems, managed care, the pharmaceutical industry, medical writing, and informatics.[1] Specialists often are involved in drug information activities that overlap with other pharmacists and healthcare professionals; however, their advanced training and expertise allows them to more efficiently retrieve, evaluate, and disseminate medication information. In the academic setting, drug information specialists are often engaged in providing didactic and experiential education of pharmacy students, precepting pharmacy residents, managing operational aspects of a formal DIC, and maintaining appropriate resources for the center and college of pharmacy. Didactic education typically includes fundamentals of drug information practice, study design and methodology, principles and clinical application of primary literature evaluation, and evidence-based practice.[10] In addition, topics such as medication safety, medication use policy, and informatics are often incorporated into drug information courses. Experiential education can involve both introductory pharmacy practice experiences (IPPEs) for pharmacy students in their first to third years and advanced pharmacy practice experiences (APPEs) for fourth-year students. These experiences are designed to allow pharmacy students to observe and/or participate in the clinical practice of drug information under the guidance of a drug information specialist. Drug information specialists in an academic setting may also precept both postgraduate year 1 (PGY1) pharmacy practice residents and postgraduate year 2 (PGY2) drug information residents on rotations of varying length and depth. Operational aspects of a formal DIC may include staffing issues, budgetary concerns, contracting, and business development. Finally, maintaining appropriate drug information resources is an area where academic drug information specialists may be heavily involved.[1] In its standards, the Accreditation Council for Pharmacy Education (ACPE) discusses the importance of maintaining adequate library and educational resources within a college of pharmacy in order to meet the needs of faculty and students.[11] The academic drug information specialist within the college is often the point person for this process, because many are intimately familiar with needed references and resources.

In the institutional health system setting, drug information specialists may also be responsible for operating a DIC and responding to drug information requests and precepting students and residents; however, many are also intimately involved in medication use policy and medication safety activities. Drug information specialists often coordinate pharmacy and therapeutics (P&T) committee activities, frequently serve as the secretary of the committee, and participate in subcommittees (e.g., anti-infective, pain, medication safety). These individuals may often be responsible for evaluating new medications for potential formulary inclusion through the development of evidence-based single drug or drug class monographs and present conclusions and/or recommendations to the P&T committee. In addition, drug information specialists in the institutional healthcare system setting may be engaged in performing medication use evaluations, developing criteria for use and treatment protocols, managing drug shortages, participating in adverse drug event reporting, and producing newsletters or other educational documents in order to continuously inform staff of medication therapy changes within the institution. Specialists may also play a role in management of the investigational drug process in some health systems through serving on institutional review boards, evaluating investigational research protocols, or disseminating information related to approved protocols to appropriate healthcare providers.[1]

Within managed care organizations, such as pharmacy benefit managers, specialty pharmacy vendors, government agencies, and health maintenance organizations, drug information specialists participate in a number of activities. Specialists may contribute to formulary management, therapeutic guideline development, prior authorization, step-care programs, disease state management, adverse drug event monitoring, and P&T committee support. In addition, drug information specialists may answer drug information requests from other employees and provide education to patients within the health plan. Counter detailing for healthcare providers and management of Medicare Part D issues may also be significant portions of day-to-day activities in a managed care environment.

Drug information specialists in the pharmaceutical industry setting are often limited to the product labeling when answering drug information requests; off-label information may be provided to healthcare providers only under specified conditions.[1] However, specialists may be involved in areas such as regulatory affairs and drug development, which are unique to industry. Activities commonly performed by drug information specialists in the pharmaceutical industry include:

- Writing and updating global response documents and medical and standard letters
- Updating compendia and drug information resources
- Developing dossiers and slide kits
- Maintaining patient support programs
- Developing direct-to-consumer programs
- Providing literature reviews and product and disease-state training to sales representatives or medical science liaisons
- Writing regulatory documents
- Developing abstracts, posters, and manuscripts from clinical study reports
- Reviewing product promotional materials for accuracy
- Providing medical information support at professional meetings

Although medical writing is an activity performed in most drug information practice settings, some specialists focus solely on medical writing as the core component of their daily practice. Companies that may employ drug information specialists as primarily medical writers include drug information resource publishers (e.g., Wolters Kluwer, Epocrates, Therapeutic Research), medical education companies, and pharmaceutical firms. These companies recognize that literature evaluation, evidence-based practice, and medical writing are skills often inherent to the clinical practice of drug information. In this practice setting, drug information specialists may update existing and develop new therapeutic content for resources, compile grant proposals, and develop manuscripts, posters, and abstracts. In addition, the medical writer may serve as a content editor and reviewer in order to ensure accuracy, appropriateness, and completeness of the written document.

The pharmacy informatics setting is a fairly new area of practice for drug information specialists. These individuals "focus on using technology to improve patient care by combining clinical and technologic skills to create useful applications in health care."[1] Drug information specialists may have a hand in various applications, including computerized physician-order entry (CPOE), electronic health records, clinical decision-support tools, automated dispensing cabinets, telehealth, robotics, barcode drug administration, and drug surveillance.[1,12] In addition, drug information specialists may review the clinical content of various databases or applications developed by informaticists (e.g., *Micromedex®*, *Clinical Pharmacology*, *Lexicomp®*) and are sometimes asked to develop databases for institutional or DIC use.

In 2009, the American College of Clinical Pharmacy (ACCP) Drug Information Practice and Research Network (DI PRN) published an opinion paper on drug information education and practice.[1] Within this opinion paper, the members of the ACCP DI PRN provided recommendations for the practice of drug information in the areas of academia, health systems, managed care, industry, medical writing, and informatics (**Table 1-3**).

| **TABLE 1-3** ACCP DI PRN Recommendations for Drug Information Practice | |
|---|---|
| **Practice Area** | **Recommendations** |
| Academia | • Drug information specialists in academic DICs should have extensive postgraduate training (i.e., pharmacy practice residency plus a drug information specialty residency or equivalent drug information practice experience). <br> • Training of drug information skills to pharmacy students, residents, and practitioners should remain a focal point for academic drug information specialists. <br> • Academic DICs should explore alternative means of financial support, such as fee-for-service activities. |
| Health systems | • Drug information specialists should continue to be intimately involved in therapeutic policy management and consult on challenging drug information inquiries. <br> • Specialists should be engaged in medication safety initiatives, purchasing of drug information resources, and drug shortage management. <br> • Drug information specialists should also evaluate patient outcomes with regard to drug-related policies and potentially become involved in investigational drug services. <br> • Other areas of potential involvement include training employees regarding the availability and use of drug information resources; developing drug alerts for software programs, such as CPOE; and handling difficult reimbursement issues. |
| Managed care | • Organizations that provide traditional drug information services to employees or members should employ a drug information specialist. <br> • Drug information specialists who participate in activities such as formulary management, medication use evaluation, and adverse event monitoring in this setting should have postgraduate training in drug information or managed care. <br> • If no "in-house" drug information or managed care specialist exists, every effort should be made to include at least one such individual in drug information–related activities. |
| Industry | • Individuals who answer drug information requests in this setting should have at least 1 year of specialized drug information residency training. <br> • Drug information specialists within the medical communications department in industry settings should collaborate with individuals within other areas to ensure that all product materials and programs are medically accurate. |

**TABLE 1-3** ACCP DI PRN Recommendations for Drug Information Practice (*Continued*)

| Practice Area | Recommendations |
|---|---|
| Medical writing | • Drug information specialists should only be medical writers if appropriately medically trained.<br>• Specialists should be considered to complete or assist in medical writing tasks. |
| Informatics | • Drug information specialists should collaborate with informaticists to develop useful healthcare applications. |

Data from Bernknopf AC, Karpinski JP, McKeever AL, et al. Drug information: from education to practice. *Pharmacotherapy.* 2009;29(3):331-346.

# PHARMACY CURRICULAR INSTRUCTION

To ensure the quality of pharmacy graduates, the ACPE sets forth standards that schools and colleges of pharmacy must satisfactorily achieve.[11] Included in these standards are 34 sections of curriculum guidance regarding subject matter to be incorporated or covered during students' didactic instruction. Of the 34 curricular guidance sections, 24% (8 of the 34 sections) are drug information competencies and other closely related topics, such as medication safety and informatics (**Table 1-4**).

This general assessment demonstrates the importance of drug information but does not preclude the necessity of other curricular areas, such as pharmacology, medicinal chemistry, and therapeutics, which establish the foundational pharmacy knowledge base.

Additionally, drug information is highly emphasized throughout the experiential education component of pharmacy education, allowing pharmacy students to apply information learned in the classroom setting to clinical practice. A sample of drug information activities requested for inclusion by ACPE into IPPEs and APPEs is provided in **Table 1-5**.[11]

Note the active language associated with the activities in Table 1-5. The tasks extend beyond memory and recall to implementation. For example, pharmacy students may initially be engaged in simple drug information question research for IPPEs while transitioning to more complex activities, such as assisting with the formulary process, during APPEs. The activities of drug information question research require a basic

**TABLE 1-4** ACPE Drug Information–Related Curricular Areas

1. Biostatistics
2. Drug information (retrieval and application of information)
3. Economics/pharmacoeconomics
4. Informatics
5. Literature evaluation and research design
6. Medication safety
7. Pharmacoepidemiology
8. Professional communication

Data from Accreditation Council for Pharmacy Education. Accreditation standards and guidelines for the professional program in pharmacy leading to the doctor of pharmacy degree. https://www.acpe-accredit.org/pdf/FinalS2007Guidelines2.0.pdf. Accessed July 15, 2014.

**TABLE 1-5**    ACPE Introductory and Advanced Pharmacy Practice Experience Drug Information–Related Activities

1. Responding to drug information inquires
2. Identifying and reporting medication errors and adverse drug reactions
3. Managing the medication use system and applying the systems approach to medication safety
4. Managing the use of investigational drug products
5. Participating in the health system's formulary process
6. Performing prospective and retrospective financial and clinical outcomes analyses to support formulary recommendations and therapeutic guideline development

Data from Accreditation Council for Pharmacy Education. Accreditation standards and guidelines for the professional program in pharmacy leading to the doctor of pharmacy degree. https://www.acpe-accredit.org/pdf/FinalS2007Guidelines2.0.pdf. Accessed July 15, 2014.

understanding of pharmacy databases and search techniques; however, reviewing a drug for formulary consideration includes performing literature searches for clinical trials and assessing the study design, statistics, outcomes, medication safety, and pharmacoeconomic data. Although drug information research is similar between IPPE and APPE activities, the knowledge and skill for information assessment increases in complexity with advanced training.

# RESIDENCY TRAINING

Postgraduate residency training offers additional opportunities for drug information skill set development and refinement. For pharmacy graduates seeking advanced training as part of a PGY1 residency, drug information–related activities are identified as components of the American Society of Health-System Pharmacists' (ASHP) educational outcomes. For instance, the first and sixth required educational outcomes focus on patient care through the provision of drug information (e.g., evidence-based medicine, reducing medication misadventures, researching drug information inquires); these outcomes focus on managing and improving the medication-use process and utilization of medical informatics.[13] PGY1 pharmacy residents are actively engaged in "on-the-job training" for clinical pharmacy practice and rely on drug information to quickly identify effective solutions to patient care issues. For example, the medication safety team at a hospital reported increased adverse events associated with vancomycin. The report prompted a medication use evaluation by the PGY1 pharmacy resident who discovered that the reactions were infusion related, because the infusion pumps were not programmed with "guardrails," or maximum infusion rate parameters. Therefore, the PGY1 resident worked with the informatics pharmacist to program the "guardrails" and performed follow-up nursing education on maximum infusion rates for vancomycin. The drug information skills utilized by the PGY1 resident included the employment of a medication use evaluation to discern the etiology of the adverse events, the implementation of a workable solution for the avoidance of subsequent medication misadventures, and the education of the healthcare team regarding the informatics pump "guardrail" solution.

A PGY2 residency in drug information further emphasizes the importance of efficient and safe medication-use processes and medical informatics through the use of drug information knowledge and skills.[14] Additionally, the practice involves a more global approach to patient care, because the PGY2 drug information resident may be involved in trending non-formulary-drug use as part of formulary management for the institution, writing newsletters or articles on drug-related topics for patients and/or healthcare providers, and meeting with pharmaceutical industry representatives as part of P&T committee activities.

# FUTURE DIRECTIONS AND CHALLENGES

As noted within the ACCP DI PRN recommendations, there is an increasing push for extensive postgraduate training for drug information specialists. More and more, potential employers are looking for drug information specialists to not only complete a specialty **drug information residency** and/or fellowship, but also a general pharmacy practice residency. These employers note that a solid clinical foundation in direct patient care, in addition to literature evaluation, medical writing, and evidence-based practice skills, is an essential component to drug information practice in most settings. Even though the pharmacy job market has become more saturated, particularly in urban areas, appropriately trained drug information specialists remain in high demand with multiple career options available. The reason for this demand is quite simple—a shortage of residency-trained drug information specialists continues to exist. Many graduates of pharmacy schools do not even consider drug information as a career path, focusing on "direct patient care" residency programs and clinical positions instead. Drug information specialists need to actively promote and share their work experiences and activities with pharmacy students and PGY1 residents in order to spur interest in this career path. Drug information specialists affect patient care on a daily basis on both individual (i.e., answering drug information requests) and population (i.e., monitoring adverse events, developing criteria for use or guidelines) levels. In addition, the skill sets of a drug information specialist can be transferable to a variety of different settings throughout a career.

As noted earlier, many formal DICs have closed over the past decade, and those that are currently in existence are looking for ways to expand and charge for services. Expansion efforts are often challenging.[9] Gaining initial access to potential clients for drug information services may be difficult, and economic changes or reorganizational efforts, particularly in the pharmaceutical industry, can affect the consistency of work from those sources. Balancing unpaid yet time-consuming teaching and other faculty requirements against client responsibilities can be daunting for specialists within an academic-based DIC. In addition, recruiting appropriately trained individuals for drug information positions can often be a complex process, with many pharmacists lacking suitable educational and training backgrounds, as mentioned earlier. In order to establish a fee-for-service DIC, drug information specialists need to take into account the amount of time and effort required to identify potential clients and develop contractual relationships. Having individuals who are comfortable networking and interacting with potential clients is key. In addition, drug information specialists need to think creatively and develop services that clients may not have even considered or that are outside the specialists' "wheelhouse" in order to be successful at transitioning to a revenue-generating DIC.

With the decline in formal DICs, drug information specialists have begun to take footholds in other areas outside traditional drug information, including medication use policy, medication safety, and informatics. The ASHP has recognized this change in drug information practice and has added required objectives related to medication use policy and medication safety to the standards for all accredited PGY2 drug information residency programs.[14] In addition, more PGY2 drug information residencies are adding electives in informatics. Drug information specialists are also starting new residency training programs that are specifically geared toward these growing areas of practice. The numbers of these programs are currently limited; however, continued expansion is almost guaranteed.

## SUMMARY

The core of the clinical practice of drug information remains the efficient retrieval, evaluation, and communication of medication information in order to enhance the appropriate use of patient-specific drug therapy and improve outcomes. Historically, drug information specialists provided services within formal DICs; however, as the number of such centers has decreased, specialists have branched out into other practice areas, including health systems, industry, managed care, medical writing, and informatics. In addition, drug information–related activities have also expanded into medication use policy and medication safety, among others. The skills of appropriately trained drug information specialists remain in high demand within the pharmacy marketplace, demonstrating the continued need for such professionals.

## REFERENCES

1. Bernknopf AC, Karpinski JP, McKeever AL, et al. Drug information: from education to practice. *Pharmacotherapy*. 2009;29(3):331-346.
2. ASHP guidelines on the provision of medication information by pharmacists. *Am J Health-Syst Pharm*. 1996;53(15):1843-1845.
3. Bond CA, Raehl CL, Franke T. Clinical pharmacy services and hospital mortality rates. *Pharmacotherapy*. 1999;19(5):556-564.
4. Parker PF. The University of Kentucky drug information center. *Am J Hosp Pharm*. 1965;22:42-47.
5. Amerson AB, Wallingford DM. Twenty years' experience with drug information centers. *Am J Hosp Pharm*. 1983;40(7):1172-1178.
6. Rosenberg JM, Martino FP, Kirschenbaum HL, Robbins J. Pharmacist-operated drug information centers in the United States—1986. *Am J Hosp Pharm*. 1987;44(2):337-344.
7. Beaird SL, Coley RMR, Crea KA. Current status of drug information centers. *Am J Hosp Pharm*. 1992;49(1):103-106.
8. Rosenberg JM, Schilit S, Nathan JP, Zerilli T, McGuire H. Update on the status of 89 drug information centers in the United States. *Am J Health-Syst Pharm*. 2009;66(19):1718-1722.
9. Gabay M. Generate revenue with drug information services. *Pharmacy Purchasing & Products*. 2013;10(5):50, 52.
10. Phillips JA, Gabay MP, Ficzere C, Ward KE. Curriculum and instructional methods for drug information, literature evaluation, and biostatistics: survey of US pharmacy schools. *Ann Pharmacother*. 2012;46(6):793-801.
11. Accreditation Council for Pharmacy Education. Accreditation standards and guidelines for the professional program in pharmacy leading to the doctor of pharmacy degree. https://www.acpe-accredit.org/pdf/FinalS2007Guidelines2.0.pdf. Accessed July 15, 2014.
12. ASHP statement on the pharmacist's role in informatics. *Am J Health-Syst Pharm*. 2007;64:200-203.
13. American Society of Health-System Pharmacists. Accreditation standard for postgraduate year one (PGY1) pharmacy residency programs. http://www.ashp.org/DocLibrary/Accreditation/ASD-PGY1-Standard.aspx. Accessed July 15, 2014.
14. American Society of Health-System Pharmacists. Educational outcomes, goals, and objectives for postgraduate year two (PGY2) pharmacy residencies in drug information. http://www.ashp.org/menu/Accreditation/ResidencyAccreditation.aspx. Accessed July 15, 2014.

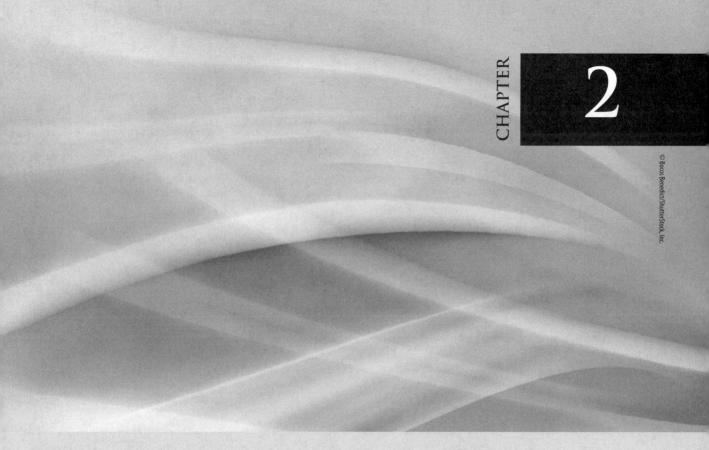

## CHAPTER 2

# THE SYSTEMATIC APPROACH TO RESPONDING TO DRUG INFORMATION REQUESTS

Jamie N. Brown, PharmD, BCPS, BCACP
Christine K. Choy, PharmD, BCPS

## CHAPTER OBJECTIVES

▸ Describe how the demographics of a requestor can affect the drug information response.

▸ Identify appropriate background questions necessary for determining the ultimate drug information question.

▸ Categorize the ultimate question of the drug information request in order to identify resources with the highest likelihood of containing appropriate information.

▸ Construct an appropriate search strategy using tertiary, secondary, and primary resources when researching a drug information response.

▸ Describe the process of prioritizing resources based on the implied strength of evidence.

> ▸ Determine the appropriate mode of communication for a drug information response and describe the characteristics of a complete response.
> ▸ Explain the purpose of follow-up after responding to a drug information request.
> ▸ Identify mechanisms to assess the quality of drug information services.

## CHAPTER OUTLINE

| | |
|---|---|
| Introduction | Legal and Ethical Considerations |
| Receive | Continuous Quality Improvement |
| Research | Summary |
| Respond | References |
| Record | |

## KEY TERMS

| | |
|---|---|
| Background information | Requestor |
| Categorization | Research |
| Demographics | Respond |
| Receive | Ultimate question |
| Record | |

# INTRODUCTION

In 1975, Watanabe and colleagues created a framework to teach student pharmacists about the process of responding to drug information requests in preparation for their clerkship rotations. The authors published a primer that outlined a five-step process, or systematic approach, for answering a drug information question.[1] In 1980, Fischer published a brief commentary about the systematic approach and recommended modifications to this process with the addition of two steps.[2] This seven-step process became known as the *modified systematic approach* and remains foundational to the practice of drug information.

The modified systematic approach is valuable in that it provides organization and consistency in the teaching and practice of drug information. However, a formulaic approach to drug information practice is not particularly useful. In response to Fischer's commentary, Watanabe wrote that answering a drug information question involves communication, which is a "dynamic process ... [and] no systematic approach can be applicable to all situations."[3] Strict adherence to the precise wording and sequence of the modified systematic approach is not necessary to capture the principles and intended outcomes of the process. It is possible to simplify the methodology to include four important and distinct actions related to the processing of a drug information request: (1) **receive**, (2) **research**, (3) **respond**, and (4) **record**. These four Rs implicitly follow the steps outlined in the modified systematic approach but retain flexibility in the application of these principles to specific pharmacy practice settings.

# RECEIVE

## RECEIVING THE DEMOGRAPHICS OF THE REQUESTOR

Drug information requests are received by a pharmacist or drug information service through different methods of communication: verbal requests via the telephone, voice mail, or verbal consults; written correspondence via email, postal mail, fax, or an electronic consult process; or personal interactions via an individual serving as an intermediary. Regardless of the mechanism of the request, the pharmacist must first obtain both the specific drug information question being asked and the demographic information of the **requestor**. The importance of successfully obtaining the **demographics** of the requestor is twofold. First, one must be able to identify the appropriate mode of communication in order to effectively respond to the drug information question. Without this key piece of information, the clinician may not be able to appropriately reply to the requestor in a timely manner, which the requestor will perceive as poor service, and the time and effort of the pharmacist will not be optimally utilized. The demographic information that should be obtained for each drug information request includes the requestor's name, department, affiliation, degree, address, email address and/or phone, fax, pager number, and any other identifiable contact information. The use of a structured drug information documentation form may be helpful in systematically obtaining this information (**Figure 2-1**).

Obtaining the requestor's affiliation, practice setting, and credentials will also identify basic descriptive information about the educational background, specialty training, and expected clinical knowledge of the requestor. This allows the pharmacist to assess the requestor's background knowledge of the drug information question submitted. For example, if the pharmacist were asked a question regarding the appropriate use of a novel inhaler device, the terminology and level of detail included in the response would vary if the requestor were a physician with advanced training in pulmonary medicine compared to a registered nurse conducting medication reconciliation in the emergency department or a patient without formal medical education. Identification of the requestor's demographic information allows the pharmacist to appropriately customize and individualize the response.

## RECEIVING THE BACKGROUND INFORMATION

After obtaining the initial question and the demographic information of the requestor, it is important to identify the requestor's specific need by obtaining pertinent **background information**. This is a critical step in the systematic process and can dramatically affect the direction of the response. This step is particularly important because the initial question posed by the requestor may not completely correspond with the true drug information need. In other words, the initial question asked may be different from the question that will ultimately be answered. This discrepancy exists for a number of reasons. For example, the requestor may miss or omit important details in the original request because the requestor may be unfamiliar with the drug information service or with how to ask the drug information question in an appropriate fashion. Or a practitioner may omit information that is vital to the drug information request in an effort to expedite the request process, whether because of the scheduling demands of a busy clinical practice or due to the inherent vulnerability associated with requesting advice from a pharmacist. Conversely, the requestor may include unnecessary details or phrase the question in an indirect or disorganized fashion. The pharmacist must identify pertinent background variables in order to define the true drug information need. Thus, it is important to obtain additional background information from the requestor through open dialogue. It is through this dialogue that the pharmacist can minimize potential discrepancies between the initial question asked and the true drug information need. In clinical practice, trainees and practitioners with limited clinical experience often have difficulty formulating a complete list of appropriate background questions. If the collected information is incomplete, it may be necessary to contact the requestor again

**Drug Information Request Form**

Reference #:_____ Date:_____ Time:_____ Phone/Pager/Email/Walk-in
Requestor Name:_____ Dept/Facility/Affiliation:_____
Contact Information: _____ Request Received by: _____

Requestor Status:
_____ Attending MD
_____ Med Student/Intern/Resident
_____ Pharmacist/Tech/Student
_____ Nurse/NP
_____ Physician Assistant
_____ Fellow
_____ Other HCP
_____ Other: _____

Request Classification:
_____ Product ID
_____ General Product Info
_____ Availability
_____ ADR
_____ Drug Interaction
_____ Therapeutic Evaluation
_____ Dose Recommendation
_____ Stability/Compatibility
_____ Pregnancy/Lactation
_____ Toxicology/Poisoning
_____ Abuse/Addiction
_____ Investigational Drugs
_____ Formulary Question
_____ Herbal
_____ Other: _____

Affiliation:
_____ Health-System
_____ Outpatient Clinic
_____ University Affiliate
_____ Other: _____

Drug Information Request:_____
_____

References requestor has already used: _____

Background Info:


Answer needed: ____Urgent; ____<24 hr ___<1 week ___no rush; Specific date/Time: _____

Response to Question: _____
_____

**References Searched:** (Please list)

**References Used in Response:** (Please list)


Researched by: _____          Research Time: _____
Response Given by: _____         Response Reviewed by: _____
Response Received by: _____    Date/Time: _____

Attempts made to contact requestor:
Date/Time                                Caller
_____                    _____
_____                    _____

**FIGURE 2-1** Sample drug information request form.

in order to inquire about additional background details related to the request. The ability to ask appropriate background questions during the initial encounter will improve as the pharmacist gains experience in this practice environment. Foundational questions used for obtaining background information are included in **Table 2-1**. Although the foundational questions listed in Table 2-1 may not universally apply to every drug information request, the pharmacist should be able to use these concepts to obtain the appropriate background information needed for each individual question.

When obtaining background information, the clinician should identify whether the drug information question is academic (for the general knowledge of the requestor) or patient specific (related to a patient-care scenario). This is an important distinction,

**TABLE 2-1** Foundational Questions Used for Obtaining Background Information for a Drug Information Request

| |
|---|
| Does this question pertain to a specific patient? If so, what is the patient-specific information (e.g., age, height, weight, past medical history, etc.)? |
| What is the context for the use of this medication (e.g., indication, strength, dosage form, etc.)? |
| How is this medication typically used in practice? |
| Are there special factors related to this question that should be considered? |
| How will the response to this question be applied in clinical practice? |
| What type of information or response is the requestor looking for? |
| What resources have already been used, and what was found in those resources? |

because a patient-specific question may require additional information, such as the patient's age, sex, weight, condition being treated, past medical history, allergies, concomitant medications, and preferred dosage form. A more complete understanding of the patient's current medical situation will allow for a more thorough and directed response to the patient-specific drug information request. In addition, questions that are not patient specific still often arise from clinical situations, and therefore a more thorough understanding of the origin of the question, as well as how it may be applied to clinical practice, will often help in determining the requestor's ultimate question. For example, it is not uncommon for a pharmacist to receive a question similar to the following: "I need to prescribe doxycycline for Ms. Smith in clinic. What dose would you recommend?" On initial inspection, the question appears to be straightforward, with a simple request for drug dosing. But upon further analysis, this question is not clearly defined. Many details are missing that are essential for assessing the ultimate question and determining the appropriate search strategy and response. Specifically, the pharmacist would need to identify background information regarding the specific indication for using doxycycline and whether the patient has any contraindications or comorbid conditions that would affect its use. This may include questions pertaining to the patient's age, allergies, interacting concomitant medications, pregnancy or breastfeeding status, or ability to swallow oral medications. If the pharmacist would have given the clinician a dose recommendation for treating inflammatory lesions of rosacea without knowing that the patient was being treated for the tick-borne infection Rocky Mountain spotted fever, the pharmacist may have given a recommendation that was incorrect and, if implemented, expose the patient to potential harm. Or there is the potential that the pharmacist may realize that there are multiple indications for the therapeutic use of doxycycline and create an expansive and comprehensive review of all possible indications for doxycycline and its respective dosing strategies. Thus, the treatment for Rocky Mountain spotted fever would have been included in the response and potentially answered the requestor's ultimate question, but this strategy would have been exceptionally inefficient and the workload associated with responding to this request could have been reduced significantly by initially obtaining the appropriate background information.

As a part of obtaining background information for a drug information request, the pharmacist should also determine if the requestor has already reviewed resources or completed background research on the topic. This information has the potential to avoid duplication of effort. Still, the pharmacist should be cautious about overestimating the value of previously conducted research. Even though a requestor may have reviewed a resource prior to contacting the pharmacist, it is often difficult to determine whether the requestor appropriately utilized the reference. If the requestor is able to verbally describe the references used and summarize the information gathered, the pharmacist will be less likely to duplicate the information when giving the response. However, the same resource may be consulted to gather additional information. For example, if the requestor conducted a prior literature search using the secondary resource MEDLINE and found one appropriate article, this does not imply that the pharmacist should not conduct an independent review of the biomedical literature. Instead, a literature review could be conducted using the MEDLINE database, but utilizing a different search strategy. Or the pharmacist may search additional secondary resources. Although the knowledge of the requestor's research strategy may have little overall impact on the pharmacist's search strategy, it does introduce an additional mechanism to further determine the baseline sophistication of the requestor. With the additional information obtained when identifying the demographics of the requestor, the pharmacist will continue to develop the direction of the drug information response, including the depth of information and technical language to use when responding to the drug information request.

Determination of the time frame for which the drug information response is needed is the final step of obtaining background information. Response time frames are typically categorized as urgent (as soon as possible), rush (< 1 day), low urgency (< 1 week), or no specific time frame requested. Regardless of the chronological order that drug information questions are obtained, determining the requested response time frame will assist in prioritizing the order of responses to best meet the needs of the individual requestors. The pharmacist should respond to drug information requests based on the urgency of need, rather than the order in which the requests were received.

## RECEIVING THE ULTIMATE QUESTION AND CATEGORIZATION

Clarifying the question asked through the procurement of background information is a critical step in the systematic approach and is essential in the development of an efficient drug information response. If one can truly answer the question, "Why is the requestor asking for this information?" then adequate background information has been obtained. A pharmacist may also utilize a structured response form that includes the use of specific background questions that may be useful in the identification of background information. When implemented in clinical practice, the use of a structured drug information response form dramatically improved the ability of trainees to obtain appropriate background information, as well as the ability to correctly identify the **ultimate question**.[4] Whether or not a structured response form is utilized, it is essential that specific and pointed questions are asked to clarify the initial question and determine the requestor's ultimate question. This will improve the efficiency of the search and may improve the quality and utility of the drug information response. Example questions used for obtaining background information for a drug information request were identified in Table 2-1. Thus, whether the question is academic or patient specific, both the requestor and the pharmacist must understand and be in agreement about the ultimate question. If possible, the ultimate question should be rephrased and repeated back to the requestor for final approval and acknowledgment. This step should be completed while in direct communication with the requestor.

After determining and confirming the ultimate question with the requestor, the drug information question should then be categorized. **Categorization** of the drug information question will aid in refinement of the search strategy and selection of the

| TABLE 2-2   Categorization Examples |
| --- |
| Abuse/addiction |
| Adverse drug reaction/contraindication |
| Cost/pharmacoeconomics |
| Drug interaction (drug/food/disease) |
| Formulary question |
| General product information |
| Herbal/alternative medicine |
| Investigational drugs |
| Legal/regulatory |
| Patient education |
| Pharmacokinetics/dose recommendation |
| Pharmacogenomics |
| Pregnancy/lactation |
| Product identification |
| Stability/compatibility |
| Therapeutic evaluation |
| Toxicology/poisoning |
| Other: _____ |

most appropriate resource. It requires assessment of the general type of question that is being asked and prompts the researcher to identify the most reputable sources of drug information for the given category. For example, a drug information request categorized as an "adverse drug reaction" would require the implementation of a different search strategy and resources than the classification of a "pregnancy" or "drug interaction" request. The ability to differentiate and categorize the drug information question is important, because no one resource is able to answer all drug information requests. Instead, the pharmacist must be able to recognize the type of information requested and accurately categorize it in order to assist in the identification of the most appropriate resources for the given question. Common categories for drug information questions are included in **Table 2–2**.

## SOLICITATION OF DRUG INFORMATION REQUESTS THROUGH INTERMEDIARIES

In a dynamic clinical environment, it is common for drug information requests to be solicited not from the originator or end user of the request, but through an intermediary such as a nurse, pharmacist, student, or healthcare support staff member. This occurs when the originating practitioner is not able to directly make the request because of the demands of clinical practice or is not aware of the services of a drug information practitioner. Although requests for drug information services through intermediaries are legitimate drug information questions, these requests often pose a special challenge. When a drug information question is asked through another individual, there is often the possibility that the information may not be correctly translated to the drug information clinician. In addition, the intermediary may not be well versed in obtaining appropriate background details or may be given an incomplete picture of the question. Lastly, the intermediary may potentially have less medical education or experience from which to make an appropriate drug information request. This is a particularly important consideration when drug information requests originate from a specific patient case.

When interacting with an intermediary, it is the responsibility of the pharmacist to receive the drug information request, obtain the appropriate background information, and determine whether additional background information is needed to adequately research and respond to the request. If additional information is necessary, and the intermediary is not able to provide this, one must decide whether to request the intermediary to obtain the additional information or to contact the originator of the drug information request directly for the additional information. This decision should be based on the type, sophistication, and quantity of information necessary, as well as the professional relationship between the drug information clinician, the intermediary, and the originator of the request. This decision must also be made on a case-by-case basis. A similar process should also be undertaken when deciding the best approach for responding to the drug information request.

## RESEARCH

After receiving the drug information question, the pharmacist should review appropriate drug information and medical resources and gather the most reputable information to inform the final recommendation. **Figure 2–2** outlines an appropriate general search strategy for the vast majority of drug information requests. The search strategy should begin with a review of the tertiary literature, including reputable drug information

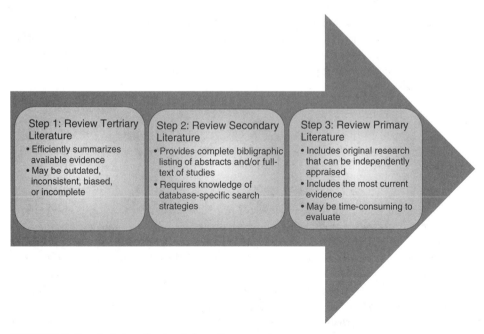

**FIGURE 2-2** Search strategy for drug information requests.

databases. Tertiary resources may provide sufficient information to answer many drug information questions and are particularly useful to inform questions related to drug identification, dosing, administration, storage, stability, equivalency, and availability. These resources are also useful to inform basic questions regarding pharmacology, pharmacokinetics, and labeled indications. In order to select the most appropriate tertiary source with which to begin the search, the pharmacist must refer to the categorization of the drug information question (established in the receive step discussed previously). Most categories are associated with a set of reliable, peer-reviewed tertiary resources, and the efficiency and effectiveness of the search will be greatly enhanced by starting with the tertiary resource that corresponds with the appropriate drug information category. It is also important to verify the accuracy and completeness of tertiary information by searching multiple tertiary sources. Because tertiary resources summarize information from primary sources, the information may be incomplete or may conflict with other sources. Searching and evaluating multiple tertiary sources of drug information will improve the quality of the review.

Information found in tertiary resources may be sufficient to completely answer a drug information question. If this is the case, research is complete, and the pharmacist may begin the process of responding to the question. However, as mentioned earlier, tertiary sources may be outdated, incomplete, or inadequate to completely answer a drug information question. If additional information is required, it is useful to transition the search to secondary resources, including databases like MEDLINE or Embase, which abstract the medical literature. The vast majority of secondary literature databases are available in electronic format, and many provide tutorials focusing on the most effective way to retrieve information from the database in order to optimize the searching technique. In addition, when the drug information question is related to a clinical or patient care scenario, the pharmacist may refine the search strategy by employing the PICO process.[5] PICO is a mnemonic that defines four key components of an answerable clinical question, and each term in the mnemonic is described in **Figure 2–3**. In order to conduct an effective search of the secondary literature, it is useful to frame the clinical question using the PICO method. For most patient-related drug information questions, it is possible to define each term in the PICO process; these terms can be used as Medical Subject Heading (MeSH) terms or keywords in the secondary database search.

A search of the secondary literature will lead to identification of published primary literature, but not all retrieved primary literature will be useful to inform the final recommendation. In order to prioritize the primary literature review, it is helpful to apply principles of evidence-based practice. Evidence-based practice is based on the

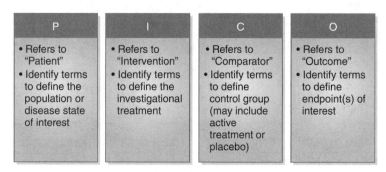

**FIGURE 2-3** PICO method of constructing an answerable clinical question.

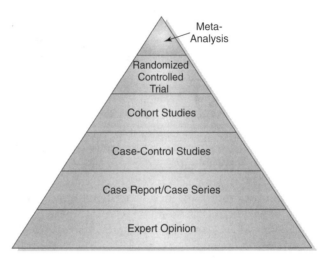

**FIGURE 2-4** Hierarchy of study types to inform clinical decisions.

principle that there is a hierarchy of study types to inform clinical decisions. As described in **Figure 2-4**, this hierarchy favors studies that (1) demonstrate causation over association and (2) minimize bias and confounding. Therefore, when reviewing the primary literature to inform a clinical decision, it is useful to prioritize experimental studies (e.g., randomized controlled trials) over observational studies (e.g., cohort studies, case-control studies), descriptive studies (e.g., case series, case reports), and expert opinion. Evidence-based practice also assumes that there is a hierarchy of study outcomes (**Figure 2-5**). Outcomes that evaluate mortality or morbidity, such as hospitalization, exacerbation of disease, or effects on quality of life, are often known as *clinical outcomes* or *patient-oriented evidence that matters* (POEMs), whereas outcomes that evaluate surrogate markers of disease are often known as *disease-oriented evidence* (DOEs).[6] Surrogate markers of disease are often laboratory values or physical signs that are substituted for clinically meaningful endpoints. Examples of surrogate markers include measures such as blood pressure, the cholesterol panel, or the minimal inhibitory concentration (MIC) of an antibacterial agent. When DOEs are found to be validated measures of disease severity, they are sometimes called *disease-oriented evidence that matters* (DOEMs).[6] In order to select the most useful primary literature to inform the clinical decision, it is useful to prioritize studies that evaluate POEMs over those that evaluate DOEMs. When evaluating primary literature to determine its usefulness in answering a clinical question, it is advantageous and practical to first review studies that evaluate POEM-level evidence (studies that evaluate morbidity and mortality) before reviewing studies that evaluate DOE/DOEM-level evidence (studies that evaluate surrogate endpoints). Other important factors to aid in the prioritization of the primary literature review are summarized in **Table 2-3**.

Overall, there are many sources of drug information that will be useful in the search process. Employing effective search strategies will improve the quality and efficiency of the research and the timeliness of the final response.

## RESPOND

After gathering the best evidence, it is necessary to critically evaluate the information and to synthesize a final response or recommendation for the drug information question. An appropriate response should not be limited to a simple summary of the research

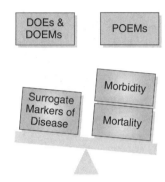

**FIGURE 2-5** Importance of study outcomes to inform clinical decisions.

or an unfiltered list of possible answers to the question. The responsibility of the pharmacist is to critically appraise the information gathered, objectively weigh the evidence, and thoughtfully articulate a well-reasoned answer. Depending on the setting and need, responses may be verbal or written. Regardless of the mode of communication, the drug information response should begin with a restatement of the ultimate question that was determined in the receive step of the systematic approach. This reorients the requestor to the question and frames the response. The response should be presented in a structured format, including an introduction or discussion of the background information on the topic, supporting evidence for any recommendations made, and a conclusion. In addition, responses should be timely, accurate, objective, well organized, concise, and complete. An appropriate response should also consider the pharmacist's scope of practice. A pharmacist practicing in a drug information center or serving in an indirect consultative role may limit the response to an objective appraisal of the data, in order to allow the requestor to make an informed decision. In contrast, pharmacists with direct patient care responsibilities often need to consider patient-related variables and provide a definitive clinical recommendation. Finally, the ideal response will anticipate associated needs and follow-up questions. For example, a response to a question about the first-line treatment options for a particular disease should also include information about monitoring parameters for the recommended treatment. Similarly, a response to a question about the identification of a foreign medication should also include information about therapeutically equivalent products that are available on the domestic market. Overall, the response should consider the pharmacist's scope of practice and address all reasonable needs of the requestor. Additional characteristics of a drug information response are included in **Table 2-4**.

| **TABLE 2-3**  Factors that Aid in Prioritization of Primary Literature Review |
| --- |
| Journal impact factor and quality of publishing journal |
| Date of publication |
| Reputation of publishing authors |
| Quality of study type |
| Importance of outcomes of interest |
| Size of the study |
| Duration of the study |

| **TABLE 2-4**   General Rules for Responding to Drug Information Requests |
|---|
| Use language appropriate to the requestor's background education and knowledge. |
| Confirm the ultimate question with the requestor when responding. |
| Format recommendations to be directly applied to clinical practice. |
| Use proper grammar and spelling. |
| Make the response look professional. |
| Avoid first person. |
| Be concise and direct. |
| Avoid uncommon abbreviations and acronyms. |
| Use high-quality references to support recommendations. |
| Summarize recommendations at the conclusion. |
| Identify any follow-up questions. |
| Document the resources and process used when formulating the response. |

# RECORD

Once a drug information response has been communicated to a requestor, it is important to verify the appropriateness of the given response. It is through direct interactions with the requestor that this step can be assessed. In particular, the pharmacist should reflect on whether the requestor readily accepts the response and recommendation or if the requestor asked additional questions or was not satisfied with the response given. In addition, it should be identified whether the response could be directly applied to clinical practice. If additional questions or follow-up research was requested, it is the responsibility of the pharmacist to complete this additional research in a timely manner using the systematic approach outlined in this chapter. In addition, the ability to verify the appropriateness of a drug information response does not just function as the quality assurance of recommendations disseminated from a drug information service, it also creates a mechanism for the pharmacist to measure the outcome of the recommendation for personal clinical development if similar clinical scenarios are encountered in the future. This is particularly true for patient-specific drug information responses. Not only does an individual have the opportunity to research and respond to the drug information question, but he or she will also be able to determine the ultimate impact of the recommendation through follow-up of the drug information request.

Next, the pharmacist should verify that the entire systematic process used to answer the drug information question has been thoroughly documented. This includes documentation of the specific drug information question, background information, response, resources utilized, follow-up information, and other logistical details, such as time the request was received or when the response was given.[7] Documentation is also an important mechanism to limit liability for the drug information services provided, to document the pharmacist's professional value to the health system, and to serve as a database of responses in the event that a similar request is identified in the future. Common documentation processes include paper forms, logbooks, or electronic or Internet databases, and Figure 2-1 includes a sample drug information documentation form. If a clinician has an opportunity to use a previous drug information response to facilitate a newly received request, it is important to consider the potential that additional references or resources may have been published since the original response was given. Therefore, it would be prudent to complete at least a modified or streamlined systematic approach to answering the drug information question prior to responding to this new request with a historic response.

Lastly, there will inevitably be circumstances when additional information or resources related to a specific drug information question is identified after the response is given. This information may either confirm or modify the recommendations made during an initial response to a drug information question. For example, an oncologist might request information on the use of a newly approved medication for an off-label indication. On initial search, the pharmacist might only identify low-level evidence such as case reports and expert opinion to support the use of the novel medication for this indication. However, a few weeks later a newly published report could prospectively study the use of this medication. Although the pharmacist may have responded to this drug information request previously, the pharmacist should contact the oncologist and provide the newly identified information. Such follow-up communication could occur in person, over the telephone, or by email correspondence. It also has the potential to improve the clinical practice of the requestor and significantly enhance the perception of quality and delivery of services by the drug information center.

---

**CASE STUDY 2-1**    **False-Positive Urine Test Clinical Scenario**

You are a pain management pharmacist and have been approached by a physician who is concerned about a patient who recently tested positive for benzodiazepines on a urine drug screen but is not currently prescribed a benzodiazepine. The physician states that the patient is adamant that he did not take any medications that were not prescribed by his doctor and wondered if the urine drug screening could be incorrect. The physician goes on to state that the patient recently came down with the common cold and had been taking cold medications obtained from the local pharmacy. He asks if this could have caused a false-positive result.

### What Are Pertinent Background Questions to Ask?

- What is the patient's current medication regimen? Have there been any recent changes? What over-the-counter medications has the patient taken recently?
- When was the urine drug test completed?
- Was further testing completed to confirm this positive test?
- What resources did the requestor consult?
- What is the urgency of this request?

### Relevant Background Information Obtained from the Requestor

Inquiring further about this patient using the background questions, you are informed that the patient is currently enrolled in the pain management clinic under the supervision of this physician. In addition, the patient has signed a pain management contract that forbids the use of illicit medications. Thus, the patient is required to undergo regular urine drug testing, which was conducted yesterday and yielded a positive result for benzodiazepines. No further testing, such as gas chromatography, was obtained to confirm this positive result. The patient's current medication profile is as follows:

- Omeprazole 40 mg orally daily
- Clonidine transdermal patch 0.3 mg/day
- Amlodipine 10 mg orally daily
- Atorvastatin 40 mg orally daily
- Sertraline 100 mg orally daily
- Morphine sustained release 15 mg orally twice daily

Recently discontinued medications:

- Trimethoprim-sulfamethoxazole 160/800 mg orally twice daily
  - Finished course last week
- Trazodone 50 mg orally as needed for insomnia
  - Discontinued 2 months prior
- Pravastatin 80 mg orally each evening
  - Discontinued at last primary care appointment because of the need for potency titration to atorvastatin

Current over-the-counter medications:

- Pseudoephedrine 30 mg orally taken with symptoms of congestion
- Acetaminophen 500 mg orally as needed for pain/headache
- Docusate 100 mg orally daily

## Differentiation of the Ultimate Question

The physician's initial drug information question focused on whether over-the-counter cold medicines could have resulted in a false-positive benzodiazepine urine drug screen. Even though this will be addressed when responding to this question, it is important to realize that the actual question that should be researched is more comprehensive. Thus, the ultimate question for this patient scenario is, "Are there any medication exposures specific to this patient that could have resulted in a false-positive urine drug screen?"

## Categorizing the Ultimate Question

Often, drug information questions may not fit perfectly within one specific category or may have aspects that apply to multiple categories. This concept is true for this drug information question. Although it could be argued that this drug information question could be categorized as abuse/addiction, because of its focus on drug testing, it is likely best to categorize this question as a drug interaction or drug–test interaction, if the drug interaction category is further subdivided. This is true because the ultimate question focuses on whether a false-positive result occurred, which is a drug interacting with a laboratory test. It was not focused on identifying if the patient was using an illicit medication.

## Research Analysis and Findings

Urine drug tests are common in the healthcare system to verify abstinence from illicit drugs and to confirm adherence to maintenance drugs with high abuse potential, such as opioids. For most urine drug tests, immunoassays using a competitive antigen-antibody reaction whereby the drug molecules that are being tested for, whether drug metabolite or parent drug, compete with a labeled version of that drug to bind with an antibody. But with such a system, there is potential for cross-reactivity when an unrelated compound conveys antibody reactivity, thus resulting in a false positive.

Upon a search of the literature, it is determined that there are multiple tertiary resources that identify potential false positives associated with urine drug screens. When reviewing these references, it is concluded that urine drug testing for benzodiazepines can be associated with a false-positive test when taking the medications oxaprozin and sertraline. No additional medications associated with a false-positive benzodiazepine result had been identified in the tertiary literature. When reviewing this patient's medication profile, it is documented that he is currently taking sertraline as a maintenance medication. Further research of the primary literature shows that false-positive testing has been confirmed in the clinical setting and is documented in the prescribing information for sertraline. Thus, the possibility of a false-positive urine drug test cannot be ruled out with the information provided. In order to be able to determine if this positive test was the result of a false-positive caused by the presence of sertraline or if it was a true-positive test for benzodiazepines, the specimen would need to undergo gas chromatography and mass spectrometry for confirmation testing.

## Opportunity for Follow-Up

Because of the variable nature of this drug information question, there is opportunity for follow-up regarding the ultimate conclusion of this case scenario. By following up with this patient's provider and obtaining the results of the gas chromatography and mass spectrometry, the pharmacist will be able to determine the true cause of the positive benzodiazepine urine drug screen. Thus, if it were truly a false-positive caused by sertraline, the clinician will be able to use this information to make better informed clinical decisions in the future.

## Take-Home Message

Without obtaining the appropriate background information, the pharmacist would have only answered the question of whether over-the-counter cold medicines could have resulted in a false-positive urine drug screen. The response to that ultimate question would have been no, but it would have overlooked the possibility that another medication that the patient was exposed to could have been associated with a positive test. In addition, the response to the question could have ended with the information that sertraline has been shown to cause false-positive tests and may have been responsible for a false-positive with this patient. But, it is important to identify the possibility of reasonable follow-up questions, which in this case would have been how to identify if it was a false-positive due to sertraline or a true-positive caused by the patient taking an illicit benzodiazepine. Thus, the information regarding gas chromatography and mass spectrometry gave the provider additional information on the drug information question and enhanced the perception of service rendered to the requestor.

## References

Brahm NC, Yeager LL, Fox MD, et al. Commonly prescribed medications and potential false-positive urine drug screens. *Am J Health Syst Pharm*. 2010;67:1344-1350.

Hammett-Stabler CA, Webster LR. A clinical guide to urine drug testing: augmenting pain management and enhancing patient care. University of Medicine and Dentistry of New Jersey, Center for Continuing and Outreach Education. Stamford, CT: PharmaCom Group, Inc.; 2008.

Nasky KM, Cowan GL, Knittel DR. False-positive urine screening for benzodiazepines: an association with sertraline? A two-year retrospective chart analysis. *Psychiatry (Edgmont)*. 2009;6:36-39.

Zoloft (sertraline) [package insert]. New York, NY: Roerig Division of Pfizer; 2012.

| CASE STUDY 2-2 | Angioedema Clinical Scenario |
|---|---|

You are the hospital's central pharmacist and you receive a call from a physician asking if it would be safe to prescribe losartan, an angiotensin II receptor blocker (ARB), in a patient recently diagnosed with angioedema due to exposure to lisinopril, an angiotensin-converting enzyme inhibitor (ACEI).

## What Are Pertinent Background Questions to Ask?

- When did the symptoms occur in relation to starting lisinopril?
- What was the severity of symptoms?
- What is the ACEI and/or ARB prescribed to treat?
- What resources did the requestor consult?
- What is the urgency of this request?

## Relevant Background Information Obtained from the Requestor

Inquiring further about this patient using the background questions, you are informed that the patient presented with lip and face swelling approximately 3 weeks after initiating lisinopril. After discontinuing lisinopril, the swelling resolved within 48 hours. The physician prescribed the ACEI for its cardioprotective effects in this patient diagnosed with hypertension, systolic heart failure, and type 1 diabetes.

## Differentiation of the Ultimate Question

For this drug information question, the relevant background did not change the ultimate question that will be answered by the pharmacist, but it did include pertinent details that will influence the final recommendations.

## Categorizing the Ultimate Question

Although there are two medications discussed in this question, the most appropriate category for this drug information question is adverse drug reaction. The drug interaction category would be inappropriate because these two agents are not influencing each other.

## Research Analysis and Findings

ACEIs have been shown to induce angioedema in 0.1–1.0% of patients, and the most common presenting symptoms include swelling of the lips, tongue, and face. Angioedema can be life threatening if it progresses to airway obstruction. Patients with angioedema caused by exposure to an ACEI should have the ACEI discontinued; symptoms generally resolve in 24–48 hours.

The use of ARBs in patients with a history of ACEI-associated angioedema is controversial. Current evidence suggests that < 10% of patients who previously developed angioedema after receiving an ACEI also develop angioedema after subsequently receiving an ARB. Thus, there is a risk of cross-reactivity in patients who receive an ARB after experiencing ACEI-associated angioedema, although this risk is thought to be relatively low. Therefore, ARBs can be considered in patients in whom an ARB offers an advantage to other antihypertensive agents or if the patient has a compelling indication for angiotensin inhibition, such as heart failure, diabetes, or chronic kidney disease.

In this patient, the symptoms of angioedema do not appear to be life threatening, and there are compelling indications that prioritize the use of an ARB over other antihypertensive agents. Thus, in this case, the use of an ARB in a patient with a history of ACEI-associated angioedema may be recommended. In addition, given the potential for negative outcomes associated with drug-associated angioedema, close monitoring is necessary to ensure that repeat angioedema does not occur.

## Opportunity for Follow-Up

Because cross-reactivity of drug-induced angioedema is low for ARBs, this is a good opportunity to follow up with this patient to identify if angioedema occurs. Although the experience of this patient may not predict the experience of future patients, it does add to the clinical experience of the pharmacist, and this knowledge may be beneficial for similar encounters in the future.

## Take-Home Message

Oftentimes, drug information questions may be controversial or not have a definite answer and may depend on the interpretation and clinical perspective of the pharmacist. This is the case for this particular drug information question—the patient's individual characteristics determined the ultimate recommendation. This further highlights the importance of the background questions and the impact they have on a drug information response.

## References

Campo P, Fernandez TD, Canto G, et al. Angioedema induced by angiotensin-converting enzyme inhibitors. *Curr Opin Allergy Clin Immunol.* 2013;13:337-344.

Caldeira D, David C, Sampaio C. Tolerability of angiotensin-receptor blockers in patients with intolerance to angiotensin-converting enzyme inhibitors: a systematic review and meta-analysis. *Am J Cardiovasc Drugs.* 2012;12:263-277.

Haymore BR, Yoon J, Mikita CP, et al. Risk of angioedema with angiotensin receptor blockers in patients with prior angioedema associated with angiotensin-converting enzyme inhibitors: a meta-analysis. *Ann Allergy Asthma Immunol.* 2008;101:495-499.

# LEGAL AND ETHICAL CONSIDERATIONS

The provision of drug information must be made with the highest regard for ethical and legal considerations. All practicing pharmacists must consider the legal and ethical implications of drug information services on patient care. As such, pharmacists should only practice under the scope of their license, and clinical recommendations should be made in the best interests of the patients. Recommendations for off-label use of medications should be appropriately documented to substantiate the recommendation in clinical practice. Patient and health information privacy should also be protected in accordance with the Health Insurance Portability and Accountability Act of 1996.[8]

In addition, it is important to consider how a drug information response will be received and affect the end user. For instance, a pharmacist may receive a question from a patient that seeks to determine whether a medication is an appropriate treatment for a particular medical condition. On the surface, this may be a simple request, and the pharmacist can provide information on the use of the medication for that disease state. But if the patient uses this information to validate or refute the recommendations of his or her healthcare provider, then it would be best to incorporate the healthcare provider into the drug information response and dialogue. Similarly, pharmacists are often asked to assist in the identification of tablets or capsules that are found without appropriate labeling, such as a loose tablet found on the ground. Although it is appropriate to identify medications for a patient or healthcare provider, it is inappropriate to identify medications that may be prescribed to a third party, because of patient confidentiality considerations. These considerations also apply to the legal guardians of children, and the ability of a pharmacist to respond to a drug information request may depend on the child's age, disease state, or medication in question. For example, the use of oral contraceptives or an antiviral for the treatment of HIV/AIDS may warrant different privacy protections than other medications or disease states. Therefore, the pharmacist should always acquire appropriate background information related to legal and ethical considerations before a drug information response is given.

If a pharmacist is establishing a formal drug information service, such as a drug information center, the founding practitioner should work with the institution's executive team and legal counsel to develop defined policies and procedures. The policies and procedures will define the scope of practice, including the type of drug information questions that will be answered, the types of requestors that may submit requests, and the charges for services, if applicable. For example, many drug information centers do not respond to urgent questions related to poisonings/exposures, but instead triage these callers to emergency management services/poison centers. Similarly, a drug information center may only offer its services to healthcare professionals of that institution, whereas others may offer their resources to all healthcare providers in a certain region, state, or country or may allow the general public or patients of that institution to utilize the services of the drug information center. Therefore, the practices of the drug information center should be based on policies that clearly define acceptable drug information practice, and all staff should be trained in accordance with these policies.

# CONTINUOUS QUALITY IMPROVEMENT

The provision of drug information services is a fundamental responsibility of the pharmacy profession and has application to all areas of pharmacy practice, including health system and community pharmacy, the pharmaceutical industry, and any other practice with a professional consultation. As licensed professionals, pharmacists have the ability to disseminate medication-related recommendations in the healthcare setting and typically do so regardless of the setting of practice. Thus, it is imperative that all pharmacists are appropriately trained and competent in the provision of drug information services and that the recommendations provided are of the highest quality and appropriate for direct implementation into clinical practice. In order to verify the quality of the drug information services provided, an assessment of the services should be incorporated into the pharmacist's clinical practice. The design of this quality assessment process will vary with differing practice settings, but it should be designed to maximize the opportunity to evaluate the quality of the drug information services and identify weaknesses and opportunities for improvements in the system.

## TRAINEES: PHARMACY STUDENTS, INTERNS, AND POSTGRADUATE RESIDENTS

It is important to establish and follow a formal quality assessment process when drug information services are provided by pharmacy students, interns, or licensed pharmacists in postgraduate training programs. Typically, this entails the review of a licensed and practicing pharmacist or preceptor prior to the dissemination of the drug information response. Thus, the reviewing pharmacist will verify the requestor's ultimate question and review the trainee's search strategy, resources and literature reviewed, and proposed response. This may occur by assessing a formal response document, with all steps formally documented in writing, or it may occur by oral presentation by the trainee if the drug information process was conducted in a patient care setting. The supervising pharmacist should evaluate the quality of the drug information response based on the pharmacist's clinical experience, background knowledge, and independent review of the available resources and literature. Once appropriate quality is met, the supervising pharmacist will give formal approval to the trainee to allow the dissemination of the drug information response.

## INFORMAL DRUG INFORMATION SERVICES

Quality assessment on the provision of drug information services in an informal drug information setting, such as in direct patient care areas, can be more difficult than that in a formal setting. This is because of the continuous communication and dialogue between practitioners that is inherent in pharmacy practice in a multidisciplinary environment. Thus, most strategies for assessing the quality of informal drug information services must be prospective or interventional in nature. Common strategies in this practice setting include concurrent observation, required documentation of drug information interactions and subsequent retrospective review, or educational opportunities and assessments of resource competence. With concurrent observation, a reviewing practitioner assesses the practicing pharmacist's ability to receive and respond to informal drug information questions in a real-time setting. Although this method can be highly effective in assessing the quality of drug information services, the additional physical presence of another practitioner in the practice environment can be distracting or obstructive to patient care and may be difficult to utilize in practices with larger numbers of pharmacists. If retrospective review is preferred, the practicing pharmacists should document drug information interactions, which can be reviewed for quality in a retrospective fashion. If employed, the practice site would need to establish the frequency of review and communicate this information to the practicing pharmacists. An example of a quality assessment tool is provided in **Table 2-5**. A final quality assessment option focuses on the drug information service establishing educational opportunities, such as introductory and advanced practices in drug information, and allowing practitioners to demonstrate proficiency in drug information through active learning principles and posteducational assessments. This final method is commonly used in many healthcare systems.

| TABLE 2-5 Quality Assurance Assessment of Drug Information Responses | | | |
|---|---|---|---|
| Pharmacist Name:_____ | | Reviewer Name:_____ | |
| Date of Drug Information Response:_____ | | Date of Review:_____ | |
| | Appropriate | Needs Improvement | Not Appropriate |
| Complete background information was obtained. | | | |
| Ultimate question was clearly recorded. | | | |
| Question was appropriately categorized. | | | |
| Appropriate resources were identified. | | | |
| Literature search was necessary and performed appropriately. | | | |
| Clear and concise evidence-based response was provided. | | | |
| Follow-up communication was clearly documented, if applicable. | | | |

## FORMAL DRUG INFORMATION SERVICES

The provision of clinical recommendations by a formal drug information service typically occurs using a more formal documentation and response process than is generally undertaken in patient care settings. As such, higher quality documentation allows for additional opportunities for quality assessment, and, with reviewable documents, quality assessment can occur in both a prospective and retrospective fashion. Review of the quality of drug information services can be undertaken by a supervising pharmacist if trainees are staffing the center, by a colleague via a peer-review process, or by a panel of reviewers. The objective of the review process is to verify the quality of drug information services provided, but it can also determine if additional resources are needed for the drug information service. Table 2-5 outlines a formal assessment tool that can be used for assessing the quality of drug information responses. Additionally, a survey study of end users may be undertaken by the drug information service, focusing on the perception of quality, and could include physicians, mid-level providers, pharmacists, and nurses. Many different quality elements can be assessed in a survey, but it is particularly important to assess the perception of completeness and accuracy of the response, the appropriateness of communication, the timeliness of the response, the ability of the end user to directly apply the response to clinical practice, and the appropriateness of any follow-up communication. Although this survey method does not directly evaluate the quality of a specific drug information response, it does evaluate the end user's perspective of overall quality and service based on his or her background, expertise, and clinical experience.

## OUTCOME TRACKING

The dissemination of drug information is a cognitive service, and pharmacists may not be directly involved in the implementation of the recommendations directly into patient care or clinical practice. Because of a lack of objective measures that are commonly seen in other clinical practices, such as reduction in blood pressure or cholesterol, morbidity, mortality, etc., it is difficult for drug information services to measure the impact of the cognitive services on the healthcare system. Thus, drug information services should be challenged to document the services provided to a healthcare system in ways that are available, such as cost avoidance and perceptions of service from end users. This can be accomplished by developing economic models to assign cost savings to individual drug information responses, identifying opportunities for formulary or dosage form conversions (e.g., IV to oral), documenting recommendation acceptance rates, or demonstrating decreased workload for requestors after consulting a drug information center.[9-11] Drug information services can also demonstrate value to the healthcare system by assessing the quality of services through direct surveys to end users of the service or through the provision of scholarly activities such as newsletters, peer-reviewed publications, or local, regional, or national presentations. Lastly, drug information services can demonstrate value by supporting student and pharmacy resident trainees, thus directly contributing to the development of future practitioners and advancing the practice of pharmacy.

## SUMMARY

The provision of drug information is a foundational responsibility of the pharmacy profession and is instrumental for achieving optimal outcomes in clinical practice. The receive, research, respond, and record (the four Rs) process outlines a systematic approach for responding to drug information requests and enhances the quality and efficiency of drug information responses. With the application of the concepts outlined in this chapter, the pharmacist will serve as a distinguished resource for the healthcare community and demonstrate continual value to any institution.

## REFERENCES

1. Watanabe AS, McCart G, Shimomura S, Kayser S. Systematic approach to drug information requests. *Am J Hosp Pharm*. 1975;32(12):1282-1285.
2. Fischer JM. Modification of the systematic approach to drug information requests. *Am J Hosp Pharm*. 1980;37(4):470, 472, 476.
3. Watanabe AS. [Letter to the Editor]. *Am J Hosp Pharm*. 1980;37(4):472, 476.
4. Lavsa SM, Corman SL, Verrico MM, Pummer TL. Effect of drug information request templates on pharmacy student compliance with the modified systematic approach to answering drug information questions. *Ann Pharmacother*. 2009;43(11):1795-1801.
5. Counsell C. Formulating questions and locating primary studies for inclusion in systematic reviews. *Ann Intern Med*. 1997;127(5):380-387.
6. Shaughnessy AF, Slawson DC, Bennett JH. Becoming an information master: a guidebook to the medical information jungle. *J Fam Pract*. 1994;39(5):489-499.
7. American Society of Health-System Pharmacists. ASHP guidelines on the provision of medication information by pharmacists. *Am J Health-Syst Pharm*. 1996;53(15):1843-1845.
8. Health Insurance Portability and Accountability Act of 1996, Pub. L. No. 104-191, 110 Stat. 1936 (1996).
9. Brown JN. Cost savings associated with a dedicated drug information service in an academic medical center. *Hosp Pharm*. 2011;46(9):680-684.
10. Hands D, Stephens M, Brown D. A systematic review of the clinical and economic impact of drug information services on patient outcome. *Pharm World Sci*. 2002;24(4):132-138.
11. Kinky DE, Erush SC, Laskin MS, Gibons GA. Economic impact of a drug information service. *Ann Pharmacother*. 1999;33(11):11-16.

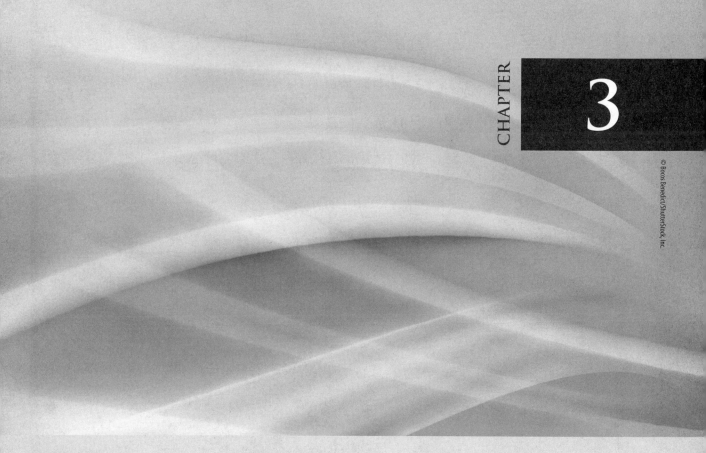

# TERTIARY SOURCES OF INFORMATION

Vicki R. Kee, PharmD, BCPS
Vern Duba, MA

## CHAPTER OBJECTIVES

▸ Define *tertiary literature*.

▸ List advantages and disadvantages of tertiary literature.

▸ Discuss methods for evaluating tertiary literature.

▸ Identify appropriate general and specialty tertiary literature sources and electronic applications for answering drug information questions.

▸ Compare and contrast the content of tertiary literature sources.

# CHAPTER OUTLINE

# KEY TERMS

Tertiary literature

# INTRODUCTION

**Tertiary literature** consists of information gathered from primary and secondary literature. Textbooks, reference books and databases, monographs, and review articles are types of tertiary literature. Tertiary resources add value by summarizing or interpreting original works. Tertiary sources can be divided into two types: general and specialty. General sources cover a wide range of topics, whereas specialty sources focus on a specific area. The primary advantages of tertiary literature are that it is convenient and easily accessible.[1] However, lag time between time of writing and time of publication, space limitations that may prevent in-depth topic discussion, the potential for author biases to be introduced, and the fact that the information may be incomplete, misleading, or inaccurate are all limitations to using tertiary literature.

This chapter will present methods of evaluating tertiary sources; review general references; discuss specialty references for drug interactions, adverse drug reactions, pregnancy and lactation, pediatrics, compatibility and stability, natural products, foreign drugs, and other specialty references; and offer an overview of electronic applications.

# METHODS OF EVALUATION

Katz and Kinder's classic review elements (accuracy, appropriateness, arrangement, authority, bibliography, comparability, completeness, content, distinction, documentation, durability, ease-of-use, illustrations, index, level, reliability, revisions, and uniqueness)[2] are still applicable today when evaluating tertiary literature. Validating tertiary literature content is important in an era of increasing information output, ease of publishing, and access to web-based information. One method of evaluation is application of the Health On the Net Foundation Code of Conduct for medical and health websites (HONcode).[3] **Table 3–1** lists key attributes of the HONcode that are specific to websites, but each can be applied to print and other online resources as well. In addition, several key pharmacy journals provide peer reviews of published tertiary literature materials (**Table 3–2**). Book reviews are considered out of scope by PubMed, making it important to search individual journals publishing book reviews that may include pharmacy-specific tertiary resources.

# GENERAL REFERENCES

## AHFS® DRUG INFORMATION (DI)™

*Publisher*: American Society of Health-Systems Pharmacists, Bethesda, Maryland.
*Editor*: Gerald K. McEvoy.

| TABLE 3-1 | The HONcode for Medical and Health Websites | |
|---|---|---|
| **Principle** | **Explanation** | **Details** |
| 1. Authoritative | Indicate the qualifications of the authors. | Any medical or health advice provided and hosted on this site will only be given by medically trained and qualified professionals unless a clear statement is made that a piece of advice offered is from a non-medically qualified individual or organization. |
| 2. Complementarity | Information should support, not replace, the doctor–patient relationship. | The information provided on this site is designed to support, not replace, the relationship that exists between a patient/site visitor and his or her existing physician. |
| 3. Privacy | Respect the privacy and confidentiality of personal data submitted to the site by the visitor. | Confidentiality of data relating to individual patients and visitors to a medical/health website, including their identity, is respected by this website. The website owners undertake to honor or exceed the legal requirements of medical/health information privacy that apply in the country and state where the website and mirror sites are located. |
| 4. Attribution | Cite the source(s) of published information, date medical and health pages. | Where appropriate, information contained on this site will be supported by clear references to source data and, where possible, have specific hypertext markup language (HTML) links to that data. The date when a clinical page was last modified will be clearly displayed (e.g., at the bottom of the page). |
| 5. Justifiability | Site must back up claims relating to benefits and performance. | Any claims relating to the benefits/performance of a specific treatment, commercial product, or service will be supported by appropriate, balanced evidence in the manner outlined above in Principle 4. |
| 6. Transparency | Accessible presentation, accurate email contact. | The designers of this website will seek to provide information in the clearest possible manner and provide contact addresses for visitors who seek further information or support. The webmaster will display his or her email address clearly throughout the website. |
| 7. Financial disclosure | Identify funding sources. | Support for this website will be clearly identified, including the identities of commercial and noncommercial organizations that have contributed funding, services, or material for the site. |
| 8. Advertising policy | Clearly distinguish advertising from editorial content. | If advertising is a source of funding, it will be clearly stated. A brief description of the advertising policy adopted by the website owners will be displayed on the site. Advertising and other promotional material will be presented to viewers in a manner and context that facilitates differentiation between it and the original material created by the institution operating the site. |

Data from Health On the Net Foundation. The HONcode of conduct for medical and health websites. http://www.hon.ch/HONcode/Pro/Conduct.html. Accessed July 15, 2014.

*Format*: Yearly print edition with online updates, online (in *Lexicomp Online*™ and *STAT!Ref*®).

*Organization*: Arranged by the American Hospital Formulary Service (AHFS®) Pharmacologic-Therapeutic Classification System©, allowing for review of drugs with similar activity and use; indexed by trade name, synonym, pharmacy equivalent names, and acronyms.

*Monograph sections*: Monograph title and synonyms, risk evaluation and mitigation strategies, introductory description, uses, dosage and administration, cautions, drug interactions, laboratory test interferences, chronic toxicity, pharmacology, mechanism of action (for anti-infectives), spectrum (for anti-infectives), resistance (for anti-infectives), pharmacokinetics, chemistry and stability, and preparations.

| TABLE 3-2 Selected Pharmacy Journals Publishing Book Reviews | |
|---|---|
| Journal | International Standard Serial Number (ISSN) |
| Canadian Journal of Hospital Pharmacy | 0008-4123 |
| American Journal of Health-System Pharmacy | 1079-2082 |
| American Journal of Pharmaceutical Education | 0002-9459 |
| Annals of Pharmacotherapy | 1060-0280 |
| Biochemical Pharmacology | 0006-2952 |
| British Journal of Clinical Pharmacology | 0306-5251 |
| Cardiovascular Drugs and Therapy | 0920-3206 |
| Drug Metabolism and Disposition | 0090-9556 |
| Fundamental and Clinical Pharmacology | 0767-3981 |
| Investigational New Drugs | 0167-6997 |
| Journal of Cardiovascular Pharmacology | 0160-2446 |
| Journal of Clinical Pharmacy and Therapeutics | 0269-4727 |
| Journal of Clinical Psychopharmacology | 0271-0749 |
| Journal of Psychopharmacology | 0269-8811 |
| Journal of the American Pharmacists Association | 1544-3191 |
| Pharmacology & Therapeutics | 0163-7258 |
| Pharmacotherapy | 0277-0008 |
| Therapeutic Drug Monitoring | 0163-4356 |
| Toxicology and Applied Pharmacology | 0041-008X |
| Trends in Pharmacological Sciences | 0165-6147 |

*Comments*: Exceptional resource for discussion of pharmacologic–therapeutic categories. Note that the AHFS® classification is not intuitive; users should rely on indexing when searching for specific drug information. It should be noted that for subscribers of the print edition, some monographs are available online only. The username and password for accessing the online-only monographs are provided at the start of the index in the print edition. Even so, the print volume is nearing 4,000 pages. *AHFS DI® Essentials™*, a summarized highlights version of *AHFS DI®*, is no longer in print, but is available electronically in *Lexicomp Online™*, *Pepid™*, and *STAT!Ref®*.

## DRUG FACTS AND COMPARISONS®

*Publisher*: Facts & Comparisons, Wolters Kluwer Health, St. Louis, Missouri.
*Editors*: Renee M. Wickersham and Kirsten K. Novak.
*Format*: Yearly print edition, online (in *Facts & Comparisons® eAnswers*), CD-ROM.
*Organization*: Arranged in chapters by therapeutic use; each chapter is divided into groups and subgroups that aid in comparisons between medications with similar uses; indexed by generic and trade name, synonyms, common abbreviations, and therapeutic group names.

*Monograph sections*: Prescribing information, indications (FDA-approved and off-label uses), administration and dosage, actions, contraindications, warnings and precautions, drug interactions, adverse reactions, overdosage, and patient information.
*Comments*: Similar to *AHFS DI*®, *Drug Facts and Comparisons*® provides discussion of drug classification information. This resource is noted for extensive information arranged in table format. Listings grouped by dosage form and strength at the beginning of each monograph provide product details and cross-referencing to appropriate drug monographs.

## DRUGDEX® System

*Publisher*: Micromedex, Truven Health Analytics, Englewood, Colorado.
*Format*: Online (in *Micromedex*®).
*Organization*: The *DRUGDEX*® *System* is composed of drug evaluation monographs, patient-related drug consultations, and a product index. The product index includes trade names, manufacturers, and dosage forms for investigational, international, FDA-approved, and over-the-counter preparations.
*Monograph sections*: Dosage, pharmacokinetics, interactions, cautions, adverse effects, contraindications/precautions, comparative drug efficacy, clinical applications, comparative drug efficacy, indications, therapeutic uses, and generic names.
*Comments*: *DRUGDEX*® *System* is one component of *Micromedex*® 2.0, comprising the bulk of the drug information searchable by generic name, trade name, or indication. Each evaluation monograph is well referenced, and cross-referenced to other sources within the *Micromedex*® 2.0 suite, including, for example, *Tox & Drug Product Lookup*, *Martindale*, and *Red Book*™ listings. *DRUGDEX*® *DrugPoint*® *Summary* provides brief bulleted summaries of dosing, indications, single-drug interactions, adverse effects, name information, mechanism of action, pharmacokinetics, administration/monitoring, toxicology, and clinical teaching patient instructions.

## Clinical Drug Data

*Publisher*: McGraw-Hill, New York.
*Editors*: Kelly M. Smith, Daniel M. Riche, and Nickole N. Henyan.
*Format*: Print, full-text download for mobile devices.
*Organization*: Three sections: drug categories subdivided in therapeutic groups, clinical information chapters, and appendices.
*Monograph sections*: Drug class instructions (this heading may appear at the beginning of each drug class intended for patient instruction applying to more than one drug) followed by generic name, pharmacology, administration and adult dosage, special populations, dosage forms, patient instructions, pharmacokinetics, adverse reactions, contraindications, precautions, drug interactions, parameters to monitor, and notes. Clinical information chapters include drug-induced diseases, drug use in special populations, immunization and emergency information, nutrition support, and drug interactions and interferences. The appendices include conversion factors, anthropometrics, lab indices, drug–lab test interferences, and pharmacokinetic equations.
*Comments*: Purchase of the print volume includes a full-text download code for mobile devices.

## DRUG INFORMATION HANDBOOK

*Publisher*: Lexicomp, Wolters Kluwer Health, Hudson, Ohio.

*Format*: Yearly print edition, online (in *Lexicomp Online*™), mobile application.

*Organization*: Alphabetical by generic name.

*Monograph sections*: Alerts/warnings, pronunciation, brand names, pharmacologic category, dosages, uses, clinical practice guidelines, administration and storage issues, medication safety issues, medication guides, warnings and precautions, pregnancy and lactation, adverse reactions, interactions, patient and therapy management, preparations, pharmacology and pharmacokinetics, dental information, pearls and related information, and references.

*Comments*: Well referenced with a range of detail depending on the drug monograph. *Drug Information Handbook* is available with or without the International Trade Names Index. In addition to drug monographs, this resource contains several appendices, including abbreviations and measurements, assessments of liver and renal functions, comparative drug charts, cytochrome P450 and drug interactions, immunization and therapy recommendations, and miscellaneous items (e.g., oral dosages not to be crushed). *Lexicomp*® drug monographs are integrated into *UpToDate*®.

## CLINICAL PHARMACOLOGY

*Publisher*: Elsevier/Gold Standard, Tampa, Florida.

*Format*: Online, mobile website.

*Organization*: In addition to browsing monographs alphabetically by generic name, the database is searchable by drug name, indication, contraindication/precaution, adverse reaction, classification, national drug code (NDC), manufacturer, and product classification. It is also possible to execute an advanced search using multiple criteria.

*Monograph sections*: Description/classification, mechanism of action, pharmacokinetics, indications/dosage, administration, contraindications/precautions, pregnancy/breastfeeding, interactions, adverse reactions, IV compatibility, how supplied, and monitoring parameters.

*Comments*: *Clinical Pharmacology* has several features that make it appealing for clinical practitioners. Drop-down tabs allow viewing of reports, patient education materials, identification of physical drug products, drug class overviews, laboratory values, clinical calculators, and manufacturer contact information. Many of these reports are also available as embedded links directly from the drug monograph.

## PHYSICIANS' DESK REFERENCE

*Publisher*: PDR Network, Montvale, New Jersey.

*Format*: Yearly print edition, online database, mobile application.

*Organization*: FDA-approved drug labeling information is arranged by manufacturer; indexed by brand and generic name, prescribing category, and manufacturer.

*Monograph sections*: Exact FDA-approved labeling format.

*Comments*: Note that this resource is a not a complete listing of all FDA-approved drugs. Drug manufacturers pay for inclusion of their selected products. This, in addition to other issues, has created controversy regarding its limitations.[4,5] In addition to the Product Information section, the Product Identification Guide displays full-color photos of products arranged by manufacturer. Other useful sections include contact information for the FDA and poison control centers, controlled substance category information, FDA pregnancy risk ratings, and alphabetical listings of drugs that should not be crushed and those causing photo-sensitivity. Each volume includes MedWatch and vaccine adverse event reporting forms.

## TEXTBOOKS

Textbooks serve as a solid starting point for therapeutic evaluation, drugs of choice, and other foundational information. Therapeutics textbooks are generally organized by organ system and include basic concepts about drug therapy. The following selected textbooks are useful for the clinical pharmacist (the publisher's name is in parentheses):

- *ACP Medicine: Principles and Practice* (Decker Publishing)
- *Applied Therapeutics: The Clinical Use of Drugs* (Lippincott Williams & Wilkins)
- *Conn's Current Therapy* (Saunders/Elsevier)
- *Goldman's Cecil Medicine* (Saunders/Elsevier)
- *Goodman and Gilman's The Pharmacological Basis of Therapeutics* (McGraw-Hill)
- *Harrison's Principles of Internal Medicine* (McGraw-Hill)
- *Merck Manual of Diagnosis and Therapy* (Merck)
- *Pharmacotherapy Handbook* (McGraw-Hill)
- *Pharmacotherapy: A Pathophysiologic Approach* (McGraw-Hill)
- *Pharmacotherapy: Principles & Practice* (McGraw-Hill)
- *Principles and Practice of Infectious Diseases* (Churchill Livingstone)
- *Textbook of Therapeutics: Drug and Disease Management* (Lippincott Williams & Wilkins)

# SPECIALTY REFERENCES

## DRUG INTERACTIONS

A drug interaction results when a drug interacts with another drug (including dietary supplements), a food, a disease state, and/or a laboratory test. A drug interaction occurs when the effects of a drug are modified by the administration of another drug or dietary supplement (drug–drug interaction) or by the consumption of a food or food group (drug–food interaction). A drug–disease state interaction occurs when a drug unmasks or worsens a disease. When a drug interferes with a laboratory test, it is considered a drug–laboratory test interaction. Not all drug interactions are undesirable. For example, the drug–drug interaction between penicillin and probenecid (probenecid increases penicillin serum concentrations) may be desirable in patients being treated for diseases such as meningitis that require that a high penicillin serum concentration be maintained.

Most drug–drug interactions can be classified as pharmacokinetic or pharmacodynamic interactions. Pharmacokinetic drug interactions occur when one drug affects the absorption, distribution, metabolism, or excretion of another.[6] Pharmacodynamic drug interactions occur when two drugs have additive or antagonistic effects.[6] Additive effects occur when two or more drugs with similar effects cause excessive response and toxicity.[6] Antagonistic effects occur when two drugs with opposing effects reduce the response to one or both drugs.[6]

## Specialty Sources of Information

Specialty sources of drug information often rate the level of interaction and the documentation to support the interaction using a unique rating system.

### Drug Interaction Facts™

*Publisher*: Facts & Comparisons, Wolters Kluwer Health, St. Louis, Missouri.
*Editor*: David S. Tatro.
*Format*: Yearly print edition, online (in *Facts & Comparisons® eAnswers*), CD-ROM.
*Organization*: Alphabetical by generic name or drug class.
*Monograph sections*: Significance rating, onset, severity, documentation, effects, mechanism, management, discussion, and references.
*Rating system*: A significance rating from 1 to 5 is assigned based on the interaction's severity and documentation. A significance rating of 1 is a severe and well-documented interaction, whereas a significance rating of 5 is the least severe and not well documented. There are three levels of severity: (1) major, the interaction is life threatening or may cause permanent damage; (2) moderate, the interaction may cause the patient's clinical status to deteriorate and additional treatment, hospitalization, or an extended hospital stay may be necessary; and (3) minor, the interaction usually has mild effects that may be bothersome or unnoticeable but should not affect the therapeutic outcome and more treatment is usually not necessary. Documentation represents the quality and clinical relevance of the primary literature supporting the occurrence of the interaction. The five documentation levels are (1) established (well-controlled studies have proven that the interaction exists), (2) probable (the interaction has not been proven clinically but is likely), (3) suspected (there is some good data that the interaction may occur but more study is needed), (4) possible (could occur, but data are limited), and (5) unlikely (there is no good evidence of the interaction, and it is doubtful that one exists). The onset is classified as rapid (occurring within 24 hours and immediate action is required to avoid the effects of the interaction) or delayed (occurring within a period of days or weeks and immediate action is not required).
*Comments*: This resource includes drug–drug and drug–food interactions. It includes more than 1,800 monographs covering 20,000 drugs.

### Drug Interactions Analysis and Management

*Authors*: Philip D. Hansten and John R. Horn.
*Publisher*: Facts & Comparisons, Wolters Kluwer Health, St. Louis, Missouri.
*Format*: Yearly print edition.
*Organization*: Alphabetical by generic name.
*Monograph sections*: Significance rating, summary, risk factors, mechanism, clinical evaluation, related drugs, management options, and references.
*Rating system*: A significance rating from 1 to 5 is assigned based on management options. A significance rating of 1 means that the combination should be avoided because the risk always outweighs the benefit, 2 means that the combination should usually be avoided and only used under special circumstances, 3 means to take action as necessary to minimize risk, 4 means that no action is needed because the risk of adverse outcomes appears small, and 5 means that evidence suggests that there is no interaction.

*Comments*: This resource contains more than 2,500 interactions. It includes prescription, nonprescription, and herbal medications. This resource is often referred to as *Hansten and Horn*, the authors' last names. The two authors are pharmacists.

### Stockley's Drug Interactions

*Publisher*: Pharmaceutical Press, London, UK.
*Editors*: Karen Baxter and Claire L. Preston.
*Format*: Yearly print edition, online.
*Organization*: Alphabetical by drug class. Monographs within each drug class are organized alphabetically.
*Monograph sections*: Clinical evidence, mechanism, importance, management, and references.
*Comments*: This resource contains approximately 4,200 monographs. It includes drug–herbal interactions that have available clinical evidence.

## Tools in General References

*Facts & Comparisons® eAnswers* has a drug interaction tool to search for drug–drug interactions (including herbs and supplements) and other types of interactions (e.g., drug–food/alcohol, drug–pregnancy, and drug–lactation). The tool is useful when screening more than two drugs for interactions (the monographs in *Drug Interaction Facts*™ contain interacting pairs only). The monographs use the same significance ratings as *Drug Interaction Facts*™, but caution should be exercised, however, because the resulting monographs produced by the tool are not the same as those in *Drug Interaction Facts*™. In addition, the significance ratings found using the tool also may be different from those in *Drug Interaction Facts*™.

*Lexi-Interact* is a tool available in *Lexicomp Online*™. Users can use *Lexi-Interact* to enter a single drug and see all drugs that can interact with it, or they can enter multiple drugs and run a report to see which drugs interact. The risk ratings in *Lexi-Interact* are A–D and X (A = no known interaction, B = no action needed, C = monitor therapy, D = consider therapy modification, X = avoid combination). Monograph sections include risk rating, summary, severity, reliability, patient management, similar drugs with the interaction, exceptions, discussion, and footnotes (references).

*Clinical Pharmacology* has a drug interaction report tool that can be used to create a report that summarizes interactions for prescription and nonprescription drugs, herbals, and nutritional agents. Users can also search for interactions with caffeine, enteral feedings, ethanol, food, grapefruit juice, and tobacco. The tool also checks for therapeutic duplications. Monographs include one of four severity ratings: level 1 = severe, avoid using these drugs together, which means that the use of the medications is contraindicated; level 2 = major, which means that using the medications together may be contraindicated in certain patients, the patient should be monitored, and further therapy and/or a change in therapy may be necessary; level 3 = moderate, which means that using the medications together may have unintended clinical effects, the patient should be monitored, and changes in therapy may be necessary; and level 4 = minor, which means that using the medications together does not usually result in clinically significant interactions and monitoring or changes in therapy are not usually required. It also provides a discussion of the interaction and references. A professional or a consumer interaction report can be run.

*Micromedex®* has a drug interaction tool that lets users enter a single drug and search for interactions with that drug or enter multiple drugs and see if they interact or have interactions with the other criteria the tool checks. The tool automatically checks for allergies (if any are entered), interactions with food, ethanol, lab tests, tobacco, pregnancy and lactation, and ingredient duplications. The monographs include clinical management, onset, one of five severity levels (contraindicated = the drugs are contraindicated for concurrent use; major = the interaction may be life threatening and/or require medical intervention to minimize or prevent serious adverse effects; moderate = the interaction may result in exacerbation of the patient's condition and/or require alteration in therapy; minor = the interaction would have limited clinical effects and generally would not require a major change in therapy; and unknown), one of four documentation ratings (excellent = controlled studies have clearly established that the interaction exists; good = well-controlled studies are lacking but documentation strongly suggests the interaction exists; fair = available documentation is poor but the interaction is suspected or documentation is good for a similar drug; and unknown), a summary, literature review, and references.

## Adverse Drug Reactions

An adverse drug reaction (ADR) has been defined in several ways by different organizations. The World Health Organization (WHO) defines an ADR as "any response to a drug that is noxious and unintended, and that occurs at doses normally used in man for prophylaxis, diagnosis, or therapy of disease or for the modification of physiologic function." Karch and Lasagna argued that the WHO definition of an ADR could be interpreted to include a therapeutic failure of a drug. They did not think that a therapeutic failure should be considered an ADR, so they proposed to define an ADR as "any response to a drug that is noxious and unintended, and that occurs at doses used in humans for prophylaxis, diagnosis, or therapy, excluding failure to accomplish the intended purpose."[7]

Other organizations have defined an ADR on the basis of significance or severity. The American Society of Health–System Pharmacists (ASHP) defines a significant ADR as:

> Any unexpected, unintended, undesired, or excessive response to a drug that (1) requires discontinuing the drug (therapeutic or diagnostic), (2) requires changing the drug therapy, (3) requires modifying the dose (except for minor dosage adjustments), (4) necessitates admission to a hospital, (5) prolongs stay in a healthcare facility, (6) necessitates supportive treatment, (7) significantly complicates diagnosis, (8) negatively affects prognosis, or (9) results in temporary or permanent harm, disability, or death.[8]

The U.S. FDA uses the term *adverse event* rather than ADR and defines an adverse event as "any undesirable experience associated with the use of a medical product in a patient." The FDA considers a serious adverse event as one in which the patient outcome is death, a life-threatening condition, initial or prolonged hospitalization, disability or permanent damage, or congenital anomaly/birth defect; intervention is required to prevent permanent impairment or damage; or it does not fit the other outcomes but is a serious, important medical event that may jeopardize the patient and may require medical or surgical intervention to prevent one of the other serious adverse events.[9]

The term *side effect* is often used interchangeably with ADR, although technically they are not the same. ASHP defines a side effect as an "expected, well-known reaction resulting in little or no change in patient management" that has "a predictable frequency and an effect whose intensity and occurrence are related to the size of the dose."[10]

ADRs may be classified as type A or type B reactions.[11] Type A reactions are an extension of a drug's pharmacologic effects.[11,12] They are predictable and dose dependent. Type A reactions may result from a therapeutic effect carried beyond a desired limit (e.g., a hangover after benzodiazepine use), or they may be a pharmacologic result of therapy unrelated to the objective (e.g., galactorrhea with phenothiazine use). Type A reactions have a high incidence and morbidity but have a low incidence of mortality. In many cases, adjusting the dose alleviates the reaction.[12] Type B reactions, in contrast, have a low incidence and morbidity but have a high incidence of mortality. Type B reactions are unpredictable and dose independent. These reactions include idiosyncratic and hypersensitivity reactions.[11,12] Examples of type B reactions include a reaction to an excipient (e.g., sulfite) or hemolysis in a patient with a G6PD deficiency who receives a sulfa drug. Treatment of a type B reaction includes discontinuation of the drug.[12]

There are four types of hypersensitivity reactions: type I (immunoglobulin E [IgE]-mediated; e.g., penicillin-induced anaphylaxis), type II (cytotoxic; e.g., heparin-induced thrombocytopenia), type III (immune complex; e.g., hydralazine-induced systemic lupus erythematosus), and type IV (delayed hypersensitivity; e.g., sulfamethoxazole-induced Stevens-Johnson syndrome).[11]

## Specialty Sources of Information

### *Meyler's Side Effects of Drugs: The International Encyclopedia of Adverse Drug Reactions and Interactions*

*Publisher*: Elsevier, Oxford, UK.

*Editor*: Jeffrey K. Aronson.

*Format*: Print (two volumes; updated sporadically), online.

*Organization*: Alphabetical by generic name.

*Monograph sections*: General information, organs and systems (e.g., respiratory system effects), long-term effects (e.g., drug withdrawal), second-generation effects (e.g., teratogenicity), susceptibility factors (patient-specific factors such as age or sex), drug administration (e.g., dose and route), drug–drug interactions, food–drug interactions, drug–smoking interactions, other environmental interactions, interference with diagnostic tests, diagnosis of ADR, management of ADR, monitoring therapy, and references.

*Comments*: First published in 1952, the title of this book still bears the name of its original author, Leopold Meyler, a physician who pioneered the study of ADRs. The current editor is a physician and clinical pharmacologist. This book includes approximately 1,500 individual drugs. It also includes some drug class monographs. Some major interactions are classified according to the dose at which they occur, time course over which they occur, and susceptibility factors that make them more likely to occur. The print edition contains two indexes—one by drug name and one by adverse reaction. It is international in scope; most drug names are the International Nonproprietary Name (INN) or proposed INN (pINN). This resource is often referred to simply as *Meyler's*.

### Side Effects of Drugs Annual

*Publisher*: Elsevier, Oxford, UK.

*Editor*: Jeffery K. Aronson.

*Format*: Yearly print edition, online.

*Organization*: Drug class.

*Chapter sections*: General information about organ/system ADRs of the class as a whole, information about organ/system ADRs of specific drugs within the class, and references.

*Comments*: This book is published annually as a complement to *Meyler's Side Effects of Drugs: The International Encyclopedia of Adverse Drug Reactions and Interactions*. It reviews significant new information on ADRs since the previous annual publication.

## Tools in General References

*Clinical Pharmacology* contains two tools for running adverse reaction reports, the Adverse Reaction Report and the Find/List by Adverse Reaction Report. With the Adverse Reaction Report, users can enter one drug and view all of its ADRs or enter multiple drugs to see what adverse reactions they may cause. The Find/List by Adverse Reaction Report allows users to enter an adverse reaction and search for drugs that may cause it.

*Facts & Comparisons® eAnswers* has an interactive tool called Drug Search by Disease/Symptom that can be used to find drugs that may cause one or more particular adverse reactions.

In *Lexicomp Online™*, a specific adverse reaction can be entered into the main search field, limiting the results to adverse reactions. *Lexicomp Online™* also contains a *Drug Allergy and Idiosyncratic Reactions* database. The monographs in this database include the range of the reaction, timing, cross-reactivity, assessment, patient management considerations in patients with a previous allergic reaction to the drug, and references.

# PREGNANCY AND LACTATION

A systematic review of population-based studies found that 82% of privately insured women in the United States had taken at least one prescription drug, including vitamins and minerals, during pregnancy (64%, excluding vitamins and minerals).[13] A small study at a single center in the United States found that that 96% of the subjects reported taking a medication while breastfeeding.[14] Women reported taking an average of 4.9 medications (1.1 medications per month), including vitamins, minerals, iron, and folic acid, while breastfeeding (4.0 medications, or 0.9 medications per month, excluding vitamins, minerals, iron, and folic acid).[14]

Drugs are transferred from the mother to the fetus via the placenta. The placenta is a lipid barrier between the maternal and fetal circulations. Nearly all drugs will cross the placenta to some degree. The degree to which a drug will cross the placenta is based on several drug factors, including the drug's molecular weight, lipid solubility, protein binding, degree of ionization at physiologic pH, and polarity.[15,16] Drugs that have a low molecular weight (< 500 Da), are highly lipophilic, have low protein binding, are unionized at physiologic pH, and have limited polarity cross the placenta more easily.[15,16] The maternal drug concentration is the most important factor that determines the fetal drug concentration.[15] Near term, the maternal and fetal drug concentrations of most drugs are approximately the same.[15]

Just as there are several factors that affect drug passage across the placenta, there are also several factors that affect drug passage from the maternal blood and tissues into breast milk. Drug factors include molecular weight, lipid solubility, protein binding, degree of ionization at physiologic pH, and pKa.[15,16] Drugs that have a low molecular weight (< 300 Da), are highly lipophilic (breast tissue and milk are fatty), have low protein binding, are unionized at physiologic pH, and have a high pKa are more likely to transfer into breast milk.[15,16] The maternal plasma concentration determines the amount of drug that is available to transfer into the breast milk.[16] Drug factors such as bioavailability and half-life play an important role in determining maternal plasma concentration. Drugs with high bioavailability or a long half-life will generally result in higher concentrations in the milk.[16] Selecting drugs or dosage forms that are less likely to result in low plasma concentrations in the mother will usually mean that the concentration in the breast milk will be lower.[16]

Two calculations are particularly useful for predicting drug safety in lactation: the milk/plasma (M/P) ratio and the relative infant dose (RID). The M/P ratio is the concentration of the drug in the breast milk versus the concentration of the drug in the maternal plasma.[16] A ratio of 1.0 means that the concentration is the same in the breast milk and maternal plasma, a ratio of < 1.0 means that the concentration in the breast milk is lower than the concentration in the maternal plasma, and a ratio of > 1.0 means that the concentration in breast milk is higher than the concentration in the maternal plasma. Most drugs have an M/P ratio of < 1.0. The RID is calculated by dividing the absolute infant dose (mg/kg/day) via breast milk by the maternal dose (mg/kg/day).[16] In general, an RID of ≤ 10% is considered a safe level, but factors such as the infant's age and the toxicity of the drug also should be taken into account.[16]

To minimize drug exposure in pregnancy and lactation, nonpharmacologic therapy should be recommended as initial therapy when appropriate. For example, for nausea and vomiting in pregnancy, women should be advised to avoid exposure to nausea triggers (e.g., odors, food, supplements), to eat small amounts of food several times a day, to drink fluids between meals, and to eat bland, dry, high-protein foods.[17] As another example, for constipation in pregnancy, increasing dietary fiber, liquid intake, and exercise and avoiding foods that can cause constipation should be advised.[18]

In 1979, the FDA established a system for determining the risks associated with a drug during pregnancy.[19] This system has five pregnancy categories: A, B, C, D, and X. Category A drugs have the least risk of fetal injury, and category X drugs are contraindicated during pregnancy. The pregnancy risk factors and their definitions are shown in **Table 3–3**.

In 2008, the FDA proposed eliminating these categories because they are limited in their ability to convey risk and benefit accurately and consistently.[20] The new proposed labeling would have a subsection for pregnancy and a subsection for lactation. Each subsection would include a risk summary, clinical considerations to support patient care decisions and counseling, and a data section with more detailed information. This rule is currently in the writing and clearance process.[20]

## Specialty Sources of Information

### *Drugs in Pregnancy and Lactation: A Reference Guide to Fetal and Neonatal Risk*

> *Publisher:* Lippincott Williams & Wilkins, Philadelphia, Pennsylvania.
> *Authors:* Gerald G. Briggs, Roger K. Freeman, and Sumner J. Yaffe.
> *Format:* Triennial print edition, online, mobile application.
> *Organization:* Alphabetical by generic name.

| TABLE 3-3 FDA Pregnancy Risk Categories and Definitions | |
|---|---|
| **Pregnancy Risk Category** | **Definition** |
| A | Controlled studies in women fail to demonstrate a risk to the fetus in the first trimester (and there is no evidence of a risk in later trimesters), and the possibility of fetal harm appears remote. |
| B | Either animal-reproduction studies have not demonstrated a fetal risk but there are no controlled studies in pregnant women or animal-reproduction studies have shown an adverse effect (other than a decrease in fertility) that was not confirmed in controlled studies in women in the first trimester (and there is no evidence of a risk in later trimesters). |
| C | Either studies in animals have revealed adverse effects on the fetus (teratogenic or embryocidal or other) and there are no controlled studies in women or studies in women and animals are not available. Drugs should be given only if the potential benefit justifies the potential risk to the fetus. |
| D | There is positive evidence of human fetal risk, but the benefits from use in pregnant women may be acceptable despite the risk (e.g., if the drug is needed in a life-threatening situation or for a serious disease for which safer drugs cannot be used or are ineffective). |
| X | Studies in animals or human beings have demonstrated fetal abnormalities or there is evidence of fetal risk based on human experience or both, and the risk of the use of the drug in pregnant women clearly outweighs any possible benefit. The drug is contraindicated in women who are or may become pregnant. |

Data from Federal Register. 1979;44:37434-37467.

*Monograph sections*: Pharmacologic class, pregnancy recommendation, breastfeeding recommendation, pregnancy summary, fetal risk summary, breastfeeding summary, and references.

The pregnancy recommendations are:

Compatible
No (limited) human data—probably compatible
Compatible—maternal benefit >> embryo-fetal risk
Human data suggest low risk
No (limited) human data—animal data suggest low risk
No (limited) human data—animal data suggest moderate risk
No (limited) human data—animal data suggest risk
No (limited) human data—animal data suggest high risk
Contraindicated—first trimester
Contraindicated—second and third trimesters
Contraindicated
No (limited) human data—no relevant animal data
Human data suggest risk in first and third trimesters
Human data suggest risk in second and third trimesters
Human data suggest risk in third trimester
Human (and animal) data suggest risk

The breastfeeding recommendations are:

> Compatible
> Hold breastfeeding
> No (limited) human data—probably compatible
> No (limited) human data—potential toxicity
> No (limited) human data—potential toxicity (mother)
> Contraindicated

*Comments*: This resource contains approximately 1,200 monographs. The pregnancy and breastfeeding recommendations were developed by the authors. Beginning with the 11th edition, the monographs no longer include the FDA risk categories. This book is sometimes referred to by the last name of the first author, *Briggs*. He is a clinical pharmacy specialist and has written numerous books and articles about drug therapy in pregnancy and lactation. Links to the monographs in this publication are accessible from the Pregnancy/Lactation section of *Drug Facts and Comparisons®* in *Facts & Comparisons® eAnswers*.

## Medications and Mothers' Milk

*Publisher*: Hale Publishing, Amarillo, Texas.
*Author*: Thomas W. Hale.
*Format*: Biennial print edition.
*Organization*: Alphabetical by generic name.
*Monograph sections*: Trade names (U.S. and foreign), drug category, discussion, pregnancy risk category, lactation risk category, drug properties (half-life, M/P ratio, volume of distribution, protein binding, time to maximum absorption, oral bioavailability, molecular weight, pKa), adult concerns, pediatric concerns, drug interactions, relative infant dose, adult dose, alternatives, and references. There are five lactation risk categories: L1 = safest, L2 = safer, L3 = moderately safe, L4 = possibly hazardous, L5 = contraindicated.
*Comments*: This book contains more than 1,300 drugs, vitamins, herbs, and vaccines. The lactation risk categories were developed by the author, who is a pharmacist and clinical pharmacologist. This book is sometimes referred to by the last name of the author, *Hale*. The drug properties are contained in a table within each monograph. One appendix contains information on the use of radiopharmaceuticals in lactation. The other appendix contains several tables, including pediatric immunization schedules, contraceptive methods that are acceptable or should be avoided during lactation, normal growth during development for boys and girls, normal range for thyroid function tests, therapeutic drug levels, pediatric laboratory values, drugs to avoid in lactation, drugs that are potentially hazardous in breastfeeding mothers, drugs that are usually contraindicated in lactating women, symptoms of a cold versus the flu, properties of neuromuscular blocking agents, safety of topical corticosteroids, herbal drugs to avoid in lactation, iodine content from various natural sources, environmental pollutants and toxins, and over-the-counter products listed by brand name with the lactation risk category provided.

## Drugs and Lactation Database (LactMed)

*Publisher*: U.S. National Library of Medicine, Bethesda, Maryland.
*Format*: Online, mobile application.
*Monograph sections*: Chemical structure, Chemical Abstracts Service (CAS) regis-

try number, summary of use in lactation, maternal drug levels, infant drug levels, effects in breastfed infants, possible effects on lactation, alternate drugs to consider, and references.

*Comments*: This database is one of the databases in the *Toxicology Data Network (TOXNET)*, which is published by the U.S. National Library of Medicine. *LactMed* contains several hundred peer-reviewed monographs. It was developed by a pharmacist who has authored books and publications on drug use during breastfeeding.

### Information in General References

Most drug monographs in general references include at least the FDA pregnancy risk category of the drug. Some general references contain more specialized information.

*Lexicomp Online*™ contains the *Pregnancy and Lactation, In-Depth* database. This database contains monographs of the most commonly used drugs for women of reproductive age and pregnant women. This database is evolving.

As mentioned previously, links to *Drugs in Pregnancy and Lactation: A Reference Guide to Fetal and Neonatal Risk* are accessible from the Pregnancy/Lactation section of drug monographs in *Drug Facts and Comparisons*® in *Facts & Comparisons*® *eAnswers*.

The *DRUGDEX*® *System* monographs in *Micromedex*® contain a section titled Teratogenicity/Effects in Pregnancy/Breastfeeding under Cautions. In addition to the FDA pregnancy risk category, this section contains information on whether the drug crosses the placenta, the American Academy of Pediatrics rating in breastfeeding, a *Micromedex*® lactation rating, clinical management in pregnancy and breastfeeding, and literature reports about use of the drug in pregnancy and breastfeeding.

The *REPRORISK*® *System* is a suite of four databases available through *Micromedex*®. *REPROTEXT*® *Reproductive Hazard Reference* contains information on the reproductive effects of industrial chemicals commonly encountered in the workplace. *REPROTOX*® *Reproductive Hazard Reference* contains information about the impact of the physical and chemical environment on human reproduction and development. *Shepard's Catalog of Teratogenic Agents* contains information on teratogenic agents, including chemicals, food additives, household products, environmental pollutants, pharmaceuticals, and viruses. *Teratogen Information System (TERIS)* provides current information on the teratogenic effects of drugs and environmental agents. Access to some of these databases is available at other websites.

## Pediatrics

Relatively few drugs have indications for use in pediatric patients, although most drugs that have been approved by the FDA are used in the pediatric population.[21] Relatively little data are available on the pharmacokinetics, pharmacodynamics, efficacy, and safety of drugs in children. Children are not simply small adults, so dosing in pediatric patients cannot be extrapolated from adult dosing.[21] Another consideration with pediatric patients is that the available dosage forms of a drug may not be suitable for infants and children, so extemporaneous dosage forms may have to be prepared.[21]

### Specialty Sources of Information

#### The Harriet Lane Handbook, The Johns Hopkins Hospital

*Publisher*: Mosby/Elsevier, Philadelphia, Pennsylvania.
*Editors*: Megan M. Tschudy and Kristin M. Acara.

*Format*: Print (every 3–4 years), online (in *MD Consult*), mobile application.

*Organization*: This book has four main parts: pediatric acute care, diagnostic and therapeutic information, reference, and formulary. The drug monographs are in the formulary section and are arranged alphabetically by generic drug name.

*Monograph sections*: Pregnancy risk category, breastfeeding category (1 = compatible, 2 = use with caution, 3 = unknown with concerns, X = contraindicated, ? = safety not established), need for caution or dose adjustment in hepatic or renal impairment (yes or no), trade name and other names, drug category, how supplied, drug dosing, comments about adverse effects, drug interactions, precautions, therapeutic monitoring, and other relevant information.

*Comments*: This is one of the most widely used pediatric resources. It is written by doctors completing their residency in pediatrics at The Johns Hopkins Hospital.

## Pediatric & Neonatal Dosage Handbook

*Publisher*: Lexicomp, Hudson, Ohio.

*Authors*: Carol T. Taketomo, Jane Hurlburt Hodding, and Donna M. Kraus.

*Format*: Yearly print edition, online (in *Lexicomp Online*™ as *Pediatric and Neonatal Lexi-Drugs*), mobile application.

*Organization*: Alphabetical by generic name.

*Monograph sections*: Pronunciation, medication safety issues, U.S. and Canadian brand names, therapeutic category, generic availability, use, pregnancy risk factor, pregnancy considerations, lactation information, breastfeeding considerations, contraindications, warnings, precautions, adverse reactions, interactions, stability, mechanism of action, pharmacokinetics (adult unless noted), pharmacodynamics, dosing, dosage adjustments, dosage forms, prescribing and access restrictions, administration, stability, compatibility, monitoring, and references.

*Comments*: Some monographs contain a link to more information about shortages of the drug if the drug is in short supply or unavailable. Recipes for extemporaneous preparation are provided for some drugs. The appendix contains more than 250 pages and includes charts, tables, and other supporting information. The appendix includes immunization guidelines; calculations and conversions; dosages of inhaled corticosteroids; treatment of HIV in neonates, children, and adolescents; an enteral nutrition product comparison; and information on several other topics. All of the authors are pharmacists.

## Pediatric Injectable Drugs (The Teddy Bear Book)

*Publisher*: American Society of Health-System Pharmacists, Bethesda, Maryland.

*Editors*: Stephanie J. Phelps, Tracy M. Hagemann, Kelley R. Lee, and A. Jill Thompson.

*Format*: Triennial print edition, online (in *STAT!Ref*® and *MedicinesComplete*).

*Organization*: Alphabetical by generic name.

*Monograph sections*: Brand names, medication error potential, contraindications and warnings, infusion-related cautions, dosage, dosage adjustments in organ dysfunction, maximum dosage, additives, suitable diluents, maximum concentration, preparation and delivery, IV push, intermittent infusion, continuous infusion, other routes of administration, comments, and references.

*Comments*: This book is called *The Teddy Bear Book* because it has a teddy bear on the cover. It only contains information about the most common intravenous and intramuscular drugs used in children. The appendices contain nomograms for determining body surface area of children and for estimating ideal body mass in children, additives and antibiotic considerations, Y-site compatibility of medications with parenteral nutrition, and extravasation treatment. All of the editors and writers are pharamcists.

### Pediatric Drug Formulations

*Publisher*: Harvey Whitney Books, Cincinnati, Ohio.
*Authors*: Milap C. Nahata and Vinita B. Pai.
*Format*: Print (updated sporadically).
*Organization*: Alphabetical by generic name.
*Monograph sections*: Dosage form being made, dosage form made from, concentration being made, stability, stability reference, storage, information for label, recipe (ingredients, strength, quantity), instructions, and notes.
*Comments*: This book contains more than 350 recipes for extemporaneous preparation of oral and parenteral dosage forms for children.

### NeoFax® Essentials

*Publisher*: Truven Health Analytics, Englewood, Colorado.
*Format*: Mobile application.
*Organization*: Alphabetical by generic name.
*Monograph sections*: Dose, administration, uses, boxed warning, contraindications/precautions, adverse effects, monitoring, pharmacology, special considerations, preparation, compatibilities with other drugs and solutions, and references.
*Comments*: This resource provides neonatal-specific drug information. In addition to the drug monographs, it includes enteral nutrition information. This resource was published in print as *NeoFax®* until 2011.

**Textbooks**   The following two textbooks are widely used in pediatrics. Both of these textbooks are organized by disease and organ system and include information on drug therapy:

- *Current Diagnosis and Treatment: Pediatrics*
  *Publisher*: McGraw-Hill, New York.
  *Editors*: William W. Hay, Myron J. Levin, Robin R. Deterding, Mark J. Abzug, and Judith M. Sondheimer.
  *Format*: Print, online (in *AccessMedicine®*).
- *Nelson Textbook of Pediatrics*
  *Publisher*: Saunders/Elsevier, Philadelphia, Pennsylvania.
  *Editors*: Robert M. Kliegman, Bonita F. Stanton, Joseph W. St. Geme, Nina F. Schor, and Richard E. Behrman.
  *Format*: Print, online (in *MD Consult*).

## COMPATIBILITY AND STABILITY

Compatibility and stability data for a single drug in a solution, two or more drugs in a solution, two or more drugs in a syringe, and Y-site injection compatibility can be found in the following resources.

**Specialty Sources of Information**

### *Trissel's Handbook on Injectable Drugs*

*Publisher*: American Society of Health-System Pharmacists, Bethesda, Maryland.
*Author*: Lawrence A. Trissel.
*Format*: Biennial print edition, online (interactive, *MedicinesComplete*, *STAT!Ref*®),
mobile application.
*Organization*: Alphabetical by generic name.
*Monograph sections*: Products, administration, stability, compatibility information (the drug in various solutions, two or more drugs in intravenous solutions
[additive compatibility], two or more drugs in syringes, Y-site compatibility),
additional compatibility, and other information.
*Comments*: This book is commonly referred to as *Trissel's*. It uses compatibility
indicators of C (compatible), I (incompatible), or ? (is not clearly compatible or
incompatible and cannot be designated as either). It contains data on approximately 350 drugs.

### *King*® *Guide to Parenteral Admixtures*

*Publisher*: King Guide Publications, Napa, California.
*Format*: Print, online (standalone and in *Lexicomp Online*™), mobile application.
*Monograph sections*: Brand names, description, pharmacokinetics, compatibility of
the uncombined drug in various solutions, Y-site compatibility, syringe compatibility, admixture compatibility, and references.
*Comments*: This resource uses four compatibility indicators (compatible, incompatible, conflicting reports, or no information). It is commonly referred to as
*King's*. It contains information on more than 500 injectable drugs, more than
18,000 drug combinations, and 12 fluids. The online product is called *New King*®
*Guide Online*. The online product can be used to check compatibility information for a single drug or multiple drugs.

**Tools in General References**

Tools in *Micromedex*® (*Trissel's*™ *2 IV Compatibility*), *Facts & Comparisons*® *eAnswers* (*Trissel's*™
*IV-Check*), and Clinical Pharmacology (*Trissel's*™ *2 Clinical Pharmaceutics Database*) enable
practitioners to check intravenous compatibility of a single drug or multiple drugs.

## NATURAL PRODUCTS

Natural products include such things as vitamins, minerals, amino acids, herbs, botanical products, bodily constituents, and other substances. The FDA does not define *natural
product*, but it defines a *dietary supplement* as a product (other than tobacco) that

- Is intended to supplement the diet;
- Contains one or more dietary ingredients (including vitamins; minerals; herbs or other botanicals; amino acids; and other substances) or their constituents;
- Is intended to be taken by mouth as a pill, capsule, tablet, or liquid; and
- Is labeled on the front panel as being a dietary supplement.[22]

About half of U.S. adults report using one or more dietary supplements, and use has
been increasing over the past 30 years.[23] Although patients may believe that "natural"
means "safe," this is not always the case.[24] Therefore, it is important to know where to
locate reliable, unbiased information about natural products.

## Specialty Sources of Information

### Natural Medicines Comprehensive Database

*Publisher*: Therapeutic Research Faculty, Stockton, California.

*Format*: Online, mobile application.

*Organization*: Alphabetical by generic name.

*Monograph sections*: Synonyms, scientific names, uses, safety, effectiveness, mechanism of action, adverse reactions, interactions (rated major, moderate, or minor), dosage, administration, comments, and references.

*Rating system*: This resource uses safety and effectiveness ratings. There are five safety ratings (likely safe, possibly safe, possibly unsafe, likely unsafe, and unsafe) and six effectiveness ratings (effective, likely effective, possibly effective, possibly ineffective, likely ineffective, and ineffective). If there is insufficient evidence to assign a safety and/or effectiveness rating, it will be stated as such in the monograph.

*Comments*: This resource uses an evidence-based approach to systematically review and critically appraise the literature. The editor is a pharmacist. Subscribers gain access to additional online tools and features, including an effectiveness checker, drug interaction checker, disease/medical conditions search, continuing education, and patient handouts. Some free content, such as a clinical management series, special reports, a nutrient depletion chart, and a chart containing the caffeine content of energy drinks, is also available at the website.

### Natural Standard

*Publisher*: Natural Standard, Somerville, Massachusetts.

*Format*: Online (for institutions), desktop (for individuals), mobile application.

*Organization*: Alphabetical by generic name or condition.

*Monograph sections*: Its Food, Herbs & Supplements database features synonyms, clinical bottom line/effectiveness, evidence grades, dosing/toxicology, precautions/contraindications, pregnancy and lactation, interactions, mechanism of action, history, evidence table, evidence discussion, product studies, author information, and references. Its Comparative Effectiveness database lists the levels of scientific evidence, organized from A to F, for specific therapies with links to the monographs for the specific therapies.

*Rating system*: This resource uses a grading system (A = strong positive scientific evidence, B = positive scientific evidence, C = unclear scientific evidence, D = negative scientific evidence, F = strong negative scientific evidence).

*Comments*: This resource contains information about complementary and alternative medicine (CAM), including dietary supplements and integrative therapies (e.g., acupressure, music therapy, meditation). The grading system is evidence based. The resource contains several separate databases: Foods, Herbs & Supplements; Health & Wellness; Comparative Effectiveness; Charts & Tables; Brands & Manufacturers; Medical Conditions; Sports Medicine; Genomics & Proteomics; Environment & Global Health; and Animal Health. The Foods, Herbs & Supplements and Comparative Effectiveness databases are probably the most relevant for pharmacists. A number of tools are available online, including interactions, depletions, adverse effects, pregnancy and lactation, symptom checkers, a therapy finder, calculators, patient handouts, a recipe finder, nutrition labels, continuing education, and news and events.

### The Review of Natural Products

*Publisher*: Facts & Comparisons, Wolters Kluwer, St. Louis, Missouri.

*Format*: Print, online (in *Facts & Comparisons*® *eAnswers*), mobile (mobile version is titled *Guide to Popular Natural Products*).

*Organization*: Alphabetical by generic name.

*Monograph sections*: Date of issue, scientific name, common name(s), clinical overview, botany, history, chemistry, uses and pharmacology, dosing, pregnancy and lactation, interactions, adverse reactions, toxicology, and references.

*Comments*: Several appendices pertain to natural products, including an appendix that contains a lengthy list of other sources of information about natural products.

### The Complete German Commission E Monographs: Therapeutic Guide to Herbal Medicines

*Publishers*: American Botanical Council, Austin, Texas, and Integrative Medicine Communication, Boston, Massachusetts.

*Editors*: M. Blumenthal, W. R. Busse, A. Goldberg, J. Gruenwald, T. Hall, C. W. Riggins, and R. S. Rister.

*Translators*: S. Klein and R. S. Rister.

*Format*: Print, online.

*Organization*: Divided into four parts: introduction and overview, monographs, therapeutic indexes, chemical and taxonomic indexes. The monographs are divided into two sections: approved herbs and nonapproved herbs. The monographs are organized alphabetically by generic name within each section.

*Monograph sections*: Date of publication/revision, name, composition, uses, contraindications, side effects, interactions, dosage, mode/duration of administration, risks (unapproved herbs), evaluation (unapproved herbs), and actions.

*Comments*: The German Commission E is a German regulatory agency that evaluated nearly 400 herbs sold in Germany for safety and effectiveness. Herbs were either approved (approximately 200) or disapproved for use in Germany. The monographs were published in English in 1998, but had been published in German before then, so some of the evidence in the monographs is outdated. The monographs of the unapproved herbs include the reasons for nonapproval and/or the risks. The monographs do not contain references.

### Herbal Medicine: Expanded Commission E Monographs

*Publishers*: American Botanical Council, Austin, Texas, and Integrative Medicine Communications, Newton, Massachusetts.

*Editors*: M. Blumenthal, A. Goldberg, and J. Brinckmann.

*Format*: Print, online.

*Monograph sections*: Overview, description, chemistry and pharmacology, uses, contraindications, side effects, use during pregnancy and lactation, interactions with other drugs, dosage and administration, references, and additional resources.

*Comments*: This resource includes about 100 of the original German Commission E monographs, but provides more details about each herb. It was published in 2000 and has not been updated since, so some of the evidence in the monographs is outdated.

## Information in General References

*Lexicomp Online*® contains a *Natural Products Database*, which was adapted from *The Review of Natural Products*. The database contains an alphabetized list of natural products monographs.

*Micromedex*® contains an alternative medicine component. The monographs within this component provide evidence-based information on herbals, dietary supplements, vitamins, minerals, and other alternative therapies. Some of the monographs are from

*AltMedDex®* (a *Micromedex®* database) and some are from *Herbal Medicines: A Guide for Health-Care Professionals*, which is published by the Royal Pharmaceutical Society of Great Britain.

*Clinical Pharmacology* contains approximately 100 CAM monographs, which can be located by using the Find/List tool.

### Websites

**Table 3–4** contains a list of useful websites for information about natural products.

## FOREIGN DRUGS

Access to international tertiary literature is vital for patient care, product identification, and availability information.

### Specialty Sources of Information

### *Martindale: The Complete Drug Reference*

*Publisher*: Pharmaceutical Press, Royal Pharmaceutical Society of Great Britain.
*Editor*: Sean C. Sweetman.
*Format*: Print, online.
*Organization*: Three main sections of drug monographs, preparations, and manufacturer information, plus general and Cyrillic indexes.

| **TABLE 3-4**  Useful Websites for Natural Products Information | | |
|---|---|---|
| **Website** | **URL** | **Comments** |
| Center for Food Safety and Applied Nutrition (CFSAN) | www.fda.gov/food/default.htm | CFSAN is the center at the FDA that is responsible for regulating dietary supplements. The website contains questions and answers about dietary supplements and tips for people who take dietary supplements. |
| Office of Dietary Supplements (ODS) | ods.od.nih.gov | The ODS is part of the National Institutes of Health. The website contains background information about dietary supplements and fact sheets. A free mobile application is available for consumers to keep track of dietary supplements. |
| National Center for Complementary and Alternative Medicine (NCCAM) | nccam.nih.gov | NCCAM is part of the National Institutes of Health. The website contains an overview of complementary and alternative medicine (CAM), research-based information on CAM, safety information, and information about uses and side effects of herbs and botanicals. |
| Dietary Supplements Labels Database | www.dsld.nlm.nih.gov/dsld/ | This website is maintained by the National Library of Medicine. It contains label ingredients for more than 8,000 dietary supplements. |
| United States Pharmacopoeia (USP) Verification Services | www.usp.org/usp-verification-services | This website contains information about the USP's verification services for dietary supplements, dietary ingredients, and pharmaceutical ingredients. It contains a link to current USP Verified products. |
| American Botanical Council | abc.herbalgram.org | This website contains news about and resources for herbal medicine. |

*Monograph sections*: General identification and physical information, adverse effects, precautions, interactions, and pharmacokinetic properties. Preparations and brand names follow the use, dose, and administration information.

*Comments*: Includes proprietary preparation information from the United Kingdom, United States, and 39 other countries/regions.

### *Index Nominum: International Drug Directory*

*Publisher*: Medpharm, Swiss Pharmaceutical Society.

*Format*: Print plus CD-ROM of manufacturers' contact information, online.

*Organization*: Drug monographs indexed by brand name, synonyms, and WHO ATC/ATCvet codes.

*Monograph sections*: Brief monographs listing synonyms, international trade names, therapeutic classification, chemical structures, and molecular weight.

*Comments*: Includes French, German, Latin, and Spanish substance names as well as international nonproprietary names.

### *Drug Product Database (DPD)*

*Publisher*: Health Canada (www.hc-sc.gc.ca).

*Format*: Online.

*Organization*: Contains searchable fields for brand name, identification number, market status, class, active ingredient, dosage form, route, and strength. The descriptive fields in the monographs include company information for both human and veterinary products.

*Comments*: Health Canada is the federal regulator of therapeutic products in Canada.

## Websites

A list of websites for identifying foreign medicines can be found in the article by Grossman and Zerilli.[25]

## OTHER SPECIALTY AREAS

The previous sections reviewed some of the more common specialty areas from which pharmacists receive questions. Pharmacists may encounter several other specialty areas. **Table 3–5** lists some of the other specialty areas and references that pharmacists may find useful.

| **CASE STUDY 3-1** | **Choosing an Appropriate Tertiary Resource** |
| --- | --- |

Joan Doe approaches you with a new prescription in hand. As she hands you the paperwork, she asks the following questions. Which tertiary resources could be consulted for answering each question?

1. I was recently diagnosed with open-angle glaucoma. The physician prescribed Xalatan. My insurance plan covers generics without added charge to me. Is this product available as a generic?
2. This is the first medication I will have to take as a long-term treatment. How and when should I use this drug?
3. How does this medication work to lower the pressure in my eye?
4. I am on no other medications, but do I need to worry about any side effects? Will my eyes hurt after I use it?
5. I have never been on any sort of eye medication before, so I do not know what to do. Should I keep it in the refrigerator while I am using it, or can I keep it on the nightstand near my bed?
6. I travel a lot and have a sabbatical planned in Prague from May 2015 until August 2016. Will I be able to buy the drug while I am there? What is the name of the drug?

| **TABLE 3-5**   Other Specialty Areas and Resources |
|---|

**Toxicology**
*Casarett & Doull's Essentials of Toxicology*. Curtis D. Klaassen and James B. Watkins III, editors. McGraw-Hill.
*Goldfrank's Toxicologic Emergencies*. Lewis S. Nelson, Neal A. Lewin, Mary Ann Howland, Robert S. Hoffman, Lewis R. Goldfrank, et al., authors. McGraw-Hill.
*Micromedex® POSINDEX® System*. Truven Health Analytics.
*Poisoning & Drug Overdose*. Kent R. Olson, editor. McGraw-Hill.

**Pharmacogenomics**
*Concepts in Pharmacogenomics*. Martin M. Zdanowicz, editor. American Society of Health-System Pharmacists.
*Pharmacogenomics: An Introduction and Clinical Perspective*. Joseph S. Bertino Jr., Angela Kashuba, Joseph D. Ma, Uwe Fuhr, C. Lindsay DeVane, editors. McGraw-Hill.
*Pharmacogenomics: Applications to Patient Care*. Howard L. McLeod, C. Lindsay DeVane, Susanne B. Haga, Julie A. Johnson, Daren L. Knoell, et al., editors. American College of Clinical Pharmacy.
*Principles of the Human Genome and Pharmacogenomics*. Daniel A. Brazeau and Gayle A. Brazeau, authors. American Pharmacists Association.

**Dosing in Renal Failure**
*Drug Prescribing in Renal Failure: Dosing Guidelines for Adults and Children*. George R. Aronoff, William M. Bennett, Jeffery S. Berns, Michael E. Brier, Nishaminy Kasbekar, et al., editors. American College of Physicians.

**Geriatrics**
*Fundamentals of Geriatric Pharmacology: An Evidence-Based Approach*. Lisa C. Hutchison and Rebecca B. Sleeper, editors. American Society of Health-System Pharmacists.
*Geriatric Dosage Handbook*. Todd P. Simla, Judith L. Beizer, Martin B. Higbee, editors. Lexicomp.

**Infectious Disease**
*Antibiotic Essentials*. Burke A. Cunha, author. Jones & Bartlett Learning.
*Johns Hopkins ABX Guide: Diagnosis and Treatment of Infectious Disease*. John G. Bartlett, Paul G. Auwaerter, Paul A. Pham, editors. Johns Hopkins Medicine.
*Mandell, Douglas, and Bennett's Principles and Practice of Infectious Diseases*. Gerald L. Mandell, John E. Bennett, Raphael Dolin, editors. Churchill Livingstone.
*The Sanford Guide to Antimicrobial Therapy*. David N. Gilbert, Henry F. Chambers, George M. Eliopoulos , Michael S. Saag, Douglas Black, editors. Antimicrobial Therapy.
*The Washington Manual of Infectious Diseases Subspecialty Consult*. Nigar Kirmani, Keith Woeltje, Hilary Babcock, editors. Department of Medicine, Washington University School of Medicine.

# ELECTRONIC APPLICATIONS

Availability and popularity of mobile devices has increased greatly. More than 50% of smartphone owners use their devices for health information.[26] This comes as no surprise considering the ease of use of affordable hardware at point of need. Clinical practitioners may encounter various methods of access, including full websites, mobile-compatible websites, and mobile applications. Desktop Internet users are familiar with full websites. Newer technologies allow browsing of uniform resource locators (URLs) from tablet devices or smartphones. Mobile-compatible websites are redesigned for handheld devices to enable content delivery to the smaller screen. Mobile applications are downloaded to the handheld device. Live connection to online content is not necessary, with the exception of downloading updates or uploading gathered data.

# SOURCES FOR MOBILE APPLICATIONS AND DIGITAL INFORMATION

## MobiHealthNews

*URL*: mobihealthnews.com
*Editor*: Brian Dolan.
*Format*: Website and twice-weekly e-mail newsletter.
*Comments*: News and information focused on digital health. The resource center offers free and fee-based state-of-the-industry reports, webinars, and other mobile health information.

## iMedicalApps

*URL*: www.imedicalapps.com
*Editor*: Iltifat Husain.
*Format*: Website and weekly e-mail newsletter.
*Comments*: News and product reviews with the ability to filter by operating system, medical specialty, and mobile application type (e.g., clinical references, drug references, procedures and simulations, textbooks). A tab is available linking to reviews and instructional videos. The "Top Apps" feature retrieves stories showcasing popular and well-rated products. The editorial staff includes physicians, a pharmacist, a medical librarian, medical residents, and students.

## Selected Tertiary Mobile Applications

See **Table 3-6** for a list of selected tertiary mobile applications.

**TABLE 3-6** Selected Tertiary Mobile Applications

| Application | URL |
| --- | --- |
| AHFS® Drug Information | www.skyscape.com/estore/ProductDetail.aspx?ProductId=1188 |
| Clinical Pharmacology | secure.goldstandard.com/subscribe |
| Epocrates® Rx Epocrates® Essentials | epocrates.com/mobile |
| Facts & Comparisons® A to Z Drug Facts™ with Auto-Updates | http://www.unboundmedicine.com/staging/news_um_dfs.html |
| Lexicomp products | webstore.lexi.com/ON-HAND |
| Medscape® | www.medscape.com/public/mobileapp |
| Micromedex® Drug Information | truvenhealth.com/products/micromedexmobile.aspx |
| mobilePDR® | www.skyscape.com/estore/ProductDetail.aspx?ProductId=2738 |
| Tarascon® Pharmacopoeia | www.tarascon.com/products/mobile |

## Mobile Applications from the National Library of Medicine

### Drug Information Portal

*URL*: druginfo.nlm.nih.gov/m.drugportal/m.drugportal.jsp
*Format*: Mobile-compatible website.
*Comments*: Acting as a meta-search engine, *Drug Information Portal* quickly searches a wide range of National Library of Medicine resources simultaneously. See **Table 3-7** for a listing of the databases included in the results.

### NLM Mobile

*URL*: www.nlm.nih.gov/mobile
*Format*: Online.
*Comments*: NLM Mobile serves as an installation launch site for various applications and mobile-compatible sites of interest for the healthcare practitioner. New items are added as they are developed.

**TABLE 3-7** List of Databases Searched by the National Library of Medicine's *Drug Information Portal*

| Summary | Database |
|---|---|
| Summary of drug information | MedlinePlusDrug |
| Summary of dietary supplement and herbal information | MedlinePlusSupp |
| Summary of consumer health information | MedlinePlusTopics |
| Summary of HIV/AIDS treatment | AIDSinfo |
| Summary of the effect on breastfeeding | LactMed |
| Summary of drug-induced liver injury | LiverTox |
| Manufacturer drug labels | DailyMed |
| Summary of ingredients and label information | Dietary Supplements Labels Database |
| Clinical trials | ClinicalTrials.gov |
| Drug identification and image | Pillbox beta |
| **Detailed Summary** | |
| Summary of reviewed biological and physical data | Hazardous Substances Data Bank |
| References from scientific journals | Medline/PubMed |
| References from toxicological journals | TOXLINE |
| Biological activities and chemical structures | PubChem |
| Biological activities against HIV/AIDS and other viruses | NIAID ChemDB |
| Toxicological and chemical resources | ChemIDplus |
| **Additional Resources** | |
| Information from the Food & Drug Administration (FDA) | Drugs@FDA |
| Information from the Drug Enforcement Administration (DEA) | DEA |
| Search engine for other government resources | www.usa.gov |

| CASE STUDY 3-2 | **Choosing an Appropriate Specialty Tertiary Resource** |

You are a pharmacist in a drug information center. You receive the following questions. Which specialty tertiary resources should you consult for each question?

1. I recently found out I am pregnant. I currently take Prozac. Can I take this while pregnant, or are there other anti-depressants that are preferred in pregnant women? If I breastfeed, can I continue taking the same antidepressant that I take during my pregnancy, or will I have to switch?
2. I want to lose weight, but I've heard that prescription drugs have bad side effects. Which natural product works best for weight loss?
3. I take warfarin, lisinopril, hydrochlorothiazide, albuterol, and montelukast. My doctor just prescribed Bactrim for me. Can I take Bactrim with my current drugs?
4. My child has just been diagnosed with multiple sclerosis. The doctor would like him to take baclofen to treat some of his symptoms. He cannot swallow pills. Can you make a liquid out of the tablets?
5. How is methylprednisolone dosed for an 8-year-old with acute spinal cord injury? Is it compatible with a 3-in-1 total parenteral nutrition admixture?
6. I recently had a major medical event and now I have to take seven drugs. I've noticed my hair is falling out. Can you tell me which drug is causing this?

## Sources for Availability of Tertiary Literature

### *Basic Resources for Pharmacy Education*

*URL*: www.aacp.org/governance/SECTIONS/libraryinformationscience/Pages/LibraryInformationScienceSpecialProjectsandInformation.aspx

*Publisher*: The Library and Information Sciences Section of the American Association of Colleges of Pharmacy.

*Editors*: Barbara Nanstiel and Sharon Giovenale.

*Comments*: This document is a service project of the Library and Information Sciences section of the AACP. Each subject section is reviewed every 3 years through two review cycles and is published semiannually. Intended as a collection development tool for pharmacy librarians, *Basic Resources* serves as a tertiary literature guide for clinical practitioners.

### *Drug Information: A Guide to Current Resources*

*Publisher*: Neal-Schuman Publishers, New York.

*Author*: Bonnie Snow.

*Format*: Print.

*Comments*: Snow's *Guide* has served health science professionals through three editions. Chapters include resource listings for drug identification, governmental regulations, source evaluation and search strategy logistics, pharmacology and therapeutics, drug analysis formulation and compounding, development, and marketing. Online resources for information retrieval are also included.

# SUMMARY

Tertiary sources summarize and interpret information derived from the primary literature and provide a concise and fairly complete overview of a topic. Tertiary references may be general or specialized in nature and are usually used as first-line resources to research a drug information request. A variety of general and specialty tertiary sources of information are available in numerous formats that are easy to use and accessible.

Although tertiary sources offer many advantages, users must also consider their disadvantages, including publication lag time, space limitations within the references, and the potential for author bias.

# REFERENCES

1. Wright SG, LeCroy RL, Kendrach MG. A review of the three types of biomedical literature and the systematic approach to answer a drug information request. *J Pharm Pract.* 1998;11(3):148-162.
2. Katz WA, Kinder R, eds. *The Publishing and Review of Reference Sources.* New York, NY: Haworth Press; 1987.
3. Health On the Net Foundation. The HON code of conduct for medical and health web sites (HONcode). http://www.hon.ch/HONcode/Pro/Conduct.html. Accessed July 15, 2014.
4. Cohen JS, Insel PA. *The Physicians' Desk Reference.* Problems and possible improvements. *Arch Intern Med.* 1996;156(13):1375-1380.
5. Mindel JS, Teich SA, Teich CM, Beam P. Editorial: limitations of the *Physicians' Desk Reference* 2007. *Surv Ophthalmol.* 2008;53(1):82-84.
6. Hansten P, Horn J. Drug–drug interaction mechanisms. http://www.hanstenandhorn.com/article-d-i.html. Accessed July 15, 2014.
7. Karch FE, Lasagna L. Adverse drug reactions. A critical review. *JAMA.* 1975;234(12):1236-1241.
8. World Health Organization. Requirements for adverse reaction reporting. Geneva, Switzerland; 1975.
9. U.S. Food and Drug Administration. What is a serious adverse event? http://www.fda.gov/safety/medwatch/howtoreport/ucm053087.htm. Accessed July 15, 2014.
10. American Society of Health-System Pharmacists. ASHP guidelines on adverse drug reaction monitoring and reporting. http://www.ashp.org/DocLibrary/BestPractices/MedMisGdlADR.aspx. Accessed July 15, 2014.
11. Wooten JM. Adverse drug reactions: part I. *South Med J.* 2010;103(10):1025-1028.
12. Beard K. Introduction. In: Lee A, ed. *Adverse Drug Reactions.* London: Pharmaceutical Press; 2001:1-17.
13. Daw JR, Hanley GE, Greyson DL, Morgan SG. Prescription drug use during pregnancy in developed countries: a systematic review. *Pharmacoepidemiol Drug Saf.* 2011;20(9):895-902.
14. Stultz EE, Stokes JL, Shaffer ML, Paul IM, Berlin CM. Extent of medication use in breastfeeding women. *Breastfeed Med.* 2007;2(3):145-151.
15. Briggs GG. Drug effects on the fetus and breast-fed infant. *Clin Obstet Gynecol.* 2002;45(1):6-21.
16. Berens PD, Hale TW. Drug principles in pregnancy and lactation. In: Borgelt LM, O'Connell MB, Smith JA, Calis KA, eds. *Women's Health Across the Lifespan: A Pharmacotherapeutic Approach.* Bethesda, MD: American Society of Health-System Pharmacists; 2010:355-370.
17. Niebyl JR. Nausea and vomiting in pregnancy. *N Engl J Med.* 2010;363(16):1544-1550.
18. Wigle PR, Kim KY. Conditions associated with pregnancy. In: Borgelt LM, O'Connell MB, Smith JA, Calis KA, eds. *Women's Health Across the Lifespan: A Pharmacotherapeutic Approach.* Bethesda, MD: American Society of Health-System Pharmacists; 2010:371-386.
19. US Food and Drug Administration. 1979. Labeling and prescription drug advertising. Content and format for labeling for human prescription drugs. *Federal Register.* 1979;44:37434-37467.
20. U.S. Food and Drug Administration. Pregnancy and lactation labeling. http://www.fda.gov/Drugs/DevelopmentApprovalProcess/DevelopmentResources/Labeling/ucm093307.htm. Accessed July 15, 2014.
21. Nahata MC, Taketomo C. Pediatrics. In: DiPiro JT, Talbert RL, Yee GC, Matzke GR, Wells BG, Posey LM, eds. *Pharmacotherapy: A Pathophysiologic Approach.* 8th ed. New York, NY: McGraw-Hill; 2011. http://www.accesspharmacy.com/content.aspx?aID=7967211. Accessed July 15, 2014.
22. Office of Dietary Supplements National Institutes of Health. Background information: dietary supplements. http://ods.od.nih.gov/factsheets/DietarySupplements-HealthProfessional. Accessed July 15, 2014.
23. Bailey RL, Gahche JJ, Miller PE, Thomas PR, Dwyer JT. Why US adults use dietary supplements. *JAMA Intern Med.* 2013;173(5):355-361.
24. National Center for Complementary and Alternative Medicine. Using dietary supplements wisely. http://www.nccam.nih.gov/health/supplements/wiseuse.htm. Accessed July 15, 2014.
25. Grossman S, Zerilli T. Health and medication information resources on the world wide web. *J Pharm Pract.* 2013;26(2):85-94.
26. Fox S, Duggan M. Mobile Health 2012: Half of smartphone owners use their devices to get health information and one-fifth of smartphone owners have health apps. http://pewinternet.org/~/media//Files/Reports/2012/PIP_MobileHealth2012_FINAL.pdf. Accessed July 15, 2014.

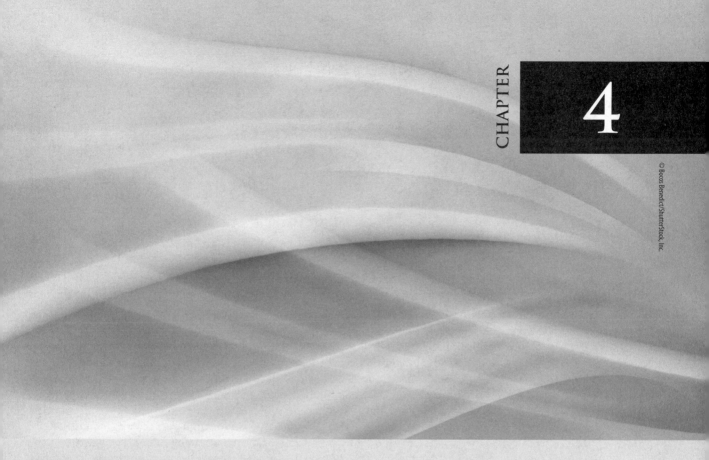

# SECONDARY SOURCES OF INFORMATION

Luigi Brunetti, PharmD, MPH, BCPS
Evelyn R. Hermes DeSantis, PharmD, BCPS

## CHAPTER OBJECTIVES

▸ List the characteristics of an ideal secondary resource.

▸ Identify the strengths and weaknesses of commonly used secondary resources.

▸ Recognize the importance of using multiple secondary resources when performing a literature search.

## CHAPTER OUTLINE

## KEY TERMS

Boolean operators

MEDLINE

MeSH

Secondary resources

# INTRODUCTION

**Secondary resources** of drug information direct the user to primary resources such as clinical trials. The user is provided a searchable database that either indexes or abstracts primary literature. The difference between indexing and abstracting is that the former only provides bibliographic information without a brief description of the primary literature. Since the invention and evolution of the Internet, the availability and usability of secondary resources has expanded dramatically. Although there are advantages to using multiple secondary resources, one of the challenges with these resources is the variability in performing a search. Clinicians should familiarize themselves with several secondary resources in order to perform an adequate search of the literature. Any comprehensive literature search should employ at least two, and preferably more, secondary resources. Utilizing multiple secondary resources is especially important when performing a systematic review. Several authors have highlighted the importance of using multiple secondary resources when reviewing the literature to identify support for a clinical practice.[1-3] In addition to using various search engines, it is important to understand that there is not one "perfect" search strategy. Each search may require a number of different terms and strategies to be able to identify appropriate results.

# SEARCH STRATEGY ISSUES

Secondary resources by their very nature need to be searched. As with any tool, the final results are dependent upon the skill of the user. Being able to design an appropriate search strategy is essential for finding the results that one is looking for. The first step in any search is defining the question that is being asked. Identification of appropriate terms is critical. As Mark Twain once said, "the difference between the right word and the almost right word is the difference between lightning and a lightning bug."[4] In addition, it is important to realize that each secondary resource has its own way of constructing a search.

To assist in selecting the best terms, it is important to frame the search question with as many specifics as possible. Specific terms may include the specific drug, disease state, patient characteristics, outcomes of interest, and so on. Again, the specific search term depends on the question being asked. It may not be important to use every term that applies, because some will be inherently applied with other terms (such as the use of "elderly" with "Alzheimer's disease"), but it is important to use terms essential to the question. Databases have two different types of vocabulary terms that they may use: open and closed. An open vocabulary allows one to search any term in the title, abstract, author listing, and so on. An advantage with the open vocabulary is that it allows the user to search for any term; a disadvantage is that it allows the user to search for any term regardless of whether it is important to the article or spelled correctly. A closed vocabulary, also known as a *thesaurus*, restricts the search to identified keywords for a given article. An example of a closed vocabulary is the Medical Subject Headings, or **MeSH**, utilized by **MEDLINE** or Emtree utilized by Embase. The closed vocabulary allows for similar topics to be grouped together. So whether the article specifically stated "high blood pressure" whereas another article mentioned "hypertension," both articles would be categorized as "hypertension" in a closed vocabulary setting.

## TREE STRUCTURE

The terms in the thesaurus are organized in a hierarchical structure known as the *tree structure*. In MeSH, there are 16 categories organized as A, anatomical terms; B, organisms; C, diseases; D, drugs; and so on. Each category then has a hierarchical listing of terms from general to most specific. Understanding the tree structure can be very helpful when searching. For example, if searching for anemia, it is helpful for the searcher to know that not only could the broad category of anemia be searched, but also the more specific types of anemia, such as hemolytic anemia, and even more specific types, such as autoimmune hemolytic anemia. Similarly, when searching for a drug, it may be helpful to use the specific term, similar agents, or the entire drug class.

## EXPLODING THE HIERARCHY

A helpful tool for searching and maximizing the utility of the tree structure is "exploding," or expanding, the term based on the hierarchy. Exploding a term allows the searcher to capture all of the more specific types of the original category. Taking the example of anemia, by exploding anemia, the searcher will also capture the more specific types of anemia, such as aplastic anemia, hemolytic anemia, hypochromic anemia, and so on. Another search where exploding can be helpful is when the user is searching for information on a class of drugs. For example, if the searcher is looking for adverse effects associated with levofloxacin or other fluoroquinolones, a more efficient search than using each individual drug is to explode fluoroquinolones. The limitation of exploding all the time is getting too many results that may not be pertinent. For example, exploding ampicillin in MEDLINE yields results not only for ampicillin, but for amoxicillin, mezlocillin, piperacillin, and other agents as well.

## FOCUSING BY MAJOR TOPIC

Another issue with searching secondary resources is having too many results that may not deal directly with the question at hand. Whereas exploding will broaden the search results, focusing allows for the refinement of the search. The focus feature is based on the search term being one of the main topics of the article. Historically, *Index Medicus*, the print version of MEDLINE, identified each article with MeSH terms and grouped the terms as major MeSH and minor MeSH. Focus only searches the major MeSH terms. In databases that utilize and list the MeSH terms, the major MeSH terms are identified by an asterisk in the MeSH listing.

## SUBHEADINGS

Another tool that assists in limiting a search is the use of subheadings. Each category of MeSH terms has unique subheadings. Subheadings allow for the refinement of a search strategy. For example, a search of thrombocytopenia secondary to contrast dye would benefit from searching "thrombocytopenia" with the subheading of "chemically induced." Not all searches and search terms benefit from using subheadings, but many, very specific searches or searches with a large number of results do benefit from the use of subheadings.

## BOOLEAN OPERATORS

Once specific terms are identified, it is important to put them into the context of the question and combine the terms. To combine terms, **Boolean operators** are utilized. The two most common are AND and OR; however, another one that can be helpful is NOT. The term AND will take the two search statements and only return results that contain both terms. The term OR will return results that have either of the two terms in them, yielding a much larger search. NOT can be helpful in limiting results from a larger search string. For example, if a user has looked at all of the review articles on a topic and wants to eliminate them from the search listing, the original results can be combined with the Boolean operator NOT, and the remaining review articles are the original results minus the review articles.

# REVIEW OF IMPORTANT SECONDARY RESOURCES

Several secondary resources are available for clinicians to search and identify relevant biomedical literature. Each has its advantages and disadvantages. Furthermore, each resource indexes different sources of information (e.g., journals, conferences, symposia, etc.). For these reasons, a good literature search will utilize more than one secondary resource. Many of the commonly used secondary resources provide tools to aid the user in performing searches, such as user guides, web tutorials, and presentations. **Table 4–1** provides a partial listing of the website addresses (URLs) for these tools.

## MEDLINE AND PUBMED

The National Library of Medicine (NLM) introduced MEDLINE in 1971 as the first interactive searchable database.[5] In 1996, OLDMEDLINE was also added to expand coverage to include publications published between 1950 and 1965. In 1997, a combination

| **TABLE 4-1**   URLs for Secondary Resource Tutorials and/or User Guides | |
|---|---|
| **Resource** | **URL for Tutorial/User Guide** |
| PubMed | www.nlm.nih.gov/bsd/disted/pubmedtutorial/cover.html |
| OvidSP | http://www.ovid.com/site/support/training.jsp |
| Google Scholar | www.google.com/intl/en/scholar/help.html |
| Web of Science | wokinfo.com/training_support/training/web-of-knowledge/ |
| Embase | www.elsevier.com/online-tools/embase/support#guides-and-manuals |
| Scopus | help.scopus.com/Content/tutorials/sc_menu.html |
| Cochrane Library | www.thecochranelibrary.com/view/0/HowtoUse.html |

*Note:* Links are current and working as of October 2014.

of both databases was launched as PubMed. As of February 2013, the MEDLINE database contained more than 19 million references to journal articles in the life sciences. The majority of these references are concentrated in biomedicine. These citations are retrieved from approximately 5,600 worldwide journals that are indexed in MEDLINE. Although the majority of publications retrieved using MEDLINE are peer reviewed, some are not (e.g., some magazines, newsletters, and newspapers).

Numerous platforms search MEDLINE, including PubMed, Ovid, EBSCO, First Search, and others. Each of these platforms varies slightly in their functionality; however, PubMed is NLM's platform, available free of charge to the public at www.ncbi.nlm.nih.gov/pubmed/, and will be the focus of this section. The primary component of PubMed is MEDLINE. PubMed provides the user an interface to search citations indexed in MEDLINE. In addition to MEDLINE citations, PubMed also contains in-process citations (a record for an article before it is indexed with MeSH terms and added to MEDLINE), citations that precede the date the journal was selected for MEDLINE indexing, some OLDMEDLINE citations, citations that are out of scope for MEDLINE, and citations that submit full-text articles to PubMed Central. Many of the citations retrieved will provide abstracts in addition to the author, title, and source. Accessibility to the full text of the citation is dependent on whether the citation is open access or requires a subscription. Many citations retrieved also contain links to the full text.

To perform a PubMed search, the user enters search topics (one or more terms) and selects the option to search. Several options for searching include the use of MeSH terms, author names, title words, keywords, phrases, journal names, or any combination of these items. Upon entering a search term in PubMed, the term will automatically be searched as a text word and a MeSH term that "best fits" the word entered. Citations fitting the search are retrieved and displayed in a list. The list may be scanned and abstracts viewed to verify relevance to the topic of interest. Users also have the option to find related articles for any citation they choose. More advanced or complex searches may be performed using filters, including but not limited to article type, age group, study type, publication year, and language. PubMed uses many of the search features discussed earlier in the search strategy section.

PubMed is a key secondary resource and is widely used by scientists and clinicians. In 2012, 2.2 billion searches were performed using MEDLINE/PubMed.[6] Several features of PubMed are advantageous to the user. First, it does not require a subscription and is easily accessible. Second, it includes a large number of journals, and the majority are peer reviewed. Finally, the search capabilities, filters, and features to quickly identify references related to retrieved citations provide the user with ample methods for expanding or narrowing a search. One disadvantage of PubMed is that it excludes a majority of "grey" literature; that is, literature that is not peer reviewed. Exclusion of grey literature may result in an incomplete search and biased findings. In fact, meta-analyses that exclude grey literature are more likely to overrepresent studies with significant findings.[7] Using MEDLINE/PubMed as a sole secondary resource may be disadvantageous because some relevant literature may be missed because all available journals are not indexed.

---

**CASE STUDY 4-1**    **Male Sterility Search Strategy**

You are completing a review of fertility and sterility issues facing patients receiving chemotherapy. As you search for specific chemotherapy agents and sterility in male patients, you hit a roadblock. Develop a search strategy and ways to overcome this roadblock using appropriate MeSH terms and other features of MEDLINE.

## CUMULATIVE INDEX TO NURSING AND ALLIED HEALTH

The Cumulative Index to Nursing and Allied Health (CINAHL) database provides comprehensive coverage of the nursing and allied health literature.[8] In addition to indexing journals, CINAHL also includes nursing conference proceedings, health-related books, educational software, and publications of the American Nurses Association and the National League for Nursing. Researchers may also find selective consumer health, alternate/complementary medicine, biomedicine, and health sciences literature as well. As of March 2013, 3,071 journals were indexed, beginning from 1981. Expanded CINAHL coverage is available (CINAHL Plus, 4,995 journals indexed, and CINAHL Complete, 5,168 journals indexed).

## INTERNATIONAL PHARMACEUTICAL ABSTRACTS

The International Pharmaceutical Abstracts (IPA) database was originally started by the American Society of Health-System Pharmacists (ASHP) in 1964 in print and electronically in 1970 and subsequently produced by Thomson Scientific since 2005.[9] IPA includes approximately 800 journals, including all U.S. state pharmacy journals, to provide worldwide coverage of pharmacology, pharmacy, and health-related literature. The citations focus on comprehensive information for drug therapy, toxicity, and pharmacy practice, as well as legislation, regulation, technology, utilization, biopharmaceutics, information processing, education, economics, and ethics, as related to pharmaceutical science and practice.

IPA utilizes an open vocabulary format. Any term can be used, and depending on the database vendor, the term can be searched in a specific field, such as all text, title, author, author affiliation, source, abstract, descriptors, chemical name, generic name, section heading, therapeutic classification, trade name, and language. In addition, all three Boolean operators can be used.

IPA includes both published articles as well as grey literature such as abstracts from various meetings, such as the ASHP Midyear Clinical Meeting, the ASHP Annual Meeting, and others. The abstract results of clinical studies in IPA include the study design, number of patients, dosage, dosage forms, and dosage schedule. The main limitation of this database is the limited scope and number of journals included.

## EMBASE

Embase was established in 1947.[10] The focus of Embase is biomedical and pharmacological scientific literature from more than 3,000 international titles. Embase includes all the articles and journals indexed in MEDLINE, plus more than 5 million records and 2,000 biomedical journals not currently covered by MEDLINE, representing more than 90 countries and 40 languages. In addition to published articles, Embase also covers approximately 1,000 conferences annually and indexes their conference abstracts. Emtree is the thesaurus used by Embase and has twice as many terms as MeSH. Unfortunately, many major medical and pharmacy school libraries do not have access to Embase because of its cost.

## GOOGLE SCHOLAR

Google Scholar was launched by its parent company, Google, in 2004.[11] This resource provides access to full-text journals, preprints, theses, books, and other "scholarly" publications. Theoretically, Google Scholar has the capability to search all literature in any language as long as it has been uploaded in electronic format onto the Internet.

Google Scholar provides an advanced search feature that enables users to narrow searches using keywords, author, subject, and/or publication date. The most important advantages of Google Scholar are the open access format and the ability to search peer-reviewed and grey literature. In general, Google Scholar offers results that are less accurate and less frequently updated compared to other databases. Additionally, results are often displayed in relation to the number of visits by users, resulting in bias toward older literature. The coverage of Google Scholar appears to be broad and identifies many relevant citations. In one analysis where Google Scholar was used to repeat searches performed in published systematic reviews, no citation would have been missed if Google Scholar was used alone.[12]

## WEB OF SCIENCE

Web of Science is published by Thomson Reuters and is only available with a subscription. Although launched in 2004 as an Internet-accessible database, the concept of Web of Science was the vision of Eugene Garfield, founder of the Institute for Scientific Information.[13,14] Web of Science includes non-peer-reviewed as well as peer-reviewed resources. Some non-peer-reviewed resources that may be useful include seminars, symposia, conference proceedings, and poster presentations. Coverage is extremely broad, including literature in areas such as agriculture, biological sciences, engineering, medical and life sciences, physical and chemical sciences, anthropology, law, library sciences, architecture, dance, music, film, and theater. Coverage includes more than 8,300 major journals in the Science Citation Index, 4,500 journals in the Social Science Citation Index, 2,300 arts and humanities journals, and selected items from more than 6,000 scientific and social sciences journals. Web of Science also provides coverage of the Conference Proceedings Citation Index, including more than 148,000 journals and book-based proceedings. Researchers may also search content in Index Chemicus and Current Chemical Reactions using Web of Science. Web of Science also includes some grey literature. In April 2011, 49.4 million records were reported in Web of Science.[14]

## SCOPUS

Scopus is owned by Elsevier and requires a subscription in order to access the online portal. Approximately 19,500 citations from more than 5,000 international publishers are included in Scopus.[15] The reach of this secondary resource is extensive, and coverage includes 8,500 peer-reviewed journals, 425 trade publications, 325 book series, conference coverage, articles in press, 375 million scientific web pages, and 24.8 million patents, in addition to all citations indexed in MEDLINE. The resource is updated daily and provides subscriber alerts such as RSS and HTML feeds to maintain up-to-date information.

## COCHRANE LIBRARY

The Cochrane Library, launched in 1996, consists of several databases, including the Cochrane Database of Systematic Reviews, Cochrane Central Register of Controlled Trials, Cochrane Methodology Register, Database of Abstracts of Review of Effects, Health Technology Assessment Database, NHS Economic Evaluation Database, and About The Cochrane Review Collaboration Database.[16] The most popular of the databases in the Cochrane Library is the Cochrane Database of Systematic Reviews (CDSR). This database is the leading resource for systematic reviews and meta-analyses. CDSR and Cochrane Central are updated monthly, whereas the remaining databases are updated quarterly. Although access to the systematic reviews in the CDSR is free in some low- and middle-income countries, in the United States full access requires a subscription. As of March 2013, the CDSR included 7,819 records, 5,449 reviews, and 2,370 protocols. The Cochrane Library may be searched and abstracts viewed without a subscription. Although the Cochrane Library does not direct the user to non-Cochrane primary literature, it remains an important resource in retrieving systematic reviews and meta-analyses.

## OTHER SPECIALTY RESOURCES

### Iowa Drug Information System

The Iowa Drug Information System (IDIS) is a bibliographic indexing service for more than 200 premier English-language medical and pharmaceutical journals from 1966 to the present.[17] Only 1988 to the present is available online; older articles are available via microfiche. The database includes pivotal drug studies, case reports, clinical practice guidelines, systematic reviews, comparative effectiveness studies and reviews, Food and Drug Administration (FDA) new drug approval packages and advisory committee reports, reports from the Agency for Healthcare Research and Quality (AHRQ), and guidelines and appraisal reports from the National Institute for Health and Care Excellence (NICE). IDIS utilizes a closed vocabulary for searching. One main advantage of IDIS is access to full-text articles for all of the citations listed.

### Journal Watch

Journal Watch is from the publishers of the *New England Journal of Medicine* and selects and summarizes the most important research and guidelines.[18] Although not a traditional searchable secondary resource, Journal Watch can add value to a search. Specifically, this resource highlights primary literature deemed to be of the highest clinical relevance. There are 13 specialties covered by Journal Watch. One major benefit of Journal Watch is that it provides, through either the website or email updates, a quick summary of recent articles.

### Reactions Weekly

Reactions Weekly, from Springer, is a weekly publication of information related to adverse effects.[19] Information includes labeling changes, drug withdrawals due to safety issues, adverse reaction research, and current issues in drug safety. This information is pulled from journals, scientific meetings, media releases, regulatory agency websites, and bulletins from the national centers that participate in the World Health Organization (WHO) International Drug Monitoring Programme. Searching the publication is limited to text word (open vocabulary). The availability of Reactions Weekly is somewhat limited based on library subscriptions and expense. Similar to Journal Watch, Reactions Weekly is not a traditional secondary resource in that it provides an abstraction of select primary literature. Nonetheless, this resource can direct clinicians to pertinent primary literature related to drug-related iatrogenic events.

### Clin-Alert

Clin-Alert, from SAFE Publications, is a semi-monthly newsletter that summarizes reports about adverse drug reactions (including those related to dietary supplements), drug-drug interactions, medication errors, and market withdrawals from more than 100 key journals and cites the original source. Initial reports of an adverse drug reaction are noted and the editor of Clin-Alert is a pharmacist.

| CASE STUDY 4-2 | Nebulized Morphine Search Strategy |
|---|---|

Your research team is asked to perform a systematic review of the literature to identify whether the use of nebulized morphine is beneficial for the treatment of dyspnea in end-stage chronic obstructive pulmonary disease. What search strategy would you recommend (i.e., search terms, databases, etc.)?

# COMPARISON OF SECONDARY RESOURCES

Several characteristics may be used to define an "ideal" secondary resource; however, user preference is also a key factor in resource selection.[20] A secondary resource should be inclusive and contain all (peer-reviewed and non–peer-reviewed) available information. When performing a search, the ideal resource should return only the most relevant literature. Another important characteristic is tools for filtering search results. Other important characteristics include linking to full-text articles and citation analysis. Finally, availability of a secondary resource without a subscription is desirable. Direct comparisons between secondary resources are difficult because the functionality and scope of the databases differ.[21] Different databases search different sets of information; therefore, one should expect different results. Nonetheless, several authors have attempted to provide a comparison of currently available databases. **Table 4-2** provides a general overview of the more common databases/search engines utilized when performing drug information queries. Overall, each database has its inherent advantages and disadvantages.

Falagas and colleagues compared PubMed, Scopus, Web of Science, and Google Scholar.[22] They concluded that each database had its own strengths and weaknesses. For example, Google Scholar and PubMed are free to access, whereas the other databases evaluated require a subscription. Scopus had about 20% more coverage than Web of Science. Google Scholar was plagued with inconsistencies; however, it was useful for obtaining obscure information. In another analysis, Embase retrieved twice as many citations as MEDLINE for family medicine topics.[23] A comparison of Scopus and Web of Science found that although the scope of coverage was greater with the latter database, the databases complement each other.[24] IPA has been compared to MEDLINE and was found to provide far fewer search results.[25] However, the quantity of results should not be the basis of success. The goal of any search should be to identify all relevant literature. Many of the aforementioned comparisons also reported that search results had some (not complete) overlap. Although there is overlap in the retrieved citations, some search results are unique. Thus, using multiple secondary resources decreases the likelihood of missing key references.

Given the popularity and ease of use of Google Scholar, several authors have attempted to evaluate its effectiveness versus other secondary resources. A comparison of PubMed and Google Scholar using 10 test searches revealed that the latter database provided more search results.[21] Although the secondary resource providing a larger number of results may suggest a robust search method, it should be noted that the quality of search results is more important. PubMed appears to provide more precise results compared with Google Scholar. In a study comparing Google Scholar and PubMed for locating primary literature to answer drug-related questions, both resources performed well.[26] PubMed retrieved fewer citations, but was more specific for primary literature. Anders and colleagues reported similar findings when these two databases were compared in their ability to retrieve relevant respiratory care topics.[27] The authors concluded

| **TABLE 4-2** | Comparison of Major Databases/Search Engines | | | | | |
|---|---|---|---|---|---|---|
| **Characteristic** | **Embase** | **Google Scholar** | **International Pharmaceutical Abstracts** | **PubMed** | **Scopus** | **Web of Science** |
| Launch date | 1947 | 2004 | 1970 | 1996 | 2004 | 2004 |
| Platform | Searchable database | Search engine | Searchable database | Search engine | Search engine | Search engine |
| Number of peer-reviewed journals indexed[a] | > 8,000 | Unlimited[b] | 800 | 6,000 | 19,500 | > 12,000 |
| Coverage period | 1947-present | Unlimited[a] | 1970-present | 1950-present | 1966-present | 1900-present |
| Includes "grey" literature | ++ | +++ | ++ | – | ++ | ++ |
| Update frequency | Daily | Monthly | Monthly | Daily | Daily | Weekly |
| Citation analysis | Yes | Yes | Yes | No | Yes | Yes |
| Subscription required? | Yes | No | Yes | No | Yes | Yes |

Data from Falagas ME, Pitsouni EI, Malietzis GA, Pappas G. Comparison of PubMed, Scopus, Web of Science, and Google Scholar: strengths and weaknesses. *FASEB J.* 2008;22:338-342.
[a] As of April 2013.
[b] No information is provided by Google Scholar; theoretically covers all journals available electronically.
++ Includes selected grey literature.
+++ Includes a wide array of grey literature.
– No grey literature included.

that PubMed appeared better at performing valid searches for constructing patient care policies, guiding patient care, and developing education materials.

Another consideration when evaluating secondary resources is citation analysis; that is, an evaluation of the frequency with which a contribution to the literature has been cited in published works. Citation counts are used to evaluate the impact of a piece of literature and are often incorporated in academic advancement decisions. Web of Science, Scopus, and Google Scholar provide this feature. Several authors have reported that citation counts may differ substantially between secondary resources.[28,29] In order to get a comprehensive citation analysis, it is prudent to use more than one resource to identify citations.

## SUMMARY

Numerous secondary resources are available to the healthcare practitioner. Each resource has advantages, disadvantages, and nuances with regard to searching. Understanding the scope of coverage and how to search each database is essential to maximize the yield of the search. Being an efficient searcher is critical to being an effective clinician. The ability to find the information necessary to answer the question is the first step in being able to answer the question.

# REFERENCES

1. Zheng MH, Zhang X, Ye Q, Chen YP. Searching additional databases except PubMed are necessary for a systematic review. *Stroke.* 2008;39(8):e139.

2. Higgins JPT, Green S, eds. Cochrane Handbook for Systematic Reviews of Interventions Version 5.1.0 [updated March 2011]. The Cochrane Collaboration, 2011. http://handbook.cochrane.org. Accessed July 18, 2014.

3. Schuman AL. For literature searches, is Medline enough? Perception of an adequate literature search. *Lab Anim (NY).* 2004;33(8):15-16.

4. Twain M. Letter to George Bainton, October 15, 1888. http://www.twainequotes.com. Accessed August 1, 2013.

5. National Library of Medicine, National Institutes of Health. Factsheet MEDLINE®. http://www.nlm.nih.gov/pubs/factsheets/medline.html. Accessed July 18, 2014.

6. National Library of Medicine, National Institutes of Health. Key MEDLINE® Indicators. http://www.nlm.nih.gov/bsd/bsd_key.html. Accessed July 18, 2014.

7. Conn VS, Valentine JC, Cooper HM, Rantz MJ. Grey literature in meta-analyses. *Nurs Res.* 2003;52(4):256-261.

8. Cumulative Index to Nursing and Allied Health Literature. http://www.ebscohost.com/academic/the-cinahl-database. Accessed July 18, 2014.

9. International Pharmaceutical Abstracts. http://www.csa.com/factsheets/ipa-set-c.php. Accessed July 18, 2014.

10. Embase. http://www.elsevier.com/online-tools/embase. Accessed July 18, 2014.

11. Google Scholar. http://www.google.com/intl/en/scholar/about.html. Accessed July 18, 2014.

12. Gehanno JF, Rollin L, Darmoni S. Is the coverage of Google Scholar enough to be used alone for systematic reviews. *BMC Med Inform Decis Mak.* 2013;13:7. doi: 10.1186/1471-2148-13-7.

13. Web of Science. http://thomsonreuters.com/content/science/pdf/Web_of_Science_factsheet.pdf. Accessed July 18, 2014.

14. Web of Knowledge. Real facts: real numbers: real knowledge. http://wokinfo.com/realfacts/qualityandquantity/. Accessed April 13, 2013.

15. SicVerse Scopus facts and figures. http://www.info.sciverse.com/UserFiles/2508.SciVerse.Scopus_Facts_Figures(LR).pdf. Accessed April 13, 2013.

16. Cochrane Library. About the Cochrane Library. http://www.thecochranelibrary.com/view/0/AboutTheCochraneLibrary.html. Accessed July 18, 2014.

17. Division of Drug Information. IDIS Drug Database. http://itsnt14.its.uiowa.edu. Accessed July 18, 2014.

18. NEJM Journal Watch. About NEJM Journal Watch. http://www.jwatch.org/misc/about.dtl. Accessed July 18, 2014.

19. Adis. Reactions Weekly. http://www.springer.com/adis/journal/40278. Accessed July 18, 2014.

20. Kejariwal D, Mahawar KK. Is your journal indexed in PubMed? Relevance of PubMed in biomedical scientific literature today. *WebmedCentral.* 2012;3(3):WMC003159.

21. Schultz M. Comparing test searches in PubMed and Google Scholar. *J Med Libr Assoc.* 2007;95(4):442-445.

22. Falagas ME, Pitsouni EI, Malietzis GA, Pappas G. Comparison of PubMed, Scopus, Web of Science, and Google Scholar: strengths and weaknesses. *FASEB J.* 2008;22(2):338-342.

23. Wilkins T, Gillies RA, Davies K. EMBASE versus MEDLINE for family medicine searches. *Can Fam Physician.* 2005;51:848-849.

24. Burnham JF. Scopus database: a review. *Biomedical Digital Libraries.* 2006;3:1.

25. Fishman DL, Stone VL, DiPaula DA. Where should the pharmacy researchers look first? Comparing International Pharmaceutical Abstracts and Medline. *Bull Med Libr Assoc.* 1996;84(3):402-408.

26. Freeman MK, Lauderdale SA, Kendrach MG, Woolley TW. Google Scholar versus PubMed in locating primary literature to answer drug-related questions. *Ann Pharmacother.* 2009;43(3):478-484.

27. Anders ME, Evans DP. Comparison of PubMed and Google Scholar literature searches. *Respir Care.* 2010;55(5):578-583.

28. Kulkarni AV, Aziz B, Shams I, Busse JW. Comparisons of citations in Web of Science, Scopus, and Google Scholar for articles published in general medical journals. *JAMA.* 2009;302(10):1092-1096.

29. Li J, Burnham JF, Lemley T, Britton RM. Citation analysis: comparison of Web of Science®, Scopus™, SciFinder®, and Google Scholar. *JERML.* 2010;7:196-217.

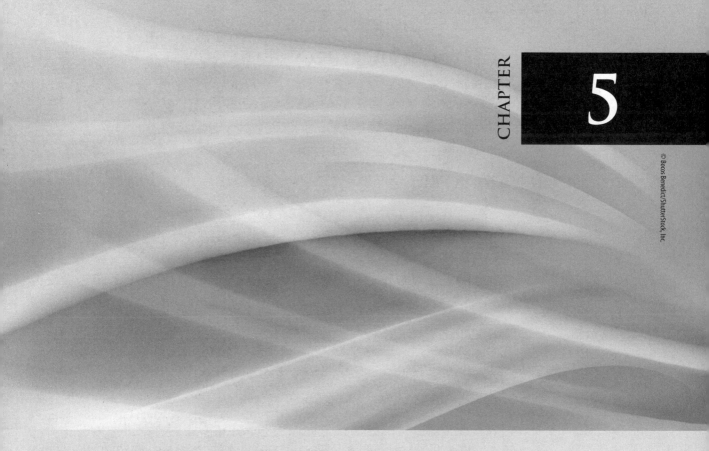

# PRIMARY SOURCES OF INFORMATION

Joshua L. Conrad, PharmD

## CHAPTER OBJECTIVES

▸ Define and identify various types of primary literature.

▸ Compare and contrast primary and tertiary literature, including their relative advantages, disadvantages, and principal uses.

▸ Explain factors contributing to the quality of primary scientific literature.

▸ Chronicle the customary process for peer-reviewed primary scientific literature publication.

▸ Identify the standard sections of a research article and describe the content typically presented in each section.

## CHAPTER OUTLINE

## KEY TERMS

Abstract

*h* index

Impact factor

Peer review

Primary literature

Refereeing

## INTRODUCTION

In addition to tertiary and secondary sources of information, there is also primary literature. **Primary literature** consists of written accounts of original thought or discovery
directly derived from firsthand observation or research. The two key requirements are
that the information is derived firsthand (i.e., it is primary) and that it is in the form
of a written work (i.e., it is literature). Original thought and discovery may be presented orally or may not be presented at all. Although these would be primary sources
of information if witnessed or otherwise acquired, they are not literature. Alternatively,
information derived from secondhand sources may be presented in writing in another
context. Although this would be literature, it would not be primary. With acknowledgment that primary information can be obtained through sources other than literature,
this chapter will focus largely on primary literature.

Primary medical literature is commonly published in biomedical journals, such as
*JAMA*, *The New England Journal of Medicine*, and *American Journal of Health-System Pharmacy*, in the form of original research articles. However, sources of primary literature are
not limited to such journals. For instance, many posters presented at various healthcare
conferences and meetings are primary literature. Other primary literature is published
electronically and presented only on the Internet, sometimes in association with a physi-
cally published biomedical journal and sometimes not. Published dissertations and theses can also be primary literature when they are accounts of original research. Although
most biomedical journals publish primary literature, most also publish some amount of
literature that is not primary. Therefore, one should not consider primary literature and
biomedical journals to be equivalent. Likewise, one should avoid the assumption that an
article appearing in a biomedical journal must be primary literature. Indeed, the widely
circulated journal *American Family Physician* seldom includes primary literature, prefer-
ring instead to publish high-quality review articles. Although most primary medical
literature is published in biomedical journals, it is important to recognize that primary
literature is defined by its content, not its manner or place of publication.

As a general rule, original published reports describing the methods and results of
clinical trials, cohort studies, case-control studies, cross-sectional studies, case reports
and series, survey research, economic studies, animal studies, in vitro studies, bench
research, and meta-analyses are all considered primary literature. In contrast, systematic reviews and other review articles are tertiary literature, even when published
in biomedical journals. Published clinical guidelines and drug, biologic, and medical
device prescribing information are also forms of tertiary literature. Other written works

commonly published in biomedical journals, such as editorials and letters to the editor, are usually tertiary literature. However, there are instances in which editorials and letters can be considered primary literature. For instance, if an editorial or letter is a presentation of original thoughts or ideas that are derived directly from observations the author has made in the course of clinical practice, this can be a form of primary literature. Likewise, letters to the editor will occasionally present original results of small clinical studies conducted by the authors or descriptions of firsthand observations of the authors' own patients. These would also be considered primary literature. The important point here is that, regardless of the label that the journal places on the article, if the author is describing his or her own experiences and direct observations, and thus introducing new evidence into the body of scientific knowledge, not simply commenting on or critiquing others' observations or published work, the article should be considered to be primary literature.

In order to support or contextualize the methods and results of the original research described in a work of primary literature, it is relatively common for such works to reference previous publications. This should not be inferred to make them tertiary literature. If a publication describes original research or introduces novel evidence, it is considered primary literature, even if references to previous works are also included.

# ADVANTAGES AND DISADVANTAGES OF PRIMARY LITERATURE

When compared with other types of literature, primary literature is generally more detailed. This is probably the most prominent advantage of primary literature. Most works of primary literature include thorough descriptions of the methods used to collect the data that are presented and extensive exhibition of the results obtained. Such detail allows consumers of this information to scrutinize and evaluate the validity of the evidence for themselves, as opposed to relying on the interpretation of others. In contrast, works of tertiary literature typically consist of selected results from a number of related works of primary literature, presented in the context of one another with significantly less detail. This limits the reader's ability to make his or her own judgments about the validity with which the evidence was gathered. Of course, the consumer of primary literature must have an adequate understanding of research methodologies in order to perform independent assessments of validity, which can be a disadvantage of primary literature. In addition, it can take significantly more time to acquire, read, analyze, and synthesize primary literature than tertiary literature, which can also be a disadvantage when limited time is a factor.

Another advantage of primary literature is that it is relatively quick to publish, making the information contained therein timelier than in other types of literature. Indeed, good tertiary scientific literature is based on primary literature. So, it is obvious that primary literature must be published first. In a practical context, it is simply easier to publish smaller works of literature, such as an issue of a biomedical journal, than it is to publish larger works, such as a textbook. One of the most widely respected and circulated biomedical journals, *JAMA*, reports median submission-to-publication time for articles appearing in its print version to be 75 days, and even less time for electronic versions of articles published online by the journal.[1] In contrast, the publication process for textbooks is typically counted in months to years. Given the rapidity of change in modern medicine, certain content appearing in a medical textbook can be outdated by the time the textbook is available for general consumption.

One of the major disadvantages of primary literature is that each work is limited in scope. Although most works of primary literature will cite some works that have been previously published and that are directly related to the topic, this is not the purpose of primary literature, and cited works do not usually represent the entirety of published literature on the topic. Thus, it is often required that the reader must contextualize the content of a work of primary literature. This typically requires gathering and evaluating additional literature on one's own.

Another disadvantage of primary literature is its availability relative to tertiary literature. Most textbooks cover wide areas of interest and can be purchased by anyone at relatively reasonable prices. Furthermore, most medical product prescribing information and nationally recognized clinical guidelines are available free of charge on the Internet. In contrast, the costs associated with subscribing to biomedical journals can be very high, usually limiting their availability to those with access to academic or large medical institution libraries. Individuals who are not affiliated with such organizations may find it particularly challenging to access some primary literature, especially if access to a number of journals in a given field is desired. Fortunately, the practice of publishing electronic versions of journals on the Internet and allowing purchase of individual articles through this medium is becoming more prevalent, making access for individuals more convenient than obtaining print copies and more affordable than maintaining regular subscriptions. Using the National Library of Medicine's Loansome Doc service can reduce the cost for individual articles even further and can provide access to journal articles that have not been published electronically. Some biomedical journals are open access, meaning that they allow electronic access to all content to anyone via the Internet free of charge. Flying Publisher curates a list of such journals. In addition, some journals that require paid subscriptions offer select articles free in electronic form on the Internet (open-access articles) or release for free access most articles after a period of time (open-access archives).

Even when available free of charge, some primary literature is simply difficult to discover and obtain. For instance, posters presented at healthcare conferences are not generally indexed in MEDLINE or other large secondary medical literature databases. It may be necessary to consult more focused secondary literature resources, such as the International Pharmaceutical Abstracts (IPA) or the Iowa Drug Information Service (IDIS), to locate posters or proceedings presented at pharmacy conferences. Of course, such secondary resources are not available freely and many clinicians do not have access to them. Even when the existence of less conventional primary literature is discovered, obtaining full-text versions of these can prove difficult. When a poster has been presented at a scientific or professional conference, one may be able to track down the corresponding author in order to obtain a copy. If the poster was on a medical product, the product manufacturer's medical affairs department may be able to provide an individual with a copy on request. Manufacturers of drugs, biologics, and medical devices can often provide other published primary literature and sometimes even unpublished primary information free of charge. Because biopharmaceutical industry communication is highly regulated, however, such companies may be reticent to provide information beyond what is included in the prescribing information for their products. When requesting information from a medical product manufacturer that is beyond what is contained in the prescribing information for the product, it is advisable for the requestor to specify that he or she is making an unsolicited request for off-label information in accordance with the Food and Drug Administration's guidance documents on responding to unsolicited requests for off-label information and distributing scientific and medical publications on unapproved uses (both currently in draft form).[2,3]

# PRIMARY LITERATURE QUALITY

As of March 2014, the MEDLINE database indexes 5,669 biomedical journals, many of which include primary literature pertaining to drugs.[4] IPA indexes nearly 400 journals just related to the areas of pharmacy and drugs.[5] In 2013, the American Association of Colleges of Pharmacy (AACP) recommended no fewer than 214 specific journals to be included in collections of libraries serving pharmacy schools in the United States.[6] With so much being published on a regular basis, it is not difficult to imagine that the quality of primary literature can vary widely. It is often left to the reader to evaluate the quality of any given work of primary literature on his or her own. Fortunately, this chapter provides many tools that can be used to evaluate the quality of primary literature. It should be noted that the use of the term "quality" in this chapter refers only to the scientific merit of the literature, not to its production values, grammatical correctness, or other nonscientific aspects.

Part of the process of evaluating a work of primary literature can include an evaluation of the medium in which it is published. If the work is published independently on the Internet, one will likely need to bring a more critical eye to its appraisal than if the work was submitted and accepted for presentation in poster form at a medical conference. Likewise, if the work is published in a well-regarded biomedical journal, one may generally expect that it has undergone more scrutiny than a poster presentation has.

Because most primary medical literature is published in biomedical journals, evaluating the quality of a work of primary literature may also involve an evaluation of the quality of the journal in which it appears. Identifying and evaluating the quality of each individual journal in which drug and pharmacy information can be found is well beyond the scope of this text. However, there are some aspects of journals that one can look to when undertaking such evaluations.

## PEER REVIEW

Probably the most important aspect affecting the quality of a biomedical journal is whether it is peer reviewed. **Peer review** is a structured process by which persons who have similar competence to the authors of a work of literature and knowledge in the work's subject matter evaluate submitted manuscripts and supply feedback to the authors before the work is published. Because the members of the editorial staff of a biomedical journal seldom possess the qualifications or knowledge to undertake thorough scientific evaluations of every article that might be considered for publication in the journal, peer review is an excellent method for ensuring that articles published in the journal meet a minimum quality standard. Although a biomedical journal may be referred to as "peer reviewed," it is actually only certain articles considered for publication in the journal that undergo this process. For instance, editorials and letters to the editor are seldom formally peer reviewed. Peer review usually plays a role in the acceptance or rejection of major manuscripts submitted for publication, such as systematic reviews and original research articles. In addition, the content of the final article of an accepted manuscript is often subject to recommendations by peer reviewers. Peer review of scientific literature is sometimes referred to as **refereeing**, and peer reviewers can be called *referees*. Regardless of the terminology, the process is essentially equivalent.

## JOURNAL AFFILIATIONS

Other aspects of a biomedical journal that one can look to when assessing its quality are its affiliations, such as its publisher, its editorial staff, and the organizations with which it is associated. If a journal is produced by a publisher focused on scholarly or scientific literature, one may generally expect higher quality content than a journal produced by a publisher more aligned in the marketing and communications sector. The credentials of the editorial staff, in particular the editor-in-chief, can also provide some insight into the quality of its content. The editorial staff of a higher quality journal is typically led by an individual with credentials in the journal's discipline or field. In addition, if the journal is affiliated with a well-regarded professional organization, this tends to increase the quality of the articles it includes.

Let us compare two pharmacy-related journals, *Pharmacotherapy* and *Pharmacy Times*, with regard to these aspects. *Pharmacotherapy* is the official peer-reviewed journal of the American College of Clinical Pharmacy (ACCP), a professional pharmacy organization, and is produced by Wiley-Blackwell, a company that publishes hundreds of scientific, medical, and scholarly journals. This journal's current editor-in-chief holds a doctorate in pharmacy with board certification, is a fellow of ACCP, and has an academic appointment as a professor at a major U.S. medical school.[7] In contrast, *Pharmacy Times* is produced by Intellisphere, which is a division of a larger company focused on promotion of products to the healthcare sector. This journal is not affiliated with any professional organizations, it does not claim to be peer reviewed, and its current editorial leadership does not appear to have any credentials specific to the area of pharmacy.[8] Although both journals may provide readers with valuable information, one can expect the general scientific quality of the content appearing in *Pharmacotherapy* to be greater than that in *Pharmacy Times*.

## IMPACT FACTOR

One frequently reported surrogate for the influence of a biomedical journal is its impact factor. **Impact factor** is the average number of times each article appearing in a journal during a given period of time was cited during a subsequent period of time. Impact factor is intended to provide an objective rating that relates to the importance the scientific community places on articles published in a journal. A higher impact factor suggests greater scientific influence. The general equation for impact factor is shown in **Figure 5-1**.

The impact factors of thousands of scientific journals are published annually in Thomson Reuters' *Journal Citation Reports*. The specific time periods used by this publication for the variables in the equation are the reporting year for period Z and the immediately preceding two years for period Y. Thus, when calculating a journal's impact factor for 2013, the articles of reference would be taken from 2011 and 2012 (period Y, a 2-year period) and the number of times they were cited would be taken from 2013 (period Z).[9,10] As a reference point, 2-year impact factors for 2012 and 2013 for some journals familiar to the field of pharmacy are listed in **Table 5-1**.[9-12] (Note that 2013 data were the most recently published at the time of writing this text.)

It is important to acknowledge that the validity of impact factor has been called into question for a number of reasons. As has been discussed, the availability of primary literature can vary widely by journal. It is easy to see how open-access journals or those that offer electronic versions of certain articles to nonsubscribers at low or no cost might

$$\text{impact factor} = \frac{\text{total number of citations to journal X's articles from period Y during period Z}}{\text{total number of articles published in journal X during period Y}}$$

**FIGURE 5-1** Impact factor equation.

**TABLE 5-1** Two-Year Impact Factors for 2012 and 2013 for Selected Journals Related to Pharmacy, Pharmacology, and Therapeutic Drugs

| Journal | 2012 | 2013 |
|---|---|---|
| Advanced Drug Delivery Reviews | 12.888 | 12.707 |
| American Journal of Geriatric Pharmacotherapy | 2.627 | 2.651 |
| American Journal of Health-System Pharmacy | 1.984 | 2.205 |
| American Journal of Pharmaceutical Education | EX | 1.188 |
| American Journal of Psychiatry | 14.721 | 13.559 |
| Annals of Internal Medicine | 13.976 | 16.104 |
| Annals of Pharmacotherapy | 2.567 | 2.923 |
| Annual Review of Pharmacology and Toxicology | 21.543 | 18.523 |
| Antimicrobial Agents and Chemotherapy | 4.565 | 4.451 |
| Basic & Clinical Pharmacology & Toxicology | 2.124 | 2.294 |
| Biopharmaceutics & Drug Disposition | 2.090 | 2.178 |
| British Journal of Clinical Pharmacology | 3.578 | 3.688 |
| British Journal of Pharmacology | 5.067 | 4.990 |
| British Medical Journal | 17.215 | 16.378 |
| Canadian Journal of Hospital Pharmacy | NL | NL |
| Canadian Journal of Physiology and Pharmacology | 1.556 | 1.546 |
| Cancer Chemotherapy and Pharmacology | 2.795 | 2.571 |
| Cardiovascular Drugs and Therapy | 2.673 | 2.952 |
| Chest | 5.854 | 7.132 |
| Circulation | 15.202 | 14.948 |
| Clinical Infectious Diseases | 9.374 | 9.416 |
| Clinical Neuropharmacology | 1.815 | 1.836 |
| Clinical Pharmacokinetics | 6.109 | 5.486 |
| Clinical Pharmacology & Therapeutics | 6.846 | 7.390 |
| CNS Drugs | 4.826 | 4.376 |
| Current Neuropharmacology | 2.031 | 2.347 |
| Drug Information Journal | 0.401 | 0.490 |
| Drug Metabolism and Disposition | 3.361 | 3.334 |
| Drug Metabolism and Pharmacokinetics | 2.071 | 2.863 |
| Drug Safety | 3.408 | 2.620 |
| Drugs | 4.633 | 4.133 |
| Drugs & Aging | 2.646 | 2.503 |
| European Journal of Clinical Pharmacology | 2.741 | 2.697 |
| European Journal of Drug Metabolism and Pharmacokinetics | 0.944 | 1.312 |
| European Journal of Pharmacology | 2.592 | 2.684 |
| Experimental and Clinical Psychopharmacology | 2.545 | 2.626 |
| Food and Drug Law Journal | 0.373 | 0.340 |

*(continues)*

**TABLE 5-1**  Two-Year Impact Factors for 2012 and 2013 for Selected Journals Related to Pharmacy, Pharmacology, and Therapeutic Drugs *(Continued)*

| Journal | 2012 | 2013 |
| --- | --- | --- |
| Formulary | 0.208 | 0.370 |
| Hospital Pharmacy | NL | NL |
| International Journal of Clinical Pharmacology and Therapeutics | 1.200 | 1.044 |
| International Journal of Clinical Pharmacy | 0.859 | 1.250 |
| International Journal of Neuropsychopharmacology | 5.641 | 5.264 |
| International Journal of Pharmaceutical Compounding | NL | NL |
| JAMA Internal Medicine (formerly Archives of Internal Medicine) | NL | 13.246 |
| JAMA: Journal of the American Medical Association | 29.978 | 30.387 |
| Journal of Cardiovascular Pharmacology | 2.383 | 2.111 |
| Journal of Cardiovascular Pharmacology and Therapeutics | 2.380 | 3.072 |
| Journal of Child and Adolescent Psychopharmacology | 2.773 | 3.073 |
| Journal of Clinical Oncology | 18.038 | 17.960 |
| Journal of Clinical Pharmacology | 2.841 | 2.472 |
| Journal of Clinical Pharmacy and Therapeutics | 2.104 | 1.533 |
| Journal of Clinical Psychopharmacology | 3.513 | 3.761 |
| Journal of Managed Care Pharmacy | 2.414 | 2.682 |
| Journal of Natural Medicines | 1.516 | 1.447 |
| Journal of Pharmaceutical Sciences | 3.130 | 3.007 |
| Journal of Pharmacokinetics and Pharmacodynamics | 1.808 | 1.458 |
| Journal of Pharmacology and Experimental Therapeutics | 3.891 | 3.855 |
| Journal of Pharmacy and Pharmaceutical Sciences | 2.198 | 1.681 |
| Journal of Pharmacy and Pharmacology | 2.033 | 2.161 |
| Journal of Psychopharmacology | 3.374 | 3.396 |
| Journal of the American College of Cardiology | 14.086 | 15.343 |
| Journal of the American Medical Informatics Association | 3.571 | 3.932 |
| Journal of the American Pharmacists Association | 1.156 | 0.929 |
| Lancet | 39.060 | 39.207 |
| Medical Letter on Drugs and Therapeutics | 0.557 | 0.407 |
| Molecular Pharmacology | 4.411 | 4.120 |
| Neuropharmacology | 4.114 | 4.819 |
| Neuropsychopharmacology | 8.678 | 7.833 |
| New England Journal of Medicine | 51.658 | 54.420 |
| Pediatric Drugs | 1.884 | 1.721 |
| Pediatrics | 5.119 | 5.297 |
| Pharmaceutical Research | 4.742 | 3.952 |
| PharmacoEconomics | 2.861 | 3.338 |
| Pharmacoepidemiology and Drug Safety | 2.897 | 3.172 |
| Pharmacogenetics and Genomics | 3.608 | 3.450 |

**TABLE 5-1** Two-Year Impact Factors for 2012 and 2013 for Selected Journals Related to Pharmacy, Pharmacology, and Therapeutic Drugs *(Continued)*

| Journal | 2012 | 2013 |
|---|---|---|
| *Pharmacogenomics* | 3.857 | 3.425 |
| *Pharmacogenomics Journal* | 5.134 | 5.513 |
| *Pharmacognosy Magazine* | 1.525 | 1.112 |
| *Pharmacological Reports* | 1.965 | 2.165 |
| *Pharmacological Research* | 4.346 | 3.976 |
| *Pharmacological Reviews* | 22.345 | 18.551 |
| *Pharmacology* | 1.788 | 1.603 |
| *Pharmacology & Therapeutics* | 7.793 | 7.745 |
| *Pharmacopsychiatry* | 2.109 | 2.168 |
| *Pharmacotherapy* | 2.311 | 2.204 |
| *Pharmacy Times* | NL | NL |
| *Psychopharmacology* | 4.061 | 3.988 |
| *Pulmonary Pharmacology & Therapeutics* | 2.543 | 2.570 |
| *Therapeutic Drug Monitoring* | 2.234 | 1.926 |
| *US Pharmacist* | NL | NL |
| *Xenobiotica* | 1.984 | 2.101 |

Data from Thomson Reuters. 2012 Journal Citation Reports. New York, NY: Thomson Reuters; 2013; Thomson Reuters. 2013 Journal Citation Reports. New York, NY: Thomson Reuters; 2014.Thomson Reuters. Journal Citation Reports Notices Web site. http://admin-apps.webofknowledge.com/JCR/static_html/notices/notices.htm. Accessed March 15, 2014. Thomson Reuters. Journal Citation Reports Notices Web site. http://admin-apps.webofknowledge.com/JCR/static_html/notices/notices .htm. Accessed October 10, 2014. EX: excluded due to anomalous citation patterns. NL: Not listed in reference.

have a higher impact factor than more cost-prohibitive and less accessible journals. If authors do not have access to certain literature, they are not likely to cite that literature in their own works. Articles appearing in less accessible journals, however, are not necessarily less important or of lower quality. So, one must be careful not to confuse influence, which more accurately describes what impact factor measures, with importance or quality. If more people have access to a given work of medical literature, it may very well be more influential on clinical practice than is a work of greater importance or higher quality that, unfortunately, is not seen by as many people.

One other major criticism of impact factor is that it is highly variable between disciplines and fields. One need only look at the sampling of journals presented in Table 5-1 to see some patterns. For instance, among healthcare journals, those of broader medical interest, such as *The New England Journal of Medicine*, *JAMA*, and *The Lancet*, consistently have the highest impact factors, with the highest among these ranging from about 30 to greater than 50. Comparatively, the highest impact factors among specialty medical journals generally only range into the teens, with those related to oncology and cardiology consistently ranking higher than those related to most other medical fields. In contrast, few pharmacy-related journals achieve an impact factor greater than 5.0, and the only three of those listed in Table 5-1 with 2013 two-year impact factors above 10—*Advanced Drug Delivery Reviews*, *Annual Review of Pharmacology and Toxicology*, and *Pharmacological Reviews*—are journals that focus more on systematic reviews than on primary literature.

Impact factor disparities between disciplines and fields probably occur for a number of reasons. For instance, research in certain disciplines and fields is naturally more reliant on more recent research than on older research. Thus, articles in these areas would systematically be more likely to cite works from the preceding 2 years than articles in other areas. The important thing to remember is that impact factor may be less useful when attempting to make interdisciplinary comparisons or even when making comparisons between journals focusing on different fields within a single discipline. It can be a good surrogate, however, for comparing relative influence of journals covering similar subject matters.

## HIRSCH'S *H* INDEX

Another less widely known value that could be used when evaluating the quality of a work of primary literature is the **h index**. Developed by Jorge Hirsch and published in 2005, the *h* index is a surrogate for the cumulative impact and relevance of an individual researcher's published work.[13] Whereas impact factor assigns a numeric value to a journal, the *h* index assigns a numeric value to an individual researcher. Like impact factor for journals, the determination of the *h* index for an individual accounts for both the number of publications and the number of times those publications have been cited in other works. Publications authored by researchers with higher *h* indices may be of higher quality, or at least be more influential. Although Hirsch developed the *h* index for his own field, physics, he noted that it could be extended to any scientific field, but that *h* indices for individuals in different fields but with similar scientific impacts would likely be incomparable. (This is similar to the pattern we see for impact factor.) As a frame of reference for individuals in fields related to health care, Hirsch offered that the median *h* index for 2005 inductees into the National Academy of Sciences in the biological and biomedical sciences was 57 ($\sigma = 22$), which is significantly higher than comparable individuals in physics and probably other nonlife sciences.[13] Although the *h* index is not in widespread use in the biomedical sciences at this time, it could serve as another quality indicator for works of primary literature in the future.

## PUBLICATION IN PEER-REVIEWED JOURNALS

The processes for getting works of primary literature published in peer-reviewed biomedical journals can vary from journal to journal. However, such processes usually follow a similar pattern, which is presented in **Figure 5-2**.

The road to primary literature publication in biomedical journals always begins with submission of a manuscript to a journal for consideration. Most biomedical journals have specific requirements for manuscript submission, ranging from the content of the proposed article to the format in which the manuscript and any auxiliary materials are provided. Most reputable journals require that named authors have contributed significantly to the overall work effort supporting the written manuscript. In other words, for primary literature, all named authors should have played a significant role in the

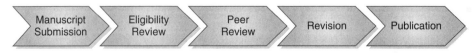

**FIGURE 5-2** Typical peer-reviewed journal publication process.

planning or conduct of the original research described in the manuscript, not necessarily in the act of composing of the manuscript. In addition, most journals require that submitted manuscripts have not been previously published in any medium and that they are not under consideration for publication by any other entity. Other common requirements involve disclosure of funding sources and potential conflicts of interest, registry of certain clinical research with a recognized nonprofit public study registry, and adherence to an internationally recognized code of conduct for clinical research.

Once a manuscript has been submitted to a journal, it will undergo an initial review for eligibility. Eligibility review always involves an assessment by the journal's editorial staff for basic criteria, such as whether the subject matter of the proposed article is appropriate for the journal and if the manuscript meets the journal's minimum criteria and format. Depending on the complexity or specificity of its content, the manuscript may be sent to peer reviewers for an initial screening. If the manuscript does not pass the eligibility review, the corresponding author will be notified and usually informed of the reason for rejection.

If a manuscript meets the initial eligibility requirements, it will next be sent to peer reviewers for a more formal review. Peer reviewers will provide detailed feedback about the scientific content and merit of the manuscript to the publisher. Usually, these comments will eventually be given to the corresponding author of the manuscript. However, the identities of the peer reviewers are often kept confidential. The outcome of peer review will typically be one of three results. First, the peer review may establish that the manuscript is not suitable for publication in the journal, even if it were to be extensively revised. Second, the review may establish that the manuscript is suitable for publication in the journal, but only after major revision. If this is the case and the authors make revisions, the revised manuscript may be sent back to the peer reviewers to ensure that the revisions were appropriate and sufficient. Third, the peer review may establish that the manuscript is suitable for publication in the journal with only minimal or no changes.

Once the manuscript has undergone peer review and any required revisions have been made, it is formally accepted for publication. The journal's editorial staff will commonly make nonsubstantive edits, such as for style, grammar, spelling, syntax, etc., and the authors will usually have one final opportunity to review and approve the version to be published. Finally, the manuscript will be published as an article in the journal, making its content available for general consumption by the scientific community.

# FORMAT OF ORIGINAL RESEARCH ARTICLES

Most works of primary literature appearing in scientific journals are presented in structured formats. Formats can differ between journals and between types of articles within a given journal. For instance, the format used for articles describing larger studies, such as clinical trials, cohort studies, and case-control studies, will often differ from the format used for smaller studies, such as case reports and series, even within a single journal. However, the formats used for larger studies usually follow a generally accepted structure, which will be discussed here.

## TITLE/AUTHORS

At the beginning of most articles will be included a title of the work and the named authors. The title will often include the independent variables, some reference to the primary dependent variable, and the population or condition under study. The title, or subtitle if used, will also commonly include the type of study conducted (e.g., randomized clinical trial, case-control study, meta-analysis). The authors will also generally be listed at the beginning of the article. Sometimes, an organization or group will be identified instead of or in addition to individual authors. Authors' terminal academic degrees may or may not be listed with their names here. Occasionally, citation numbers will be given with authors' names. When this is the case, these are references to affiliation listings in the acknowledgments section, not to literature in the references section.

## ABSTRACT

Also located at the beginning of the article, the **abstract** is a short overview or summary of the most important aspects of the article. Indeed, this section is alternatively named *summary* or *overview* in some journals. An abstract, itself, may be structured or unstructured. An unstructured abstract is simply a small section, generally consisting of a paragraph or two, that summarizes the article. The use of unstructured abstracts for major original research articles, such as those describing larger studies, is relatively uncommon in contemporary scientific journals. Unstructured abstracts are now usually reserved for less structured articles, such as those describing case reports and series. Structured abstracts contain separate subsections devoted to the most important information about specific aspects of the article. The subsections of the structured abstract will usually be similar or equivalent to the major sections in the body of the article: background, methods, results, and conclusions. The typical length of an abstract for a major article is 200–400 words. Shorter articles will generally have more stringent word count limits for their abstracts.

Abstracts are intended to give the reader a quick feel for the major aspects of an article in order to facilitate a decision as to the reader's potential interest in its full contents. It can be tempting to forgo reading an entire article in favor of simply relying on the information presented in its abstract. It cannot be cautioned enough, however, to avoid this temptation when the information is intended to be used as evidence in support of a clinical decision. An abstract is seldom sufficient to present all the information and context necessary for truly evaluating the merit and applicability of study findings. In addition, content presented in an abstract can sometimes simply be unsupported by the data presented in the main body of the article. Indeed, one study that compared abstracts from articles in six major medical journals to their respective bodies reported content discrepancies in 18–68% of articles.[14]

## BACKGROUND

Sometimes called the *introduction*, the background section of an article describes the study's context. The background will often include information on the pathophysiology and epidemiology of the condition of interest, history and pharmacology of the study drug or biologic intervention or description of the procedure, currently accepted standards of care, and rationale for the current study. The background will generally also include or conclude with the stated objective or purpose of the study. It is completely acceptable, and usually desirable, to cite previously published literature that adequately contextualizes the current study in the background section of an original research article. The purpose of the background section is to set the stage and present the rationale for the study to the reader.

## METHODS

The section of an original research article in which are described the design of the study, the subject selection procedures, any interventions to be used and how they are to be used, the measurements to be taken and in what manner, the planned statistical analyses, and the oversight of the study is commonly called the methods section. Different journals frequently have different names for this section, such as *materials and methods*, *patients and methods*, or simply *study design*. They are all essentially the same thing. This section should describe practically everything that a reader may wish to know about how the study was planned. Given the desire to limit journal articles to a reasonable size, it is relatively common these days for the methods section to refer to another document, published as another journal article or electronically, that more completely describes the study methods in greater detail. Except for references to such documents and to publications that support or describe the methods used in the current study, the methods section should be relatively free from citations to other works. The purpose of the methods section is to present a clear picture to the reader of exactly what was planned to occur in the course of the study.

## RESULTS

Occasionally referred to by other names, such as *findings* or *observations*, the results section of an original research article describes what actually occurred and was observed in the study. In a clinical study report, the results section usually starts with a description of the disposition and demographics of the subjects that were actually enrolled in the study. Following this is a detailed description of the data collected and direct observations from the study, frequently accompanied by tables, graphs, figures, and other visuals. In interventional study reports, data on both efficacy and safety should be presented in this section. The results section of an original research report should be free from commentary, conjecture, or theory about the data. In addition, it is generally inappropriate to reference other publications in the results section. The purpose of the results section is to present in an unbiased manner the data collected during the study and the statistical analyses of these data.

## DISCUSSION/CONCLUSION

The last section of the main body of an original research article is the discussion. This section is sometimes called the *comments* section. This is the section in which the authors describe what they believe to be the impact of the study. The discussion section will commonly refer to other similar studies in order to synthesize and contextualize the findings of the current study with the findings of other studies. The discussion section is also where authors can present strengths and limitations of the study, theorize about unusual or unexpected findings, and suggest directions for future research. This section will also usually include or end with a statement of conclusion that summarizes what the authors believe to be the ultimate impact of the study. Some journals include the conclusion as a separate final section. The purpose of the discussion section is to allow authors to present their opinions about the study and their reactions to its outcomes.

## REFERENCES

Although an original research article should focus primarily on the study it presents, citations to other literature are appropriate in certain sections. The compilation of the works cited in an article appears in the references. (Although this section is occasionally called a *bibliography*, this term is incorrectly applied if the section contains a numeric list of works, each of which is specifically cited in the text of the article, as is the case with most articles appearing in biomedical journals.) Most journals set a specific limit to the number of other works that may be cited in an original research article.

## ACKNOWLEDGMENTS

The acknowledgments section of a journal article is where one will find additional information about individuals involved in the preparation of the article or in the planning or conduct of the research it describes. Sometimes this information is presented without a section title. Nonetheless, it will generally include similar content. Information that is commonly presented in the acknowledgments or equivalent section are identification of the corresponding author, the corresponding author's contact information, the authors' affiliations and disclosures, descriptions of the authors' individual contributions to the research and manuscript, others whom the authors wish to acknowledge or thank, and identification of the funding sources and sponsors and their roles in the research and manuscript.

# USING THE PRIMARY LITERATURE

Many routine clinical questions can be adequately answered using only tertiary literature. In these cases, it is seldom necessary to delve into the primary literature. However, there are also some relatively common instances in which consulting the primary literature can be beneficial or necessary. It is not uncommon to consult multiple tertiary references when faced with a clinical question or situation with which one is unfamiliar. Sometimes, the information found in these tertiary references differs from one another. In such cases, it may be prudent to conduct one's own evaluation of the primary literature to guide the clinical decision. In addition, tertiary literature is often focused on routine cases and scenarios. Thus, it may be inadequate when one is faced with a clinical situation that is abnormal, unusual, or otherwise falls outside the standard course or presentation. Likewise, the content in tertiary literature may be outdated if developments in the field are rapid. Primary literature can be useful or necessary in all these situations. Finally, if one is tasked with developing standardized procedures, protocols, or guidelines for clinical decisions, such as are often used in hospitals and health systems, it will usually be necessary to gather and review as much of the primary literature on the topic as possible.

It is important to remember that evaluating and extrapolating information from primary literature requires excellent critical-thinking skills and a solid comprehension of research methods.

# SUMMARY

Primary literature consists of written accounts of original thought or discovery directly derived from firsthand observation or research. Primary medical literature is commonly published in biomedical journals, but may also appear as posters presented at healthcare conferences and meetings, as dissertations and theses, and as electronic articles on the Internet. Original published reports describing the methods and results of clinical trials, cohort studies, case-control studies, cross-sectional studies, case reports and series, survey research, economic studies, animal studies, in vitro studies, bench research, and meta-analyses are all considered primary literature, as are some editorials, letters, and other written works that introduce information gathered firsthand to the body of scientific knowledge.

One major advantage of primary literature is that it is usually more detailed than tertiary literature. Another advantage of primary literature is that it is relatively quick to publish, making it timelier than tertiary literature. Some distinct disadvantages of primary literature when compared to tertiary literature are that primary literature requires the consumer to have a better understanding of research methodologies in order to assess its validity; primary literature can take more time to acquire, analyze, and synthesize; each work of primary literature is relatively limited in scope; and some primary literature is more difficult to discover and costly to acquire.

As with any literature, the quality of primary medical literature can vary widely. One aspect that can be used to gauge the quality of a work of primary literature is the medium in which it is published. In addition, when a work of primary medical literature is published in a biomedical journal, the quality of the journal can be an indicator of the general quality of the work. Articles that are published in peer-reviewed journals and in journals that have trusted affiliations are often of higher quality than those published in journals that are not peer reviewed and that are not affiliated with well-established organizations, publishers, or individuals. Peer review is a process by which persons who have similar competence to the authors of a work of literature and knowledge in the work's subject matter evaluate submitted manuscripts and supply feedback to the authors before the work is published. Impact factor can serve as a representation of a journal's influence, and may reflect the quality of primary literature published therein. However, it is important to remember that comparisons of impact factors for journals targeted at different professions or specialties are often unreliable.

The process for getting a work of primary literature published can vary between journals, but usually follows a standard pattern consisting of manuscript submission, eligibility review, peer review, revision, and publication. Likewise, the format required for works of primary literature can vary between journals and between types of articles. However, most original research articles contain the following components, even if called by different names: title and authors, abstract, background, methods, results, discussion/conclusion, and acknowledgments.

It is not always necessary to consult the primary literature to answer a clinical question. However, some circumstances in which it is common or preferred to look to primary medical literature are when tertiary references provide differing or conflicting information, when one is investigating evidence for an abnormal or unusual case, when the tertiary literature is outdated, and when one is developing a protocol that will be used by others for standardized patient care.

# REFERENCES

1. American Medical Association. *JAMA* instructions for authors. *JAMA*. http://jama.jamanetwork.com/public/instructionsForAuthors.aspx. Accessed March 15, 2014.
2. U.S. Food and Drug Administration. Guidance for industry: responding to unsolicited requests for off-label information about prescription drugs and medical devices: draft guidance. Rockville, MD: U.S. Food and Drug Administration, U.S. Department of Health and Human Services; December 2011.
3. U.S. Food and Drug Administration. Guidance for industry: distributing scientific and medical publications on unapproved new uses—recommended practices: revised draft guidance. Rockville, MD: U.S. Food and Drug Administration, U.S. Department of Health and Human Services; February 2014.
4. U.S. National Library of Medicine. Number of titles currently indexed for *Index Medicus* and MEDLINE on PubMed. http://www.nlm.nih.gov/bsd/num_titles.html. Accessed March 15, 2014.
5. ProQuest. International Pharmaceutical Abstracts (IPA)—current serials source list. http://www.csa.com/factsheets/supplements/ipa.php. Accessed March 15, 2014.
6. Beckett RD, Bickett S, Cole SW, et al. *AACP Core List of Journals for Libraries that Serve Schools and Colleges of Pharmacy.* 5th ed. Alexandria, VA: American Association of Colleges of Pharmacy; 2013.
7. Pharmacotherapy. http://www.pharmacotherapy.org. Accessed March 15, 2014.

8. Intellisphere, LLC. Contact Us. Pharmacy Times. http://www.pharmacytimes.com/contact_us. Accessed March 15, 2014.

9. Thomson Reuters. *2012 Journal Citation Reports*. New York, NY: Thomson Reuters; 2012.

10. Thomson Reuters. *2013 Journal Citation Reports*. New York, NY: Thomson Reuters; 2013.

11. Thomson Reuters. Journal Citation Reports Notices website. http://admin-apps.webofknowledge .com/JCR/static_html/notices/notices.htm. Accessed March 15, 2014.

12. Thomson Reuters. Journal Citation Reports Notices website. http://admin-apps.webofknowledge .com/JCR/static_html/notices/notices.htm. Accessed October 10, 2014.

13. Hirsch JE. An index to quantify an individual's scientific research output. *Proc Natl Acad Sci U S A*. 2005;102(46):16569-16572.

14. Pitkin RM, Branagan MA, Burmeister LF. Accuracy of data in abstracts of published research articles. *JAMA*. 1999;281(12):1110-1111.

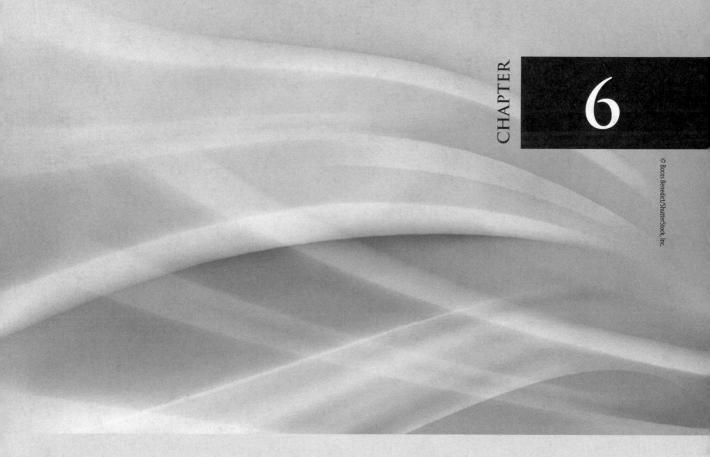

# 6

# INTRODUCTION TO CLINICAL STUDY DESIGN

Joshua L. Conrad, PharmD
Heather A. Pace, PharmD

## CHAPTER OBJECTIVES

▸ Define *clinical research*, *independent* and *dependent variables*, and *study hypotheses* and *outcomes*.

▸ Evaluate study outcome meaningfulness and measurability, instrument precision and accuracy, negative and positive predictive values, and sensitivity and specificity.

▸ Compare and contrast clinical studies with regard to orientation to time, researcher role, subject distribution, and comparative analyses.

▸ Describe various methods for and purposes of sampling, screening, randomizing, and blinding in clinical research.

▸ Understand factors affecting internal and external validity of a clinical study.

▸ Identify ethical issues germane to clinical research and common safeguards used to avoid improper treatment of human subjects.

# CHAPTER OUTLINE

Introduction
Study Hypotheses
Study Objectives
Outcome Measurement and Meaning
Types of Study Designs
Populations and Sampling

Study Groups and Subject Allocation
Blinding
Study Validity
Ethics in Clinical Research
Summary
References

# KEY TERMS

A posteriori
A priori
Accessible population
Accuracy
Active control
Active treatment group
Alternative hypothesis
Baseline characteristics
Blinding
Blocked randomization
Clinical research
Clinical significance
Cluster randomization
Cluster sampling
Combined outcome
Composite outcome
Concordance
Control
Control group
Convenience sampling
Crossover study
Data dredging
Data mining
Data and safety monitoring board
Data monitoring committee
Dependent variable
Direct outcome
Disproportional allocation
Double-blind trial
Double-dummy
Dummy
Effectiveness
Efficacy
Efficacy outcome
Endpoint
Equivalency study
Ethical review board
Exclusion criteria
Experimental study
External validity
False negative

False positive
Gold standard
Head-to-head trial
Identical placebo
Inclusion criteria
Independent research ethics committee
Independent variable
Informed consent
Institutional review board
Instrument
Internal validity
Inter-rater reliability
Intervention
Interventional study
Maneuver
Matched placebo
Matched study
Meaningfulness
Measurement
Negative predictive value
Noninferiority study
Nonprobability sampling
Nonrandom sampling
Null hypothesis
Objective measurement
Observational study
One-sided superiority study
One-tailed superiority study
Open label trial
Outcome
Parallel study
Placebo
Placebo-controlled trial
Population
Positive predictive value
Post-hoc analysis
Precision
Primary outcome
Probability sampling
Prospective study
Purposive sampling

Quota sampling
Random allocation
Random sampling
Randomization
Repeatability
Retrospective study
Safety analysis
Sample
Sampling
Secondary outcome
Sensitivity
Simple random sampling
Simple randomization
Single-blind trial
Specificity
Standard of care
Stratified random sampling
Stratified randomization
Study group
Study hypothesis
Study objective

Study orientation
Study population
Subgroup analysis
Subject allocation
Subjectivity
Superiority study
Surrogate outcome
Systematic sampling
Target population
Tertiary outcome
Test-retest reliability
Triple-blind trial
True negative
True positive
Two-sided superiority study
Two-tailed superiority study
Unblinding
Validation

# INTRODUCTION

The Declaration of Helsinki, a preeminent code of conduct for ethical clinical research, states, "Medical progress is based on research that ultimately must include studies involving human subjects."[1] In this chapter, we will introduce you to some of the most important concepts and methods used when conducting modern research in humans. In its broadest sense, **clinical research** refers to original investigations in living subjects that are intended to provide insight into an aspect of biology, health, or medical care in the same types of subjects as the investigation is conducted. For the purposes of this chapter, we will assume that those subjects and the population are human, although clinical research can be conducted in and for any living population. The key is that the subjects being studied are from the same species to which the results will be extrapolated. Thus, investigations in nonhuman animals are not considered to be clinical research when the results of those investigations are intended to be extrapolated to humans. Types of research that are not considered to be clinical research when the results are to be extrapolated to humans are laboratory (or "bench") research, animal research, and most health economics research.

The purpose of conducting clinical research is to answer a clinical question that will provide support and guidance for decisions in health and medicine. Often, the clinical question involves the effect of a medical intervention or **maneuver**, such as conducting a diagnostic test, administering a drug, or performing a procedure. However, the clinical question can also involve the effect of a variable not controlled by the researcher, such as the effect of cigarette smoking on cardiovascular disease or the effect of having a particular genetic abnormality on development of breast cancer. Whether it is controlled by the researcher or not, the intervention or contributing factor under study is termed the **independent variable**. The effect of the independent variable that is being studied is termed the **dependent variable**. For example, if a study is conducted to determine if administration of a drug to subjects with high plasma levels of low-density lipoprotein cholesterol (LDL-c) results in fewer cardiovascular-related deaths, administration of the drug is the independent variable, whereas the effect on cardiovascular-related death is the dependent variable. Ultimately, the researcher wishes to establish evidence that the dependent variable is associated with or caused by (or not associated with or not caused by) the independent variable. Clinical research can be conducted in many different ways, from the simplest of case reports, wherein an observed phenomenon in a single subject is described and attempted to be explained, to the most elaborate randomized controlled clinical trials. This chapter will introduce you to several of the most important concepts and commonly employed methods in clinical research.

## STUDY HYPOTHESES

As previously mentioned, clinical research is intended to answer clinical questions. However, one clinical study is seldom sufficient to definitively answer any given question. In more practical terms, a single clinical study simply provides some evidence to support one answer to a clinical question. It may require multiple studies in support of a particular answer before the scientific community accepts that answer as truth. Indeed, in the United States, the Food and Drug Administration (FDA) usually requires multiple clinical studies demonstrating favorable results before it will approve a new drug for general use. In addition to providing evidence in support of an answer to a clinical question, most clinical studies also generate more new questions based on novel observations made during the study. Thus, there is no shortage of research questions, or hypotheses, to study. Although a researcher may attempt to answer several questions in a single study, each question may be examined individually.

In most clinical studies, the researcher wishes to investigate whether an **intervention** or factor (the independent variable) is associated with or results in a particular effect (the dependent variable). This gives rise to a dichotomous set of answers; either the independent variable resulted in a change to the dependent variable or it did not. Regardless of what the researcher expects the answer to be, the circumstance in which the independent variable does not affect the dependent variable is called the **null hypothesis**, or the hypothesis of no difference (in statistics, abbreviated $H_0$). The circumstance in which the independent variable does affect the dependent variable is then called the **alternative hypothesis**, or the hypothesis of difference (in statistics, abbreviated $H_1$). The alternative hypothesis is often referred to as the **study hypothesis**.

Consider a study of the effects of administration of a drug on cardiovascular-related death. Let us say that the drug will be compared against giving no drug, represented by giving a matching counterpart that does not contain the active drug ingredient, known as a **placebo**. Even if the researcher expects that administration of the drug will result in fewer cardiovascular-related deaths, the null hypothesis is that there will be no statistical difference in the number of cardiovascular-related deaths between the group of subjects receiving the drug and the group receiving the placebo. The alternative hypothesis is that there will be a difference. Thus, the term "alternative" in relation to this hypothesis does not necessarily imply that it is unexpected. It merely refers to the alternative to "no difference." If a researcher aims to answer multiple questions through a single study, each question will have its own null and alternative hypotheses.

## STUDY OBJECTIVES

No single study can address the myriad questions that can exist about a given topic. However, a researcher will often wish to use a single study to examine multiple related questions. Given the expense and complexity of larger clinical studies and the desire not to expose more subjects than necessary to variables with unproven effects and potentially unknown risks, it makes sense to attempt to maximize the knowledge that can be gained through a single study. The result of each hypothesis examined is referred to as a study **outcome** (sometimes referred to as an **endpoint**). Most of the outcomes to be examined in a clinical study should be determined before the initiation of the study, or **a priori**, literally translated as "from the one before." However, it is sometimes important to examine some outcomes that are identified after the study has started, or **a posteriori**, literally translated as "from the one behind."

## PRIMARY OUTCOMES

For every outcome that is examined in a clinical study, there is risk that the answer provided by the study will be erroneous. For instance, the results of a clinical study demonstrate that a drug does not reduce cardiovascular-related death compared to placebo, when in reality the drug actually does reduce cardiovascular-related death. This might occur for a number of reasons, not the least common of which is simply chance. As the number of outcomes examined increases, so does the chance that an error in at least one of them will occur. Because we have no way of knowing for absolute certain which results from a clinical study are true for the entire population to which they will be extrapolated and which are not, it is important to apply a structure, or hierarchy, to the outcomes in order to minimize the chance of drawing false conclusions from them.

First, the researcher should determine a priori which outcome is the main outcome being studied, and focus largely on that. This is referred to as the **primary outcome**, and is often cited as the "purpose" of the study. (Although a researcher may identify multiple primary outcomes, these should still be ranked in order of importance for the purposes of the statistical analyses.) The primary outcome represents the answer to the key question that the study is conducted to obtain and is the outcome around which the study is fundamentally designed. When a clinical study involves some intervention made on the part of the researcher, the primary outcome is most often related to the efficacy of that intervention in terms of preventing, improving, or curing some health or medical condition. However, the primary outcome could involve the relative safety of two interventions. Returning to our example, the primary outcome of the study would be the difference in cardiovascular-related deaths between subjects receiving the drug and subjects receiving placebo. Because the drug is intended to prevent cardiovascular-related death, this would be an **efficacy outcome**.

It is important to distinguish between efficacy and effectiveness when referring to clinical study outcomes. **Efficacy** is the ability of an intervention to elicit a specific desired effect. Efficacy can be established through clinical research. In contrast, **effectiveness** is a measure of how well an intervention works for a condition outside the boundaries of clinical research. Effectiveness takes into account such factors as the efficacy, safety, and accessibility of an intervention. For example, a drug can be found to be highly efficacious for slowing Alzheimer's disease. But, the drug's poor safety profile, high cost, or limited availability may decrease its overall effectiveness. Clinical research is much better suited to determining the efficacy of an intervention than it is to determining the effectiveness of an intervention.

## SECONDARY OUTCOMES

As we mentioned, there may be multiple outcomes that are appropriate to examine in a single clinical study. Those outcomes that are deemed important to examine, but that are not the primary purpose of the study, may be classified as **secondary outcomes**.

Secondary outcomes should also be determined a priori, and planning to examine them may significantly affect the design of the study. Continuing with our previous example, the researchers conducting the clinical study may also wish to determine the drug's effects on the number of deaths from all causes (i.e., all-cause mortality), its effects on plasma LDL-c levels, and its effects on the number of serious nonfatal cardiovascular occlusive events, such as ischemic stroke and myocardial infarction (MI). Because these outcomes are important and may require changes to how the study is conducted, they would be named as secondary outcomes.

## TERTIARY OUTCOMES

Additional outcomes that may be part of a study, but that are not deemed to be as important as the primary or secondary outcomes, may be classified as tertiary outcomes. It is not uncommon for even a large clinical study to have no identified **tertiary outcomes**. Often, tertiary outcomes are more exploratory in nature and are intended to answer peripheral questions or provide initial evidence upon which to base future studies. As with primary and secondary outcomes, tertiary outcomes are generally determined a priori. However, the requirements that are necessary to examine a tertiary outcome should not affect the design of the study to a great extent or put subjects through significantly more discomfort or risk. Otherwise, the researcher should determine whether the outcome should be considered a secondary outcome or if the outcome is even worth examining in the study.

In our previous example, one tertiary outcome could be the drug's effects on plasma C-reactive protein (CRP) levels. Because this parameter has not been as closely associated with actual patient outcomes as plasma LDL-c has, monitoring plasma CRP is not as important as monitoring plasma LDL-c. Furthermore, because subjects are already undergoing phlebotomy for the purposes of monitoring plasma LDL-c, monitoring plasma CRP introduces relatively no additional discomfort or risk to subjects. Having this additional data, however, may guide future studies involving this parameter. Thus, it is a good candidate for inclusion as a tertiary outcome. Another possible tertiary outcome could be subject-reported quality of life (QOL). In addition, the researcher may identify the differences in MIs and ischemic strokes, separately, as individual tertiary outcomes, contingent on the results of the secondary outcome of serious nonfatal cardiovascular occlusive events being statistically significant. Like monitoring plasma CRP, these other potential tertiary outcomes are not likely to be as important as the secondary outcomes, and examining them poses little additional inconvenience or risk to subjects, as QOL is typically assessed using a harmless standardized questionnaire and MIs and ischemic strokes are already being tracked.

## SAFETY ANALYSES

In addition to outcomes related to efficacy, most clinical studies should include some evaluation of adverse effects. This is especially true when the independent variable is an intervention or carries some inherent risks, such as administering a drug or performing a procedure. Such evaluations take the form of **safety analyses**. If the researcher has some foreknowledge of the kinds of adverse effects that are reasonably likely to occur with the intervention, such as might be gathered from previous studies with the intervention and past experience with similar interventions, these should generally be screened for and analyzed in the study. Unexpected significant adverse effects that occur should also be analyzed, a posteriori. For instance, if earlier studies with the drug in our example indicate that it may cause elevations in plasma levels of liver enzymes, it would be important for the researcher to plan safety analyses of the drug's effects on this parameter in any new study of the drug. Likewise, if other drugs with the same mechanism of action as the study drug have been previously associated with muscle deterioration, the researcher should plan to assess this potential effect in any study of the new drug. In addition, if reports begin to arise during a study of subjects experiencing a particular new type of adverse effect not previously identified as associated with the intervention, the researcher should start analyzing these for their potential association with the intervention, even though it was not planned a priori to do so. All serious adverse effects occurring in a clinical study should be examined individually and analyzed in aggregate, as should adverse effects resulting in subjects voluntarily or involuntarily withdrawing from the study.

## SUBGROUP ANALYSES

It is often desirable to determine if the outcomes observed in the entire pool of subjects in a clinical study apply to subsets of those subjects to the same degree. To accomplish this, the researcher may perform additional analyses on smaller groups of subjects from the larger pool. These subsets should be selected based on factors that have a relatively significant chance of altering the results or are in some other way deemed important. Such analyses are called **subgroup analyses**. Many subgroup analyses to be conducted can be determined a priori. These are commonly referred to as *prespecified subgroup analyses*. However, unexpected signals observed during a study may warrant conducting subgroup analyses that are identified a posteriori. Any outcomes (e.g., primary, secondary, safety) examined in the entire pool of subjects may be appropriate to examine in smaller groups of subjects, but it is important to remember that each additional analysis increases the risk that some results will be erroneous. Thus, the researcher must balance the desire to examine every possible outcome and subgroup with the risk of arriving at false conclusions. In our example study, subgroup analyses could be appropriate for a myriad of subject subsets, such as those based on sex, age, weight, baseline plasma LDL-c levels, drug dose, history of prior cardiovascular occlusive events, etc. Any of these could be designated a priori. Alternatively, if unexpected signals occurred during the study that indicated that the results of one or more outcomes could likely be different in any of these subgroups, a posteriori analyses could be warranted if they were previously unplanned.

## POST-HOC ANALYSES

Any a posteriori analyses that are conducted on the data derived from a clinical study are termed **post-hoc analyses**, whether they are related to efficacy, safety, or another aspect of the study. We have already mentioned some of the circumstances under which a posteriori analyses are commonly warranted. However, it is often suspect when post-hoc analyses are conducted, and with good reason. There is a widely accepted belief that the more one looks for anything, the more likely that something will be found. However, as we have mentioned, with each additional analysis that is conducted, there is increased risk that some of the answers will be erroneous. When conducting multiple analyses on the data from a single clinical study, there is a point beyond which the risk of making a false conclusion based on these analyses outweighs the benefit of looking further. This point usually comes well before any post-hoc analyses have been conducted. For this reason, the practice of conducting post-hoc analyses, especially when such analyses are numerous or in the absence of strong signals or rationale, has often been likened to **data mining** or **data dredging**. At best, post-hoc analyses should serve to inform new research questions that can be examined more adequately in future clinical studies. They should rarely be the sole basis for conclusions or clinical decision making.

# OUTCOME MEASUREMENT AND MEANING

We have previously defined study outcomes and discussed the relative hierarchy of those outcomes within a clinical study. Now, we will look at some other aspects of outcomes and their effects on how clinical studies are conducted and the conclusions that can be drawn from them. Determining appropriate study outcomes is one of the most important aspects of planning and conducting clinical research. To be useful, study outcomes must be both measurable and meaningful. **Measurement** involves assigning a value to an observation. When we envision measuring something, we often think of numeric scales, such as plasma LDL-c levels or amount of pain. However, measurement of an outcome can also include assignment of subjects to nominal values or dichotomous groups, such as death versus no death. **Meaningfulness** relates to the importance of an outcome both within and beyond the clinical study. To be meaningful, an outcome must represent a significant effect or circumstance in the subject. The term **clinical significance** is often used in reference to the meaningfulness of a clinical study outcome and informs the degree to which the outcome can be extrapolated beyond the study to the "real world." If an outcome is measureable but has limited meaning, there is little value in measuring it. Conversely, if an outcome is meaningful but its measurement is unreliable, it will be difficult to have confidence in that outcome. The concepts of measure and meaning are integral to understanding and extrapolating clinical study outcomes.

Depending on the nature of an outcome, its measurement may be made using a variety of methods or tools. Plasma LDL-c levels can be measured using a nuclear magnetic resonance spectrometer, or they can be estimated from an equation using total cholesterol, high-density lipoprotein cholesterol (HDL-c), and triglyceride levels as variables. Adjudication of death as related to cardiovascular causes can be determined by following a set of guidelines or an algorithm. QOL can be measured using a questionnaire. In all measurements, the methods and tools used, whether they involve equipment, calculations, algorithms, or surveys, are referred to as **instruments**.

## PRECISION AND ACCURACY

Let us examine some aspects that predominantly relate to the measurability of a study outcome. One such aspect is the precision of the instrument used to measure it. Each outcome in a clinical study must be able to be measured (or adjudicated) for each subject. **Precision** refers to the relative proximity to one another of measurements of a characteristic that are taken from different subjects in whom that characteristic is actually identical (or that are taken from the same subject at the same time). It is the measurement's consistency or reproducibility. The measurement of an outcome is said to be more precise when individual subjects with identical actual outcomes are recorded as having the same or very similar outcomes to one another. In contrast, the measurement of an outcome is said to be less precise when individual subjects with identical actual outcomes are recorded as having significantly different outcomes from one another.

Let us examine this concept in the context of the primary outcome from our example clinical study, cardiovascular-related death. For each subject who dies in the study, a determination (i.e., measurement) must be made as to whether the death was related to cardiovascular causes. For some subjects, this may be relatively straightforward. For other subjects, it may be less so. If two subjects actually died of an identical cardiovascular-related cause, but one was adjudicated as being related to cardiovascular causes and the other was not, this would make the outcome less precise. It would be better (i.e., more precise) if these two subjects' outcomes were adjudicated in the same way, whether that was both related to cardiovascular causes or both unrelated to cardiovascular causes. Although it might seem counterintuitive to describe it as "better" if both cardiovascular-related deaths were adjudicated as not being related to cardio-vascular causes than one of them being correctly assigned and one not, it is generally important for like events to be adjudicated in a similar manner across the entire study to maintain the integrity of the data. Of course, getting the data correct is also important, which will be examined in a bit, when we discuss accuracy.

When examining the precision of an outcome, it is especially helpful to assess the subjectivity of the instrument used to measure that outcome. **Subjectivity** refers to the amount of interpretation required in taking a measurement, and directly affects the precision of an outcome. An outcome is generally said to be subjective when a reason-able portion of its measurement requires human interpretation. In contrast, when the measurement of an outcome is relatively free from human interpretation, it is said to be **objective**.

To illustrate the concept of subjectivity, let us examine the adjudication of an MI. A patient presents to an emergency department with chest pain, dyspnea, pallor, and dia-phoresis. Although all of these symptoms suggest MI, a diagnosis based solely on these observations would clearly be subjective, because the same symptoms could be attribut-able to other conditions, such as pulmonary embolism. A 12-lead electrocardiograph (ECG) is attached to the patient and blood is drawn for chemistries. The clinician reads ST elevation in multiple leads of the ECG. This also points to MI. However, although a diagnosis of MI based on the ECG is more objective than on the symptoms alone, read-ing an ECG often requires a significant amount of human interpretation. Finally, the blood chemistry results return, showing elevated creatine kinase (CK), CK-MB, and troponin, which are highly specific for MI, and the suspected diagnosis is confirmed by objective data. If adjudication of MI in a clinical study was to be allowed solely on the basis of symptoms, the outcome would likely be less precise than if ECG and/or highly specific blood chemistries were required for such adjudication.

Even some measurements that utilize a scale and are thought of as being relatively objective can have some degree of subjectivity, and thus imprecision. Consider, for instance, measuring subjects' blood pressure. A number of factors may lead to impre-cise blood pressure measurements between subjects, such as if some were taken using a manual sphygmomanometer and stethoscope, which requires human interpretation, whereas others were taken using an electronic machine, which does not require such interpretation. So, although we generally think of blood pressure as being an objective measurement, it can still have an element of subjectivity to it.

Clearly, subjective outcomes are inherently less precise than objective outcomes. Despite this, it is still acceptable to use a subjective outcome when it is deemed more meaningful than any reasonable objective outcome available. For instance, subject-answered questionnaires can be highly subjective, because individual subjects may inter-pret questions or responses very differently. However, using a questionnaire may still be the most meaningful or only reasonable way to measure certain outcomes, such as amount of pain or degree of depression. When using subjective outcomes, it is especially important to make them as precise as possible. Some common methods employed to increase the precision of subjective outcomes are using a clearly defined and standard-ized set of parameters for each possible measurement, giving adjudicators and subjects timely and detailed descriptions and informing them of possible nuances between dif-ferent responses, using a single person or committee to adjudicate all cases to ensure that similar cases are treated in a similar manner, and using the same laboratory and equip-ment to analyze all specimens.

Another important aspect of an outcome is the accuracy of the instrument used to measure it. **Accuracy** refers to the relative proximity of a measurement to the real value.

Whereas precision is the consistency of a measurement, accuracy is the measurement's correctness or truthfulness. The measurement of an outcome is said to be more accurate when the outcomes recorded for individual subjects are close to the outcomes they actually experienced. In contrast, the measurement of an outcome is said to be less accurate when the outcomes recorded for individual subjects are not as close to the outcomes they actually experienced.

Let us again examine this in the context of the primary outcome from our example clinical study, cardiovascular-related death. For obvious reasons, it is important for each death in this study to be correctly adjudicated as related versus unrelated to cardiovascular causes. As we previously saw, high precision does not necessarily address this; it is addressed by the instrument's accuracy. As with a measurement's precision, subjectivity of the measurement plays a role in its accuracy, albeit to a lesser extent if the measurement has been sufficiently established as credible through rigorous testing.

Let us examine precision and accuracy together in another example. Consider three electronic instruments, A, B, and C, used to measure cardiac QT interval. Each instrument is used to measure the QT interval in 10 subjects, each with an actual QT interval of exactly 400 milliseconds (msec). The measurements taken by the three instruments are shown in **Table 6-1**.

To assess the accuracy of each of these instruments, we can look at the distance of each measurement from its actual value and take the averages of these for the 10 measurements. A perfectly accurate instrument would measure each subject's QT interval as 400 msec, and would thus have an average distance between actual and measured values of 0 msec. As an instrument's accuracy decreases, the average distance between actual and measured values moves farther from this value. For the three instruments, A, B, and C, the average distances of their measurements from the actual values of 400 msec are 0 msec, 13.4 msec, and −1 msec, respectively. Thus, instruments A and C are quite accurate, whereas instrument B is less so.

To assess the precision of each of the instruments, we can look to the average distance of each measured value from each other measured value made by the same instrument. Because the actual QT intervals of all 10 subjects were exactly the same, a perfectly precise instrument would measure all 10 subjects' QT intervals as exactly the same as one another, and would thus have an average distance of each measured value to each other value measured by the same instrument of 0 msec. For the three instruments, A, B, and C, the average distances of each measured value from each other measured value made by the same instrument are 4.44 msec, 0.76 msec, and 1.02 msec, respectively. Thus, instruments B and C are quite precise, whereas instrument A is less so. In this way, we can see that instrument A is relatively accurate, but not very precise; instrument B is relatively precise, but not very accurate; and instrument C is both relatively accurate and relatively precise.

Whenever possible, it is preferential to use instruments that have both high accuracy and high precision when taking measurements in clinical studies. Assessment of the impact of a study should take into consideration the accuracy and precision of the

**TABLE 6-1** QT Interval Measurements of 10 Subjects Taken with Three Instruments

| Instrument | Measurements (milliseconds) |
|---|---|
| A | 394, 396, 396, 399, 400, 401, 402, 403, 404, 405 |
| B | 412, 413, 413, 413, 413, 414, 414, 414, 414, 414 |
| C | 398, 398, 398, 398, 399, 399, 399, 400, 400, 401 |

instruments used to measure the study's outcomes. When one of these aspects must be sacrificed, it may seem that high accuracy is always preferential to high precision. But, this is not necessarily the case. Consider a study that examines the change in a subject's QT interval from a baseline measurement to a measurement taken after some intervention has been given. The measurements can be taken with an instrument having higher accuracy and lower precision (instrument A) or with an instrument having lower accuracy and higher precision (instrument B). Imagine that the subject's baseline and postintervention QT intervals were actually 400 msec and 420 msec, respectively. This is an increase of 20 msec. Baseline and postintervention measurements taken with instrument A could be 397 msec and 424 msec, respectively. Although these measurements are relatively accurate, they would indicate an increase of 27 msec, 7 msec more than actually occurred. In contrast, baseline and postintervention measurements taken with instrument B could be 415 msec and 436 msec, respectively. Although these measurements are relatively inaccurate, they would indicate an increase of 21 msec, only 1 msec more than actually occurred. This is because instrument B is more precise. (Although instrument B is inaccurate, it is consistently inaccurate, resulting in a consistent interval with regard to the baseline and postintervention measurements.) This example illustrates that accuracy is not always more important than precision.

When an instrument is first developed, it will generally undergo some testing to validate it by assessing in a quantitative way the precision and accuracy of that instrument for a given measurement. Using instruments that have been validated for high precision and accuracy to measure outcomes in clinical studies is extremely important. Because the assessment of an instrument's accuracy requires knowledge of the actual values of what is being measured, **validation** of accuracy requires another, preferably a gold standard, method of measuring the outcome of interest. (Recall that in our previous examples with measuring QT interval, we assumed that we knew what the subjects' actual values were. This represents the application of a gold standard method of measuring the value, which may or may not, itself, be 100% accurate.) A **gold standard** is an instrument or method for taking a measurement that is considered to be the best available at a given time and under a given set of conditions. Assessments of precision do not always require an alternate measurement method. But, they do often require that the instrument be used by multiple different individuals in order to assess **inter-rater reliability**, or **concordance**, and by the same individual multiple times in order to assess **test–retest reliability**, or **repeatability**. So, instrument validation can be an arduous task in and of itself. When a validated instrument is unavailable, it is acceptable to take measurements using a method that is generally recognized as a standard of care.

The number of statistical methods that can be used to assess the accuracy and precision of instruments that measure all manner of outcomes is too great to allow for them all to be examined in this chapter. However, we will discuss some specific parameters that are commonly used to quantitatively describe the precision and accuracy of instruments used to measure dichotomous outcomes. Before we get to the specific parameters, however, let us take a moment to visit some broad concepts about dichotomous outcomes.

For a given dichotomous outcome, there exist the circumstances of having the condition of interest and of not having the condition of interest. At any single point in time, a given individual has one and only one of those circumstances. If we use the example of ischemic stroke, any given individual either has or has not suffered this condition. The proportion of all individuals in a defined population who have the condition of interest, in this example all those who have had an ischemic stroke, is called the prevalence of that condition. Because there are obvious factors that prevent us from knowing the true and exact proportion of all individuals who have a given condition in a large population, most reports of prevalence in such populations are merely estimations. For the purposes

| TABLE 6-2    Possible Measurements for Dichotomous Outcomes | | | |
|---|---|---|---|
| | | **Condition Actually Present** | |
| | | **NO** | **YES** |
| **Condition Measured** | **NO** | True negative | False negative |
| **as Present** | **YES** | False positive | True positive |

of our discussions, however, we will assume that the prevalence is accurately characterized among a well-defined population.

When using any instrument to measure a dichotomous outcome in a given individual, four possible circumstances exist. If the individual actually has the condition of interest and the instrument measures the individual as having that condition, the result is a **true positive**—true because the measurement was correct and positive because the measurement identified the condition as present. If the individual actually does not have the condition of interest and the instrument measures the individual as not having that condition, the result is a **true negative**—true because the measurement was correct and negative because the measurement identified the condition as absent. However, if the individual actually has the condition of interest but the instrument measures the individual as not having that condition, the result is a **false negative**—false because the measurement was incorrect and negative because the measurement identified the condition as absent. Finally, if the individual actually does not have the condition of interest but the instrument measures the individual as having that condition, the result is a **false positive**—false because the measurement was incorrect and positive because the measurement identified the condition as present. **Table 6–2** shows these concepts graphically.

## NEGATIVE AND POSITIVE PREDICTIVE VALUES

Two quantitative expressions relating to the precision of an instrument that measures dichotomous outcomes are its **negative predictive value** (NPV) and **positive predictive value** (PPV). Predictive values are expressed as probabilities and are calculated by dividing the number of true results of the given type (negative or positive) measured by an instrument by the total number of true and false results of that same type measured by the instrument.

The NPV of an instrument is equal to the number of true negatives measured by the instrument divided by the total number of true and false negatives measured by the instrument, yielding a probability from 0% to 100%. NPV represents the probability that a negative result measured by an instrument actually represents a truly negative case. For example, an instrument to diagnose ischemic stroke has a 95% NPV. If a given individual is measured as having not had an ischemic stroke by that instrument, then we can have 95% confidence that the individual indeed did not have an ischemic stroke. Alternatively, out of every 100 individuals measured as having not had an ischemic stroke using the instrument, 95 actually have not had an ischemic stroke (and 5 actually have had one). If every negative result that an instrument measures is truly negative, its NPV is equal to 100%. As the instrument increasingly classifies positive cases as negatives, its NPV diminishes proportionally.

The PPV of an instrument is equal to the number of true positives measured by the instrument divided by the total number of true and false positives measured by the instrument, yielding a probability from 0% to 100%. PPV represents the probability that a positive result measured by an instrument actually represents a truly positive case.

For example, an instrument to diagnose ischemic stroke has 95% PPV. If a given individual is measured as having had an ischemic stroke by that instrument, then we can have 95% confidence that the individual indeed had an ischemic stroke. Alternatively, out of every 100 individuals measured as having had an ischemic stroke using the instrument, 95 actually have had an ischemic stroke (and 5 actually have not had one). If every positive result that an instrument measures is truly positive, its PPV is equal to 100%. As the instrument increasingly classifies negative cases as positives, its PPV diminishes proportionally.

PPV has sometimes been referred to as *precision rate*. However, this is somewhat deceptive, as PPV alone does not provide a complete picture of an instrument's overall precision. Take, for instance, an instrument that is used to measure ischemic stroke in a group of 100 individuals, 20 of whom have actually had an ischemic stroke and 80 of whom have actually not had an ischemic stroke. The instrument classifies 10 individuals as having had ischemic strokes (positives) and 90 individuals as having not had ischemic strokes (negatives). Of the 10 positives identified, all 10 truly had an ischemic stroke (true positives). The PPV would be 100% (10 true positive results ÷ 10 total positive results), despite the fact that there were another 10 positive cases that were misclassified by the instrument as not ischemic strokes. If there are a total of 20 individuals who had ischemic strokes and the instrument classifies 10 individuals as having had an ischemic stroke and 10 as not having had an ischemic stroke, the instrument overall is not precise, despite a 100% PPV. This example emphasizes the importance of examining PPV and NPV in the context of one another. If taken individually, either can be misleading. The PPV for this instrument was 100%, meaning that 100% of the positive results identified were true positives. However, of the 90 negative results, 10 were false. So, the NPV would only be 89% (80 true negatives ÷ 90 total negatives). If the PPV were the only value reported for the instrument, we could not truly assess its overall precision. When the 100% PPV and 89% NPV are presented together, we see that the instrument is very reliable when a positive case is identified, but not as reliable when a negative case is identified.

## SENSITIVITY AND SPECIFICITY

Even PPV and NPV together are not sufficient to fully assess an instrument for measuring dichotomous outcomes. The accuracy of an instrument that measures dichotomous outcomes can also be quantitatively expressed in terms of its sensitivity and specificity. Like predictive values, sensitivity and specificity are also expressed as probabilities. However, whereas PPV and NPV are calculated by dividing the number of true results of the given type measured by an instrument by the total number of true and false results of that same type measured by the instrument, sensitivity and specificity are calculated by dividing the number of true results of the given type (positive or negative, respectively) by the actual total number of cases of that type.

The **sensitivity** of an instrument is equal to the number of true positives measured by the instrument divided by the number of actual positive cases in the population screened (i.e., the prevalence of the condition). Sensitivity represents the probability that any actual positive case will be classified as such by the instrument. Another way of saying this is that sensitivity is the probability that a false negative will not occur. Sensitivity can also be expressed as the proportion of actual positive cases that will be identified by the instrument. For example, an instrument to diagnose ischemic stroke has 95% sensitivity. If an individual has suffered an ischemic stroke, the instrument is 95% likely to identify that. Alternatively, out of every 100 individuals who have suffered an ischemic stroke, the instrument will identify 95 of them (and miss 5 of them). If an instrument identifies every positive case, its sensitivity is equal to 100%. As the instrument increasingly fails to identify positive cases, its sensitivity diminishes proportionally.

The **specificity** of an instrument is equal to the number of true negatives measured by the instrument divided by the number of actual negative cases in the population screened. Specificity represents the probability that any actual negative case will be classified as such by the instrument. Another way of saying this is that specificity is the probability that a false positive will not occur. Specificity can also be expressed as the proportion of actual negative cases that will be identified by the instrument. For example, an instrument to diagnose ischemic stroke has 95% specificity. If an individual has not suffered an ischemic stroke, the instrument is only 5% likely to identify that he has. Alternatively, out of every 100 individuals who have not suffered an ischemic stroke, the instrument will identify 95 of them as such (and falsely identify 5 of them as having suffered an ischemic stroke). If an instrument identifies every negative case, its specificity is equal to 100%. As the instrument increasingly fails to identify negative cases, its sensitivity diminishes proportionally.

Note that sensitivity does not account for individuals in whom the condition being measured is not actually present, even when the instrument incorrectly classifies these individuals as having the condition (i.e., false positives). Likewise, specificity does not account for individuals in whom the condition being measured is actually present, even when the instrument incorrectly classifies these individuals as not having the condition (i.e., false negatives).

To illustrate this, let us again look at an instrument used to diagnose ischemic stroke. Assume that 20 out of 100 individuals screened actually had an ischemic stroke, and 80 of them have not had an ischemic stroke. If the instrument correctly identified all 20 of the individuals who actually had an ischemic stroke (true positives) and correctly identified all 80 of the individuals who did not actually have an ischemic stroke (true negatives), the sensitivity of the instrument would be 100% (20 true positives ÷ 20 actual positive cases). Likewise, its specificity would be 100% (80 true negatives ÷ 80 actual negative cases).

Now, let us imagine that, in addition to correctly identifying the 20 individuals who actually did have an ischemic stroke (20 true positives), the instrument also misclassified 20 individuals who did not actually have an ischemic stroke as having had one (20 false positives). This would leave 60 individuals who did not have an ischemic stroke and were identified as such (60 true negatives). The sensitivity of the instrument would still be 100% (20 true positives ÷ 20 actual positive cases). This is because the equation for sensitivity does not factor in false positives. However, the specificity of the instrument would fall to 75% (60 true negatives ÷ 80 actual negative cases).

As with PPV and NPV, we can see that sensitivity and specificity are most useful when presented in the context of one another. For an outcome to be truly accurate, it must be measured using an instrument that has both high sensitivity and high specificity. Indeed, we can quantify accuracy in terms of both sensitivity and specificity by using the following equation:

$$\text{Accuracy} = (\text{Sensitivity} \times \text{Prevalence}) + [(\text{Specificity} \times (1 - \text{Prevalence})]$$

where sensitivity, specificity, and prevalence are expressed as proportions. In this equation, more weight is given to sensitivity when the prevalence is high because the sensitivity equation is already diluted for conditions with a high prevalence. Likewise, more weight is given to specificity when the prevalence is low because the specificity equation is already diluted for conditions with a low prevalence.

In practice, it is sometimes necessary to screen for conditions with two separate instruments because one instrument with both high sensitivity and high specificity is not known to exist. In such cases, one of the instruments will typically have a high sensitivity and the other a high specificity. These may be used concurrently, or one may be used only in the instance of a specific result from the other. For instance, the instrument with a high specificity may be used only to confirm positive cases detected by using the instrument with high sensitivity, because the high-sensitivity instrument has a tendency to identify false positives.

Given the same sampling (100 individuals, 20 of whom actually have had an ischemic stroke and 80 of whom have not), think about what would happen to PPV, NPV, sensitivity, and specificity if the instrument identified 15 true positives and the remainder of the subjects as negative. What about if the instrument identified 20 positives, but 5 of them were false? What about an instrument that identified 35 positives, 15 of which were true, and 65 negatives, 60 of which were true?

## SURROGATE AND DIRECT OUTCOMES

We have previously discussed the hierarchy used when a clinical study includes multiple outcomes. This hierarchy is often established based on the relative meaningfulness of the outcomes. We will now examine some additional concepts relating to the meaningfulness of outcomes.

The most meaningful, and thus the most useful, outcomes are those that relate to significant and important events or aspects of an individual's life. Such outcomes are referred to as **direct outcomes** because they directly alter the individual in some meaningful way. Examples of direct outcomes include things like death, change in subject-reported QOL, diagnosis of diabetes, nonfatal MI, shift in ability to perform activities of daily living (ADLs), hospitalization, etc. Each of these examples represents an event that will significantly change an aspect of the individual's life, either temporarily or permanently.

In many instances, a researcher may wish to substitute a more convenient measurement in place of a direct outcome. Such substitute outcomes are known as **surrogate outcomes**. Surrogate outcomes are not meaningful in and of themselves. Rather, to be a meaningful outcome, a surrogate outcome must in some way predict or be directly associated with one or more meaningful events or effects. The relationship between the surrogate outcome and its more meaningful event or effect should have been sufficiently established through previous research. For instance, having consistently high plasma LDL-c levels is not necessarily meaningful, in and of itself, to a given individual if that individual never experiences an event or effect related to having high plasma LDL-c levels. In other words, if that individual lives an entire life and never develops heart disease or suffers a stroke, MI, or any other condition related to having high plasma LDL-c levels, what his or her plasma LDL-c levels actually were is meaningless. So, plasma LDL-c level is not a direct outcome. However, having consistently high plasma LDL-c levels has been shown through numerous studies to be a risk factor for heart disease, MI, and other meaningful cardiovascular events, which are themselves meaningful. So, plasma LDL-c level is a good surrogate outcome for these events.

Whenever possible, it is preferential for the primary outcome of a clinical study to be a direct outcome. Indeed, the FDA often requires multiple clinical studies with direct outcomes to be conducted with a new drug before they will approve it for general use. That said, it is sometimes impossible, unethical, or highly inconvenient to conduct a study with a direct primary outcome. In such cases, the researcher may opt to use a surrogate outcome instead. For instance, early clinical studies of new drugs for chronic conditions seldom have direct primary outcomes because studies with direct outcomes generally require greater numbers of subjects enrolled for longer periods of time than do studies with surrogate outcomes. Thus, the use of surrogate outcomes in these earlier studies minimizes subject exposure to drugs with relatively unknown risks.

## COMPOSITE OUTCOMES

It is not uncommon for a single independent variable to affect multiple dependent variables. For instance, lowering plasma LDL-c levels can reduce the risk of several different conditions, such as heart disease, MI, ischemic stroke, and peripheral vascular disease (PVD). The researcher may wish to examine the effects of the independent variable on some or all of these dependent variables grouped together as a single outcome. Such grouped outcomes are called **composite outcomes**, also sometimes referred to as **combined outcomes**.

A researcher may wish to use composite outcomes for a variety of reasons, and it may be appropriate to do so. If the respective incidence rates of multiple individual dependent variables are expected to be relatively low, a clinical study to adequately examine these outcomes individually may require enrollment of more subjects for a longer period of time than is desirable. However, rolling up these effects into a single composite outcome may allow the study to be reasonably conducted using fewer subjects for a shorter duration.

The practice of using composite outcomes is not without its pitfalls. Combining outcomes can sometimes lead to inflated results, especially if individual dependent variables are used in multiple composite outcomes. In other instances, combining outcomes can lead to diluted results if a study intervention has little or no effect on one or more of the individual dependent variables in the composite outcome. Combining outcomes can also lead to results that are more difficult to interpret or apply beyond the study. Furthermore, if the individual dependent variables included in a composite outcome are too disparate with regard to their causes or impacts on subjects, the composite outcome loses meaning. For this reason, the individual dependent variables that are examined as part of a composite outcome should be similar with regard to their causes and clinical impacts. The more similar these aspects are, the more suited the dependent variables are to be grouped together in a single composite outcome. For the most part, only dichotomous outcomes should be included as components of a composite outcome. For instance, it would be inappropriate to merge numeric values for plasma LDL-c levels and plasma triglyceride levels into a single composite outcome. Although potentially similar with regard to their causes and the impact of their effects on an individual, these parameters are measured on scales and are not dichotomous variables.

In our example, clinical study of a drug that is expected to lower plasma LDL-c levels, one of the secondary outcomes was the number of serious nonfatal cardiovascular occlusive events, which included MI and ischemic stroke. Because the risks for MI and ischemic stroke are both increased in individuals with high plasma LDL-c levels and the impacts of these events on individuals are both relatively high, they are good candidates for grouping together in a composite outcome. However, it would be less meaningful to group MI and cancer together in a composite outcome, because their risk factors (at least as they pertain to this study) do not significantly overlap. Likewise, it would be less meaningful to group MI and erectile dysfunction (another possible effect of high plasma LDL-c levels) together in a composite outcome, because their relative clinical impacts are so different. In our example study, we also identified all-cause mortality as a secondary outcome. Because death can occur from multiple causes, this outcome could technically be thought of as a composite outcome as well.

A researcher may also examine the effects from a composite outcome in separate individual analyses. In our example study, the numbers of MIs and ischemic strokes were identified as individual tertiary outcomes contingent on the results of the composite outcome of serious nonfatal cardiovascular occlusive events. In other words, if the composite outcome was found to be insignificant, then the individual tertiary outcomes would not be analyzed. However, if the composite outcome was found to be significant, its individual components would be analyzed separately as well. In this context, we must again emphasize the increased risk of erroneous results and false conclusions inherent in conducting numerous analyses.

# TYPES OF STUDY DESIGNS

Until now, the majority of what we have examined with regard to clinical research has been relatively abstract and conceptual. Now, we will transition into discussing some of the more practical aspects of conducting clinical studies. The first of these considerations is given to the various types of clinical study designs.

## RETROSPECTIVE AND PROSPECTIVE STUDIES

Clinical studies can be divided into two orientations with regard to time: those that look back at things that have already happened and those that look forward to what will happen. Studies that look back in time and examine events that have already occurred are called **retrospective studies**. Retrospective studies may examine data that were already collected for other purposes, such as in the normal care of patients. Alternatively, the researcher may examine recorded events and their circumstances in an attempt to create meaning around and gain more understanding about those events. In contrast, **prospective studies** are planned in a forward-looking manner. They examine circumstances as they begin and events as they progress in real time.

Both **study orientations** have advantages and disadvantages. For instance, the resource expenditure for conducting retrospective studies is generally less than for prospective studies. The sponsor of the study generally need not incur costs for implementing interventions, ordering and interpreting assessments, etc., because these have typically already been done. In addition, because the researcher will usually not be exposing subjects to new risks, retrospective studies have the added benefit of not typically requiring voluntary participation from those subjects. The major drawback of retrospective studies is that the researcher has less control over the subjects and their circumstances. Thus, significant amounts of data may be missing and there is a greater risk that uncontrolled and potentially unidentifiable variables will alter the results. In prospective studies, the researcher can increase the potential that all data that will be required for proper analyses will be collected from all subjects. In addition, prospective study designs afford the opportunity for the researcher to plan for and control many aspects of the subjects' circumstances that could potentially alter the results. However, conducting prospective studies typically requires more resources to plan and execute. In addition, all potential prospective study subjects must give voluntary approval to be included.

In general, prospective studies are considered to provide stronger evidence for clinical decision making than retrospective studies. However, it may not always be appropriate or feasible to conduct a prospective study.

## OBSERVATIONAL AND INTERVENTIONAL (EXPERIMENTAL) STUDIES

Clinical studies can also be divided into two types based on the role the researcher plays in them. The researcher can be a passive witness to the events of the clinical study, or he or she can take an active part by controlling or altering certain circumstances. If the researcher merely bears witness to events and describes their circumstances, the study is an **observational study**. However, if the researcher actively alters the normal course of events, the study is an **interventional study**, also called an **experimental study**.

Clearly, interventional studies must be prospective in orientation because the researcher cannot go back in time and make changes to the events that occurred. However, observational studies may be oriented retrospectively or prospectively. That is, the researcher may simply look backward in time to examine events as they already happened, or he or she may follow events forward in time without actively altering them. Thus, by combining the study orientation with the researcher role, we can describe any given clinical study design as retrospective (which implies an observational role), prospective observational, or interventional (which implies a prospective orientation).

Some of the more common types of retrospective clinical studies are case studies and series, case-control studies, and meta-analyses. The most common type of prospective observational clinical study design is the cohort study, although the cohort study design can also be applied retrospectively. In addition, a special type of observational study, called a cross-sectional study, exists somewhat outside the framework of time orientation because it generally examines circumstances neither retrospectively nor prospectively, but rather as they exist at an instant in time. Interventional clinical studies are also called clinical trials, which can be further defined by certain other aspects that we will discuss later in this chapter, such as study purpose, subject distribution, allocation, blinding, and control modalities. **Table 6-3** shows the most commonly employed types of clinical studies in the context of orientation to time and researcher role.

In many ways, the clinical question that a researcher endeavors to answer will guide the type of clinical study that is required. Some clinical questions lend themselves to retrospective study designs, whereas others require prospective approaches. Some clinical questions can be answered purely through observation, whereas others necessitate active intervention.

## PARALLEL, MATCHED, AND CROSSOVER STUDIES

Not only can clinical studies be classified by the role of the researcher, they can also be categorized by the distribution of subjects and how they are compared to one another. The most basic pattern of a clinical study is that subjects are identified from a population, they are assigned to groups based on a naturally occurring or artificially created difference in a specific exposure, all other circumstances between groups are attempted to be held identical, an outcome of interest is measured in each subject at an appropriate interval thereafter, and these data are pooled in groups and analyzed to see if the outcome changed differently between the groups. This is a description of a **parallel study**. In a parallel study, each subject is assigned to a single group and his or her data are pooled with others in the same group. These pooled data are then analyzed against the pooled data from one or more other groups in the study. The design is called "parallel"

| TABLE 6-3 | Common Types of Clinical Studies | | |
|---|---|---|---|
| | | **Orientation to Time** | |
| | | Retrospective | Prospective |
| **Researcher Role** | **Observational** | Case studies/series<br>Case-control studies<br>Meta-analyses (Cohort studies) | Cohort studies |
| | **Interventional** | N/A | Clinical trials |

because subjects in different groups follow parallel paths through the study, but are never exposed to what the other groups' subjects are exposed. For instance, in a parallel study comparing drug A versus drug B, subjects in the drug A group will only receive drug A during the study, never drug B. Likewise, drug B subjects will never receive drug A.

Similar to a parallel study, subjects in a **matched study** never leave their initially assigned groups. The difference is in how their data are compared. Whereas in a parallel study with two groups the data from all subjects in one group are pooled and then compared in that form to the pooled data from the other group, in a matched study with two groups each subject in one group is paired with a similar subject in the other group. Their data are directly compared to one another, rather than simply being added to the pooled group data, and then used in aggregate. A matched study can be very powerful because paired subjects are presumably similar to one another. Studies in twins are often designed as matched studies.

Who can serve as a better **control** for a given subject than her twin? She can, herself. To allow subjects to serve as their own controls, a study can be designed in a crossover fashion. In a **crossover study**, each subject receives each study intervention or exposure in a sequential order, with a sufficient period between each to allow for lingering effects from the previous experience to dissipate. Like matched studies, crossover studies can be powerful, because each subject is compared with himself or herself, and then those data used in aggregate. They also offer the advantage of requiring half as many subjects as matched studies (when studying two interventions), because each crossover study subject serves double duty. However, crossover studies are only feasible when the same prestudy condition can be recreated between receiving one intervention or exposure and receiving the next. For instance, one could not use a crossover study to compare the efficacy of two antibiotics for an acute infection because the condition will no longer exist, or at least not exist to the same degree, after the subject has completed the first antibiotic regimen.

## SUPERIORITY, EQUIVALENCY, AND NONINFERIORITY STUDIES

We have previously discussed that clinical research endeavors to answer clinical questions. In many clinical studies, this question involves the comparison of two or more interventions (the independent variable) against one another to see how they affect an outcome (the dependent variable). The appropriate statistical methods to be used in answering a question involving the comparison of multiple interventions are in large part dictated by how the dependent variable is measured. How the statistical analyses are planned and how the data may be interpreted are dependent upon the hypothesis set forth by the researcher. Although there are more complex methodologies appropriate for examining more than two interventions at the same time, in order to simplify matters we will restrict our examples to the comparison of two interventions, because this is the most common scenario. Three basic questions can be considered when comparing two interventions (or comparing one intervention to no intervention), and these questions give rise to three different types of analyses that are commonly employed, each with its own uses and sets of conclusions that can be drawn.

The first question that can be asked is whether one intervention is "better" than another intervention (or no intervention) with regard to a specific outcome. This outcome is commonly about the relative efficacy of the interventions for a given disease or condition. If this is the clinical question being asked, the study will be a **superiority study**. Superiority studies often involve the comparison of an unestablished intervention to no intervention (or a placebo). However, sometimes the comparator intervention is an established intervention that has already been shown to have a positive impact on the outcome of interest and the study intervention is a newer intervention that has not been so established. Alternatively, the positive impacts of both interventions could already be established and the study intended to determine if either has a greater positive impact.

As with all studies, the null hypothesis in a superiority study is that there is no difference between the two interventions with regard to the outcome of interest. The alternative hypothesis is that one intervention is superior to the other with regard to that outcome. If the null hypothesis is rejected, it can be concluded that one intervention is statistically superior to the other with regard to the study outcome. In a superiority study, the boundary of acceptance for the null hypothesis is set at absolute equivalence. That is to say that if the entire confidence interval around the result is entirely above or entirely below the line of absolute equivalence, the null hypothesis is rejected and statistical superiority is demonstrated. (Simplistically, a confidence interval is a range of values within which there is relatively high probability that the true value exists.) In addition, if the magnitude of the effect is sufficient, a superiority study can also support a conclusion that the intervention is meaningfully (or "clinically") better than the other with regard to that outcome, in addition to being statistically better. It is important to note, however, that if the null hypothesis is not rejected, that is to say that the data do not support the statistical superiority of one intervention over the other, it does not necessarily mean that the two interventions are the same with regard to the outcome. It only means that there was insufficient evidence to claim that one intervention was superior to the other. Superiority studies are not designed to establish true similarity. Because they can establish one intervention as being statistically and meaningfully better than another, superiority studies are the most common types of interventional studies conducted.

Superiority studies can be one sided (or one tailed) or two sided (or two tailed) with regard to the direction of superiority examined. In a **two-sided (two-tailed) superiority study**, favor can be demonstrated for either of the interventions, or favor can be demonstrated for neither of the interventions. Thus, in a two-sided superiority study comparing interventions A and B, there are three possible results: superiority is demonstrated for intervention A over intervention B, superiority is demonstrated for intervention B over intervention A, or no superiority is demonstrated for either intervention. In a one-sided superiority study, favor is only examined for one intervention over the other, for instance intervention A over intervention B, but not for the reverse. So, in a **one-sided (one-tailed) superiority study** comparing interventions A and B, there are only two possible results: superiority is demonstrated for intervention A over intervention B, or superiority is not demonstrated for intervention A over intervention B. The possibility of superiority of intervention B over intervention A is not examined. One-sided superiority studies are only appropriate if only one intervention realistically has the possibility of being superior to the other, but the reverse is not possible. This is a very rare circumstance, and the use of one-sided superiority studies should be likewise rare. Even when an intervention is compared to no intervention, there is still usually a possibility, albeit potentially remote, that no intervention will be better than the intervention being studied.

If the clinical question being asked is whether two interventions are essentially the same with regard to a given outcome, that is to say that there is not a meaningful difference between the two interventions with regard to that outcome, the study should be designed as an **equivalency study**. As with all studies, the null hypothesis in an equivalency study is that there is no difference between the two interventions with regard to the outcome. The alternative hypothesis is that there is a difference. In an equivalency study, there are two statistical boundaries: one lower threshold, which is below the line of absolute equivalence, and one upper threshold, which is above the line of absolute equivalence. These boundaries are set closely enough to absolute equivalence as to represent a margin in which there is little to no clinical meaningfulness between them and absolute equivalence. Failing to reject the null hypothesis requires that the entire confidence interval around the result is within the area between these two thresholds and can be interpreted as the interventions being statistically and meaningfully equivalent to one another. If any portion of the confidence interval extends outside either of these thresholds, the null hypothesis is rejected and equivalency is not demonstrated. Just as failing to reject the null hypothesis in a superiority study does not necessarily mean that the two interventions are equivalent, rejecting the null hypothesis in an equivalency study does not necessarily mean that one of the interventions is superior or inferior to the other. Equivalency studies are not designed to establish true superiority. Equivalency studies are most commonly employed when it is important to establish that one intervention is not significantly different than another in either direction, such as to establish the therapeutic equivalence of a generic drug to a reference brand name drug.

There is one final relatively common type of question posed when comparing two interventions, and that is if one intervention is meaningfully worse than another with regard to an outcome of interest. Such questions are addressed by noninferiority studies. As the name implies, **noninferiority studies** are used to support a claim that one intervention is not meaningfully worse than a comparator that has already been shown to have a positive impact on the outcome of interest. The null and alternative hypotheses are the same in noninferiority studies as in other studies. That is, the null hypothesis is that there is no difference between the two interventions with regard to an outcome; the alternative hypothesis is that there is a difference. As with other studies, the differences lie in the placement of the statistical boundaries around absolute equivalence. Whereas in a superiority study, the boundary of acceptance for the null hypothesis is set at the line of absolute equivalence, the lower boundary of acceptance for the null hypothesis in a noninferiority study is set below absolute equivalence but equal to or above a value that is considered to be not meaningfully worse than absolute equivalence. This is similar to the lower boundary in an equivalency study. Unlike in equivalency studies, however, there is no upper boundary in a noninferiority study. In a noninferiority study, the intervention being studied may be slightly worse than the comparator with regard to the outcome, but the null hypothesis will still not be rejected. Because there is no upper boundary of equivalence, there is no statistical way to reject the null hypothesis in this direction, even in the event that the study intervention has an extremely greater positive effect on the outcome than the comparator. The only circumstance in which the null hypothesis is rejected in a noninferiority study is if the study intervention is potentially worse than the comparator (i.e., any portion of the confidence interval around the result extends below the noninferiority boundary).

Noninferiority studies are most appropriate when a new intervention needs to be at least as good as an existing intervention that has an established positive impact on the outcome of interest, but is unlikely to be superior to the existing intervention, and withholding the existing intervention from study subjects in the comparator group would be unethical. It is important to ensure that the dependent variable in a noninferiority study is identical to the dependent variable used in the study that initially established the comparator as efficacious. Otherwise, the results of the noninferiority study should be called into question. In addition, the comparator should be administered in the same manner as it is in current standard clinical practice. It is also desirable that the new intervention has some other potential benefit over the existing intervention, such as a lower cost, better safety profile, or less invasive method of administration. A good example of this is comparing a new antibiotic to an existing antibiotic to treat a severe infection. If

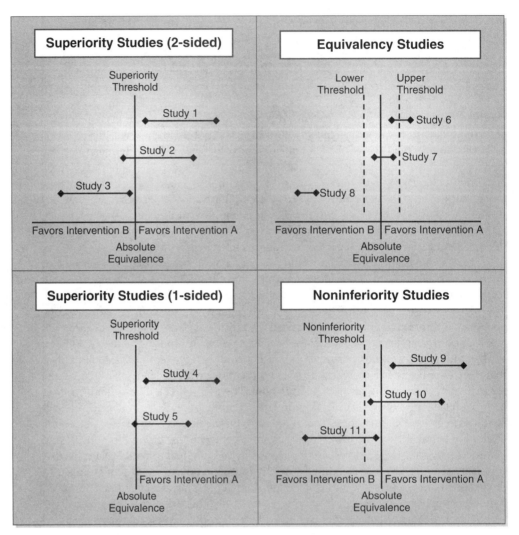

**FIGURE 6-1** Common clinical trial types.

the established antibiotic is relatively efficacious in the treatment of the infection, it is unlikely that the new antibiotic will be better enough to establish superiority in a superiority study, and it would be unethical to withhold treatment in the comparator group in order to compare the new antibiotic to placebo. Therefore, a noninferiority study would be most appropriate.

**Figure 6-1** is a graphical representation of confidence intervals from a number of theoretical equivalency, noninferiority, and one-sided and two-sided superiority studies, each involving two interventions, A and B.

Studies 1, 2, and 3 are two-sided superiority studies. In study 1, the entire confidence interval is above the superiority threshold, which is set at absolute equivalence. Thus, this study demonstrates superiority of intervention A over intervention B. In study 2, the confidence interval crosses the superiority threshold. Thus, this study demonstrates superiority of neither intervention. In study 3, the entire confidence interval is below the superiority threshold. Thus, this study demonstrates superiority of intervention B over intervention A.

Studies 4 and 5 are one-sided superiority studies. In study 4, the entire confidence interval is above the superiority threshold, which is again set at absolute equivalence.

Thus, this study demonstrates superiority of intervention A over intervention B. In study 5, the confidence interval touches the superiority threshold. Thus, this study does not demonstrate superiority of intervention A over intervention B. In one-sided superiority studies, these are the only two possible conclusions. It is not possible to determine if intervention B is superior to intervention A.

Studies 6, 7, and 8 are equivalency studies. Notice that there are now two statistical boundaries, a lower threshold and an upper threshold, and that these thresholds are relatively close to the line of absolute equivalence. In study 6, part of the confidence interval is above the upper equivalency threshold. Thus, this study does not demonstrate equivalency of the two interventions. In study 7, the entire confidence interval is between the lower and upper equivalency thresholds. Thus, this study demonstrates equivalency of the two interventions. In study 8, the entire confidence is below the lower equivalency threshold. Thus, this study does not demonstrate equivalency of the two interventions.

Studies 9, 10, and 11 are noninferiority studies. Notice that the noninferiority threshold is below the line of absolute equivalence and that this threshold is relatively close to the line of absolute equivalence. Notice also that there is only one threshold, as with superiority studies. In study 9, the entire confidence interval is above the noninferiority threshold. Thus, this study demonstrates noninferiority of intervention A to intervention B. In this study, the entire confidence interval also happens to be entirely above the line of absolute equivalence, which would seem to imply superiority of intervention A over intervention B. However, we should be careful about drawing such a conclusion, because other factors in the design of a noninferiority study may affect the results in a different way than if the study had been designed as a true superiority study. Therefore, it is probably safer simply to conclude noninferiority, and not superiority, from such a result. In study 10, the entire confidence interval is also above the noninferiority threshold. Thus, this study also demonstrates noninferiority of intervention A to intervention B, despite the fact that the confidence interval crosses the line of absolute equivalence. In study 11, the confidence interval crosses below the inferiority threshold. Thus, this study does not demonstrate noninferiority of intervention A to intervention B.

# POPULATIONS AND SAMPLING

Much of the determination of the quality of a clinical study is related to the population and sampling of the subjects for the trial. The selection of subjects for participation in a clinical study can affect the degree to which the results can be applied in practice and is a pivotal part of the design process. It is important to understand how subjects are chosen for study participation and the various methods that can be used to choose the **study population** and samples. A **population** is defined as "a group of individual persons, objects, or items from which samples are taken for statistical measurement," whereas a **sample** is a subset of the population.[2] Because access to an entire population is difficult and can rarely ever be confirmed, it is much easier to choose a sample of a given population. In our example study, the appropriate population to test the clinical question would be enormous to say the least, and it would be impossible to ensure that all possible individuals have been included. Instead, we choose a sample from that given population. Findings in the sample are then generalized to the population, so it is important to ensure that the sample is representative and has similar heterogeneity as the general population to which the conclusions will be applied. Effective **sampling** ensures that the study population will have the characteristics necessary to accurately answer the clinical question and ultimately minimize the chance of error. This, in turn, increases the likelihood that the outcome will be attributed to the independent variable rather than to differences in the population studied. Researchers usually do not have access to the whole population; therefore, they need to identify a target population for which the clinical question is to be tested. The **target population** depends on the research question to be answered. The researchers must have a specifically defined research question to accurately identify the specific characteristics of subjects that are needed to answer the research question.

Once the target population characteristics are identified, an **accessible population** needs to be identified. The accessible population takes into consideration geographic location as well as necessary logistical characteristics for participation and completion of the study. The accessible population is the group from which the subjects will be recruited for participation in the study using a variety of sampling techniques. Following screening and enrollment, these subjects will comprise the study population. For example, if a researcher was interested in studying men and women with a diagnosis of type 2 diabetes mellitus, with a predefined hemoglobin A1c (HbA1c) of 7–10%, he would have an extremely large population to sample, and it would be very difficult to ensure that all eligible individuals were screened for inclusion. Instead, he might select all patients enrolled in the diabetes clinics affiliated with his healthcare institution. The resulting population would be the accessible population. Using this population ensures that all eligible individuals were screened for inclusion and ultimately creates a relatively homogenous study population.

## PROBABILITY (RANDOM) SAMPLING

Sampling techniques can fall into one of two categories: probability or nonprobability methods. **Probability sampling** allows each member of the accessible population an equal chance of being randomly selected for the actual study sample. The most basic form of probability sampling is random sampling. With **random sampling**, each member of the accessible population is available for selection to be included in the study sample with equal chances of selection. Random sampling follows no systematic method for selection. To decrease the risk of error in random sampling, it is important that all eligible members of the accessible population are identified and included in the selection process. Any omission may introduce error in the selection process.

**Simple random sampling** requires enumerating all possible selections from the accessible population and selecting numbers at random to obtain the sample. One technique to accomplish random sampling is by using a table of random numbers (**Table 6-4**). Such tables can be generated by computers to create numbers representing all potential selections in no particular order or systematic method. Selections are made at random, and each number selected would correlate with a number on the participant list. This particular sampling technique requires a numbered list of all eligible participants and a rather laborious selection process.

**Systematic sampling** is another form of probability sampling that can reduce the burden of nonsystematic sampling, particularly with a large accessible population. In systematic sampling, the sample is chosen by a periodic or systematic process to select subjects from the larger population using a preidentified sampling interval and a randomly selected starting point. For example, the first selection is chosen at random and subsequent selections will be made at every 10th interval. It is even more important with systematic sampling that the accessible population is representative of the larger population with no underlying bias so that inherent differences in characteristics are not introduced with the systematic sampling. Any recurring pattern in the accessible population or listing can also potentially be carried over with the systematic sampling process.

| TABLE 6-4 Example Table of Random Numbers Used for Simple Random Sampling | | | | | |
|---|---|---|---|---|---|
| Row # | A | B | C | D | E |
| 1 | 79 | 235 | 355 | 66 | 261 |
| 2 | 89 | 212 | 126 | 145 | 328 |
| 3 | 119 | 19 | 322 | 331 | 50 |
| 4 | 167 | 28 | 346 | 101 | 44 |
| 5 | 424 | 170 | 315 | 273 | 38 |
| 6 | 82 | 106 | 112 | 120 | 103 |
| 7 | 341 | 21 | 306 | 181 | 269 |
| 8 | 426 | 233 | 493 | 478 | 475 |
| 9 | 411 | 159 | 309 | 125 | 21 |
| 10 | 410 | 207 | 339 | 163 | 476 |

**Stratified random sampling** can reduce the risk of study error by evenly distributing specific characteristics in the original accessible population. This allows relevant characteristics (e.g., gender or race) to be divided into subgroups so that specific populations are fairly represented and can be evaluated separately. In stratified random sampling, subjects are divided into groups by specified characteristics and samples are randomly selected from the specific groups. This approach can strengthen study design, because it often provides a more representative sample of a specific population than random sampling does.

**Cluster sampling** allows for more manageable sampling of large dispersed populations by allowing successive random sampling of a series of units in the population that fall into natural groupings. Clusters are often created based on geographic locations, and cluster sampling is typically accomplished in stages. The first stage involves the selection of a random sample or cluster based on geographic location. The second stage then involves selecting a random sample from the groups selected in the first stage and then further randomly selecting a sample from the identified clusters. Although this technique can offer conveniences, it does not always produce independent samples due to clusters being chosen based on preidentified characteristics, and efforts should be made to ensure selection of generalizable clusters and minimization of potential study errors.

## NONPROBABILITY (NONRANDOM) SAMPLING

In contrast to probability sampling, **nonprobability sampling** is executed in a more systematic, nonrandom manner. The most common form of **nonrandom sampling** is **convenience sampling**, in which subjects are chosen based on availability. Convenience sampling has many advantages, including ease and decreased cost. Unfortunately, self-selection becomes a concern as a potential source of bias because subjects are targeted based on availability to the researcher. In this type of sampling technique, a researcher wishing to look at pharmacy student perceptions on prescriptive authority might post recruitment flyers in the school of pharmacy down the street. Although this method would target pharmacy students, it is questionable as to how heterogeneous of a population would result as compared to all pharmacy schools in the United States.

**Purposive sampling** is accomplished with a purpose or defined population and methods are then targeted to achieve predefined populations. Although this method will ensure an abundance of samples from the target population that has been identified, it in no way ensures an accurate representation of the general population and often will result in extremely limited populations because of predefining and choosing specific characteristics of the desired population. Although this helps increase the sample size for studies of relatively rare conditions, it also introduces study error risk in the selection process and decreases heterogeneity. However, it may be a necessary sampling process for particularly specific research questions aimed at specific populations. For example, if a researcher wanted to test our example study hypothesis specifically in men from central Texas, aged 40–50 years, he might need to use purposive sampling to achieve an appropriate study population.

**Quota sampling** is a type of purposive sampling accomplished by choosing participants based on a fixed quota. This technique can be either proportional, resulting in equal numbers of subjects between groups, or nonproportional, in which one group will have more participants than the other in a fixed ratio, such as in a 2:1 ratio. The selection of groups and subjects are chosen based on defined criteria and certain preidentified characteristics. Subjects are then screened based to match the desired characteristics until the anticipated number of participants or quota is reached.

Nonrandom sampling methods are typically more practical; however, it is difficult to ensure that the resulting sample is representative of the general population and free from bias. To further ensure that a representative sample is included in the trial, rigor in the subject screening process is imperative, thus requiring appropriate and extensive inclusion and exclusion criteria.

## SUBJECT CRITERIA AND SCREENING

Regardless of sampling methods and techniques, potential subjects need to be screened to ensure eligibility based on defined inclusion and exclusion criteria. The **inclusion criteria** will define a set of characteristics that potential subjects must meet to be included in the study, whereas **exclusion criteria** will define specific characteristics that will preclude a potential subject from study participation. In addition, should a subject develop an exclusion criterion during the course of study participation, this could lead to forced study withdrawal. Potential subjects are screened by using predefined inclusion and exclusion criteria that have been established in the early stages of the study design process.

The clinical question and study hypothesis need to be considered when defining appropriate inclusion and exclusion criteria, and the specific disease or condition in question, as well as demographics, will guide the development of the criteria. The researchers must decide what characteristics are most important to test the clinical question while allowing for an appropriate study population to be formed. Inclusion and exclusion criteria should be defined explicitly, but not so restrictively that the resulting population is so specific that application of trial results would be difficult in the general population. In the same sense, if the inclusion and exclusion criteria are too general and include a wide range of variability, it makes it difficult to control for errors within the study population, and accurate conclusions about the interventions being studied are difficult to make. The balance lies in defining a diverse population, but not so diverse that variability is introduced, making application of results to the general population difficult.

Oftentimes, exclusion criteria will include comorbid conditions or medication use that could potentially interfere with study results or compromise safety of patients.

Comorbid conditions and demographics are essential aspects for consideration when defining inclusion and exclusion criteria. The inclusion and exclusion criteria should be explicitly stated in the methods section of the research article. The inclusion and exclusion criteria need to be evaluated by those who might use study conclusions for clinical decision making. Not only should the inclusion and exclusion criteria be evaluated for completeness, but they must also be evaluated for application of study results to a particular population or setting and for identification of potential errors caused by incorrectly or incompletely defined criteria.

In the example study that we have been using throughout this chapter, we have discussed a variety of study populations that could be selected in this trial, and the results of the population selection. The subjects in these examples would have been chosen based on predefined inclusion and exclusion criteria that would outline plasma LDL-c levels, age range, any comorbid conditions that may alter the results of the trial, and possibly other factors. In the case of comorbid diseases, any individual with a condition that carries an increased risk of death within the study period might be excluded so as to not confound the results of cardiovascular-related death. Additionally, some defined parameters for blood pressure would also help control for potential errors in study results. Thus, individuals being treated for high blood pressure and those with uncontrolled high blood pressure may be excluded from participation. The question then becomes whether the inclusion and exclusion criteria allow a population sufficient to test the clinical question. Conversely, would any of the inclusion or exclusion criteria limit the ability to apply the results to the general population or compromise the safety of the subjects during the study?

# STUDY GROUPS AND SUBJECT ALLOCATION

Once subjects have been selected and screened with the inclusion and exclusion criteria, they will be assigned to a **study group**. This process is called **subject allocation**. In observational studies, subject allocation is based on presence or absence of a condition or exposure. Because the researcher does not intervene, subject allocation is prescribed by the inclusion criteria. In interventional studies, however, subjects may be assigned to groups via a number of different techniques. As we will see, most of these techniques will have some degree of randomness to them. Depending on the type of study and the design, a subject may be assigned to an **active treatment (study) group** or to the **control group**. Subjects in the study group will receive the intervention under scrutiny, as defined in the research question and hypothesis. Controls can either be active or inactive. The most common type of inactive control is the placebo. **Placebo-controlled trials** are necessary to establish efficacy of an intervention and benefit over no treatment, but do not allow comparison to other available treatment options.

Sometimes, however, a placebo control is determined to be inappropriate, because of either ethical reasons or subject reluctance. Potential subjects may be hesitant to participate in a clinical trial knowing that they could potentially receive a placebo for their condition. In the same sense, if a standard of care has been established for a particular disease state, treatment with placebo would be considered unethical, as it is akin to withholding treatment. In this case, an **active control** would be used to ensure that patients receive necessary treatment. Alternatively, all subjects in all groups can receive the current standard of care and the intervention can be examined as an adjunct or add-on to this standard of care. In this case, a placebo control would generally be acceptable.

Active-controlled trials can establish differences in efficacy between two interventions and provide additional insight regarding the comparative effectiveness of the study intervention, due to the fact that results will be directly compared to an active control. When the active control is a drug, selection of a suitable control is important not only in regard to the agent, but also in regard to dosing and regimen, to ensure appropriate comparison. Interventions that can be used for similar conditions and similar outcomes can be compared in what is called a **head-to-head trial**, in which the comparisons are made directly between the two active interventions to determine efficacy relative to each other. Many times, this will involve drugs in the same medication class, but it can also involve drugs from different classes. However, when the comparisons are not made between similar agents, it can be difficult to compensate for risks of errors due to inherent differences in mechanism of action and drug characteristics.

## RANDOMIZATION TECHNIQUES

Once subjects have been determined to be eligible for study participation based on inclusion and exclusion criteria, they are then assigned to study groups. In clinical trials, the most common method of subject allocation is via randomization. **Randomization**, also called **random allocation**, can occur in various ways. Regardless of method, however, all subjects have the same chance of being assigned to a given group in an unpredictable manner. That is not to say that subject X has an equal chance of being assigned to group A as to group B. It does mean, however, that subject X and subject Y have the same chances as one another of being assigned to group A or group B. If groups A and B are intended to be proportional with regard to subject allocation, that is, they are intended to include approximately the same numbers of subjects, then there is an equal chance of a subject being assigned to group A as to group B. However, there are circumstances in which it is preferable to allocate subjects to groups in a **disproportional** manner. In such cases, every subject will have a higher chance (but an equal chance to one another) of being assigned to one group over another. In all cases, however, the actual allocation of a given subject is still random.

Randomization attempts to ensure equal distribution of subject characteristics between groups, reducing the potential for study errors and strengthening the design of the trial. The ultimate goal of randomization is having groups with similar characteristics so that comparisons between the groups will be attributable to the independent variable. Although randomization aims to produce similar groups, it is important to verify similarities of important attributes between groups following randomization by measuring and comparing subjects' **baseline characteristics**. Randomization techniques and final resulting groups should be described by the researchers in the research report. Any differences in groups following randomization will be carried over into the study and may affect the results of the trial. The statistical analysis and tests that are applied to the results rely on and make assumptions that the groups' characteristics are similar. Next we present the most common types of clinical trial randomization techniques.

**Simple randomization** is similar to a coin toss, in that subjects are assigned with a known probability. With each toss of the coin, the subject will be assigned to a group based on the outcome of the toss. Simple randomization carries the possibility of differences between groups caused by chance, particularly in studies with fewer subjects. It is more likely that simple randomization to larger groups will result in equally distributed characteristics; however, the potential still exists for imbalances.

**Stratified randomization** is a randomization technique that attempts to balance groups based on characteristics, to achieve balance within smaller subgroups, or to maintain balance between groups in studies with fewer subjects. Subjects are randomized in blocks based on known and unknown baseline characteristics or potentially confounding disease states or attributes. Subjects are identified by a particular characteristic, for example, smoking status, and placed in respective groups. Once the respective groups are identified and formed, subjects undergo random assignment to treatment group. Subjects still have an equal chance of being assigned to either treatment group, but in the end the number of smokers and nonsmokers per group will be balanced. This technique ultimately results in more balanced groups, particularly where imbalances are inherent in the randomization process.

**Cluster randomization** involves a method in which clusters or groups of subjects, rather than individual subjects, are randomized to treatment group. This randomization method is often used in trials when it is important to keep the specific group of individuals together through the trial. An example of this would be a particular group of subjects that might be living in a specific healthcare facility where an intervention may have been implemented, compared to a neighboring healthcare facility in which the intervention has not been implemented. Due to the design of these trials, this type of technique is not ideal for establishing efficacy, but is better suited for effectiveness.

**Blocked randomization** is a method of randomization that ensures approximately equal numbers of subjects in all groups throughout the enrollment period. It is most commonly used when enrollment of subjects must be extended over a long period of time, such as in studies of rare diseases. Blocked randomization may also be used when enrollment occurs over a shorter period of time, but in which time of enrollment is important. This is common for conditions with seasonal differences, such as allergic rhinitis or influenza.

# BLINDING

Any characteristic that differs between groups in a clinical study could potentially be detected by subjects or investigators and could affect the results of the study, based on expectations of the known or suspected group assignment. Subjective outcome measures and adverse effects are more likely to be affected by such knowledge, whereas objective outcomes are less susceptible to these types of effects. If a subject is aware of a particular medication and its expected response or adverse effect, she may be more likely to affect positive results or report adverse effects differently based on her expected outcomes than if she were not aware of treatment assignment. Conversely, if subjects or investigators are aware of placebo assignments, they might be more likely to report a lack of response or adverse effects. **Blinding** attempts to ensure that subjects and/or investigators are unaware of treatment assignment and is aimed at reducing potential sources of study error.

Various techniques can be used to blind subjects and investigators to treatment, ranging anywhere from matching but inactive tablets and capsules to providing sham injections. Subjects in a placebo-controlled trial will sometimes receive a placebo treatment that is designed to be identical to the intervention in all regards except containing an active ingredient, oftentimes described as **matched placebo**. Using **identical placebos** is important to maintain blinding if certain characteristics such as smell, taste, or even route of delivery are unique or distinguishing to the intervention being tested. Subjects may be aware of or recognize the difference, and make inferences regarding the treatment, ultimately affecting results of the trial.

In situations involving two active treatments, it may be difficult to make the active treatments appear identical. In this case, a **dummy** technique may be used. **Double-dummy** describes the technique that is used to match differing dosage forms, providing a placebo that matches the active treatments dosage form. In double-dummy trials, a matching placebo would be made for each active treatment and subjects would be administered one active and one placebo treatment simultaneously. For example, in a study comparing drug A that is a tablet and drug B that is a capsule, subjects in one group would receive drug A and a placebo designed to match drug B, whereas subjects in the other group would receive drug B and a placebo designed to match drug A. Blinding and dummying are not limited to dosage form; if a particular medication has a distinctive taste or odor or even an anticipated adverse effect, the treatment assignment can be easily determined.

It may be determined that it is necessary for either the investigators or the subjects to be aware of treatment assignment, but not both. This type of trial is defined as a **single-blind trial**. Typically, this is used when it would be important for either the subject or the investigator to be aware of the risks with the treatment, so that appropriate monitoring can occur and safety can be maintained.

A **double-blind trial** conceals the treatment assignments from both the investigator and the subjects and is the most common type of blinding in clinical trials. In a double-blind trial, it is still important to be sure that there is no indication of **unblinding** that may have occurred based on characteristics of the medications or anticipated adverse effects with one treatment over the other.

In all of the blinding techniques discussed so far, additional personnel, aside from subjects and investigators, who are involved in the data analysis of the trial are aware of treatment assignment. Because these additional personnel may develop an opinion or have a bias regarding treatment that could potentially affect the analysis of the treatment if not blinded as well, a **triple-blind trial** can be used, which ensures that all persons involved in the conduct of the trial and data collection and analysis are unaware of treatment. For example, if a particular medication is known to have an increased effect on dizziness and headache, monitoring for that particular response may be heightened in those subjects that are known to be receiving that particular treatment.

In certain trials, depending on the types of intervention and **study objectives**, it may be difficult to blind, and an open label trial is the only option. An **open label trial** describes a trial in which all subjects and personnel involved in the trial are aware of treatment assignment. Ideally, open label trial outcomes consist of objective measures rather than subjective outcomes, although adverse effect reporting could potentially be affected regardless. One example of a circumstance in which blinding would not be feasible is a trial investigating surgical procedures. It would be extremely difficult to blind the intervention or provide a "sham procedure" to maintain the blinding. As another example, if the objective of a trial was to investigate differences in titration schedules of a medication (e.g., one-step vs. two-step titration), blinding of the titration could be difficult to establish and maintain, and an open label might be a more appropriate trial design. It becomes important to determine what areas of a trial may have been affected by an open label design and evaluate the results for any indication that they may have been affected in order to determine if any errors resulted from the lack of blinding.

# STUDY VALIDITY

In this chapter thus far, we have defined clinical research and established its purposes. We have discussed clinical questions and the role these play in determining study hypotheses and independent and dependent variables. We have described study outcomes and factors contributing to their measurability and meaningfulness. We have compared and contrasted a variety of clinical study models and identified methods for sampling, controlling, randomizing, and blinding. In essence, we have examined numerous considerations and concepts that, when taken on the whole, can be used to assess the validity of a clinical study or, more properly, the validity of the conclusions drawn from a clinical study. The concepts that contribute to a study's validity, as they pertain to clinical research, can be divided into two groups: those that relate to what occurred in the study and those that relate to what can be extrapolated from the study.

## INTERNAL AND EXTERNAL VALIDITY

**Internal validity** describes how effectively and appropriately a study examined what it was intended to examine. It addresses the issues of how well the study was designed and conducted and how confident we can be in the results obtained. Although there are many things that can damage a study's internal validity, common contributors to low internal validity include poor study design, use of inappropriate statistical methods, absence of subject data and how that was managed, use of imprecise or inaccurate measurements, and unblinding of subjects or investigators.

When assessing the internal validity of a study, anything that could have caused what happened in the study, or how what happened in the study was interpreted, to differ from what would have occurred and how that would have been interpreted under the same conditions outside the study are taken into account. We would assign a high internal validity to a clinical study that was designed well, employed proper statistical methods, examined measurable outcomes, had few subjects drop out, and managed other potential sources of error adequately. However, if a study failed to accomplish all of these things, its internal validity would diminish correspondingly.

In contrast to internal validity, **external validity** describes the extent to which the results of a study can be extrapolated to a population beyond the study. It addresses the issue of how extensive and important the findings are to the "real world." We have noted that internal validity is concerned with how much confidence we can have in the results obtained within the study. It would stand to reason that extrapolation of conclusions drawn on the results of a study are subject to our confidence in those results as well. Thus, a study cannot have a great degree of external validity without having high internal validity. That is, external validity is contingent upon high internal validity. That does not mean, however, that high internal validity automatically translates to extensive external validity. A soundly conducted study could have limited external validity if, for instance, the population sampled was narrow or the outcomes examined were of limited clinical impact.

To illustrate this, let us put the concept of external validity in the context of the example study that we have used throughout this chapter. Let us assume that the study was conducted well (i.e., has high internal validity). If the researchers only included 40- to 50-year-old Caucasian males who lived in central Texas and who had baseline plasma LDL-c levels > 200 mg/dL, the study's external validity would be relatively limited despite its high internal validity because the results can only be extrapolated to individuals with similar characteristics as those sampled. If the researchers included 40- to 80-year-old males and females of any race from multiple countries who had baseline plasma LDL-c levels > 130 mg/dL, but the primary outcome was a decrease of at least 10 mg/dL in plasma LDL-c levels, the study's external validity would still be limited, even if its internal validity was just as high, because the threshold for plasma LDL-c level decrease is not likely to be clinically meaningful.

In addition to the dependency of external validity on internal validity, these two types of validity can often affect one another in an inversely relational manner. That is to say that some actions taken to increase internal validity can decrease external validity, and vice versa. For instance, expanding the population from which subjects are sampled from one country to multiple countries can increase the external validity of a study.

However, this expansion also inherently decreases the control that the researcher can exhibit over the actual conduct of the study, which increases the risk that study methods will be imprecisely translated, measurements will be taken differently, and more subject data will be lost after enrollment, all of which decrease internal validity. Likewise, having a single surgeon perform all of the procedures in a clinical study conducted to examine the effects of using a novel surgical technique with which he is proficient can increase the consistency with which the procedures are conducted, thus increasing internal validity. However, the results will have limited external validity, at least until other surgeons can become proficient with the technique as well.

Internal and external validity are not measured on numeric scales and are generally not explicitly stated in articles describing clinical studies. Rather, they are concepts that are applied, more or less subjectively, by those who might use the results of a clinical study to make decisions affecting individuals beyond the study. The fact that they are conceptual, however, does not diminish their importance; internal and external validity can and should be assessed for any clinical study conducted. It should be noted that there are other types of clinical study validity, such as conclusion validity, construct validity, and ecological validity. For our purposes, we consider that these other types of validity are subsumed under the larger concepts of internal and external validity.

# ETHICS IN CLINICAL RESEARCH

No discussion of clinical research would be complete without addressing some of the myriad ethical considerations that must be taken into account when conducting studies in human subjects. It should not be inferred that the position of this topic at the end of this chapter means that it is any less important than the other concepts discussed. To the contrary, ethical considerations should be given the utmost priority and consideration throughout the process of planning and conducting a clinical study. However, to fully appreciate the ethical concerns that exist when conducting studies in humans, one must first comprehend many of the concepts we have previously discussed.

As a general concept, ethics concerns itself with the moral principles of right and wrong. When extending this concept to clinical research, however, ethics loses some of its abstraction in favor of practical actions to be taken (or not to be taken) on the part of the researcher in order to protect study subjects from harm while maximizing the potential greater good that may be gained as a result of their participation. To be certain, interventional clinical studies require the most oversight and planning where ethics is concerned, because these studies often involve intentionally exposing subjects to an independent variable with some unproven effects and unknown risks. But, even observational clinical studies have some ethical considerations to take into account.

Numerous publications provide guidelines and recommendations on individual aspects or the entire topic of ethics in human clinical research, and the literature on this subject is too extensive to completely cover in the portion of this chapter allotted for this topic. Therefore, we will focus only on key publications and concepts.

## PRINCIPAL PUBLICATIONS

Two preeminent international guidelines, or "codes of conduct," for the ethical treatment of human subjects in clinical studies currently exist: the Declaration of Helsinki and the International Conference on Harmonisation of Technical Requirements for Registration of Pharmaceuticals for Human Use (ICH) Guideline for Good Clinical Practice (GCP Guideline E6).[1,3] Although other notable guidelines and codes have been developed over the years concerning ethical conduct of human clinical research, such as the Nuremberg Code and the Belmont Report, the Declaration of Helsinki and the ICH GCP Guideline E6 both incorporate the major principles set forth in these other documents. It is important to note that the Declaration of Helsinki and the ICH GCP Guideline E6 are not, themselves, instruments of law. However, many concepts presented in them have been established as laws in numerous countries. Furthermore, most reputable biomedical journals require studies to have complied with at least one international ethical guideline for articles about those studies to be accepted for publication. In the United States, the Code of Federal Regulations (CFR) includes a policy on protection of human subjects involved in research that is conducted, supported, or regulated by the federal government or one of its departments or agencies.[4,5] The subsection of this regulation that primarily addresses ethical treatment of human research subjects is entitled "The Common Rule for the Protection of Human Subjects" and is often referred to colloquially as the *Common Rule*. We will focus our ethical discussion on the aforementioned two codes of conduct and the CFR subsection.

The Declaration of Helsinki was established in 1964 by the World Medical Association, an international organization representing physicians and whose purposes include achieving the highest standards for international medical science.[1] It has been updated numerous times, most recently in 2013, and emphasizes that the care of individual human research subjects should take precedence over all other interests, including the greater good that comes from conducting clinical research. Despite its enormous impact on the manner in which clinical research in humans is conducted, the document is only a few pages in length. Yet, within those pages are statements addressing almost every major concept considered to comprise the backbone of ethical treatment of human subjects in clinical research.

In 1991, the U.S. federal government adopted 45 CFR 690 (and 45 CFR 46, which is essentially identical), Subpart A of which is informally known as the Common Rule, and which establishes regulations pertaining to the treatment of human research subjects.[4,5] The Common Rule was based in large part on some of the principles set forth in the Declaration of Helsinki, as well as by the Belmont Report. Developed in 1978, the Belmont Report was commissioned primarily in response to ethical issues raised during the Tuskegee syphilis studies conducted by the U.S. Public Health Service in which black men with syphilis living in rural Alabama were studied without being told that they had the disease or that they were being treated for it. Although the Belmont Report was published in the *Federal Register*, it had never been formally codified as a federal regulation.

Finalized in 1996, the ICH GCP Guideline E6 was developed to compile into a single document both the ethical considerations for conducting studies with human subjects that were set forth in prior codes of conduct and the regulations governing human data collection for medical product approval in the United States, Japan, and the European Union.[3] This document, which is significantly longer than both the Declaration of Helsinki and the Common Rule, is a practical guideline for conducting ethical clinical studies that meet the human data collection requirements of all the included countries. Its primary purpose is to assist in minimizing redundancy and risk to human subjects from studies intended to support the approval of new medical products (e.g., drugs) in multiple international jurisdictions in order to facilitate faster availability of these products globally. For ethical principles not specifically addressed by the ICH GCP Guideline E6, this document refers to and affirms the importance of compliance with the Declaration of Helsinki.

Each of the following ethical concepts is described and mandated by the Declaration of Helsinki and, where identified, the Common Rule and/or the ICH GCP Guideline E6.

# INSTITUTIONAL REVIEW BOARDS AND DATA SAFETY MONITORING COMMITTEES

The Declaration of Helsinki, the Common Rule, and the ICH GCP Guideline E6 all establish the requirement for and general composition of **institutional review boards** (IRBs).[1,3-5] (Each document may refer to such bodies by a different name, such as **independent research ethics committees** or **ethical review boards**, but they all serve essentially the same functions.) An IRB is a committee that is independent of a study's investigators and whose purpose is to review protocols for studies to be conducted in human subjects. Each institution that conducts, supports, or sanctions clinical research should have an IRB to approve such studies. Smaller institutions that do not routinely conduct clinical research may have their clinical research sanctioned by the IRB of a larger institution with which they have some affiliation.

Before the first potential subject is screened for inclusion in a clinical study, the study must first have obtained IRB approval. Any subsequent changes to a study's protocol for any reason must also be approved by the IRB. In order for a clinical study of humans to be approved, the Declaration of Helsinki and the ICH GCP Guideline E6 both mandate that the researcher supply sufficient evidence that the potential benefits of conducting the study are not outweighed by the expected risks.[1,3] This risk-benefit assessment may require data from nonhuman studies to adequately predict risk. Human studies should not be approved if the expected risks outweigh the potential benefits.

For a long clinical study, the IRB is also tasked with ensuring that periodic monitoring of the risks and benefits of the continuing the study is conducted. The IRB itself may conduct this monitoring, or it may delegate this task to a **data and safety monitoring board** (DSMB), sometimes referred to as a **data monitoring committee** (DMC). During the course of the study, if the IRB or DSMB determines that sufficient evidence exists that the risks of continuing the study outweigh the benefits, the study should be terminated early. Likewise, if sufficient evidence is collected before the planned conclusion of the study that clearly and overwhelmingly supports the benefit of an intervention, the study may also be terminated early in support of making that intervention available to all study participants and possibly to the general public. In either case, the evidence may be obtained from interim assessments of the data collected within the study, or it may be the result of evidence obtained from other sources, such as from concurrent studies on the same intervention. In the case of evidence supporting greater risks, the study should be terminated immediately. However, in the case of evidence supporting benefits of an intervention, care should be taken not to terminate a study too early if there is reason to suspect that the magnitude of initial benefit could decrease over time or insufficient time has passed to adequately discover less frequent, but major safety concerns. The ICH GCP Guideline E6 specifically addresses what should be reported when a study is terminated early and to whom this should be reported, including to the study subjects.[3]

# STANDARDS OF CARE

The Declaration of Helsinki mandates that new interventions must be tested against the established **standard of care** in order to ensure that all study subjects, including those in the control group, are receiving the same care to which they would otherwise be entitled if they were not participating in the clinical study.[1] The use of placebos or no treatment in control groups is only justified in specific circumstances, such as when no standard of care exists or when subjects receiving placebo or no treatment are not at risk for enduring serious or permanent harm. A placebo or no additional treatment may also be used when the new intervention is being tested as an augmentation to a standard of care if that standard of care is given to all subjects in all study groups. Furthermore, the ICH GCP Guideline E6 mandates that researchers plan and provide for the medical care of subjects who experience adverse effects that are a direct result of participation in a clinical study, regardless of whether such adverse effects were foreseeable.[3]

## INFORMED CONSENT

The Declaration of Helsinki, the Common Rule, and the ICH GCP Guideline E6 all also set forth requirements for obtaining informed consent from study subjects.[1,3-5] **Informed consent** is the process by which a potential study subject is presented with information about the study and willingly volunteers to participate as a subject in that study.

Although this may sound relatively straightforward, the preparation and process for obtaining informed consent is demanding and complex. The potential subject must be adequately informed, in a language and manner understandable to him or her, the purpose of the study, the methods that will be employed to conduct the study, the expected benefits of the study to the subject and to society, the anticipated inconveniences and discomforts the subject will be expected to endure, the potential temporary and permanent risks to the subject, any contingent compensations the subject can expect, all reasonable alternatives to which the subject is entitled, the subject's right to withdraw from the study at any time without reprisal, and other considerations. The Declaration of Helsinki further mandates that all potential conflicts of interest with regard to the sponsors that are funding and investigators who are conducting a clinical study be identified in the study protocol and to potential study subjects.[1] The ICH GCP Guideline E6 notably does not use the term "conflict of interest."[3]

The researcher must ensure that all the information given as part of informed consent is fully understood by the potential subject. Contingencies do exist for enrolling subjects that are temporarily or permanently incapable of understanding the information or granting voluntary consent, such as unconscious or mentally incapacitated individuals. In addition, the researcher is required to ensure that informed consent is obtained from subjects or their legal representatives in the absence of coercion, undue influence, or duress. The absence of duress, in particular, can be difficult to determine in certain circumstances, such as when immediate and serious threats to an individual's health or life exist.

The Declaration of Helsinki and the ICH GCP Guideline E6 also stress the importance of maintaining the respect and privacy of study subjects.[1,3] The study protocol and informed consent should contain information about the extent to which individual subject data will be exposed and to whom, as well as a summary of the methods that will be employed to ensure this. Individually identifiable subject data should never be exposed to the public or even to anyone involved in the study that does not have a necessity to identify specific subjects or link specific data to specific individuals.

For certain types of retrospective studies that do not involve further exposure of subjects to experimental methods and do not pose a significant threat to subject confidentiality, the requirement to obtain informed consent from subjects may be waived. However, it is often desirable to obtain informed consent from individuals who are to be the subject of published case studies, even though their individually identifiable data will be withheld from the publication.

## SPECIAL POPULATIONS

Primarily because of the atrocities imposed on unwilling human subjects during World War II, the Declaration of Helsinki includes specific language regarding disadvantaged and vulnerable populations, such as incarcerated individuals and those particularly susceptible to coercion or undue influence.[1] Inclusion of subjects from such a population is only justified when the research directly addresses a specific need in that population and when there is a reasonable likelihood that the population will directly benefit from the research. The ICH GCP Guideline E6 also suggests extra care to safeguard such populations.[3] It is important to recognize the difference between disadvantaged and vulnerable populations versus underrepresented populations, such as minorities, children, and the elderly. Indeed, newer guidance for conducting clinical research in humans addresses the need for increased efforts to include subjects from underrepresented populations, in order to expand the external validity of clinical research to these populations.

## REPORTING RESULTS

When the results of clinical research are made publicly available, such as in the form of a published biomedical journal article or as part of an application for general approval of a medical product, the Declaration of Helsinki calls for complete and accurate reporting.[1] Biomedical journals are encouraged to reject any article submissions describing studies not conducted in accordance with the Declaration. In addition, researchers and biomedical journal publishers are reminded of the importance of publishing results from studies that do not demonstrate differences between groups.

# SUMMARY

Clinical research refers to original investigations in living subjects that are intended to provide insight into an aspect of biology, health, or medical care in the same types of subjects as the investigation is conducted. The purpose of conducting clinical research is to answer a clinical question that will provide support and guidance for decisions in health and medicine.

Whether it is controlled by the researcher or not, the intervention or contributing factor under study is termed the independent variable. The effect of the independent variable that is being studied is termed the dependent variable. Ultimately, the researcher wishes to establish evidence that the dependent variable is associated with or caused by (or not associated with or not caused by) the independent variable. Regardless of what the researcher expects the answer to the clinical question to be, the circumstance in which the independent variable does not affect the dependent variable is called the null hypothesis ($H_0$), and the circumstance in which the independent variable does affect the dependent variable is then called the alternative hypothesis, ($H_1$).

The result of each hypothesis examined is referred to as a study outcome or endpoint. The primary outcome is determined a priori and is the main outcome being studied. Those outcomes that are deemed important to examine, but that are not the primary purpose of the study, may be classified as secondary outcomes. Additional outcomes that may be part of a study, but that are not deemed to be as important as the primary or secondary outcomes, may be classified as tertiary outcomes. Most clinical studies should include some evaluation of adverse effects, which are called safety analyses. Subgroup analyses may be conducted to determine if the outcomes observed in the entire pool of subjects also apply to subsets of those subjects. Finally, any a posteriori analyses that are conducted on the data derived from a clinical study are termed post-hoc analyses.

To be useful, study outcomes must be both measurable and meaningful. Measurement involves assigning a value to an observation. Precision and accuracy relate to the measurability of a study outcome. Precision refers to the relative proximity to one another of measurements of a characteristic that are taken from different subjects in whom that characteristic is actually identical (or that are taken from the same subject at the same time), and can be quantitatively expressed for dichotomous outcomes in terms of negative and positive predictive values. Accuracy refers to the relative proximity of a measurement to the real value, and can be quantitatively expressed for dichotomous outcomes in terms of sensitivity and specificity.

Meaningfulness relates to the importance of an outcome both within and beyond the clinical study, and is often referred to as "clinical significance." The most meaningful, and thus the most useful, outcomes are those that relate to significant and important events or aspects of an individual's life, which are referred to as direct outcomes. A surrogate outcome is a substitute for a direct outcome that is more convenient to measure. Direct outcomes can also be grouped together to form composite, or combined, outcomes.

Clinical studies can be divided into two orientations with regard to time—those that look back at things that have already happened, called retrospective studies, and those that look forward to what will happen, called prospective studies. Clinical studies can also be divided into two types based on the role the researcher plays in them—those in which the researcher actively alters the normal course of events, called interventional or experimental studies, and those in which the researcher merely bears witness to events and describes their circumstances, called observational studies. Common types of retrospective clinical studies include case studies and case series, case-control studies, and meta-analyses. The most common type of prospective observational clinical study design is the cohort study, although the cohort study design can also be applied retrospectively. Interventional clinical studies are also known as clinical trials. Cross-sectional studies exist somewhat outside the framework of time orientation because they generally examine circumstances as they exist at an instant in time, neither retrospectively nor prospectively.

Clinical studies can also be categorized by the distribution of subjects and how they are compared to one another. In a parallel study, each subject is assigned to a single group and his or her data are pooled with others in the same group. These pooled data are then analyzed against the pooled data from one or more other groups in the study. In a matched study with two groups, each subject in one group is paired with a similar subject in the other group; the data are not pooled, as in a parallel study. In a crossover study, each subject receives each study intervention or exposure in a sequential order, with a sufficient period between each to allow for lingering effects from the previous experience to dissipate, allowing each subject to serve as his or her own control.

Finally, clinical studies can be categorized by the primary question that is being asked and the manner in which the data will be analyzed to support the answer to this question. Studies that attempt to determine if one intervention is "better" than another intervention (or no intervention) with regard to the primary outcome are superiority studies. Superiority studies can be one-sided or two-sided with regard to the direction of superiority examined. Studies that attempt to determine if two interventions are essentially the same with regard to the primary outcome are equivalency studies. Studies that attempt to determine if one intervention is or is not meaningfully worse than another with regard to the primary outcome are noninferiority studies.

Clinical studies endeavor to use samples from a population to provide evidence that reflects circumstances as they are or will be in that population. Techniques for sampling populations can fall into two categories: probability methods and non-probability methods. Probability sampling allows each member of the accessible population an equal chance of being randomly selected for the actual study sample. Common techniques for probability sampling include simple random sampling, systematic sampling, stratified random sampling, and cluster sampling. In contrast to probability sampling, non-probability sampling is executed in a more systematic, non-random manner. Common techniques for non-probability sampling include convenience sampling, purposive sampling, and quota sampling.

Potential subjects for a clinical study need to be screened to ensure their eligibility to participate. Inclusion criteria define a set of characteristics that potential subjects must meet to be included in a study, while exclusion criteria define specific characteristics that will preclude a potential subject from study participation.

Once subjects have been selected and screened with the inclusion and exclusion criteria, they will be assigned to a study group, a process called subject allocation. Most interventional studies allocate subjects via randomization, a process through which all subjects have the same chance as one another of being assigned to a given group in an unpredictable manner. Common randomization techniques include simple randomization, stratified randomization, cluster randomization, and blocked randomization.

Blinding methods can be used to increase the potential that study participants and personnel are unaware of treatment assignment. The most common type of blinding design is double-blind, which conceals subjects' group assignments from both the investigators and the subjects. Single-blind studies conceal subjects' group assignment either from subjects or from investigators, but not from both. Triple-blind studies conceal subjects' group assignment from all persons involved in the study, including subjects, investigators, and data analysts. Open label studies do not conceal subjects' group assignments from anyone.

The validity of a clinical study can be described in terms of how effectively and appropriately the study examined what it was intended to examine, referred to as internal validity, and in terms of the extent to which the results of the study can be extrapolated to a population beyond the study, referred to as external validity.

In addition to maintaining good design principles, individuals who plan and conduct clinical studies must also adhere to strict ethical principles. The two most widely accepted international guidelines for the ethical treatment of human subjects in clinical studies are the Declaration of Helsinki and the International Conference on Harmonisation of Technical Requirements for Registration of Pharmaceuticals for Human Use Guideline for Good Clinical Practice. In the United States, the Common Rule codifies some ethical principles in the Code of Federal Regulations. These documents discuss, among other topics, considerations for utilizing institutional review boards, using standards of care, obtaining informed consent, including and protecting special populations, and reporting results.

# REFERENCES

1.  World Medical Association. World Medical Association Declaration of Helsinki: ethical principles for medical research involving human subjects. *JAMA*. 2013;310(20):2191-2194.
2.  Merriam-Webster, Inc. Population. http://www.merriam-webster.com. Accessed July 18, 2014.
3.  International Conference on Harmonisation of Technical Requirements for Registration of Pharmaceuticals for Human Use. Guideline for good clinical practice E6 (R1). http://www.ich.org/products/guidelines/efficacy/article/efficacy-guidelines.html. Published June 10, 1996. Accessed July 18, 2014.
4.  National Science Foundation. Federal policy for the protection of human subjects 45 CFR §690. http://www.nsf.gov/bfa/dias/policy/docs/45cfr690.pdf. Revised January 15, 2009. Effective July 14, 2009. Accessed July 18, 2014.
5.  Department of Health and Human Services. Protection of human subjects 45 CFR §46. http://www.hhs.gov/ohrp/policy/ohrpregulations.pdf. Revised January 15, 2009. Effective July 14, 2009. Accessed July 18, 2014.

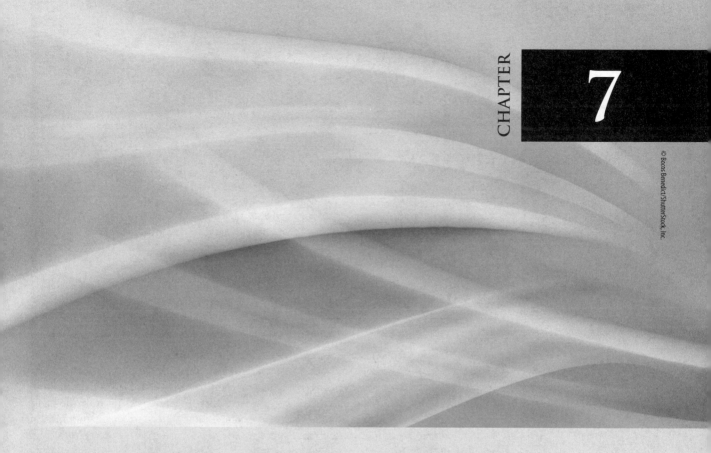

© Bocos Benedict/ShutterStock, Inc.

# RESEARCH STUDY DESIGN

Lara K. Ellinger, PharmD, BCPS

## CHAPTER OBJECTIVES

- ▶ Differentiate between analytical and descriptive studies.
- ▶ List the major differences between observational and interventional studies.
- ▶ Describe what various observational study designs can and cannot establish.
- ▶ Identify what niche various observational and interventional study designs have in evidence-based medicine (EBM).
- ▶ Describe situations in which meta-analyses are helpful tools for answering a research question.

# CHAPTER OUTLINE

# KEY TERMS

Analytical study

Descriptive study

Evidence-based medicine

Interventional study

Meta-analysis

Observational study

Prospective cohort study

Randomized controlled trial

Retrospective cohort study

Systematic review

# INTRODUCTION

Clinical research study designs are often categorized based on action and time.[1-3] When an intervention (action) is applied, studies are **interventional**. When no intervention is applied (no action), studies may be **observational** or **descriptive**. Additionally, studies can be categorized as prospective (looking forward in time) or retrospective (looking backward in time). Some consider the broadest categories of study design to be descriptive or analytical. Descriptive studies aim to characterize a patient or patient population and include cross-sectional studies and surveys, case series, and case reports. **Analytical studies** attempt to identify associations between a characteristic and an event or outcome. When using this classification, observational and interventional studies fall under the analytical umbrella.[4] This chapter will describe both descriptive and analytical studies. Regardless of the classification system used, it is important to understand what each type of study design can and cannot establish. It is also important to keep in mind that trial design is not always straightforward and that design types may overlap. Understanding clinical trial design begins with the research question, as it will dictate study design. Other factors that will dictate study design include feasibility, cost, available data, and ethics.

Knowledge on trial design is important for the application of results of published studies in one's practice in order to practice **evidence-based medicine** (EBM). Because pharmacists' responsibilities include providing optimal patient care, assessing and improving practices at the institutions in which they work is a crucial aspect of their careers. Understanding observational and interventional trial design is imperative to this. Although pharmacists may be involved in interventional trials, it is more common that they are involved in designing and implementing observational or descriptive studies. This is especially true for pharmacy residents, as they will commonly collect patient data from medical records at their institutions in order to characterize a patient population or identify a characteristic associated with an outcome for their mandatory research project.

# DESCRIPTIVE STUDIES

## CASE REPORTS AND CASE SERIES

Two of the weakest forms of evidence are case reports and case series.[1,2] These are descriptions of unique events that occur in a patient (case report) or two or more similar patients (case series). No comparison group is included. The described events may be new findings that lead to the discovery of a new disease state (e.g., opportunistic infections in men with cellular immunodeficiency—the first report of what is now known as AIDS), unexpected adverse events that have not been reported before (e.g., amantadine associated with dropped head syndrome in a patient with Parkinson's disease), or a new way to manage a disease state (e.g., the use of gabapentin for the treatment of intractable chronic cough).[5-7] The report or series should contain a detailed description of the patient's clinical course, including the timeline of events, lab values, medications and interventions, follow-up, and so on. The description should be detailed enough so that a clinician would be able to identify the event in a similar patient population. For a case series, the authors should explicitly define what constitutes a "case." It should also include a discussion on how the event or phenomenon can be further investigated through other study designs.

## Case Reports and Case Series in Evidence-Based Medicine

Case series and case reports provide anecdotal evidence that may lead to hypotheses on disease etiologies and discovery of new diseases, novel treatment of diseases, and unexpected or adverse events.[1,2] Some authors may include a literature review on similar reported cases, describing how their case differs. They may suggest how the case or hypothesis can be studied further through a specific study design.

When the report is for an event, case reports cannot provide incidence or prevalence estimates, because the single patient or series of patients may not be representative of all patients at risk for the event. The included cases may be patients who are more likely to seek treatment or medical advice or those who have access to it and/or have greater disease severity.[2] Cases may not represent patients who do not seek treatment or have access to it, or they may not represent those with mild disease. Therefore, the generalizability of findings from these reports is low. Publication of case reports is easy and rapid in comparison to trials or studies, and clinical pharmacists are uniquely positioned to be involved in the identification and publication of case reports or case series.

# CROSS-SECTIONAL STUDIES

Cross-sectional studies are used to identify prevalence of a disease or event in a patient population at one point in time.[1,2] All variables are measured at once, creating a "snapshot" in time of a disease in a defined patient population. There is no follow-up period. This study design can answer questions such as "What was the prevalence of whooping cough in the United States in 2013?" and "What is the average LDL cholesterol level of all patients taking atorvastatin at an ambulatory care clinic in Rockford, Illinois?" If it is not possible for the investigator to study the entire population, a representative convenience sample may be used. When the question is regarding prevalence of a disease, all patients will be included in the disease count regardless of whether it is a chronic condition for them or recently developed. Because cross-sectional studies do not measure new cases of a disease over a given time period, they cannot measure incidence. Depending on what data are collected, associations between variables may be determined. In this case, cross-sectional studies may be categorized as analytical rather than descriptive. For example, a cross-sectional study assessed the associations between oral contraceptive (OC) use, bone mineral density (BMD), and fractures in women aged 50 to 80 years.[8] The investigators used computer-generated random numbers to randomly identify a sample of women from a database of older adults in Tasmania. The participants' bone mass was measured and they were given questionnaires on OC use ("Have you ever used the oral contraceptive pill?" and "How many years in total have you ever taken the oral contraceptive pill?"), hormone replacement therapy (HRT) use, menstrual cycle patterns, history of gynecologic surgery, and general lifestyle. There was a statistically significant positive association between OC use and total body and spine BMD. However, significance was lost after adjusting for confounders (age, body mass index, pedometer steps, alcohol consumption, menopause, and use of HRT). The results led the authors to hypothesize that OC use may have a protective effect on spinal bone health. Further exploration of this hypothesis could be performed through cohort or case–control studies, which are discussed later in this chapter.

### Cross-Sectional Studies in Evidence-Based Medicine

In contrast to case reports or series, cross-sectional studies are more representative of the general population because they include a larger sample size, and those affected by the disease or event are included regardless of access to medical care, desire to seek medical care, or disease severity.[2] However, one must consider the database from which the data are obtained (medical records, public records, etc.) and what limitations it may have. It should also be considered that those who refuse participation may be more likely to have (or not have) the disease or event, which could lead to over- or underestimates of prevalence. Cross-sectional studies are not ideal for studying rare diseases, because it may not be feasible to reach a large enough sample size to obtain adequate data. Diseases with a short duration or those associated with certain times during the calendar year (e.g., influenza and "flu season") may not be accurately identified in a cross-sectional study. Temporal relationships between variables are not reliably established, so cause and effect cannot be determined. However, cross-sectional studies are very useful for epidemiologic purposes and can advise decision making at the public health level.

# ANALYTICAL STUDIES

## OBSERVATIONAL STUDIES

Observational studies, which may be prospective or retrospective, attempt to establish an association between a characteristic (or exposure) and an outcome.[1-3] In this design, a group of individuals are observed and evaluated over time in a natural setting. Investigators are not attempting to influence the individuals or their environment by applying an intervention.[2] Because no intervention is applied, cause and effect cannot be determined. If an association is found, the inference that the characteristic caused the individual to experience the outcome or protected them from experiencing the outcome is strengthened. In this way, observational studies can be used to generate hypotheses. If, for example, investigators identify a certain risk factor for mortality through an observational study, they may hypothesize that reduction of this risk factor by administration of a certain intervention or treatment could also reduce mortality. They could then perform an interventional trial to establish cause and effect (i.e., the intervention reduces mortality). Differences among and characteristics of observational study designs are highlighted in **Table 7-1**.

### Prospective Cohort Studies

In a **prospective cohort study**, the investigators first identify a population of interest (the cohort) and measure characteristics that could be predictive of an outcome *before* the outcome occurs.[1-3] These study designs can determine the incidence of an outcome or

**TABLE 7-1**  General Characteristics of Observational Study Designs

| Type of Study | What the Study Can Establish | General Limitations | Generalizability | Cost and Time | Bias | Variable Measurement |
|---|---|---|---|---|---|---|
| *Prospective cohort* | Risk/protective factors for a disease or outcome<br>Incidence of a disease or outcome<br>Possible etiologies of a disease or outcome<br>Factors that precede a disease or outcome | Identifies associations, not cause and effect<br>Not ideal for studying rare outcomes<br>Cannot control for confounders | High (real-world population) | Expensive Time-consuming | Selection bias Recall bias | Can be complete and accurate |
| *Retrospective cohort* | Risk/protective factors for a disease or outcome<br>Incidence of a disease or outcome<br>Possible etiologies of a disease or outcome (good for rare outcomes)<br>Factors precede an event or outcome (although not always as reliably as a prospective cohort) | Identifies associations, not cause and effect<br>Investigator has limited control over design<br>Cannot control for confounders | High (real-world population) | Low cost Time efficient | Selection bias Recall bias | May be incomplete, inaccurate, or mismeasured |
| *Case control* | Etiologies of rare diseases or events | Cannot estimate incidence or prevalence<br>Investigator has limited control over design/study groups<br>Cannot study multiple outcomes | High, if cases are representative of all patients who develop the disease and controls are representative of a healthy, disease-free population | Low cost Shorter observation period than prospective cohort | Selection bias Recall bias | May be incomplete, inaccurate, or mismeasured |

event within a population and investigate potential causes or protective factors. The time frame of a prospective cohort study begins in the present, with measurements of predictive characteristics and confounders taken at baseline and periodically in the future. Individuals are followed over a specified period of time while outcomes are measured. In this way, the investigators can establish that a characteristic or variable preceded an outcome. Because the outcome has yet to occur, a prospective study design allows the investigators to determine not only *what* they will measure, but *how* and at *what frequency* they will measure it. They are not limited to data that have already been recorded, which could be incomplete, inaccurate, and/or measured inappropriately. At study completion, rates of individuals who experienced the outcome and who had the characteristic of interest are compared to those who experienced the outcome but did not have the characteristic of interest. These associations are measured through relative risk.

An example of a prospective cohort study is the Cancer Prevention Study II that was initiated in 1982 by the American Cancer Society. This study investigates lifestyle and environmental effects on the etiology of cancer in Americans.[9] A population within this cohort was selected in order to investigate the ingestion of coffee and tea (the characteristic or exposure) and incidence of oral/pharyngeal cancer (the outcome).[10] The investigators had the participants complete a questionnaire at baseline on daily intake and amounts of caffeinated and decaffeinated coffee, as well as tea. Data on changes in coffee/tea drinking habits were also collected. Participants who already had the outcome of interest at baseline (prevalent cancer) were excluded, as were those who were missing information on beverage intake and confounders (e.g., smoking status, alcohol use). Deaths from oral/pharyngeal cancer during follow-up were recorded, and data from 968,432 participants were available at study completion in 2008. It was found that participants who drank more than 4 cups of caffeinated coffee daily had a 42% reduction in the risk of death from oral/pharyngeal cancer compared to those who drank no coffee or tea, and those who drank more than 4 cups of caffeinated coffee in addition to decaffeinated coffee or tea daily had a 55% reduction compared to those who drank no coffee or tea. These calculations were also adjusted for age, sex, smoking status, alcohol use, and other confounders.

This prospective cohort study showed a protective effect of caffeinated coffee consumption on the risk of fatal oral/pharyngeal cancer.[10] Because of the prospective nature, the investigators had the ability to collect detailed information on hot beverage consumption, as well as alcohol consumption and tobacco use. Imagine the recall bias that would have been involved if this were a retrospective study and participants were asked to remember decades of information on the amount of caffeinated/decaffeinated coffee and tea they drank! This is why this research question is not conducive to a retrospective cohort design, which is discussed in further detail in the next section of this chapter.

Although alcohol consumption and tobacco use were recorded, their confounding potential could not be controlled for because of the observational study design.[10] Statistical analyses were applied to adjust for these confounders, but this does not make the study as robust as an interventional trial design, which can better control for confounders. As with all prospective cohort studies, the investigators were able to determine that the characteristic (coffee/tea consumption) preceded the outcome (oral/pharyngeal cancer) and ensured this through exclusion of those who already had the outcome at baseline. However, the possibility exists that outcomes could have been present at baseline but were undetectable because they had not progressed to a detectable stage.

### Prospective Cohort Studies in Evidence-Based Medicine

Prospective cohort studies are excellent designs for establishing risk factors and protective factors for a disease or outcome, as well as calculating incidence of a disease or outcome.[11] One of the most notable prospective cohort studies is the Framingham Heart Study, established in 1948.[12] The objective of this study was to identify common risk factors for the development of cardiovascular disease. The original cohort comprised 5,209 men and women and has expanded to include multiple cohorts, including a third generation of the first cohort. This study has resulted in over 1,200 publications and has led to the creation of multiple risk score algorithms for various cardiovascular events. Much of what we know today about risk factors for cardiovascular diseases was established through this study.

Prospective cohort studies can be very time-consuming, as illustrated in the examples provided.[10,12] They are also very costly and are not ideal for studying outcomes that occur infrequently.[1-3] However, they are considered to be the strongest type of observational study design because of their ability to establish a temporal relationship between characteristics and an outcome.

## Retrospective Cohort Studies

Similar to a prospective cohort study, a **retrospective cohort study** (sometimes referred to as TROHOC or a noncurrent or historical cohort study) is able to make associations between characteristics and an outcome and can establish incidence of an outcome.[2] Investigators of a retrospective cohort study will first identify a population of interest and measure characteristics that could be predictive of an outcome.[1,11] However, all aspects of the study have *already* occurred; the cohort has already been assembled (in some fashion), and outcomes and measurements have already occurred (or occur in the present). In contrast to a prospective cohort study, the time frame of a retrospective cohort study begins in the past, observing a cohort over time with completion in the present. Investigators may still be able to establish that a characteristic or variable preceded an outcome, but the data may not always be conducive to this. Because data have already been recorded, information may be incomplete, inaccurate, and/or measured inappropriately. As with prospective cohort studies, rates of outcomes in individuals with or exposed to the characteristic of interest are compared to those not exposed in order to determine if any association can be made between the characteristic and an outcome. The results are measured through relative risk.

A retrospective cohort study found that use of zolpidem in the inpatient setting was associated with an increased risk for falls, even when confounding variables, such as delirium, age, and higher fall risk scores, were adjusted for.[13] The investigators of this study utilized the pharmacy database at the Mayo Clinic in Rochester, Minnesota, to identify and collect data on 16,320 patients who were admitted to the Mayo Clinic in 2010 and who had orders for zolpidem. This cohort included patients who were prescribed zolpidem and received it, as well as those who were prescribed zolpidem and did not receive it. The database had detailed information on the dosing and administration of the zolpidem orders. Because the hospital utilized electronic medical records, automated dispensing cabinets, and barcode technology, the investigators were confident in the accuracy of the information they were collecting. Had some of this technology not been in place, the data may have been lesser quality, and the results may have not been as robust or meaningful. However, the data were not necessarily void of error, as many of the confounding variables were identified through International Classification of Diseases-9 codes (ICD-9 codes), which are subject to misclassification. In comparison to a prospective cohort study, the time to complete this study was only the time involved to review the patient data and perform the analyses. The investigators did not have to follow the patients for a number of years for the results, because the outcome (falls) had already occurred. Also, costs involved in this study were likely minimal because only data collection and statistical analyses were involved.

### *Retrospective Cohort Studies in Evidence-Based Medicine*

Retrospective cohort studies are efficient and inexpensive designs to answer a research question.[2] They rely on outcomes that have already occurred and data that have already been recorded. Large databases serve as reservoirs of information conducive to performing retrospective cohort studies. Pharmacists and pharmacy residents often utilize this study design when performing research. Although investigators are less able to control for confounding variables due to the retrospective nature of these studies, retrospective cohort studies are still able to identify associations that have implications for clinical practice. For example, the Food and Drug Administration (FDA) issued a safety alert in May 2012 regarding the potential for QT prolongation with azithromycin.[14] Initially, it was thought that azithromycin was not associated with the same cardiovascular risks as other macrolide antibiotics. Results of a retrospective cohort study performed on a Tennessee Medicaid cohort challenged this belief by finding that 5 days of azithromycin use resulted in a small but significant increase in the risk of cardiovascular death.[15] The investigators used two types of controls: patients who received no antibiotic but were matched based on a cardiovascular risk score and patients taking other antibiotics who had an established cardiovascular risk. This study was large enough to detect a small difference in the outcome (cardiovascular death) between those who had the exposure (azithromycin) and those who did not (matched controls). Because of this study, greater vigilance should be taken for prescribing of azithromycin, especially for those with baseline QT prolongation and other risk factors for cardiovascular death.

## Case-Control Studies

Case-control studies attempt to identify the etiology of a disease or risk factors for it.[16] The case-control methodology differs from cohort studies in that the population sample is chosen based on individuals who have experienced the outcome of interest, rather than on those who have had the exposure. The controls have not experienced the outcome of interest. The investigator then compares characteristics or exposures between groups. An identified association between an exposure and outcome (through the measure of an odds ratio) could strengthen the inference that the exposure is a risk factor or cause of the outcome. Although only one outcome can be studied in this design, it allows for possible multiple etiologies to be investigated.[2] However, what the case-control design cannot provide is the incidence or prevalence of a disease or of the risk factors.

One of the greatest concerns with case-control studies is sampling bias (a type of selection bias).[2,16] In cohort studies, those who develop the outcome and those who do not are derived from the same sample population.[17] This is not always true for case-control studies because the controls can be derived from a different sample population. Using the same population to select cases and controls helps to reduce sampling bias.[2,16] A nested case-control study always selects controls from the same cohort from which the cases are obtained.[17] The case control is "nested" because both cases and controls are derived from an established population, usually within a prospective cohort study. This may also be referred to as "sampling within the cohort." However, attempts should also be made to ensure that the cases are representative of those who have the outcome and controls are representative of those who do not have the outcome. This may not always be feasible in a nested case-control design. Historical controls may also be used, with consideration for effects that time may have had on the evolution of the outcome or how treatment/prevention associated with the outcome may have changed over time.

In general, controls are matched for potential confounders, which often include age, gender, and/or race.[16] Singh et al. investigated the risk for acute pancreatitis with use of exenatide or sitagliptin through a case-control study.[18] The cases (patients who had pancreatitis) and controls (those who did not) were both identified from a population of patients who had Blue Cross Blue Shield Association insurance plans. They were matched for age (± 10 years), sex, insurance plan site, and diabetes severity. Any of these characteristics could have affected the outcome had they not been evenly distributed, or "matched," between the cases and controls. The use of exenatide and sitagliptin was found to be associated with significantly greater odds for development of acute pancreatitis as compared to the control group.

### Case-Control Studies in Evidence-Based Medicine

The case-control study design is appropriate to use when determining risk factors or etiologies of outcomes that occur infrequently.[16] Alternatively, if a cohort design were used, a much larger number of individuals and/or a much longer time period would be needed to compare the two groups. This would also be more costly than a case-control design.

Like cohort studies, case-control studies can be used to generate hypotheses.[16] A case-control study was responsible for identifying the association between short-acting calcium channel blockers and the risk for myocardial infarction.[19] In patients with hypertension, the adjusted risk ratio of experiencing a myocardial infarction was significantly higher with short-acting calcium channel blockers than with beta-blockers or diuretics. This case-control study led to the development of robust, prospective studies that have confirmed this finding.[20,21]

## INTERVENTIONAL STUDIES AND RANDOMIZED CONTROLLED TRIALS

Interventional studies allow investigators to apply an intervention and follow patients prospectively to investigate its effects on outcomes.[4,22,23] Investigators define the patient population through narrow inclusion/exclusion criteria, and patients follow a treatment protocol in order to ensure similar treatment and processes in each group. Efficacy of a therapeutic intervention is commonly studied through this design. In contrast to observational studies, cause and effect can be determined by an appropriately designed interventional trial. Randomization and the use of controls are two important characteristics of interventional trials and are necessary to establishing causality. Controls allow for the comparison of efficacy and safety of an intervention to a standard of care or placebo. Randomization ensures that all individuals have an equal chance of receiving either the intervention or the control and helps to eliminate confounders. Ideally, the intervention and control groups should be demographically similar except for the intervention they are receiving. When an interventional trial utilizes both randomization and controls, it is called a **randomized controlled trial** (RCT). Such studies allow for greater confidence in attributing differences seen between groups solely to the intervention. When both patients and investigators are blinded to which group the patient is in, this further reduces bias and substantiates that a difference in response is due to the biological action of the drug, as opposed to a psychological response the patients may have from knowing they are assigned to a certain intervention. Other forms of bias may arise from nonblinded or open-label studies. Generally, RCTs are considered the gold standard for determining efficacy of an intervention, and are further classified as described in the following discussion and depicted in **Table 7-2**.[4,23] The CONSORT group (CONsolidated Standards Of Reporting Trials) developed guidelines for how RCTs should be reported in order to establish transparency and standardization.[24] A recommended flow diagram is available for investigators to use in order to show the progress of patients within the trial from eligibility

**TABLE 7-2**   Characteristics of Randomized Controlled Trials

| Type of Randomized Controlled Trial | Basic Design | Design Depiction |
|---|---|---|
| Parallel arm | • Individuals are randomized to a group in which they remain in until study completion.<br>• Individuals receive one intervention or one control. | A vs. B |
| Factorial | • Individuals are randomized to a group in which they remain until study completion.<br>• Individuals receive one intervention, one control, or a combination of interventions or controls. | A vs. B vs. AB vs. C |
| Crossover | • Individuals are randomized to a group and then cross over to the other group(s) prior to study completion.<br>• Individuals receive both the intervention and the control. | AB/BA |

assessment to analysis. This checklist of information is useful when assessing an RCT and can be accessed online (http://www.consort-statement.org/).

## Parallel Arm Design

The most common and simplest type of RCT is the parallel arm trial.[25,26] In this design, individuals are randomized to an exclusive group and remain in that group for the duration of the study, receiving only one treatment. The trial may have multiple intervention and control arms, but all individuals receive their treatments concurrently and are followed forward in time until study completion.

### Parallel Arm Design in Evidence-Based Medicine

The parallel design is good for studying treatments for acute conditions.[25,26] Relative to other RCT types, this design may require less time to complete and be less burdensome on the investigators. Because of possible variability between groups, this design may require more patients to ensure a balance of characteristics. A parallel arm design is appropriate to use when comparing interventions and between-group differences are minimal. If between-group differences are present in this design, they could confound the results and make it difficult to attribute any differences in efficacy to the intervention.

## Factorial Design

The factorial design is used to address more than one research question through examining the effects of two or more interventions used concomitantly.[25-27] In this design, there are at least two interventions and two levels of the intervention, with $2 \times 2$ being the most common factorial design. The groups are all possible combinations of the interventions, so the number of groups can be determined by multiplying the number of interventions by the number of levels. Lonn and colleagues utilized a $3 \times 2$ factorial design for a study on the effects of both ramipril and vitamin E on cardiovascular events in patients at high cardiovascular risk.[28] They investigated the effects of ramipril at two doses (2.5 mg and 10 mg) and the effects of vitamin E at one dose (400 International

| **TABLE 7-3** SECURE Trial Study Groups | | | |
|---|---|---|---|
| | **Ramipril 2.5 mg** | **Ramipril 10 mg** | **Placebo** |
| **Vitamin E 400 IU** | Ramipril 2.5 mg + vitamin E 400 IU | Ramipril 10 mg + vitamin E 400 IU | Placebo + vitamin E 400 IU |
| **Placebo** | Ramipril 2.5 mg + placebo | Ramipril 10 mg + placebo | Placebo + placebo |

Data from Lonn E, Yusuf S, Dzavik V; SECURE Investigators. Effects of ramipril and vitamin E on atherosclerosis: the study to evaluate carotid ultrasound changes in patients treated with ramipril and vitamin E (SECURE). *Circulation*. 2001;103(7):919-925.

Units [IU]). Because there were two interventions, one at three levels (ramipril 2.5 mg, 10 mg, and placebo /0 mg) and the other at two levels (vitamin E 400 IUs and placebo/0 IUs), patients were randomized to one of six groups, as shown in **Table 7-3**.

The investigators were able to assess the effects of ramipril and vitamin E in combination and alone on the progression of atherosclerosis.[28] They determined that both doses of ramipril had a beneficial effect, whereas the addition of vitamin E had no effect, regardless of being administered alone or in combination with ramipril.

## *Factorial Design in Evidence-Based Medicine*

Although the factorial design is efficient in investigating more than one intervention simultaneously, consideration needs to be made for interactions between interventions in this design.[25,26] Some interventions may have an additive or multiplicative effect when used together, and, alternatively, some could inhibit the effects of other interventions. This same concept applies to their safety profiles. One advantage of a factorial design is that it requires a smaller sample size than if each question were to be investigated through separate parallel studies. Also, when interactions between interventions are minimal, the trial has increased power. Factorial designs are often used for determining appropriate doses for combination therapies when safe and effective doses for each individual therapy have already been established.

## Crossover Design

A crossover trial design differs from parallel and factorial designs in that individuals receive more than one intervention consecutively.[25,26,29] They first receive one intervention and later "cross over" to receive another intervention. In effect, they serve as their own controls so there is no between-group variability. It is assumed that the order of administration does not have an effect on the outcomes being studied. Each of the interventions should be administered over an adequate period of time to capture their effects. As such, crossover designs can require longer periods of time to assess the research question as compared to other RCTs. The crossover design commonly studies two interventions requiring two periods, but this design can also study multiple interventions and has the potential to become very complex.

One consideration for the crossover design is the possibility of treatment effects carrying over from one period to the next.[25,26,29] This can be eliminated by the use of a "washout" period. This period should be long enough to allow for the drug to be effectively cleared by the individual, which is related to the drug's half-life. Another technique for eliminating carryover effects is to take measurements only during the latter part of the periods, when any carryover effects are likely to have diminished. This strategy was utilized in a crossover trial that compared the efficacy of controlled-release (CR) tramadol and immediate-release (IR) tramadol in patients with chronic noncancer pain.[30] Patients were randomized to receive either active CR tramadol with placebo IR tramadol as needed or placebo CR tramadol with active IR tramadol as needed. They continued this treatment for 4 weeks for period 1, then immediately were switched to the opposite group for another 4 weeks for period 2. Although there was no washout period between the two study periods, the primary endpoint of pain intensity was only measured for the last 2 weeks of each period, therefore bypassing any carryover effects that may have been present.

An advantage of the crossover design is that fewer patients are required to reach the same power as would be needed by a parallel design.[25,26,29] The patients are paired with themselves, so outcomes are not affected by between-group variability. However, this also makes a crossover design more sensitive to dropout rates, because each patient is responsible for a larger portion of the data than if he or she were in a parallel design trial.

### Crossover Design in Evidence–Based Medicine

Crossover designs are useful for studying interventions for chronic diseases over relatively short periods of time.[25,26,29] Fluctuations in disease symptoms or progression/improvement in the condition could confound results, so it is also important that the disease or condition be stable. The effects of the intervention should not permanently alter the disease state (i.e., they should not be curative interventions). Symptomatic treatments are often investigated through this design, as in the case of tramadol for chronic, stable pain.[30]

## SYSTEMATIC REVIEWS AND META-ANALYSES

Sometimes a research question is investigated through many trials that have conflicting or unclear results.[31,32] A method of systematically combining trial results to ascertain a more definitive answer to a research question is a **systematic review**. The application of statistical analyses to this method is called a **meta-analysis**. Systematic reviews and meta-analyses include trials of the same design that investigate the same research question, such as "Is St. John's wort effective for treating depression?" or "Are colloids more effective than crystalloids in reducing mortality in the critically ill?" RCTs are the most common trial design used in systematic reviews, although other designs may be used as well.

Much like a clinical trial, the methods of a systematic review should be explicitly stated and reproducible.[31,32] At least two investigators should independently perform the search for articles and use stringent criteria for inclusion. A thorough search is done in multiple secondary references, and manufacturers and investigators should be contacted for unpublished results. Investigators have to be transparent in the number of articles identified and the number of articles excluded and for what reasons. Similar to the CONSORT diagram that is used for reporting of RCTs, the PRISMA statement (Preferred Reporting for Systematic Reviews and Meta-Analyses) is a checklist and flow diagram for reporting of systematic reviews and meta-analyses.[33] Ideally, trials included in a systematic review or meta-analysis will be of the same design, ask the same question, measure the same outcome variable, have similar patient populations, and be conducive to calculating the same effect size measures.[31,32] This is not always the case, however, and there are tools that can be used to assess possible variability and biases present.

Commonly applied statistical methods in a meta-analysis are the fixed effects and random effects models.[31,32] The model used is chosen based on how heterogeneous or homogeneous the included studies are. When the studies are homogeneous (i.e., have comparable effect sizes), the results will be similar regardless of which analysis is applied. The random effects model is commonly used when the included studies are heterogeneous. The $I^2$ statistic may be used to assess heterogeneity, with values < 25% representing a homogeneous group of studies and > 75% representing a heterogeneous group of studies.

Publication bias is also a concern in meta-analyses.[30,31] This occurs when studies with positive results are published more frequently than studies with negative or no statistically significant results. This bias can be assessed through development of a funnel plot, which is a graph that displays each trial according to its effect size (*x*-axis) and weight (*y*-axis). The weight may be based on the precision of the data. The assumption is that if there is no publication bias, the trials will be plotted near the average effect size, with more precise trials clustered at the top and smaller trials spread out near the bottom in a symmetrical fashion about the mean effect size. The resulting graph resembles an upside-down funnel. If publication bias is present, negative studies may not have been published and the graph will be asymmetrical.

## SYSTEMATIC REVIEWS AND META-ANALYSES IN EVIDENCE-BASED MEDICINE

When study results for a research question conflict, it may be helpful for investigators to perform a meta-analysis in order to identify a more precise effect of an intervention.[31,32] Meta-analyses are also able to better characterize treatment effects in subpopulations of patients. One example is a 1995 meta-analysis that pooled results from nine RCTs that had conflicting information on the use of corticosteroids for sepsis.[34] The investigators found that corticosteroids were not beneficial overall in patients with sepsis, and in fact may result in increased mortality in patients with overwhelming infection. These conclusions were unable to be reached through individual RCTs. Another point to consider is that systematic reviews and meta-analyses provide a comprehensive evaluation of therapy among potentially thousands of published trials on a topic.[31,32] Many clinicians do not have enough time to read through all of the published primary literature on a particular topic, nor do they always have enough time to differentiate between well-designed and poorly designed clinical trials. Systematic reviews and meta-analyses provide an alternative option to reviewing all the literature, provided they are done well and the reader understands their limitations.

## SUMMARY

Observational and interventional trial designs complement each other with the type of information they can provide on disease state risk factors and protective factors, as well as efficacy and safety of therapeutic interventions. Both observational and interventional studies have led to important findings relevant to the practice of pharmacy in a variety of settings. Although RCTs can determine cause and effect and are considered the gold standard for assessing efficacy and safety of an intervention, they are not always appropriate for the research question or possible to conduct. Results of observational studies are more generalizable to "real-world" practice because the included individuals are not as narrowly defined as they are in RCTs. Systematic reviews and meta-analyses allow one to form a better idea of the safety and efficacy of an intervention in general or in a subgroup of patients by pooling results of similarly designed trials. All of these design types have a niche in the practice of EBM, and a basic level of knowledge on clinical trial design is important for all pharmacists to have.

## REFERENCES

1. DiPietro NA. Methods in epidemiology: observational study designs. *Pharmacotherapy*. 2010;30(10):973-984.
2. Johnson LL. Design of observational studies. In: Gallin J, Ognibene FP, eds. *Principles and Practice of Clinical Research*. 3rd ed. Amsterdam: Elsevier Inc; 2012:207-223.

3.  Hulley SB, Newman TB, Cummings SR. Getting started: the anatomy and physiology of clinical research. In: Hulley SB, Cummings SR, Browner WS, Grady DG, Newman TB, eds. *Designing Clinical Research*. 3rd ed. Philadelphia, PA: Lippincott Williams & Wilkins; 2007:1-15.

4.  Koretz RL. Considerations of study design. *Nutr Clin Pract*. 2007;22(6):593-598.

5.  Gottlieb MS, Schroff R, Schanker HM, et al. *Pneumocystis carinii* pneumonia and mucosal candidiasis in previously healthy homosexual men. *N Engl J Med*. 1981;305(24):1425-1431.

6.  Kataoka H, Ueno S. Dropped head associated with amantadine in Parkinson disease. *Clin Neuropharmacol*. 2011;34(1):48-49.

7.  Mintz S, Lee JK. Gabapentin in the treatment of intractable idiopathic chronic cough: case reports. *Am J Med*. 2006;119(5):e13-e15.

8.  Wei S, Venn A, Ding C, Foley S, Laslett L, Jones G. The association between oral contraceptive use, bone mineral density and fractures in women aged 50-80 years. *Contraception*. 2011;84(4):357-362.

9.  Current cancer prevention studies. American Cancer Society website. http://www.cancer.org/research/researchprogramsfunding/cancer-prevention-study-overviews. Accessed November 17, 2014.

10. Hildebrand JS, Patel AV, McCullough ML, et al. Coffee, tea, and fatal oral/pharyngeal cancer in a large prospective US cohort. *Am J Epidemiol*. 2013;177(1):50-58.

11. Cummings SR, Newman TB, Hulley SB. Designing a cohort study. In: Hulley SB, Cummings SR, Browner WS, Grady DG, Newman TB, eds. *Designing Clinical Research*. 3rd ed. Philadelphia, PA: Lippincott Williams & Wilkins; 2007:98-107.

12. About the Framingham Heart Study. Framingham Heart Study website. https://www.framinghamheartstudy.org/about-fhs/index.php. Accessed July 7, 2014.

13. Kolla BP, Lovely JK, Mansukhani MP, Morgenthaler TI. Zolpidem is independently associated with increased risk of inpatient falls. *J Hosp Med*. 2013;8(1):1-6.

14. Zithromax (azithromycin): FDA statement on risk of cardiovascular death. Food and Drug Administration website. http://www.fda.gov/Safety/MedWatch/SafetyInformation/SafetyAlertsforHumanMedicalProducts/ucm304503.htm. Accessed November 17, 2014.

15. Ray WA, Murray KT, Hall K, Arbogast PG, Stein CM. Azithromycin and the risk of cardiovascular death. *N Engl J Med*. 2012;366(20):1881-1889.

16. Newman TB, Browner WS, Cummings SR, Hulley SB. Designing cross-sectional and case-control studies. In: Hulley SB, Cummings SR, Browner WS, Grady DG, Newman TB, eds. *Designing Clinical Research*. 3rd ed. Philadelphia, PA: Lippincott Williams & Wilkins; 2007:109-126.

17. Essebag V, Genest J, Suissa S, Pilote L. The nested case-control study in cardiology. *Am Heart J*. 2003;146(4):581-590.

18. Singh S, Chang HY, Richards TM, Weiner JP, Clark JM, Segal JB. Glucagonlike peptide 1-based therapies and risk of hospitalization for acute pancreatitis in type 2 diabetes mellitus [published online ahead of print February 25, 2013]. *JAMA Intern Med*. doi: 10.1001/jamainternmed.2013.2720.

19. Psaty BM, Heckbert SR, Koepsell TD. The risk of myocardial infarction associated with antihypertensive drug therapies. *JAMA*. 1995;274(8):620-625.

20. Borhani NO, Mercuri M, Borhani PA, et al. Final outcome results of the Multicenter Isradipine Diuretic Atherosclerosis Study (MIDAS): a randomized controlled trial. *JAMA*. 1996;276(10):785-791.

21. Furberg CD, Psaty BM, Meyer JV. Nifedipine. Dose-related increase in mortality in patients with coronary heart disease. *Circulation*. 1995;92(5):1326-1331.

22. Cummings SR, Grady D, Hulley SB. Designing a randomized blinded trial. In: Hulley SB, Cummings SR, Browner WS, Grady DG, Newman TB, eds. *Designing Clinical Research*. 3rd ed. Philadelphia, PA: Lippincott Williams & Wilkins; 2007:147-161.

23. Greenhalgh T. Getting your bearings (what is this paper about?). In: Greenhalgh T, ed. *How to Read a Paper: The Basics of Evidence Based Medicine*. 2nd ed. London: BMJ Books; 2001:46-58.

24. CONSORT transparent reporting of trials. CONSORT website. http://www.consort-statement.org. Accessed November 17, 2014.

25. Chin R, Lee BY. Periods, sequences, and trial design. In: Chin R, Lee BY, eds. *Principles and Practice of Clinical Trial Medicine*. Oxford, UK: Elsevier; 2008:95-117.

26. Chang M. Clinical trial design. In: Chang M, ed. *Classical and Adaptive Clinical Trial Designs Using ExpDesign Studio*. Hoboken, NJ: John Wiley & Sons; 2008:14-26.

27. Grady D, Cummings SR, Hulley SB. Alternative trial designs and implementation issues. In: Hulley SB, Cummings SR, Browner WS, Grady DG, Newman TB, eds. *Designing Clinical Research*. 3rd ed. Philadelphia, PA: Lippincott Williams & Wilkins; 2007:163-182.

28. Lonn E, Yusuf S, Dzavik V; SECURE Investigators. Effects of ramipril and vitamin E on atherosclerosis: the study to evaluate carotid ultrasound changes in patients treated with ramipril and vitamin E (SECURE). *Circulation*. 2001;103(7):919-925.

29. Louis TA, Lavori PW, Bailar JC, Polansky M. Crossover and self-controlled designs in clinical research. *N Engl J Med*. 1984;310(1):24-31.

30. Beaulieu AD, Peloso P, Bensen W, et al. A randomized, double-blind, 8-week crossover study of once-daily controlled-release tramadol versus immediate-release tramadol taken as needed for chronic noncancer pain. *Clin Ther*. 2007;29(1):49-60.

31. Leucht S, Kissling W, Davis JM. How to read and understand and use systematic reviews and meta-analyses. *Acta Psychiatr Scand*. 2009:119(6):443–450.

32. Ried K. Interpreting and understanding meta-analysis graphs: a practical guide. *Australian Fam Physician*. 2006;35(8):635-638.

33. PRISMA transparent reporting of systematic reviews and meta-analyses. PRISMA website. http://www.prisma-statement.org. Accessed November 17, 2014.

34. Cronin L, Cook DJ, Carlet J, et al. Corticosteroid treatment for sepsis: a critical appraisal and meta-analysis of the literature. *Crit Care Med*. 1995;23(8):1430-1439.

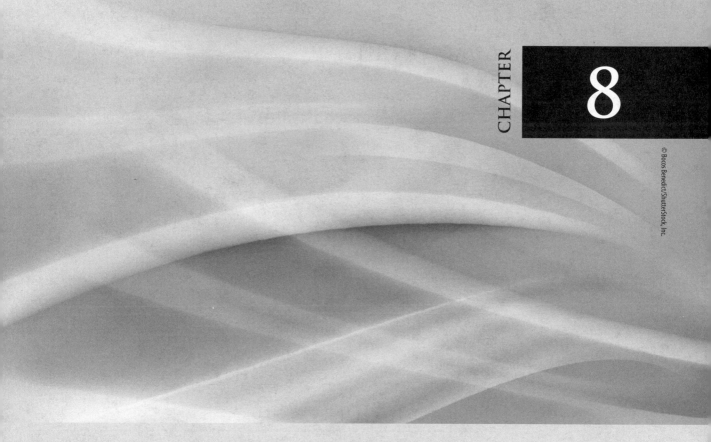

© Bocos Benedict/ShutterStock, Inc.

CHAPTER

8

# DESCRIPTIVE STATISTICS

Jennifer Phillips, PharmD, BCPS
Kristina E. Ward, PharmD, BCPS

## CHAPTER OBJECTIVES

▸ Define *dependent variable* and *independent variable*.

▸ Determine if a variable is qualitative or quantitative in nature and distinguish between the types of graphical presentations used for each.

▸ Identify if a variable is nominal, ordinal, interval, or ratio.

▸ Define and calculate the following: mean, median, and mode.

▸ Differentiate between standard deviation and standard error of the mean.

▸ Identify when it is appropriate to use the interquartile range (IQR).

## CHAPTER OUTLINE

## KEY TERMS

Bar diagram
Box plot
Dependent variable
Dichotomous variable
Histogram
Independent variable
Interquartile range
Interval data
Mean
Median
Mode
Nominal data

Normal distribution
Ordinal data
Pie chart
Polychotomous variable
Probability distribution
Qualitative variable
Quantitative variable
Ratio data
Skewed distribution
Standard deviation
Standard error of the mean
Variance

# INTRODUCTION

As part of their research, investigators collect many types of information. To convey that information to others, the data must be summarized in some meaningful way. Statistics can be defined in several ways, but it ultimately involves summarizing and analyzing data. Statistics can be divided into two broad categories: descriptive statistics and inferential statistics. This chapter explores descriptive statistics. Descriptive statistics involves summarizing and describing data.[1] The methods used for summarizing and describing data depend on the scale of data measurement and the variables being measured. Presentation of descriptive statistics can occur in tabular or graphical form. The goal of this chapter is to discuss the role of the scale of measurement, type of variable, measures of central tendency, data distributions, and methods of data presentation in descriptive statistics, as these form the basis for inferential statistics.

# VARIABLES: DEPENDENT VERSUS INDEPENDENT

When designing a study, a researcher is usually trying to ascertain the effect of a selected variable on a particular outcome. To do this, the researcher randomizes participants in the study to receive a different intervention and then measures the effect of that intervention on a predetermined outcome. The intervention chosen by the researcher is called the **independent variable**.[1] This variable is chosen in advance and is controlled by the researcher. The outcome that is measured at the end of the study is called the **dependent variable**.[1] In graphs, the independent variable is typically displayed on the $x$-axis and the dependent variable on the $y$-axis.

For example, a researcher interested in whether students learn better with traditional live lectures or through self-paced online interactive lectures designs a study to

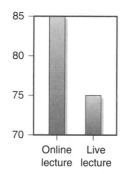

**FIGURE 8-1** Example plot of independent vs. dependent variables.

determine this. After obtaining student consent to participate, she chooses to randomize half of the students in the class to a traditional live lecture and the other half to an online interactive lecture. To determine impact on learning, she administers a quiz to both groups and measures the mean score in each group. In this case, the method of content delivery (online lecture vs. traditional live lecture) is the independent variable. The outcome measured in this study (mean quiz score) is the dependent variable, because if a difference is found between the groups, the researcher would conclude that the mean quiz score depends on the intervention group, the students were assigned to. When visually displaying this data, the researcher would have the mean quiz score on the *y*-axis and the groups on the *x*-axis, as shown in **Figure 8-1**.

Sometimes, dosage might be the independent variable of interest. A researcher might be interested in determining if the dose of a new drug has an impact on clinical and safety outcomes. An example of this is a phase II dose-ranging study that evaluated various doses of an antifactor Xa inhibitor, rivaroxaban. In this study, researchers randomized patients undergoing elective knee replacement to one of six treatment arms: 2.5 mg, 5 mg, 10 mg, 20 mg, or 30 mg twice daily of rivaroxaban, or 30 mg twice daily of enoxaparin.[2] The primary safety outcome measured in this study was major postoperative bleeding.[2] What would be the independent and dependent variables in this study?

In this example, each of the treatment arms that the patient was randomized to would be considered the independent variable; the dose and treatment selected were determined before the study began and were controlled by the researcher. The safety outcome measured in this study (major postoperative bleeding) would be considered the dependent variable. In this study, the researchers concluded that the frequency of major postoperative bleeding increased as the dose of rivaroxaban increased.[2] Therefore, we could conclude that the risk for bleeding depends on the dose of rivaroxaban.

When analyzing the results of any research study, a researcher makes many assumptions. One of the assumptions made is that one can infer that the results seen in the sample of patients selected for the study are the same results that would be seen if a different sample was selected. Use of inferential statistics helps determine if that assumption is valid. Another assumption that is made is that the results seen in the sample of patients selected are due exclusively to the intervention that was applied. Sometimes, however, other factors besides the researchers' interventions (independent variable) influence the outcome of the study (dependent variable), and these factors are called confounding variables.[1] Researchers should take care to recognize potential confounding variables and adjust for them by modifying the inclusion or exclusion criteria for a study or through the application of statistical tests designed to adjust for confounding variables.

In summary, independent variables are chosen by the researcher before a study begins. They are presumed to be the *cause* of some effect or outcome and are controlled by the researcher during the experiment. Dependent variables are the resulting outcomes, or effects, of the independent variables.

## SCALES OF MEASUREMENT

Categorizing variables appropriately is essential, because the type of statistical test used to analyze a dataset depends on the type of variables selected. The first step in categorizing a variable is determining whether it is qualitative or quantitative.

### Qualitative (Discrete) Variables

**Qualitative variables** are sometimes referred to as *categorical variables*. With this type of data, outcomes or measurements are classified into categories that are discrete; for example, gender (male/female), ethnicity (African American, Native American, Caucasian, Latino), recurrence of stroke (yes/no), or a pain score of 1–5 (1 = no pain, 2 = slight pain, 3 = moderate pain, 4 = moderate-severe pain, and 5 = severe pain). Although numbers can be used to represent qualitative data (as in the pain score example), the numbers are arbitrary and are used to show direction rather than express an absolute quantity.[3] Qualitative data are often expressed as frequency distributions (e.g., 30% of the population is male, 45% of subjects experienced a recurrent stroke, 25% of patients reported a pain score of 3). Qualitative variables may be measured with the following types of data:

- *Ordinal data*: If there is a scale or direction associated with the categories, then the categorical variable is classified as **ordinal**.[3] For example, a pain scale would be considered ordinal data. A pain score of 5 ("severe pain") is worse than a pain score of 1 ("no pain"), but it is not necessarily five times as worse. The numbers used in the scale are arbitrary and are used to show direction among the categories and are not an absolute quantity of pain. In addition to frequency distributions, the median and the mode can be used to represent ordinal data.[4]
- *Nominal data*: With **nominal data**, the categories are unrelated and no scale or direction is implied. Returning to our earlier examples, gender, ethnicity, and recurrence of stroke would be considered nominal variables. Variables that have only two possible outcomes (e.g., yes/no, male/female) are oftentimes referred to as **dichotomous variables**.[3] Variables with more than two possible outcomes are referred to as **polychotomous**. Similar to ordinal data, frequency distributions are typically used to represent nominal data. The mode can also be used for this variable type.[4]

### Quantitative (Continuous) Variables

With **quantitative variables**, outcomes are represented by a number. A quantitative variable may also be referred to as a continuous variable. Unlike ordinal data, where the value of the number is arbitrary, the numbers used to represent quantitative variables represent the magnitude of a particular outcome.[3] Examples of quantitative variables include blood pressure (e.g., 110/70 mm Hg), weight (e.g., 135 lbs), or temperature (e.g., 98.1°F). Specific subtypes of quantitative data include interval and ratio data:

- *Interval data*: With **interval data**, the difference between each unit of a measurement scale is equal, but there is no absolute zero.[1] An example of interval data would be temperature expressed in degrees Fahrenheit. Because there is no absolute zero, ratios cannot be accurately calculated. For example, 60°F is not twice as warm as 30°F because 0°F does not really represent the lowest possible temperature.

- *Ratio data*: In contrast, **ratio data** does have an absolute zero, and therefore ratios are meaningful and can be used to express this type of data.[1] Examples include weight, blood pressure, and pulse. A pulse of 120 beats per minute (bpm) is twice as fast as one that is 60 bpm because a pulse rate of zero is not arbitrary but rather represents no heartbeat.

In summary, categorizing variables is important because the type of statistical test required to analyze datasets is dependent upon the type of variable used. Qualitative variables are used to represent data that fits into discrete categories; ordinal and nominal data are two types of qualitative variables. Quantitative variables are expressed with a number and include interval and ratio data.

## MEASURES OF CENTRAL TENDENCY

### Mean

The **mean** of a dataset is calculated by summing the values associated with each individual data point and dividing by the total number of data points. It is often represented by the equation

$$\bar{X} = \frac{\sum X_i}{n}$$

where $\bar{X}$ is the mean of the dataset, $X_i$ is each individual data point, and $n$ is the total number of data points.[4] To illustrate, let us use a hypothetical example. Suppose there were five pharmacy students enrolled in an evidence-based medicine elective course that met on a Friday evening at 7:00 p.m. Now suppose that a final exam was administered and the instructor wished to determine the mean score on this exam. The final exam scores for all five students are listed in **Table 8-1**.

To calculate the mean final exam score for the five students enrolled in this course, the instructor would add up all of the scores (total = 408) and divide by the number of students ($n = 5$). In this case, the mean final exam score was 81.6%. One thing that is readily apparent when examining the dataset is that the mean score does not seem to represent the class very well. Four out of the five students scored higher than the mean. If the instructor were to report only the mean final exam score, it would underestimate the performance of the class as a whole. In this example, the reason the mean final exam score was lower than four of the five students' scores is because unlike other measures of central tendency (i.e., median, mode) the mean is sensitive to outliers.[4] An outlier is any extreme value in a dataset. In this case, the outlier was student number 5, who achieved a score of 58% on the exam, which was much lower than the other four students.

One way to mitigate the effects of outliers is to add more data points to the dataset. To demonstrate this, assume that the same instructor from the previous example decides to change the scheduled time for the evidence-based medicine elective to Wednesday

**TABLE 8-1** Example of Final Exam Scores

| Student | Final Exam Score |
| --- | --- |
| 1 | 90 |
| 2 | 88 |
| 3 | 86 |
| 4 | 86 |
| 5 | 58 |

**TABLE 8-2**  Example with Increased Number of Final Exam Scores

| Student | Final Exam Score (%) | Student | Final Exam Score (%) |
|---------|---------------------|---------|---------------------|
| 1 | 90 | 11 | 86 |
| 2 | 90 | 12 | 86 |
| 3 | 90 | 13 | 86 |
| 4 | 90 | 14 | 86 |
| 5 | 88 | 15 | 86 |
| 6 | 88 | 16 | 86 |
| 7 | 88 | 17 | 86 |
| 8 | 88 | 18 | 86 |
| 9 | 86 | 19 | 86 |
| 10 | 86 | 20 | 58 |

at 1:00 p.m. the subsequent year. This change resulted in 20 students enrolling in the course. The final exam scores for all 20 students are shown in **Table 8-2**. Once again, there was one outlier, who achieved a score of 58. However, with 20 students enrolled in the class, the mean final exam score was 85.8, which was much more representative of how the class did as a whole. As can be seen in Table 8-2, 19 out of the 20 students had a score of 86 or higher on the exam. This is a good demonstration of how adding more data points to a dataset helps mitigate the effect of outliers.

When evaluating data published in clinical trials, a reader can look at the range and standard deviation that are reported with the mean to determine if one or more outliers were present in the dataset. This will be covered in an upcoming section (Measures of Variability).

### Median

The **median** is the value of the data point that is in the middle or the 50th percentile of the dataset distribution.[4] Half of the dataset values are above the median and half of the dataset values are below the median. When determining the median one must first arrange all of the data points in ascending or descending order. In Table 8-1, the median is 86. When outliers are present, the median may be a better choice to represent the data, because it is not as sensitive to outliers as the mean. The median may also be a better choice when data are not normally distributed or for ordinal data.[1] When there is an even number of data points, the median is determined by taking the average of the two middle-most numbers.[1]

### Mode

Within a dataset, the **mode** is the most frequently occurring value. In Table 8-1, the mode would be 86, because it is the value that occurs most often in that dataset. Note that for the dataset in Table 8-2 the mode is also 86. In some datasets, there can be more than one mode. These distributions are called bimodal.[1]

## DISTRIBUTION OF THE DATA

### NORMAL DISTRIBUTION

When data are displayed as a frequency distribution, it can have several shapes. A **normal distribution** has the appearance of a bell-shaped curve, as depicted in **Figure 8-2**. Both sides of the curve are symmetric about the middle part of the curve. When data are

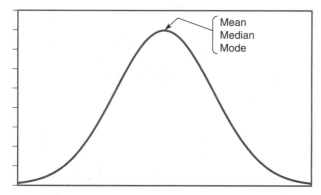

**FIGURE 8-2** Normal distribution and measure of central tendency.

normally distributed, the mean, median, and mode are all the same number, as shown in Figure 8-2. Certain statistical tests are only valid for data that are normally distributed.[1]

For data that are not normally distributed, the mean, median, and mode do not represent the same number. These types of distributions are said to be **skewed**.

## PROBABILITY DISTRIBUTIONS

In contrast to frequency distributions, **probability distributions** involve a visual representation of the probability that an event will or will not occur. The binomial distribution and Poisson distribution are both probability distributions. When a researcher is more interested in the occurrence of an event as opposed to the magnitude of the outcome, a binomial distribution can be used.[5] This type of distribution is used when an experiment is conducted multiple times and there are only a finite number of possible outcomes.[5] An example would be flipping a coin 100 times. There are only two possible outcomes each time—heads or tails. In this case, the categories are independent (i.e., getting heads on a flip does not influence the risk of getting tails on the next flip) and mutually exclusive (i.e., the coin can only land with one side up). The Poisson distribution is another type of probability distribution that is used when considering rare outcomes.[5]

# MEASURES OF VARIABILITY

## VARIANCE AND STANDARD DEVIATION

**Variance** and **standard deviation** (SD or σ) are closely related and are both measures of dispersion around the mean for interval- or ratio-level data that are normally or near-normally distributed.[4,6,7] Within a given study sample, individual data points are scattered both above and below the mean, resulting in differences from the mean that are positive and negative values; the sums of these differences always equal zero.[4,6] To determine the variance, each data point ($X_i$) is subtracted from the mean ($\bar{X}$), summed, and then squared, and finally divided by the total number of data points ($n$) minus one:

$$\text{Variance } (s^2) = \frac{\sum_{i=1}^{n}(X_i - \bar{X})^2}{(n - 1)}$$

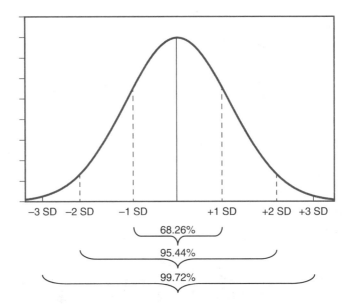

**FIGURE 8-3** Standard deviation of the normal distribution.

Because the variance is squared, the resulting value is expressed as the square of the original units used. The standard deviation is obtained by taking the square root of the variance, which expresses dispersion of the data on the original scale of measurement:[4,6]

$$SD = \sqrt{\text{Variance}}$$

For normally distributed data, 68% of data points will fall within ± 1 SD from the mean, whereas ± 2 SD from the mean accounts for 95% and ± 3 SD accounts for 99.7% of the data points. **Figure 8-3** shows a bell–shaped curve for a set of normally distributed data with the first, second, and third standard deviations noted.[4,6,7]

   **Table 8-3** shows the procedure for calculating the variance and corresponding standard deviation of the data initially presented in Table 8-2. To begin, first subtract

| TABLE 8-3 | Example Table for Variance Calculation | | | | |
|---|---|---|---|---|---|
| **Student** | $(X_i - \bar{X})$ | $(X_i - \bar{X})^2$ | **Student** | $(X_i - \bar{X})$ | $(X_i - \bar{X})^2$ |
| 1 | 4.2 | 17.64 | 11 | 0.2 | 0.04 |
| 2 | 4.2 | 17.64 | 12 | 0.2 | 0.04 |
| 3 | 4.2 | 17.64 | 13 | 0.2 | 0.04 |
| 4 | 4.2 | 17.64 | 14 | 0.2 | 0.04 |
| 5 | 2.2 | 4.84 | 15 | 0.2 | 0.04 |
| 6 | 2.2 | 4.84 | 16 | 0.2 | 0.04 |
| 7 | 2.2 | 4.84 | 17 | 0.2 | 0.04 |
| 8 | 2.2 | 4.84 | 18 | 0.2 | 0.04 |
| 9 | 0.2 | 0.04 | 19 | 0.2 | 0.04 |
| 10 | 0.2 | 0.04 | 20 | −27.8 | 772.84 |
| *Sum* | | 90 | *Sum* | | 773.2 |
| **TOTAL** $(X_i - \bar{X})^2$ | | | | | 863.2 |

the mean exam grade (85.8%) from each individual exam grade and then square the result. This results in a value of 863.2 Note that the result of summing all of the $(X_i - \bar{X})$ values would equal zero. Calculations for variance and standard deviation are shown below. Most of the time, computer software programs are used to perform these calculations.

$$\text{Variance } (s^2) = \frac{\sum_{i=1}^{20}(863.2)}{(19)} = 45.4$$

$$\text{SD} = \sqrt{45.4} = 6.74$$

## STANDARD ERROR OF THE MEAN

**Standard error of the mean** (SEM) is often confused with SD because they are expressed as mean ± SD and mean ± SEM, but they differ in important ways. Whereas SD describes the variability within a given sample from a population, the SEM is an estimate of the true mean of the underlying population. In an individual study, a sample is chosen from a population and, when normally distributed, a mean ± SD can be calculated as a way to describe the variability of the data around the mean. Conceptually, if the study were repeated many times over with sampling from the original population each time, different study samples would be chosen each time. The SEM represents the variability of the theoretical means of all the potential samples from a given population and describes how the sample means vary around the true, but unknown, population mean. In other words, the SEM describes how well the sample mean represents the population mean from which the sample was obtained.[4,7,8]

The appropriate use of the SEM is for construction of the confidence interval, which includes the estimate of the true population mean. However, the SEM can be misleading because it is always smaller than the SD, as evidenced by its mathematical formula:

$$\text{SEM} = \text{SD}/\sqrt{n}$$

Presenting data as a mean ± SEM when it should be presented as mean ± SD may mislead the reader, who could assume that the variability in the data sample is smaller than it actually is. Continuing with the example presented in Tables 8-3 and 8-4, the SEM of that dataset would be calculated as:

$$\text{SEM} = \frac{6.74}{\sqrt{20}} = 1.51$$

Use of the SEM to describe data dispersion occurs commonly and is well documented; the reader must be aware and be prepared to convert an SEM to an SD by multiplying the SEM by the $\sqrt{n}$.[8-11]

## RANGE AND INTERQUARTILE RANGE

As a measure of spread, the range is the simplest method, representing the difference between the highest and the lowest data values. Because only the highest and lowest values are considered, the range can be influenced by outliers.[4,6]

The **interquartile range** (IQR) is used to describe the middle 50% of data values. The values between the 25th and 75th percentiles represent the IQR; the median is the 50th percentile. IQRs are usually used to describe data on the ordinal scale or interval or ratio data that that do not fit the normal distribution.[3,4,6]

# METHODS OF DATA PRESENTATION

Graphical presentation of data should supplement written text and can be useful when presenting complex data to help the reader gain greater understanding of the results being presented. Types of graphic presentations vary depending on the type of data and the scale of measurement.

## DISPLAY OF QUALITATIVE (DISCRETE) DATA

Discrete data can be described using frequencies and proportions (as percentages), which can then be presented in tabular form listing the number (count) and percent for each variable of interest. The data can also be presented using bar diagrams or pie charts. Use of bar diagrams to describe discrete data is most common.[6,12]

**Bar diagrams** are constructed by placing the discrete variable on the $x$-axis and the count or frequency on the $y$-axis. Direct comparisons between the bars on the diagram are possible. **Pie charts** are commonly used in marketing materials and magazines; some have described pie charts as being useless.[6,12] Pie charts assign each discrete variable a slice of the "pie." The size of each slice is determined by the proportion of each relative to the total of the pie. In **Figure 8-4**, fictitious data are presented for the number and frequency of patients with different stages of heart failure. Based on these data, a bar graph and a pie chart can be created.

## DISPLAY OF QUANTITATIVE (CONTINUOUS) DATA

Continuous data can be quantifiably measured and can also be summarized (along with its associated measure of dispersion) in tabular form. Graphical representations commonly used to depict continuous data include the histogram and the box plot (box-and-whiskers). Other less commonly used techniques include the stem-and-leaf diagram and frequency polygons.[6,12,13]

**Histograms** are frequently used to display the distribution of a dataset. From the histogram, the visual representation of the data makes it easier to observe a bell-shaped

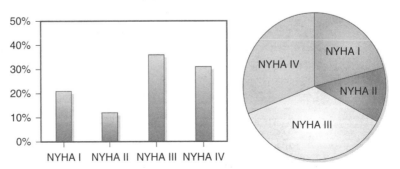

**FIGURE 8-4** Graphical presentations: bar graph and pie chart.

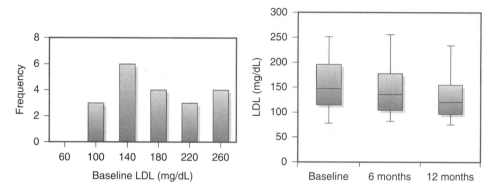

**FIGURE 8-5** Graphical presentations: histogram and box plot.

(Gaussian) distribution or to see if the data distribution is skewed or bimodal.[12] The *x*-axis provides the measurement range of the variable of interest (divided into equal units or class intervals); the *y*-axis represents frequency or relative frequency.[3,6,13] When creating a histogram, many computer programs generate *x*-axis units of equal size automatically.[13]

**Box plots** are also known as *box-and-whiskers plots*. Box plots offer a visual representation of the IQR, the middle 50% of values. To create a box plot, the median, the 25th percentile, and the 75th percentile are needed. The continuous variable is represented on the *y*-axis; time or another measurement point is usually represented on the *x*-axis. The 25th and 75th percentiles are plotted, a box drawn to include both points, and the median is denoted by a line drawn in the middle; this box includes the middle 50% of values.[3,6,13,14] The vertical lines extending out from above and below the box are the whiskers, and the values that lie outside the whiskers can be considered outliers. Whiskers may have different meanings, so it is critical to read the legend to determine their definition. In some cases, the whiskers could represent the 5th and 95th percentiles or the 10th and 90th percentiles, or they could merely represent 1.5 times the IQR or the minimum and maximum data values.[3,6,12] **Figure 8-5** presents a histogram and box plot using fictitious data on low-density lipoprotein measurements in 20 patients.

# SUMMARY

Descriptive statistics are used to summarize and describe data. Various methods are used, including measures of central tendency (i.e., mean, median, mode) and measures to indicate data spread (i.e., standard deviation, range, IQR). Distributions of data are important because they affect how data are analyzed. When a distribution is deemed "normal," the mean and standard deviation are commonly used to summarize and describe the data. If a distribution is skewed or not normal, the assumptions of the normal distribution cannot be upheld. In this situation and with ordinal data, the mean becomes less meaningful; the median provides a more informative assessment of central tendency because it is affected less by outliers than the mean. Graphical presentation of data often helps the reader understand the data being presented. Different types of graphical representations are used based on the type of data (qualitative vs. quantitative).

# REFERENCES

1. DeMuth J. *Basic Statistics and Pharmaceutical Statistical Applications*. New York, NY: Marcel Dekker; 1999.
2. Turpie AG, Fisher WD, Bauer KA, Kwong LM, Irwin MW. BAY 59-7939: an oral, direct factor Xa inhibitor for the prevention of venous thromboembolism in patients after total knee replacement. A phase II dose-ranging study. *J Thromb Haemost*. 2005;3(11):2479-2486.
3. Nick T. Descriptive statistics. *Methods Mol Biol*. 2007;404:33-52.
4. Gaddis ML, Gaddis GM. Introduction to biostatistics: part 2, descriptive statistics. *Ann Emerg Med*. 1990;19(3):309-315.
5. Kier KL. Clinical application of statistical analysis. In: Malone PM, Kier KL, Stanovich JE, eds. *Drug Information: A Guide for Pharmacists*. 3rd ed. New York, NY: McGraw-Hill; 2006:350-352.
6. Dawson B, Trapp RG. Chapter 3. Summarizing data and presenting data in tables and graphs. In: Dawson B, Trapp RG, eds. *Basic and Clinical Biostatistics*. 4th ed. New York, NY: McGraw-Hill; 2004. http://www.accesspharmacy.com/content.aspx?aID=2046198. Accessed July 21, 2014.
7. Overholser BR, Sowinski KM. Biostatistics primer: part I. *Nutr Clin Pract*. 2007;22(6):629-635.
8. Nagele P. Misuse of standard error of the mean (SEM) when reporting variability of a sample. A critical evaluation of four anaesthesia journals. *Br J Anaesth*. 2003;90(4):514-516.
9. Bunce H 3rd, Hokanson JA, Weiss GB. Avoiding ambiguity when reporting variability in biomedical data. *Am J Med*. 1980;69(1):8-9.
10. Robinson PM, Menakuru S, Reed MW, Balasubramanian SP. Description and reporting of surgical data—scope for improvement? *Surgeon*. 2009;7(1):6-9.
11. Al-Benna S, Al-Ajam Y, Way B, Steinstraesser L. Descriptive and inferential statistical methods used in burns research. *Burns*. 2010;36(3):343-346.
12. Stengel D, Calori GM, Giannoudis PV. Graphical data presentation. *Injury*. 2008;39(6):659-665.
13. Sonnad SS. Describing data: statistical and graphical methods. *Radiology*. 2002;225(3):622-628.
14. Spriestersbach A, Röhrig B, Du Prel JB, Gerhold-Ay A, Blettner M. Descriptive statistics: the specification of statistical measures and their presentation in tables and graphs. *Dtsch Arztebl Int*. 2009;106(36):578-583.

CHAPTER

# 9

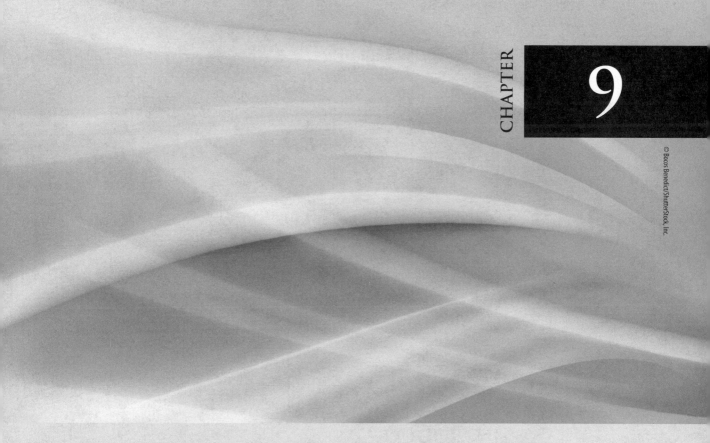

# INFERENTIAL STATISTICS

Erin M. Timpe Behnen, PharmD, BCPS
McKenzie C. Ferguson, PharmD, BCPS

## CHAPTER OBJECTIVES

▸ Describe the purpose of inferential statistics.

▸ Evaluate statistical and clinical significance utilizing alpha values, *p*-values, descriptive statistics, and confidence intervals.

▸ Explain the key factors to analyze in a study in order to choose an appropriate statistical test.

▸ Describe common statistical tests by study design and data type.

## CHAPTER OUTLINE

## KEY TERMS

Alpha

Analysis of covariance

Analysis of variance

Chi-square

Clinical significance

Confidence interval

Covariates

Fisher's exact test

Independent data

Inferential statistics

Kruskal-Wallis

Mann-Whitney U

McNemar

Nonparametric tests

Paired data

Paired *t*-test

Parametric tests

Probability value

Repeated measures ANOVA

Statistical significance

Student's *t*-test

Type I error

Type II error

Wilcoxon rank sum

Wilcoxon signed rank

# INTRODUCTION

An *inference* is a generalization made about a population based on the response illustrated by a sample of the population. Sample populations and inferences are necessary in biomedical literature due to the impracticality of studying an entire population of interest. To take inferences a step further, we use **inferential statistics** to determine the probability that our generalization, or our hypothesis, is correct versus the probability that the generalization may be due to chance. Inferential statistics differ from descriptive statistics in that descriptive statistics provide only a summary of the data found in the study. Descriptive statistics may be sufficient for small pilot studies and are necessary to later perform inferential statistics. Inferential statistics utilize the descriptive statistics and information about the population to help determine the ability to extrapolate the data to the general population. For example, if I notice several third-year pharmacy students staying late studying, I might infer that the third-year class has an exam the following day. It is possible that my inference could be flawed. Perhaps the students I saw were all in an elective rather than a class that all students were enrolled in or the students were staying late for an organization activity. We could utilize inferential statistical tests in this example to help distinguish the likelihood that the hypothesis, that the third-year pharmacy students have an exam the following day, is correct. When inferential statistics are applied to an experimental clinical trial example, we can conclude whether all patients with a disease state may be likely to respond in the same way to a new medication as the sample of patients included in our study. Inferential statistics rely heavily on an appropriate sample having been selected for study. Common inferential statistical tests used in clinical trials include Student's *t*-test, analysis of variance (ANOVA), analysis of covariance (ANCOVA), Mann-Whitney U, Wilcoxon signed rank, Kruskal-Wallis, chi-square, Fisher's exact, and McNemar.[1] This chapter will describe important factors in determining the appropriateness of common inferential statistical tests in experimental clinical trials.

# STATISTICAL SIGNIFICANCE

A **probability value**, or *p*-value, is the value provided as a result from inferential statistical tests and represents the probability of a **type I error** (erroneously rejecting the null hypothesis) and the probability that the result was due to chance.[2] When evaluating study results, both statistical significance and clinical significance of the data must be considered. Assessing for **statistical significance** involves comparing the *p*-value to the predetermined **alpha** value (significance level or threshold for accepting the null hypothesis) that is established by researchers. This will then determine whether to reject the null hypothesis or accept (i.e., fail to reject) it.[2] This value is commonly set at 0.05, meaning that any *p*-value less than or equal to this value can establish statistical significance. In other words, researchers are usually willing to take a 5% chance (1 in 20) or less of committing a type I error.[3] However, it is incorrect to interpret a smaller *p*-value as more meaningful than a larger *p*-value that is still statistically significant (e.g., 0.0001 vs. 0.001); *p*-values do not reflect the importance or magnitude of the difference noted between groups.[4] The smaller *p*-value only represents that there is less probability that the result is due to chance. Any *p*-value greater than the established significance level (e.g., $p = 0.07$ when alpha is set at 0.05) will lead to conclusions that the data are not statistically significant. This implies that the likelihood the results could be due to chance alone are too great to establish a reliable conclusion that the intervention studied caused the outcome. Once a decision is made to accept or reject the null hypothesis, the chance for error must also be considered. Type I error should be investigated if a statistically significant difference is found (i.e., the null hypothesis is rejected). This type of error is often considered as a false positive. The possibility of a **type II error** should be investigated when the null hypothesis is accepted (i.e., no statistically significant difference is found). This type of error is often considered a false negative.

Statistical significance can also be established through evaluation of a **confidence interval** (CI). Descriptive statistics (e.g., mean ± standard deviation [SD]) and calculations of odds or risk refer to the actual result seen in a sample population, whereas the confidence intervals and the standard error of the mean are estimations regarding the reliability or precision of the results in order to generalize results to a larger population.[2,4] In other words, a confidence interval provides an estimate that the result seen in the study will be what is observed in clinical practice. When set at 95%, it means that if the study were repeated 100 times, 95 of those times the true parameter value would be found within the reported interval of values. Thus a full evaluation of the entire range within the confidence interval becomes very important, because this is the range of outcomes that we could likely expect to occur clinically.

Standard deviation describes the variability of the data from the sample mean, whereas the SEM (SD/$\sqrt{n}$) measures the precision of the sample mean. Confidence intervals are often calculated via use of the SEM. Most often CIs are set to 95%, meaning that if we conducted the same study with 100 repeated samples, 95 of those times the outcome would likely fall within the reported range.[2,5] Interpretation of a CI varies based on whether the CI is describing means versus proportions. To establish statistical significance for continuous data (means) the CI must not cross zero. For example, if a study evaluated the ability of a new drug to lower blood pressure compared to another drug and presented the data as a mean change in blood pressure of −8.6 mm Hg (95% CI: −2 to −12), then we could conclude that there was a statistically significant decrease in mean blood pressure from baseline because the CI range did not include zero. If a zero value was included within the confidence interval, there is a possibility that if the study was repeated a 0 mm Hg change (i.e., no change) in blood pressure would be found, and thus the conclusion would be made that the result is not statistically significantly different. The confidence interval here tells us that if the study is repeated with 100 samples, we estimate that 95 of those times the overall mean change in blood pressure will be anywhere from −2 mm Hg to −12 mm Hg. For data presented as a ratio (e.g., hazard ratio, relative risk, odds ratio), the interval must not cross 1 in order to establish statistical significance. For proportion data, when a value of 1 is reported (e.g., 1:1 ratio), there is no difference between the groups. For example, researchers evaluating cardiovascular death when comparing the new blood pressure drug as compared to another drug might present their data as a hazard ratio (HR) 0.89 (95% CI: 0.65 to 1.45). This would be evaluated as not statistically significant given that the CI includes 1. In other words, if we were to repeat this study, there could be a chance that no difference would be observed (i.e., HR = 1.0).

# CLINICAL SIGNIFICANCE

**Clinical significance** is the ability to establish whether a result is meaningful enough to be able to incorporate a change in patient care. As opposed to the dichotomous determination of statistical significance (results are either statistically significant or not), clinical significance takes more careful evaluation of not only the data but also other factors, such as the overall magnitude of difference, cost, absolute benefit to the patient, number needed to treat, safety, and so on. Researchers should specify what they have determined as the minimum clinically important difference as part of their power calculation for the study.[4,6] When evaluating a power calculation, readers should scrutinize the estimated treatment effect size to determine if this difference would be considered to be a clinically significant difference in their practice as well. A study investigating a new first-in-class drug against placebo for treating high LDL cholesterol that aims to detect a 15% reduction in LDL cholesterol and finds that a statistically significant difference may be weak clinically if we compare it to the more robust lowering (up to 50%) that can already be achieved with existing statins. Not every statistically significant result is clinically significant; likewise, results that are nonstatistically significant can also be clinically meaningful.[2]

Confidence intervals can establish both statistical significance and clinical significance. For evaluating clinical significance, the size and range of the CI should be evaluated. A narrow CI generally indicates more precision in the point estimate representing the true population effect. The range of the CI should also be assessed for any value that does not offer much clinical benefit.[2] For example, in the example presented previously, the mean blood pressure reduction was 8.6 mm Hg (95% CI: −2 to −12). Although this result conveys statistical significance, it is difficult to justify putting someone on a newer, more expensive agent for the potential of only seeing a 2 mm Hg reduction in blood pressure. Additionally, consideration should be given to drug safety (e.g., drug-related side effects, drug interactions) and adherence issues (e.g., dosing, monitoring for efficacy and/or safety), among other factors, when establishing clinical significance. For example, if the new blood pressure drug demonstrated good blood pressure lowering, with a mean decrease of 12 mm Hg (95% CI: −8 to −20) that was both statistically and clinically significant, but the safety analysis presented some concerns, such as more patient deaths or arrhythmias (95% CI: 0% to 12%) in comparison to the placebo group, this should also be considered clinically. This may be illustrative of a clinically important safety concern with up to 12% of patients experiencing arrhythmias despite a lack of statistical significance due to a low number of reported events. Additionally, if the concerns related to development of serious arrhythmias warranted frequent monitoring, that would also need to be taken into clinical consideration.

# CHOOSING THE APPROPRIATE STATISTICAL TEST

Appropriate statistical analysis is dependent on having a clear understanding of what the study hypothesis is asking, characteristics of the research design, the levels of measurement of independent and dependent variables, and how the data are distributed. This may seem overwhelming at first, but we can begin by breaking down the unknown by answering six questions that can assist in determining the most appropriate inferential statistical test to be used. These questions include:

1. Are the data parametric or nonparametric?
2. What type(s) of data are being analyzed: continuous, ordinal, nominal, or measures of risk or survival?
3. How many samples are being compared?
4. Are the data paired or unpaired?
5. Are confounding variables incorporated into the analysis?
6. Is the hypothesis one-tailed or two-tailed?

## PARAMETRIC VERSUS NONPARAMETRIC TESTS

Parametric statistical analysis is used for continuous data that are normally distributed. If continuous data are skewed or non-normally distributed, data may be transformed to the logarithm or square root to produce a distribution to approach normality so that they can be evaluated with a **parametric test**.[7] Ordinal and nominal data and data that are not symmetrically bell shaped are assessed with **nonparametric tests**.[8] Nonparametric tests are less powerful and are not as specific as parametric tests because there are fewer underlying assumptions and the analysis relies on ranked and categorized data rather than more specific continuous measures. This potential decrease in accuracy may increase the risk of type II error (accepting a false null hypothesis). Even though nonparametric tests are less efficient, they are the most appropriate tests for ordinal and nominal data.[8,9] Qualls et al. reported an example of nonparametric data inappropriately assessed as parametric data when they evaluated studies investigating emergency department length of stay (ED LOS). The ED LOS is a continuous variable (minutes); however, it is most often non-normally distributed due to the potential for skewness from a few outlying patients who are in the ED for a much greater time than most of the other patients. This skews the mean to be higher than if the data were transformed to a normal distribution and could potentially lead to a type II error.[10]

## TYPES OF DATA

Statistical methods to be used are centered primarily on the level of measure or the type of data that are generated. For the purpose of most inferential statistical tests, the focus is on continuous, ordinal, and nominal data types. Continuous data include interval or ratio measurements where the distance between each measurement unit is equivalent; however, both ratio and interval data are evaluated using the same statistical tests. A specific systolic blood pressure measurement measured in mm Hg would be an example of continuous data.[11] Ordinal data include data that are ranked in a specific order. Likert scales or stages of hypertension would be examples of ordinal data. Ordinal scales are often associated with numbers that can be added and commonly are assessed as continuous data. For example, a survey may be conducted asking a series of 10 questions with Likert scale (e.g., 5 = strongly agree, 4 = agree, 3 = neutral, 2 = disagree, 1 = strongly disagree) answers, and the mean response for each question and the 10-question total may be reported. If an average of 3.42 is reported for a question in this case (a value that is not present on the scale), can we be sure what that actually means? Controversy exists surrounding whether statistical tests for ordinal or continuous data are most appropriate in these cases. Assessing these data as continuous is generally considered to be acceptable when there are a large number of divisions on the ordinal scale (i.e., five or more) or when there are a large number of samples. Nominal data are data assigned to a distinct and mutually exclusive category, such as presence or absence of hypertension. Nominal data should never be assessed with tests meant for continuous or ordinal data.[1]

## NUMBER OF SAMPLES

The number of samples is simply the number of groups that are being compared in the study. We are most interested in knowing if a study is comparing two groups or more than two groups. If a study is comparing a new drug to placebo, then two groups are being compared. If the study is a dose-finding study that is comparing groups assigned to more than two different doses of a new drug to each other and to placebo, then more than two groups are being compared. Statistical tests are designed to compare either two groups or multiple groups. Tests designed to compare multiple groups are based on tests comparing two groups, but allow for a correction for multiple analyses. If tests meant to compare only two groups are used repeatedly to compare multiple groups, the risk of committing a type I error is significantly increased. For example, when three groups are compared with three paired comparisons, the error rate is compounded, and the corrected alpha level would increase to 0.14, meaning that there is a 14% chance of inappropriately rejecting the null hypothesis in at least one of the comparisons, compared to the 5% chance that is most commonly accepted. The corrected alpha level is calculated as follows:

$$\text{Corrected alpha value} = 1 - (1 - \text{alpha})^{\text{\# of comparisons}}$$

In the example, there are three paired comparisons, and the corrected alpha level of 0.14 is calculated from $1 - (1 - 0.05)^3$. A statistical test designed for the multiple analyses should be used instead of the multiple paired analysis so that the increased risk of type I error is avoided.[8]

## PAIRED VERSUS INDEPENDENT DATA

A paired analysis is used when the test statistic is measuring individual subject differences rather than differences between groups. This occurs in pretest-posttest and crossover study designs where an individual's data are in both groups. Data in a parallel study, where individuals are assigned to only one group and remain in that group, are considered unpaired or **independent data**. Fewer subjects may be necessary in a paired analysis than in an independent analysis because patients serve as their own controls. Also, variability of the groups is decreased because the same subjects are utilized in the groups being compared.[7]

## CONFOUNDING VARIABLES

Confounding variables are factors that may predict outcomes or that may imbalance treatment groups. Age, gender, and presence of a disease state are common confounding variables. Most confounding variables are able to be balanced between treatment groups through randomization and stratification or are controlled for by inclusion in the statistical analysis as a covariate. **Covariates** are variables that are measured and accounted for in the statistical analysis in addition to the primary variables as factors that may affect the outcome. As an example, in clinical trials that assess the impact of interventions on cardiovascular disease outcomes (e.g., stroke), patients with diabetes may be stratified between the groups to ensure that a similar number of patients with diabetes are enrolled in each group. The reason for this is due to the increased risk of cardiovascular disease in patients with diabetes compared to patients who do not have diabetes. If one group had a greater percentage of patients with diabetes, and that group was found to have more cardiovascular outcomes overall, we would be unsure if the increased outcomes were truly a factor of the intervention or if differences in the sample populations may have affected the outcome. Stratification is used to control for that factor so that the groups are similar; however, the factor that was stratified for (diabetes in this example) should then be controlled for as a covariate in the statistical analysis as well to further investigate its impact on the outcome. Baseline characteristics are not generally assessed as covariates, but they may be assessed if they may potentially affect the outcome. Various inferential statistical tests are designed to adjust for one or more identified confounding variables as covariates.[12]

## ONE-TAILED VERSUS TWO-TAILED TESTS

A two-tailed hypothesis is one in which the researcher is looking to determine whether the groups are different, either better or worse. This is common in medication studies in which researchers are comparing a new medication to a current standard therapy and are looking to see if it is better or worse. In this case, the inferential test used divides alpha equally at both ends of the data distribution to test the statistical significance in each direction. If alpha is set at $0.05$, a two-tailed test distributes the rejection region as $0.025$ in the upper tail (e.g., better than) and $0.025$ in the lower tail (e.g., worse than). For this reason, most studies utilize a two-tailed test in order to lessen the risk of type I error. A one-tailed hypothesis is looking for a difference in one direction, either better or worse (i.e., superiority or noninferiority), but not both. If a new medication is hypothesized to be superior to a current standard therapy and alpha is $0.05$, the entire rejection region would be applied only at the upper tail of the distribution. However, many one-tailed studies set alpha at $0.025$ to avoid type I error. There must be a reason to justify looking in only one direction to avoid an inappropriate conclusion. For example, if a noninferiority study is conducted, there must be some advantage to the new intervention (e.g., decreased side effects, decreased monitoring, easier route of administration, etc.) to justify the one-sided analysis. If a superiority study is conducted, preliminary studies should have been conducted to prove noninferiority or equivalence.[7]

# COMMON STATISTICAL TESTS BY DATA TYPE

This section describes some of the most common inferential statistical tests that are used in biomedical research. The tests are organized by type of data—continuous, ordinal, and nominal—and not all statistical tests are presented. Many other statistical tests may be used and appropriate when considering additional factors. **Table 9-1** presents common statistical tests based on criteria presented in the previous section.[8,13]

The following clinical trial example will be used to illustrate the applicability of statistical tests: a double-blind, placebo-controlled clinical trial is conducted comparing the effects of an over-the-counter fever-reducing medication, ibuprofen, to placebo.

| TABLE 9-1 | Common Tests for Inferential Statistics | | | | | |
|---|---|---|---|---|---|---|
| | **Parametric** | | **Nonparametric** | | | |
| | **Continuous Data** | | **Ordinal Data** | | **Nominal Data** | |
| | **Unpaired** | **Paired** | **Unpaired** | **Paired** | **Unpaired** | **Paired** |
| **2 samples** | Student's *t*-test | Paired Student's *t*-test | Wilcoxon rank sum or Mann-Whitney U | Wilcoxon signed rank | $\chi^2$ or Fisher's exact | McNemar |
| **> 2 samples** | ANOVA | Repeated measures ANOVA | Kruskal-Wallis ANOVA | Friedman ANOVA | $\chi^2$ with Bonferroni correction | Cochran Q |
| **Covariates** | ANCOVA | ANCOVA or regression | ANCOVA ranks | Regression | Mantel-Haenszel, $\chi^2$ with Bonferroni correction or regression | |

Data from Gaddis GM, Gaddis ML. Introduction to biostatistics: part 4, statistical inference techniques in hypothesis testing. *Ann Emerg Med.* 1990;19(7):820-825; and Gaddis GM, Gaddis ML. Introduction to biostatistics: part 5, statistical inference techniques for hypothesis testing with nonparametric data. *Ann Emerg Med.* 1990;19(9):1054-1059.
ANOVA = analysis of variance; ANCOVA = analysis of covariance.

Temperature is measured by mouth 30 minutes after administration of medication or placebo.

## TESTS FOR CONTINUOUS DATA

Statistical tests for continuous data are the most powerful statistical tests available and result in a decreased risk of type II error compared to statistical tests for ordinal or nominal data.[8] The independent variables from the example scenario would be ibuprofen and placebo. The dependent variables for a continuous data analysis could be recorded as the temperature measured in degrees Fahrenheit 30 minutes after ibuprofen or placebo administration. The data should be analyzed to determine if the groups are of equal variances and are normally distributed prior to proceeding with the following statistical tests.

A **Student's *t*-test** (commonly referred to also as a *t*-test) is the most common statistical test used to evaluate two groups with continuous data. It is calculated using the mean, standard deviation, and variability of the data. This test is appropriate when the data meet the assumptions for the *t*-test, which are that the data are normally distributed and there are only two independent groups being compared, as in the ibuprofen and placebo parallel trial example. A one-tailed or two-tailed *t*-test may be conducted depending on the study hypothesis. A **paired *t*-test** should be used when the two groups being compared are paired rather than independent. For example, if the fever-reducing study was a crossover study in which patients received either ibuprofen or placebo for the first temperature $\geq 100°F$, and then received the opposite intervention for a second temperature $\geq 100°F$ at least 6 hours later, then a paired *t*-test would be more appropriate than the Student's *t*-test. Or, if the study evaluated individuals' change in temperature from baseline (i.e., before and after the intervention or pre- and posttest where patients serve as their own controls), again, a paired *t*-test would be more appropriate than the Student's *t*-test.[8]

Occasionally, *t*-tests have been used inappropriately in the literature when comparing more than two groups. For example, in the fever-reducing study, we might decide to also study an acetaminophen group in comparison to the ibuprofen and placebo groups. If multiple *t*-tests are used to compare acetaminophen to ibuprofen, acetaminophen to

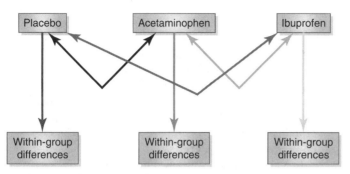

**FIGURE 9-1** Between- and within-group differences for ANOVA.

placebo, and ibuprofen to placebo, it would inappropriately increase the risk of committing a type I error, as described previously in the "Number of Samples" section.[8]

When comparing continuous outcomes in more than two groups, **analysis of variance** (ANOVA) is the appropriate statistical test to use. If acetaminophen were added as a third group to the fever-reducing study, evaluating temperature 30 minutes after administration, ANOVA could be conducted to determine if there is a difference within and between the groups (see **Figure 9-1**). This means that the groups would be evaluated to determine if there is a difference from baseline to the end of the study within each group as well as a comparison of the endpoint between each group (e.g., ibuprofen vs. acetaminophen, etc.).[8] If a statistically significant difference is reported with an ANOVA test, the result only reports that there is a difference somewhere; it does not specify exactly which groups are different from each other. A multiple comparison test is then necessary to determine where exactly that difference is. These tests are discussed in further detail later in this chapter.

A variety of different types of ANOVA tests can be used based on the number of confounding variables and other factors, such as repeated measures. **Analysis of covariance** (ANCOVA) is used to evaluate differences between three or more groups when controlling for confounding variables that are continuous data. Similar to ANOVA, a multiple comparison test must be done if the null hypothesis is rejected to determine where exactly the difference lies.[7] In the fever-reducing study, if the investigators had stated that they were comparing the temperature in degrees Fahrenheit 30 minutes after administration and controlled for factors of treatment assignment (acetaminophen, ibuprofen, or placebo), underlying cause of the fever, and patient age, an ANCOVA analysis would be appropriate. **Repeated measures ANOVA** is used when an outcome is studied in the same individual but under different conditions or multiple time periods. For example, if the fever-reducing study was used to evaluate the change in temperature for each intervention at baseline, 30 minutes, and 1, 2, 3, 4, 5, and 6 hours after the intervention in order to evaluate which one results in the greatest change in temperature for the longest duration, a repeated measures ANOVA could be used. Many studies include assessments of outcomes at multiple time points (e.g., 6 months and 12 months); however, a repeated measures ANOVA is only used for **paired data** when the data are assessed at different points in time in relation to the outcome.[7]

## TESTS FOR ORDINAL DATA

The independent variables from the example scenario again would be ibuprofen and placebo. The dependent variables for an ordinal data analysis could include a self-assessment asking how the patient feels (e.g., 1 = much better, 2 = better, 3 = about the same, 4 = worse, 5 = much worse) 30 minutes after ibuprofen or placebo administration. With ordinal data, numbers are usually assigned to each of the categories to order the responses and then the responses are ranked. It is the rank order that is then used by the statistical tests for ordinal data to determine statistical differences.

The Mann-Whitney U, Wilcoxon rank sum, Wilcoxon signed rank, and Kruskal-Wallis tests are commonly used to evaluate ordinal data or continuous data that are not normally distributed. The **Mann–Whitney U** and **Wilcoxon rank sum** tests are used when there are two independent samples and compare the distribution of ranked results between the groups. These tests are considered to be interchangeable and will provide similar results. For the self-assessment described in the parallel fever-reducing study, the overall rankings of the responses for each group are compared.[7,13,14]

The **Wilcoxon signed rank** test is similar to the paired *t*-test discussed previously and is used when paired ordinal or non-normally distributed continuous data are being compared. For the fever-reducing study, this test would be used if self-assessments are compared between ibuprofen and placebo in a crossover study (i.e., one intervention for the first temperature ≥ 100°F, then the opposite intervention for a second temperature ≥ 100°F at least 6 hours later). The **Kruskal-Wallis** test is similar to an ANOVA test and is used to compare more than two groups of independent, ordinal, or non-normally distributed data. If acetaminophen is added as a third group to the fever-reducing study and self-assessment results are compared between the groups, a Kruskal-Wallis test could be used to evaluate the results. Similar to ANOVA, a post hoc analysis is necessary to determine where the difference lies.[7,13,14]

## TESTS FOR NOMINAL DATA

The independent variables from the example scenario again would be ibuprofen and placebo. The dependent variables for a nominal data analysis would be temperature recorded as fever (temperature ≥ 100°F) or no fever (temperature < 100°F) 30 minutes after ibuprofen or placebo administration.

A **chi-square** ($\chi^2$) test is the most common statistical test used to evaluate nominal data. It is best used to report information about rates, proportions, or frequencies of outcomes and could be used in our example scenario. Data are reported in a 2 × 2 or larger table, as shown in the example in **Table 9-2**.

The observed frequencies reported from the study are compared to determine if they are different from what would be expected to occur due to chance. A **Fisher's exact test** would also be appropriate to use in this scenario; however, this test is used either when the total sample size is less than 20 or if the expected number of observations for any one of the cells would be less than 5. Therefore, a Fisher's exact test would be more appropriate than a chi-square test if the study is very small, such as if only 15 people were recruited for the fever-reducing study, or if few events are expected, such as in the case of a rare side effect when analyzing the safety of a medication in a clinical trial. However, because a Fisher's exact test is based on the expected frequency, it is not inappropriate if more observations are noted in the study. The chi-square and Fisher's exact tests are not appropriate for paired data analysis or when analyzing stratified data. The **McNemar** test should be used for nominal data that are paired, and the

| **TABLE 9-2**    Chi-Square Example Table | | |
|---|---|---|
| | **Fever** | **No Fever** |
| **Ibuprofen** | 18 | 82 |
| **Placebo** | 73 | 27 |

Mantel-Haenszel or regression test should be used for nominal data that incorporate covariates.[13,14]

## MULTIPLE COMPARISON TESTS

ANOVA and the Kruskal-Wallis test will identify whether there is a statistically significant difference somewhere among the groups compared. If the null hypothesis is rejected with ANOVA, either a planned analysis or a post hoc analysis with a multiple comparison test may then be used to determine which groups are different. The Bonferroni adjustment or tests such as the Dunn, Scheffé, Tukey, Newman-Keuls, and Dunnett's tests are commonly used to identify where exactly the difference is while controlling for type I error. These tests are not used on their own in place of ANOVA or Kruskal-Wallis because they are not as powerful, and they should only be used when a significant difference between the groups has already been found. The choice of an appropriate multiple comparison test depends on multiple factors, including whether the data are being compared to a control group, how many comparisons are being made, and whether the groups have equal variance. The tests differ in how conservative they are, and the decision to use one test over another is often determined by the investigator. Multiple comparison methods are different from multiple $t$-tests in that the multiple comparison tests evaluate the groups in a pairwise fashion while controlling for multiple error rates, unlike what occurs with multiple $t$-tests.[7,14] Using the fever-reducing study, an ANOVA test could be used to identify that a difference exists between the three groups; however, a multiple comparison test may then be used to determine if the statistically significant difference occurred between an active medication and placebo or between the two active medications.

## SUMMARY

Inferential statistics allow for study results to be generalized to a larger population. Which statistical test to use depends on several factors, including the study hypothesis, the type of data being analyzed, the study design, and the presence of confounding variables. Correct interpretation and evaluation of outcome data for both statistical and clinical significance is paramount to making evidence-based recommendations to improve patient care.

## REFERENCES

1. DeMuth JE. Preparing for the first meeting with a statistician. *Am J Health-Syst Pharm*. 2008;65(24):2358-2366.
2. Anderson HG, Kendrach MG, Trice S. Understanding statistical and clinical significance: hypothesis testing. *J Pharm Pract*. 1998;11(3):181-195.
3. Gaddis GM, Gaddis ML. Introduction to biostatistics: part 3, sensitivity, specificity, predictive value, and hypothesis testing. *Ann Emerg Med*. 1990;19(5):591-597.
4. Braitman LE. Confidence intervals assess both clinical significance and statistical significance. *Ann Intern Med*. 1991;114(6):515-517.
5. Altman DG, Bland JM. Standard deviations and standard errors. *BMJ*. 2005;331(7521):903.
6. Lang TA, Secic M. *How to Report Statistics in Medicine*. Philadelphia, PA: BMJ Publishing Group; 1997.
7. DeMuth JE. *Basic Statistics and Pharmaceutical Statistical Applications*. 2nd ed. Boca Raton, FL: Chapman & Hall/CRC; 2006.

8. Gaddis GM, Gaddis ML. Introduction to biostatistics: part 4, statistical inference techniques in hypothesis testing. *Ann Emerg Med*. 1990;19(7):820-825.

9. DeMuth JE. Overview of biostatistics used in clinical research. *Am J Health-Syst Pharm*. 2009;66(1):70-81.

10. Qualls M, Pallin DJ, Schuur JD. Parametric versus nonparametric statistical tests: the length of stay example. *Acad Emerg Med*. 2010;17(10):1113-1121.

11. Gaddis ML, Gaddis GM. Introduction to biostatistics: part 1, basic concepts. *Ann Emerg Med*. 1990;19(1):86-89.

12. Pocock SJ, Assmann SE, Enos LE, Kasten LE. Subgroup analysis, covariate adjustment and baseline comparisons in clinical trial reporting: current practice and problems. *Stat Med*. 2002;21(19):2917-2930.

13. Gaddis GM, Gaddis ML. Introduction to biostatistics: part 5, statistical inference techniques for hypothesis testing with nonparametric data. *Ann Emerg Med*. 1990;19(9):1054-1059.

14. Elenbaas RM, Elenbaas JK, Cuddy PG. Evaluating the medical literature part II: statistical analysis. *Ann Emerg Med*. 1983;12(10):610-620.

# EPIDEMIOLOGY AND MEASURES OF ASSOCIATED RISK

**Allison Bernknopf, PharmD, BCPS**

## CHAPTER OBJECTIVES

▸ Define *epidemiology*, *pharmacoepidemiology*, *prevalence*, and *incidence*.

▸ Given a specific example or set of study data, explain the clinical and statistical significance of the following: odds ratio, relative risk, hazard ratio, absolute risk, number needed to treat, and number needed to harm.

▸ Given a specific example or set of study data, calculate the absolute risk difference, relative risk difference, number needed to treat, and number needed to harm.

## CHAPTER OUTLINE

## KEY TERMS

Absolute risk difference                            Number needed to treat
Incidence                                           Odds ratio
Incidence rate                                      Prevalence
Number needed to harm                               Relative risk

# INTRODUCTION

Epidemiology is the field of study that evaluates how diseases and health-related states are distributed and factors that can cause or affect diseases and health-related states.[1-3] Epidemiology studies are used to determine how diseases and conditions are spread, their risk factors, their course or presentation, and how they can be prevented or controlled.[1,2] Therefore, epidemiology is focused on public health as a whole rather than looking at the individual patient. One classic medical example is the Framingham Heart Study. This prospective epidemiological cohort study was started in 1948 to help understand the risk factors for developing cardiovascular disease (CVD).[4] This research led to the discovery of the common CVD risk factors that we now know today.

The reason the Framingham study was able to answer so many questions about CVD risk factors was due to the large number of patients who were included in the study. Answering these types of questions often requires a large sample of patients, sometimes tens of thousands, and several years of study. This is one of the biggest benefits of epidemiological studies. The manner in which these studies are conducted allows for large sample sizes and longer durations.

Due to the need for larger sample sizes and longer durations, much of the research done in epidemiology is observational in design. The three main observational study types used in epidemiology are cohort, case-control, and cross-sectional studies.[5,6] One main reason for this, as was the case with the Framingham study, is that sometimes investigators do not know exactly what they are looking for with some diseases or health-related states. Therefore, an observational design allows them to collect data on patients over long periods of time to identify the course a disease takes as well as risk factors associated with the development of the disease or its complications. Investigators cannot conduct a randomized controlled trial if they do not even know what factors are involved in the disease. Additionally, some questions just cannot be answered or are unethical to study in an experimental design. For example, suppose investigators want to find out if exposure to a toxin leads to the development of cancer. It would not be ethical to give the toxin to individuals if the investigators suspect it leads to cancer. They could, however, find a group of patients who were already exposed to the factor and then find a group of similar patients who were not exposed to the factor to determine if there were more cases of cancer in the exposed group compared to the nonexposed group.

Another large benefit of observational study designs is the cost savings associated with them.[5,6] Keeping in mind that such studies often require thousands to tens of thousands of patients and that it can sometimes take decades to answer these questions, it would be cost prohibitive to study these patients in an experimental design. Patient retention becomes more of an issue in experimental design than with observational design. This problem becomes more pronounced the longer patients are expected to be in the controlled environment of an experimental design than when the patients are simply being observed.

Epidemiology is a large field that has multiple subsets. One subset that is of particular interest to the pharmacy profession is pharmacoepidemiology. This area of epidemiology is focused on the study of medications (prescription and over the counter), vaccines, and medical devices for the diagnosis, treatment, and prevention of diseases on a public health scale.[2,7,8] Questions raised in this field of study are answered using the same principles that epidemiologists use. In other words, observational studies, rather than traditional experimental models, are the main study designs used. This area of epidemiology looks at questions like the following: Does vaccination lead to the development of autism? Is treatment with venlafaxine a risk factor for teratogenicity? Can vaccination lead to a decrease in the incidence of cancer? Although these questions could potentially be answered using traditional experimental study designs, pharmacoepidemiologists are generally concerned with looking at a more global, real-world setting.[8] This is why observational study designs are chosen to answer these questions.

The question of whether vaccinations lead to autism will be used to help explain why experimental designs will not realistically aid investigators in answering some of these questions. Vaccinations are used to help prevent communicable diseases, and it would be unethical to not give vaccinations to patients unless the patient or the patient's parents refuse vaccination. In order to determine if there is a difference in the number of patients with autism between those receiving a vaccination and those not receiving a vaccination, thousands of children over several years need to be viewed. The time and money constraints of conducting an experimental study would truly make this cost prohibitive. Therefore, the investigators can use already collected data or prospectively observe patients to answer a question that otherwise would have been impossible to address.

One major drawback of epidemiological research is the fact that it cannot be used to determine cause and effect.[1] Because researchers are only observing the patients and not controlling the exposure to the factor of interest, they cannot make any conclusions about cause and effect like they could if they were using an experimental study design. The Framingham study identified smoking, diabetes, and obesity, among others, as risk factors for the development of CVD. Because the Framingham study was only observing the patients and not controlling the environment, it is impossible to say if these risk factors actually cause CVD. The only thing that can be said for certain is that they are known to be linked to the development of CVD.

# MEASUREMENT IN EPIDEMIOLOGICAL STUDIES

Because the study designs used in epidemiological studies are observational, traditional statistical tests cannot be used to prove causation. Therefore, measures of risk and associations are used to answer clinical questions about diseases and conditions. The main measures of risk are relative risk, hazard ratio, odds ratio, absolute risk, and number needed to treat/harm. All of the measures discussed in this section can be used in experimental as well as observational study designs.

## Incidence and Prevalence

It is important to understand the difference between incidence and prevalence, because the two terms are often confused. **Incidence** is what is most often presented, and it usually represents the number of new cases of a disease, condition, or event that occur in a specific time frame (e.g., 1 year) in the individuals at risk for developing the new event, disease, or condition.[1,8] In other words, it represents the probability or likelihood that an individual will develop a new disease/condition or have a new event. Incidences are often used to track disease and event rates over the years, allowing researchers to see changes in new cases/events from year to year.[9] The Centers for Disease Control and Prevention (CDC) is a great resource to find incidences for various diseases and conditions over the years in the Unites States, and the World Health Organization (WHO) is a great resource for global incidences.

Incidence is sometimes presented as an **incidence rate** within a specified time frame. For example, the incidence rate may be presented as 25 cases per 1,000 person-years or 10 cases per 50 person-days.[8,9] This statistic is used when looking at patients who might have been observed over variable time periods within a study. For example, say that the study period is 10 years and the study followed 100,000 patients. If all of the patients complete the entire study, then that would be 1,000,000 person-years (10 years × 100,000 patients).[10] Because it is highly unlikely that all of the patients will be in the study for the entire 10 years, researchers will look at the person-years for the time patients spent in the study. In the end, the researchers may reach a total of 951,626 person-years.[10] They would tally the total number of patient-years by adding up how many years each patient was in the study. If patient 1 was in the study for 8 years, patient 2 was in the study for 3 years, and patient 3 was in the study for 8 years, then these three patients contributed 19 person-years to the study (1 × 3 years + 2 × 8 years). To continue this example, suppose there are 9,516 events over the 951,626 person-years. The incidence rate would be 0.01 events per person-year (9,516 ÷ 951,626).[10] Typically, this will be reported as 1,000 events per 100,000 person-years. This could be presented as a cumulative incidence by simply dividing the number of events by the number of patients (9,516 ÷ 100,000). Therefore, the incidence is reported as 0.09516, or 9.5%, over the 10-year period.

Prevalence is another way to look at diseases, conditions, and events. **Prevalence** looks at all of the cases or events in the population in a given time frame.[8,9] This allows researchers to look at an overall picture of the disease or condition rather than just looking at new cases/events. Prevalence is affected by the nature of the disease, meaning that diseases that become chronic or have a long duration will have a higher prevalence than those diseases that have a short duration. For example, one would expect the prevalence for diabetes to be higher than the prevalence for something like stress fractures because stress fractures are curable and typically not chronic.

One way to illustrate the difference between incidence rates and prevalence would be to look at the cases of HIV-infected patients in the United States. According to the CDC, it is estimated that there are ~50,000 new cases of HIV each year in the United States.[11] The prevalence, in contrast, was estimated at 1,148,200 patients infected with HIV in the United States at the end of 2009. This means that there were relatively few newer cases compared to the total number of cases of HIV-infected patients when looking at the same time period.

Although incidence rates and prevalence are good epidemiological markers, they do have their limitations. Some diseases are not easy to track; therefore, it is not always possible to figure out what the true incidence or prevalence of a disease is.[8,9] As with the HIV example, the CDC had to estimate what they believed were the missing diagnoses for patients, meaning that the prevalence of 1,148,200 patients infected with HIV included 207,600 patients who were estimated to have HIV but had yet to be diagnosed.[11] It is not always easy to capture patients who have HIV, because many patients at risk are not always tested. Researchers can also run into problems when tracking a disease over a number of years, particularly when the diagnostic criteria change. As the diagnostic criteria for a disease change, more patients often are diagnosed with a disease, condition, or event. Therefore, incidence rates and the prevalence could look much higher simply because clinicians' diagnostic abilities were not as good in years past rather than there being a true increase in the incidence or prevalence of the disease.

---

| **CASE STUDY 10-1** | **Identifying Incidence and Prevalence** |
|---|---|

Attention deficit hyperactivity disorder (ADHD) has been a growing problem in the United States. Looking at the national statistics reported in 2013, it is estimated that 5.9 million children between the ages of 3 and 17 in the United States have been diagnosed with ADHD, which represents roughly 9.5% of children in that age group. It has also been reported that 13.5% of boys and 5.4% of girls in the United States between the ages of 3 and 17 have been diagnosed with ADHD.

*Question*: Do these numbers represent the prevalence, incidence rates, or both of the disease?

*Answer*: These are the prevalence numbers for the disease. The numbers represent the percent of all children between the ages of 3 and 17 who have been diagnosed with ADHD. Because the focus is not just on new cases, this is the prevalence. If the case study had stated that 9.5% of children this age were newly diagnosed in 2012, then it would have been the incidence.

---

Data from FastStats: attention deficit hyperactivity disorder (ADHD). Centers for Disease Control and Prevention website. http://www.cdc.gov/nchs/fastats /adhd.htm. Updated February 28, 2014. Accessed March 13, 2014.

## MEASURES OF RISK IN EPIDEMIOLOGICAL STUDIES

Three main risk ratios are used in epidemiological studies: odds ratio (OR), relative risk (RR), and hazard ratio (HR).[8,9] Each is calculated by dividing the value in the exposed group by the value in the nonexposed (control) group (each risk ratio is explained in detail later on in the chapter). Another measure of risk that is often presented is the absolute risk. It differs from the relative risk because it is calculated by subtracting the true difference seen between the groups within the study, rather than creating a ratio of the exposed group to the treatment group. The definition of the absolute risk is presented later in the chapter, as well as a more detailed explanation of the difference between the relative and absolute risks. It is important to note that absolute risks are always smaller than the relative risks. This is why it is often more appealing for specific groups, particularly the pharmaceutical industry, to present the ratios rather than the true absolute difference between the groups.

## INTERPRETING RELATIVE RISKS, ODDS RATIOS, HAZARD RATIOS, AND ABSOLUTE RISKS

Risk ratios (including RR, OR, and HR) are calculated by creating a ratio of the exposed group to the nonexposed group.[8,9] This means that when the risks, odds, or hazards are the same in the exposed and nonexposed groups the result will be a value of 1. For example, if the odds of having the outcome occur in the exposed group is 0.5 and the odds in the nonexposed group is also 0.5, then the odds ratio will be 1 (0.5 ÷ 0.5). This means that when dealing with a ratio, 1 is the starting point. Anything less than 1 means that the odds, risk, or hazard of the event occurring are decreased, and anything greater than 1 means that the odds, risk, or hazard of the event occurring are increased.

Absolute risks are interpreted differently from risk ratios because they look at the absolute difference between groups.[8,9,12] To find the absolute difference, we need to subtract the incidence of the event occurring in the exposed group from that of the nonexposed group. This means that when the incidence in the exposed group is equal to the incidence in the nonexposed group, the result is a value of 0. For example, if the incidence is 0.4 in the exposed group and 0.4 in the nonexposed group, the absolute difference will be 0 (0.4 − 0.4). The absolute risk is always going to range between 0 and 1, and the closer the risk is to 0, the smaller the difference between the exposed and nonexposed groups.

It is very important to note the differences in interpreting ratios and absolute risks. These measures are often presented with a 95% confidence interval (CI).[8,9,12] The confidence interval is very useful in determining the statistical and clinical significance of the ratio or absolute risk. For the ratio values (OR, RR, and HR), 1 is the marker in the CI, whereas with an absolute risk it is 0. This means that the 95% CI should not include (or cross) 1 for the risk ratios and 0 for the absolute risks. If the CI crosses 1 for the risk ratios or 0 for the absolute risks, then it means that the result is not statistically significant because the possibility exists that there is no difference between the groups. For example, a study reports an OR of 1.67 (95% CI: 0.97 to 1.98). Here, the OR is > 1, but the 95% CI crosses 1, so the results should not be considered statistically significant because the possibility exists that there is no true difference in the odds of having the outcome occur between the groups. Another example is an absolute risk of 0.2 (95% CI: 0 to 0.4). Again this would not be statistically significant because 0 is in the CI, signifying that there is the possibility that there is no difference between the incidence of an event occurring in the exposed and the nonexposed groups.

## Relative Risk

The **relative risk** (RR) is a statistic that looks at the risk of an event (or incidence) occurring in an exposed group compared to the control group.[8,9,12] The RR is sometimes referred to as the *risk ratio*. The RR is an easy statistic for most individuals to interpret because it deals with probabilities. In order to calculate the RR, the incidence rate must be calculated in order for it to be a meaningful statistic.[12,13] Therefore, a prospective study design must be used because the researchers need to start with exposure to ensure that they are identifying new occurrences (i.e., the patients did not have the outcome prior to exposure). It is important to note that the term *prospective* here means that the researchers are starting with exposure and looking forward to see whether an outcome occurred. This means that researchers can use RR in a retrospective cohort study because they are starting with patients exposed or not exposed to a factor and looking forward in their records to see if the patients have had an outcome occur. In other words, an RR can be used in a retrospective cohort because the patients will not have had the outcome prior to the exposure. In a purely retrospective study (e.g., case-control), the researchers cannot be sure that the outcome did not precede the exposure because they are starting with the outcome of interest.

An RR < 1 means that there is a decreased risk of the event occurring, meaning that there is a relative risk reduction (RRR).[8,12] Because 1 is the no difference point, RR can be subtracted from 1 to get the RRR. Suppose researchers conducted a study to look at drug Z's ability to decrease the risk of cancer. They find that the RR is 0.82 with a 95% CI of 0.68 to 0.98. This means that with drug Z, the risk of developing cancer decreased by 18% (RRR = 1 − 0.82) compared to those who did not receive drug Z. Because the CI does not include 1, then the results are statistically significant and, as indicated by the range of possible values given in the 95% CI, the risk could decrease by as little as 2% up to as much as 32%.

An RR > 1 means that the risk of the event occurring has increased; that is, there has been a relative risk increase (RRI).[8,12] Again looking at 1 as the no difference mark, the RRI can be calculated by subtracting 1 from the absolute risk increase (ARI). For example, in conducting a study to see if drug Y can increase the risk of gastric cancer, researchers find an RR of 1.69 with a 95% CI of 1.07 to 1.92. This means that exposure to drug Y has increased the risk of developing gastric cancer by 69% (RRI = 1.69 − 1) compared to those who did not receive drug Y. The CI does not include 1, which means that it is statistically significant. It also shows that the risk of developing gastric cancer can be increased by as little as 7% and as much as 92%.

It is very important to look at the endpoint to ensure correct interpretation of the RR. In the gastric cancer example, the development of the cancer is a negative effect. Therefore, seeing an increased RR is actually a bad, not a good, outcome. However, sometimes an RR > 1 can be a very positive thing. For example, in a study on patients with leukemia, the endpoint is the number of patients who reach remission status. The investigators are hoping to have a larger number of patients in the drug Z group who have remission when compared to those not exposed to drug Z. In this case, an RR > 1 is a good thing because it means that there is an increased risk that patients receiving drug Z will actually reach remission. An RR < 1 in this case would be a bad thing, because it would mean that with drug Z, there is a decreased risk that patients will reach remission. Therefore, it is important to always look at the endpoint in order to determine the true clinical meaning of the results. One cannot simply say that an RR > 1 is a bad thing and an RR < 1 is a good thing. The endpoint that is being measured is going to determine if an RR > 1 is a bad thing or a good thing.

## Odds Ratio

As noted in the RR section, the **odds ratio** (OR) is a statistic that is mainly used in a case-control study when it is not possible to calculate a relative risk.[8,9] The OR is calculated by dividing the odds of having the outcome in the exposed group by the odds of having the outcome in the control group. An OR < 1 means that the odds of the outcome occurring with exposure compared to the control group are decreased, whereas an OR > 1 means that the odds of the outcome occurring are increased. Look carefully at the outcome to determine if it is desirable for the OR to be increased or decreased. If researchers suspect that a toxin is associated with the development of cancer, then they would expect to see an OR > 1. However, if they are trying to see if treating obesity can prevent the development of diabetes, then they would want to see an OR < 1.

The OR and RR are interpreted very differently. An OR of 2 means that those who were exposed to the factor had two times the odds of having the outcome compared to those who were not exposed. A big thing to note here is that one cannot say that the risk was increased, because the OR deals with odds, not risks or likelihoods. The OR is much better at estimating the RR when the control event is rare (< 10%) and the OR is between 0.5 and 2.5.[8] An OR < 0.5 will generally underestimate the RR and an OR > 2.5 will generally overestimate the RR if the incidence is > 10%.

**Tables 10-1** and **10-2** each provide three hypothetical examples in order to illustrate this point. The major difference in the three studies in each table is the baseline incidence rate (the rate in the placebo group), which will demonstrate how the OR and RR will start to diverge as the outcome being examined has a higher incidence.

As shown in the tables, when the baseline incidence rate of an event occurring begins to increase, the disparity between the OR and RR will increase. Experiment 1 in Table 10-1 shows that when the baseline incidence rate is 8% (1,200 placebo patients with the outcome ÷ 15,000 total placebo patients), the difference between the OR and RR is relatively minor (0.02). However, in experiment 3 there is a baseline incidence of 70% (14,000 placebo patients with the outcome ÷ 20,000 total placebo patients), and the disparity between the OR and RR is larger (0.14). This same trend can also be seen in Table 10-2 when there is an increase in the OR and RR. With an increased OR and RR, the disparity is often wider compared to a decreased OR and RR, as seen by looking at experiment 3 in both tables. Looking at experiment 3 in Table 10-1, there is only a difference of 0.14 between the OR and RR compared to a difference of 1.7 when looking at experiment 3 in Table 10-2. This shows that the disparity between the OR and RR is often more exaggerated when looking at an increased risk compared to a decreased risk.

Logistic regression can be used to calculate an OR. This can be very useful when adjusting for confounding variables. To determine if a drug can decrease the risk of developing diabetes, researchers would need to account for factors such as age and the presence of other disease states, such as hypertension. This is often why a prospective study might include an OR rather than an RR. Epidemiological studies often deal with larger sample sizes. However, some studies, such as those investigating rare diseases, might use smaller sample sizes. In these instances of small to moderate sample sizes, errors in the logistic regression may occur, causing overestimation of the true effect.

**TABLE 10-1**   Three Prospective Studies Showing Positive Benefits of a Drug with Varying Incidence Rates

**Experiment 1: Chronic Obstructive Pulmonary Disease (COPD)**

|  | Number of Patients Diagnosed with COPD | Number of Patients Not Diagnosed with COPD | Total Number of Patients | OR | RR |
|---|---|---|---|---|---|
| Drug group | 300 | 14,700 | 15,000 | 0.23 | 0.25 |
| Placebo group | 1,200 | 13,800 | 15,000 | | |

**Experiment 2: Heart Failure (HF)**

|  | Number of Patients Diagnosed with HF | Number of Patients Not Diagnosed with HF | Total Number of Patients | OR | RR |
|---|---|---|---|---|---|
| Drug group | 1,400 | 8,600 | 10,000 | 0.65 | 0.7 |
| Placebo group | 2,000 | 8,000 | 10,000 | | |

**Experiment 3: Diabetes (DM)**

|  | Number of Patients Diagnosed with DM | Number of Patients Not Diagnosed with DM | Total Number of Patients | OR | RR |
|---|---|---|---|---|---|
| Drug group | 8,000 | 13,200 | 20,000 | 0.43 | 0.57 |
| Placebo group | 14,000 | 10,000 | 20,000 | | |

**TABLE 10-2** Three Prospective Studies Showing Adverse Reactions to a Drug with Varying Incidence Rates

**Experiment 1: Bleeding Episode (BE)**

| | Number of Patients with BE | Number of patients without BE | Total Number of Patients | OR | RR |
|---|---|---|---|---|---|
| Drug group | 800 | 9,200 | 10,000 | 4.3 | 4 |
| Placebo group | 200 | 9,800 | 10,000 | | |

**Experiment 2: Constipation**

| | Number of Patients with Constipation | Number of Patients without Constipation | Total Number of Patients | OR | RR |
|---|---|---|---|---|---|
| Drug group | 6,800 | 13,200 | 20,000 | 2.1 | 1.7 |
| Placebo group | 4,000 | 16,000 | 20,000 | | |

**Experiment 3: Severe Nausea (SN)**

| | Number of Patients with SN | Number of Patients without SN | Total Number of Patients | OR | RR |
|---|---|---|---|---|---|
| Drug group | 21,000 | 9,000 | 30,000 | 3.5 | 1.8 |
| Placebo group | 12,000 | 18,000 | 30,000 | | |

Statistical methods are available that can account for this overestimation, but they are not employed very often. Therefore, it is important to note that with smaller sample sizes, the OR may be an overestimation of the true effect.[14]

## Hazard Ratio

The hazard ratio (HR) is a measure used in survival analysis.[5,8] The HR takes into account the risk of an individual having an event given that the patient has not had an event up to a specific point in time. The HR is most commonly calculated using the Cox proportional hazards model and is typically reported in survival analysis studies. A survival analysis is a type of analysis that looks at patients over a given period of time to assess the risk that a patient will have an event. In many instances, survival means that the patient has not had the outcome of interest (e.g., death, myocardial infarction, stroke, etc.). When a patient has an event, it is documented on the survival plot, so the number of patients who have survived in the study without having an event up to that point will decrease. In other cases, survival may be measured in a slightly different manner. In some instances, researchers are interested in how long it will take for a patient to have a positive outcome, such as time to resolution of an infection for an anti-infective agent. Therefore, it is very important to look at what the endpoint is to determine if an increased HR is a positive result (e.g., an increased HR for resolution of an infection) or a negative result (e.g., an increased HR for a drug leading to death).

Survival analyses often have some sort of plotting of patient survival throughout the course of the study. The most common form of survival plotting is the Kaplan-Meier plot, because it can be used to measure exactly when each patient reaches an event.[5] These survival curves are a very useful visual representation of how patients survive throughout the course of a study. Statistical testing must be performed to determine if the data are statistically different from each other. Regression and the Cox proportional hazards model are two common statistical methods that researchers use to determine if the survival curves between the treatment and control groups are significantly different from each other.

## Absolute Risk Differences

The **absolute risk difference** (ARD) is the actual risk difference between the groups and can be found by subtracting the proportion of patients in the exposed group with the outcome from the proportion of patients in the nonexposed group with the outcome.[8,9,12] Another way of stating this is that the ARD is the difference between the incidence in the exposure group and the incidence in the control group.[8] An ARD can be classified as an absolute risk increase (ARI) or an absolute risk reduction (ARR).

The no difference marker for an ARD is 0, because it is calculated by subtracting the difference in the incidence rates between groups.[12] This means that if the risk is the same in the exposure group and the control group, then the difference between the groups will be 0. The absolute difference is generally presented as a positive (or absolute) number. If the exposure group has a smaller proportion of patients having the outcome, then there is a decrease in the risk of the outcome occurring, or an ARR. If the exposure group has a larger proportion of patients having the outcome, then there is an increase in the risk of the outcome occurring, or an ARI.

It is very important to know the outcome that is being measured when interpreting the ARD. In most instances, an ARR is dealing with prevention of a bad thing, and an ARI is dealing with an increase in harm. In some instances, however, an ARI can be viewed as a good thing. For example, if researchers are looking at a new medication to treat ulcerative colitis, one of their outcomes might be the number of patients who have reached remission. In this case, they would want the exposure group (those receiving the new medication) to have a higher incidence than the control group. In other words, they have increased the risk of a patient reaching remission, which is a good thing.

Sometimes the ARD is presented with a 95% CI.[12] When looking at the CI, make sure that it does not cross 0. Remember that 0 means that there is no difference between the groups. A CI that crosses 0 means that the possibility exists that there is no true difference between the exposure and nonexposure groups. As an example, say that researchers are trying to determine if drug A decreases the risk of developing diabetes compared to those not receiving drug A. The results show an ARR of 0.36 with a 95% CI of 0.19 to 0.58. This means that patients who receive drug A have a 36% decreased risk of developing diabetes compared to those who did not receive drug A. Because the 95% CI does not include 0, then the result is statistically significant, and the risk of developing diabetes could be decreased by as little as 19% up to as much as 58% if patients receive drug A compared to receiving no treatment.

## Absolute Risk Difference Versus Relative Risk Difference

The ARD and the relative risk difference (RRD), which can be either an absolute or relative risk increase or reduction, are both valid statistics when looking at risks. However, differences emerge when one begins to compare an ARD to an RRD. This becomes obvious when there is a difference when outcomes are rare compared to when they are common.[15] An RRD can remain constant when the incidence rates are lower or higher, whereas the ARD can be greatly affected. **Table 10-3** shows the results from three hypothetical studies looking at the prevention of cancer.[12] The studies have the same RRDs, but their ARDs are clearly different.

| | Control Group Incidence | Exposure Group Incidence | ARD | RRD |
|---|---|---|---|---|
| **TABLE 10-3** Comparing the ARD and RRD | | | | |
| Study 1 | 30% | 15% | 15% | 50% |
| Study 2 | 2% | 1% | 1% | 50% |
| Study 3 | 50% | 25% | 25% | 50% |

Data from Schechtman E. Odds ratio, relative risk, absolute risk reduction, and the number needed to treat—which of these should we use? *Value Health.* 2002;5(5):431-436.

Due to the nature of calculating an ARD and an RRD, the RRD will always be a larger number. Therefore, pharmaceutical companies generally provide the RRR rather than the ARD because this makes their drug appear to work better. On the flip side, you will generally not see pharmaceutical companies present the RRI because it always makes the drug look worse in terms of adverse reactions. The RRD is often presented in clinical trials as well. It is important to calculate an ARD when the authors present the number or proportion of patients experiencing the particular outcome. The ARD provides a better clinical representation of the data so that the information can be applied in a more clinically meaningful way than an RRD will. Not only does the ARD give the true difference between the groups, it is also the type of difference that is used to calculate the number needed to treat/harm.

## NUMBER NEEDED TO TREAT OR HARM

The number needed to treat (NNT) and the number needed to harm (NNH) are ways to look at the number of patients who need to be treated to see a benefit or be harmed.[8] They are calculated by taking the inverse of the ARD. It is important to keep in mind that these are simply average estimates to give the clinician an idea of approximately how many patients will need to be treated to see benefit or be harmed given the specific conditions of the study.

### Number Needed to Treat

The **number needed to treat** (NNT) is the number of patients who need to be treated for a specific period of time with the intervention being studied in order for one patient to have a positive outcome or to prevent one patient from having a negative outcome.[9,15] The NNT is calculated by taking the inverse of the ARR when attempting to prevent a bad event from occurring or the ARI when dealing with a positive outcome.

### Number Needed to Harm

The **number needed to harm** (NNH) is the number of patients who need to be treated with a particular intervention over a particular period of time to see one patient harmed. Typically, NNH is used to look at adverse reactions to a medication or intervention.[9] The NNH is calculated by taking the inverse of the ARI when looking at the occurrence of harmful events.

### Interpreting the Number Needed to Treat and the Number Needed to Harm

The confidence interval of the NNT or NNH can be calculated by using the confidence interval of the ARD.[12] The inverse of the upper and lower limits of the ARD confidence interval are used to derive the upper and lower limits of the NNT or NNH confidence interval. It is important to look at the statistical significance of the ARD before calculating the NNT or NNH, because the NNT or NNH becomes a useless statistic when the ARD is not statistically significant. In those instances, the NNT or NNH may be a very good number, but the confidence interval may be extremely wide or have infinity as an upper or lower limit. This is because the inverse of 0 is infinity. The key here is that if the ARD is not statistically significant, then there is no need to calculate the NNT or NNH.

Ideally, the NNT should be as small as possible for both positive outcomes and preventing negative outcomes.[8] An NNT of 10 means that for every 10 patients treated, 1 patient will have a positive outcome or have a negative outcome prevented. In contrast, the NNH should be as large as possible because negative outcomes are undesirable. An NNH of 250 means that for every 250 patients treated, 1 patient will be harmed. It is important to examine what the harm actually is to determine if the harm can be lower. For example, nausea is a common adverse reaction for many medications and is often tolerable for many patients. Therefore, the NNH might be low because it is a frequent adverse reaction. If, however, the drug caused nausea that was so severe that patients had to stop taking the medication, then a lower NNH would be a problem. In this case, a low NNH would mean that more patients would have to stop taking the medication.

It is also important to look at the NNT compared to the NNH for an individual drug. Ideally, it is desirable to have a very low NNT with a very high NNH, especially for more serious adverse reactions. For example, say that a new drug has an NNT of 5 and an NNH of 250. This means that for every 1,000 patients treated with this drug, 200 will see a benefit while only 4 will be harmed.

To correctly interpret the NNT or NNH, it is important to consider the NNT and the NNH within the context of study. For example, say that a new cohort study seeks to determine if drug X is linked to an increase in the risk of death in a 5-year time period compared to a control group (those not receiving drug X). The NNH is calculated to be 50. This means that for every 50 patients treated with drug X during the 5-year period, 1 patient will die. The context is especially important when comparing an NNT or NNH across studies. An NNT of 4 in a 24-week study is different from an NNT of 4 in a 52-week study.

If possible, clinicians should set a comfort level when looking at the NNT or NNH.[15] In other words, how many patients are they willing to treat to see a benefit in one patient? In coming up with this number, clinicians should consider the following: how common the disease/event is; how many patients the practice sees on an annual (or other time unit) basis; what other treatment options are available; how much harm they are willing to accept; the cost of the medication; and the potential adverse events that can occur with the medication.

### Advantages and Disadvantages of the Different Measures of Risk

Each of the different risk measures has advantages and disadvantages. Often it is best to look at more than one of these measures within a study. This will generally require the calculation of one or more of the statistics. See **Table 10-4** for a comparison of the different measures of associated risk.[8,12,16]

## WHAT MEASURE OF ASSOCIATED RISK SHOULD BE PRESENTED?

As noted earlier in the chapter, in some instances investigators are limited in what they can present. Many of the measures described in this chapter cannot be used with

**TABLE 10-4** Advantages and Disadvantages of Risk Measures

| Measure of Risk | Advantages | Disadvantages |
|---|---|---|
| Relative risk | • Easy to interpret/understand<br>• Easy to calculate | • Loss of magnitude (i.e., unable to account for large and small differences between the groups)<br>• Cannot be used in case-control studies<br>• Hard to account for confounding variables |
| Odds ratio | • Can be used in retrospective or prospective studies<br>• Easier than an RR to account for confounding variables by using logistic regression | • Often mistakenly interpreted as an RR<br>• Can overestimate or underestimate the RR when the incidence is common (> 10%) and the further away from 1 it becomes |
| Absolute risk difference | • Easy to understand and calculate<br>• Includes underlying risk (measured by the control group)<br>• Can be used to calculate the RRD when an actual RR has not been calculated | • Hard to account for confounding variables<br>• Hard to compare across studies due to differences in baseline risk between samples |
| Number needed to treat and number needed to harm | • Can help give clinical meaning to the data<br>• Easy to calculate | • Can be misinterpreted<br>• Sometimes hard to compare across studies due to differences in methodology |

Data from Quartey G, Wang J, Kim J. A review of risk measures in pharmacoepidemiology with tips for statisticians in the pharmaceutical industry. *Pharm Stat.* 2011;10(6):548-553; Schechtman E. Odds ratio, relative risk, absolute risk reduction, and the number needed to treat—which of these should we use? *Value Health.* 2002;5(5):431-436; and Simon SD. Understanding the odds ratio and the relative risk. *J Androl.* 2001;22(4):533-536.

a retrospective study design. Retrospective studies will often use an OR. When evaluating prospective studies, it is important to look at the data in a number of different ways, regardless of how the authors present the information. In most studies where an RR is presented, incidence rates will be provided or the necessary data will be available to calculate them. It is important to look at the incidence rates and not just rely on the RR.

One clear example as to why one should not just rely on a single statistic comes from a study looking to see if how data are presented can influence health policy decisions.[17] Questionnaires were sent to 180 members of health authorities, health commissions, and family health services in the United Kingdom. Data from one clinical trial on efficacy of breast cancer screening and a systematic review of cardiac rehabilitation were presented as four different options. Option A presented RRRs, option B presented ARRs, option C presented incidence rates, and option D presented NNTs. Respondents were asked to rate which of the four options they would support for each program (breast cancer and cardiac rehabilitation) and were asked not to compare the different options to each other. In other words, they were asked to just look at the data for option A and rate how likely they would be to support the program, then look at the data for option B and determine how likely they would be to support the program, and so on. The response rate for completed questionnaires was 77.8%. The authors found that there was a statistically significant difference in how support for the program was rated based on the different ways the data were presented ($p < 0.001$). Support for the options with the RRRs was higher than the other data representations, followed by NNTs. Interestingly, only three respondents (2%) noticed that the different options were really just four different ways of representing the same results.

This study shows that there can be a huge impact in how the effectiveness and/or harm of an intervention or exposure can be interpreted and the level of care that should be exercised when clinicians evaluate clinical trial results. An intervention may be accepted or rejected simply because the data were presented in one manner rather than looking at the data from different perspectives. Although this study was done in the United Kingdom, it has implications in the United States as well. Direct-to-consumer advertisements are permitted in the United States, and pharmaceutical companies take full advantage of this. Sales representatives, news reports, and direct-to-consumer advertisements often present information in the form of RRD. As noted earlier in the chapter, the RRD is often larger than the ARD, and in some instances much larger. This can potentially make the medication look much more appealing than if the ARD and/or NNT were presented. When reviewing research reports or other information, it is important to consider what type of risk is being presented and how else these data can be used to provide a more global picture. This will often require some additional calculations, but the value they provide will be worth the time it takes to make them.

Another interesting thing to note with regard to presentation of data is the adverse effects of an intervention. The incidence rates or the ARIs are often given for adverse reactions rather than RRIs. This is because the RRIs are inflated compared to the ARIs, and it will make the intervention look worse. The key here is to make sure to look at the data in multiple ways when possible to develop a more well-rounded perspective.

---

## CASE STUDY 10-2    What Measure of Risk Should I Report?

You are reviewing a study for your journal club presentation.* The goal of the study was to determine if a proton pump inhibitor (PPI) will prevent stress ulcers better than $H_2$-antagoists in patients in the intensive care unit (ICU) on a ventilator. To study this, the authors identified all patients in the ICU on a ventilator who received a PPI between 2005 and 2009 and a group of similar patients who received a $H_2$-antagonist during the same period. The researchers then looked to see how many patients developed ulcers after receiving the prophylaxis therapy with the PPI or the $H_2$-antagonist. The researchers found that the odds ratio (OR) was 0.86 (95% CI: 0.73 to 0.98).

*Question*: Did the authors present the most appropriate statistic?

*Answer*: In this case, the authors could have potentially reported a relative risk (RR) because the study was prospective in nature. This is a retrospective cohort, and because they started with the exposure, we would know that the patients in the study did not have the ulcer before exposure. That being said, it is not wrong to present the OR. You can always present an OR, and if the authors used a logistic regression to run the statistics, then they would have to report an OR because that is the statistic that comes out of the logistic regression, not an RR.

*Question*: How would you interpret this OR? Is the result statistically significant?

*Answer*: The OR shows that the odds of having an ulcer for patients receiving a PPI were lower than those who received a $H_2$-antagonist. Specifically, the odds were 0.86:1. The result is statistically significant because although the upper limit was close to 1, the confidence interval does not include 1.

---

*Note: The data in this case are fictitious.

| **TABLE 10-5** Contingency Table for Calculating Measures of Associated Risk | | | |
|---|---|---|---|
| | **Number of Patients Experiencing an Event** | **Number of Patients Not Experiencing an Event** | **Total Number of Patients** |
| Exposed group | *a* | *b* | *a + b* |
| Nonexposed (control) group | *c* | *d* | *c + d* |
| Totals | *a + c* | *b + d* | *a + b + c + d* |

Data from Sackett DL, Staus SE, Richardson WS, Rosenberg W, Haynes RB. *Evidence-Based Medicine: How to Practice and Teach EBM*. 2nd ed. New York, NY: Churchill Livingstone; 2001.

# BALANCING BENEFITS AND HARM

It is very important to keep in mind that the statistics presented in this chapter should always be used as part of a risks/benefits assessment and not solely by themselves. This can become a very complicated problem, especially when there are different patients who have different risks of outcomes occurring. For example, say that a clinician is trying to determine the treatment benefit of giving patients a medication for 3 years to prevent a stroke from occurring (e.g., an anticoagulant for patients with atrial fibrillation). Patient 1 has a baseline risk of 3% (low risk) for developing a stroke compared to a 30% risk for patient 2 (high risk) if neither of them had received treatment.[15] If both patients receive the 3-year course of therapy, then patient 1 will have a 1% risk of having a stroke, whereas patient 2 will have a 20% risk of having a stroke (ARR: 1% and 10%, respectively). Digging further, the clinician finds out that both patients have a 0.6% risk of having an episode of severe gastric bleeding over a 3-year treatment period with the medication. For patient 1, the benefit of having a stroke reduction and bleeding risk are fairly close to each other. Patient 2, however, has a much larger difference in the stroke risk reduction and the risk of a severe gastric bleeding event. Therefore, the clinician is much more inclined to recommend the treatment for patient 2 than for patient 1.

## CALCULATING RISK MEASURES

Calculating these statistics requires correct interpretation of the data. The OR can be calculated for data from both retrospective and prospective studies, but the other statistics require prospective data.

The statistics can be calculated using the information from **Table 10–5**:[18]

OR = $(a \div b) \div (c \div d) = ad \div bc$
Event rate control group = $c \div (c + d)$
Event rate exposure group = $a \div (a + b)$
RR = Event rate exposure group ÷ Event rate control group
ARD = |Event rate exposure group − Event rate control group|
NNT or NNH = 1 ÷ ARD
RRD = 1 − RR (an alternative way to calculate the RRD = ARD ÷ Event rate control group)

| CASE STUDY 10-3 | Interpreting Risk Reduction and Number Needed to Treat |

You are reviewing data from a pharmaceutical company that is marketing two new medications.

**Experiment 1: Miracle Drug 1000 Versus Placebo for Breast Cancer**

| | Number of Patients with Breast Cancer | Number of Patients without Breast Cancer | Total |
|---|---|---|---|
| Miracle Drug 1000 | 140 | 220 | 360 |
| Placebo | 179 | 179 | 358 |

**Experiment 2: Miracle Drug 2000 Versus Placebo for Prostate Cancer**

| | Number of Patients with Prostate Cancer | Number of Patients without Prostate Cancer | Total |
|---|---|---|---|
| Miracle Drug 2000 | 14 | 346 | 360 |
| Placebo | 18 | 340 | 358 |

*Question*: What are the absolute and relative risk reductions, odds ratios, and relative risks?

*Answer*:

**Evidence Rates, Absolute Risk Reductions, Relative Risk Reductions, Odds Ratios, and Risk Ratios for Experiments 1 and 2**

| | Event Rate | ARR | RRR | OR | RR |
|---|---|---|---|---|---|
| Experiment 1 | Placebo: $179 \div 358 = 0.5$ Drug: $140 \div 360 = 0.39$ | $0.5 - 0.39 = 0.11$ | $0.11 \div 0.39 = 0.2$ Alt Cal: $1 - 0.78 = 0.22$ | $(140 \times 179)$ $\div (179 \times 220)$ $= 0.64$ | $0.39 \div 0.5$ $= 0.78$ |
| Experiment 2 | Placebo: $18 \div 358 = 0.05$ Drug: $14 \div 360 = 0.039$ | $0.05 - 0.039 = 0.011$ | $0.011 \div 0.039 = 0.2$ Alt cal: $1 - 0.78 = 0.22$ | $(14 \times 340)$ $\div (18 \times 346)$ $= 0.76$ | $0.039 \div 0.05$ $= 0.78$ |

*Question*: Why does experiment 1 have a difference between the OR and RR and experiment 2 has a similar OR and RR?

*Answer*: The reason there is a difference between the two experiments is the baseline risk. In experiment 2, the occurrence of prostate cancer in the placebo group is rare (< 10%), but in experiment 1, the occurrence of breast cancer in the control group is not rare (> 10%). As the baseline risk (the incidence in the control group, in this case the placebo group) increases, the OR and RR start to get farther apart. In experiment 2, if we calculate an OR, then we need to definitely speak in terms of odds, because the OR is an overestimate of the RR. In experiment 1, if we calculated the OR, then we could treat it like an RR, because we can see that it closely represents the risk.

*Question*: You are watching a news report on the results of these studies that reports that both miracle drugs reduced their respective cancers by the same percentage (20%). Did they report the correct data? Would you report the data in this manner?

*Answer*: The data are correctly reported because the relative risk reduction for each of the experiments was 0.2, which is 20%. Although factually correct, clinically it is misleading. The relative risk reduction does not show the magnitude of the difference between the two groups. When looking at the true difference between the groups, we see that Miracle Drug 1000 was able to decrease the risk of breast cancer by 11%, whereas Miracle Drug 2000 was only able to decrease the risk of prostate cancer by 1.1%. From a pure efficacy standpoint, we can be comfortable recommending Miracle Drug 1000 but not Miracle Drug 2000.

*Question*: What is the NNT for experiment 1? Describe in words what it means.

*Answer*: NNT = $1 \div 0.11 = 9$. This means that for every 9 patients we treat with Miracle Drug 1000 instead of placebo, we will prevent 1 patient from developing breast cancer. We can also say that for every 100 patients we treat with Miracle Drug 1000 instead of placebo, we will prevent breast cancer from occurring in 11 patients, and for every 1,000 patients we can prevent 111 patients from developing breast cancer.

# SUMMARY

Epidemiology is the field of study that seeks to describe diseases and conditions. Pharmacoepidemiology is a type of epidemiology that focuses on medications, vaccines, and medical devices. Most of the study designs in epidemiology are observational and are focused on answering population-level medical questions. The common statistics used to measure associated risk include RR, OR, HR, ARD, NNT, and NNH. These should be interpreted in the context of the study constraints. They should also be part of the risk/benefit assessment to help clinicians make appropriate decisions about medical care.

# REFERENCES

1. Hennekens CH, Burning JE. *Epidemiology in Medicine.* Boston, MA: Little, Brown & Company; 1987.
2. Waning B, Montagne M. *Pharmacoepidemiology: Principles and Practice.* New York, NY: McGraw-Hill; 2001.
3. Health topics: epidemiology. World Health Organization website. http://www.who.int/topics/epidemiology/en/. Accessed July 21, 2014.
4. History of the Framingham Heart Study. Framingham Heart Study website. http://www.framinghamheartstudy.org/about-fhs/history.php. Accessed July 21, 2014.
5. Szklo M, Nieto FJ. *Epidemiology: Beyond the Basics.* Gaithersburg, MD: Aspen Publishers; 2000.
6. Friis RH, Sellers TA. *Epidemiology for Public Health Practice.* 2nd ed. Gaithersburg, MD: Aspen Publishers; 1999.
7. Pharmacoepidemiology research. UNC Gillings School of Global Public Health website. http://sph.unc.edu/epid/epidemiology-research/pharmacoepidemiology-research/. Accessed July 21, 2014.
8. Quartey G, Wang J, Kim J. A review of risk measures in pharmacoepidemiology with tips for statisticians in the pharmaceutical industry. *Pharm Stat.* 2011;10(6):548-553.
9. Kier KL. Biostatistical applications in epidemiology. *Pharmacotherapy.* 2011;31(1):9-22.
10. Pearce N. What does the odds ratio estimate in a case-control study? *Int J Epidemiol.* 1993;22(6):1189-1192.
11. HIV/AIDS basic statistics. Centers for Disease Control and Prevention website. http://www.cdc.gov/hiv/topics/surveillance/basic.htm. Accessed July 21, 2014.
12. Schechtman E. Odds ratio, relative risk, absolute risk reduction, and the number needed to treat—which of these should we use? *Value Health.* 2002;5(5):431-436.
13. Schmidt CO, Kohlmann T. When to use the odds ratio or the relative risk? *Int J Public Health.* 2008;53(3):165-167.
14. Nemes S, Jonasson JM, Genell A, Steineck G. Bias in odds ratios by logistic regression modeling and sample size. *BMC Med Res Methodol.* 2009;9:56. doi: 10.1186/1471-2288-9-56.
15. Barratt A, Wyer PC, Hatala R, et al. Tips for learners of evidence-based medicine: 1. relative risk reduction, absolute risk reduction and number needed to treat. *CMAJ.* 2004;171(4):353-358.
16. Simon SD. Understanding the odds ratio and the relative risk. *J Androl.* 2001;22(4):533-536.
17. Fahey T, Griffiths S, Peters TJ. Evidence based purchasing: understanding results of clinical trials and systematic reviews. *BMJ.* 1995;311(7012):1056-1060.
18. Sackett DL, Staus SE, Richardson WS, Rosenberg W, Haynes RB. *Evidence-Based Medicine: How to Practice and Teach EBM.* 2nd ed. New York, NY: Churchill Livingstone; 2001.

CHAPTER 11

# CORRELATION AND REGRESSION

Joan Stachnik, MEd, PharmD, BCPS

## CHAPTER OBJECTIVES

- Define *correlation* and *regression*.
- Interpret a correlation coefficient and a coefficient of determination.
- Estimate the strength of a correlation between two variables from a scatterplot.
- Define the various types of regression.
- For a given set of data, select the most appropriate type of regression.
- For a given set of data and regression coefficients, develop a regression model and interpret the results.

# CHAPTER OUTLINE

# KEY TERMS

Coefficient of determination

Correlation

Correlation coefficient

Covariance

Regression

Regression coefficient

Regression model

Scatterplot

Standardized regression coefficient

Variance

$y$-intercept

# INTRODUCTION

The statistical analysis of data is an important aspect of clinical research in that it can allow an investigator to make generalizations or inferences from data obtained from a sample to a population of interest.[1] As part of these inferences, data analysis often includes a measure of the relationship between two or more variables. The type of analysis done depends, in part, on the type of data under consideration. Relationships between categorical or binary data types—data that are quantified as counts or frequencies of an event—can be examined using measures of comparative risk, such as the odds ratio and relative risk.[2,3] These measures provide information as to the changes in the risk of an outcome with an exposure versus no exposure.[3] For higher data types—specifically those measured on a continuous scale—relationships between variables can be examined using correlation and regression.[4,5]

# CORRELATION AND REGRESSION

Correlation and regression are used to describe relationships between continuous variables and are often used together in observational or experimental studies.[5] **Correlation** is used to determine the degree to which two variables change together, or "covary," where neither variable is considered dependent or independent.[4] In contrast, **regression** looks at the nature of the relationship between two variables, specifically the magnitude of change in one variable (the dependent variable, often referred to as the *response variable*) in response to a change in a second variable (the independent variable, often referred to as the *predictor variable*).[5] Additionally, regression can be used to predict the value of a response variable based on the value of one or more predictor variables.

## CORRELATION

Correlation is used to determine to what extent two continuous variables—$x$ and $y$—are linearly related or correlated to one another.[6] The primary purpose of correlation is to determine the strength of a relationship between two variables when neither variable is characterized as independent or dependent.[4]

In general, two variables may be linearly related in three ways: a positive relationship, a negative relationship, or no relationship. In correlation, this relationship is generally determined by the degree to which the variables each deviate from their respective

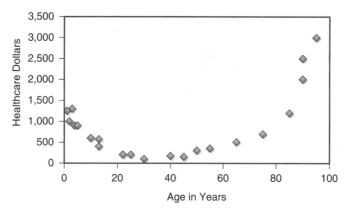

**FIGURE 11-1** Example of a curvilinear relationship.

means. A positive relationship indicates that both variables deviate from their respective means in the same direction.[6] If variables are negatively correlated, as one variable deviates from its mean, the second variable should deviate in the opposite direction. No relationship implies that there is no linear relationship between the two variables. However, a nonlinear relationship between the variables may exist, such as a curvilinear relationship. Healthcare utilization and age and physical strength and age are possible examples of curvilinear relationships. Healthcare utilization is high among the very young and the very old, but is lower in adolescents and younger adults. Similarly, physical strength is low in the very young and very old, but higher in young and middle-age adults. In these curvilinear relationships, a graph of the two variables would result in a curve rather than a straight line as seen with linear relationships (see **Figure 11-1**).[7]

The linear relationship or correlation between variables can be measured or quantified using any of three methods: covariance, the correlation coefficient, and the coefficient of determination.

## Covariance

**Covariance** is defined as a measure of the joint **variance** of two (or more) variables[7] and represents how much the two variables deviate together, on average, from their respective means.[6,8] Covariance is calculated based on the difference between each variable and its mean, similar to variance. These differences are then multiplied and summed to determine the covariance (see **Box 11-1**).

The following scenario can be used to provide an example of a covariance calculation. A study was conducted to determine if there was a correlation between the duration

**BOX 11-1** VARIANCE AND COVARIANCE

$$\text{Variance} = \frac{\sum (x_i - \bar{x})^2}{n-1}$$

$$\text{Covariance} = \frac{\sum [(x - \bar{x})(y - \bar{y})]}{n-1}$$

**TABLE 11-1**    Sample Data for Duration of Arthritis and Severity

| Observations | Duration of Rheumatoid Arthritis (years) | DAS28 |
|:---:|:---:|:---:|
| 1 | 5 | 1.6 |
| 2 | 7.5 | 2.3 |
| 3 | 3 | 1.4 |
| 4 | 2 | 1.4 |
| 5 | 15 | 6.7 |
| 6 | 6 | 2.1 |
| 7 | 9.5 | 3.0 |
| 8 | 11 | 5.3 |
| 9 | 3.5 | 1.5 |
| 10 | 22 | 8.6 |
| | $\bar{x} = 8.45$ | $\bar{y} = 3.39$ |

of rheumatoid arthritis and disease severity using disease activity scores (DAS28). Hypothetical data for 10 patients are given in **Table 11-1**.

Based on the data in Table 11-1, the covariance can be calculated as shown in **Table 11-2** and is found to be 15.57. This number can be interpreted as a positive correlation, suggesting that as the duration of rheumatoid arthritis in years increases over its average (8.45 years in this example), severity of disease based on DAS28 also increases from its average (3.39 in this example).

**TABLE 11-2**    Calculation of Covariance

| Observations | Duration of Rheumatoid Arthritis (years) | $(x - \bar{x})$ | $(x - \bar{x})(y - \bar{y})$ | $(y - \bar{y})$ | DAS28 |
|:---:|:---:|:---:|:---:|:---:|:---:|
| 1 | 5 | −3.45 | 6.1755 | −1.79 | 1.6 |
| 2 | 7.5 | −0.95 | 1.0355 | −1.09 | 2.3 |
| 3 | 3 | −5.45 | 10.8455 | −1.99 | 1.4 |
| 4 | 2 | −6.45 | 12.8355 | −1.99 | 1.4 |
| 5 | 15 | 6.55 | 21.6805 | 3.31 | 6.7 |
| 6 | 6 | −2.45 | 3.1605 | −1.29 | 2.1 |
| 7 | 9.5 | 1.05 | −0.4095 | −0.39 | 3.0 |
| 8 | 11 | 2.55 | 4.8705 | 1.91 | 5.3 |
| 9 | 3.5 | −4.95 | 9.3555 | −1.89 | 1.5 |
| 10 | 22 | 13.55 | 70.5955 | 5.21 | 8.6 |
| | $\bar{x} = 8.45$ | | $\Sigma = 140.145$ | | $\bar{y} = 3.39$ |
| | $s = 6.22$ | | | $s = 2.57$ | |
| | | | $\text{Cov}(x,y) = 140.145 \div 9 = 15.57$ | | |

Cov = covariance; s = standard deviation

| BOX 11-2 | CORRELATION COEFFICIENT |
|---|---|

$$r = \frac{Cov(x,y)}{s_x s_y}$$

However, covariance has a number of limitations in its application. It is difficult to determine how strong this relationship is (i.e., does 15.57 represent a strong or weak relationship?) or if the deviations of each variable from their respective means are similar. Additionally, this covariance is specific for one unit of measure for duration (as years of disease) and one unit of measure for disease severity (as DAS28). Covariance based on other observations where different units of measure are used cannot be compared to this covariance to help determine the relative strength of the relationship. To overcome some of these limitations, a correlation coefficient can be calculated using covariance.[6,8]

## Correlation Coefficient

The **correlation coefficient**, also known as Pearson's correlation coefficient and represented by $r$, is a standardized covariance and is calculated by dividing the covariance by the standard deviations ($s$) of both variables (see **Box 11–2**).[6,8]

Because it is a scale-free measure, the correlation coefficient is easier to interpret and allows for comparisons to be made between different units of measure. The correlation coefficient always ranges from −1 to +1 and represents both the strength and direction of a relationship.[5,9] A correlation coefficient of 1 (positive or negative) is considered a perfect linear correlation, with all data points lying in a straight line.[10] Therefore, the closer the correlation coefficient is to 1, the stronger the relationship between variables. For the sample data above, the calculated $r$ value is $15.57 \div (6.22 \times 2.57) = 0.97$, suggesting a strong, positive linear correlation between the variables. Although the strength of the correlation needs to be interpreted in the context of the data, in general, correlation coefficients greater than 0.5 can be considered moderate to strong, and those greater than 0.9 can be considered strong.[2,6] For correlation values less than 0.1, the relationship may be negligible and not clinically meaningful.

As with other statistical tests, a few assumptions are made when calculating the correlation coefficient. These include that data are measured at least on an interval scale, that a straight line or linear relationship exists between the variables, that the variables are independent, and that the underlying distribution of the data is normal.[6,9,10] When the assumption of normality does not hold true, such as with variables measured on an ordinal scale, a Spearman's rank coefficient (or Spearman's rho) or Kendall's tau can be used; both of these methods rely on the ranks of the variables rather than on continuous measurements.[6,7]

## Coefficient of Determination

The last measure of a linear correlation, the **coefficient of determination** ($r^2$), provides information on the variability shared by $x$ and $y$.[6] Although two variables may have a strong correlation, it is valuable to determine how much of the variability can be accounted for or explained by the relationship and how much cannot be explained. From the previous example of the duration of rheumatoid arthritis and its correlation with the severity of disease (based on DAS28), the correlation coefficient was 0.97. The coefficient of determination is then $0.97^2$, or 0.94. When represented as a percentage,

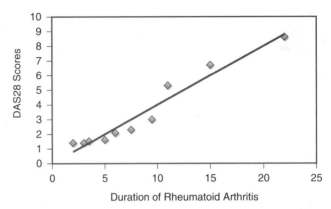

**FIGURE 11-2**  Scatterplot of rheumatoid arthritis duration and disease activity scores (DAS28).

this suggests that disease duration shares 94% of the variability in disease severity. In other words, disease duration accounts for 94% of the variability in disease severity. Therefore, only 6% of variability is unaccounted for, which could be explained by other variables, such as age, gender, or comorbidities.

## Correlation and Causality

One aspect of correlation that is important to recognize is that correlation does not indicate a cause-and-effect relationship or a direction of causality between two variables.[10] In the rheumatoid arthritis example, although disease duration and disease severity have a strong correlation and share a large percentage of variability, there is no evidence from correlation that disease duration causes disease severity or vice versa. A third, unmeasured variable may influence one or both of these variables.[2,6] This is sometimes referred to as the *third-variable problem*.

## Scatterplots

Correlation can also be represented graphically using **scatterplots**, or scatter diagrams. Each pair of data points for an observation (i.e., every value of $x$ and its corresponding $y$ value) is plotted on a graph, and the resulting pattern can be an indication of both the strength and the direction (positive or negative) of the relationship.[7] The stronger the relationship between variables, the closer the data points will be to a straight line drawn through the data points. The more the data are scattered away from a straight line, the weaker the relationship between the variables. When no linear correlation exists between two variables, a distinct linear pattern will not be apparent.

For the hypothetical data from the 10 patients with rheumatoid arthritis, a scatterplot can be made using the duration of arthritis on the $x$-axis and the DAS28 on the $y$-axis (**Figure 11-2**). The resulting scatterplot shows a near-perfect correlation, with the data points close to the straight line going through the scatterplot, as would be expected with a correlation coefficient of 0.97.

Small changes to the dataset can change the strength of a linear relationship. Using the sample data in Table 11-1, an increase in the DAS28 for two patients with short-duration disease and a decrease in the score for one patient with long-term arthritis changes the strength of the linear relationship, resulting in greater scatter of data, as shown in **Figure 11-3**. A recalculation of the correlation coefficient results in a value of 0.50, indicating a much weaker correlation than the original dataset. Examples of scatterplots showing a negative relationship and no linear relationship are provided in **Figures 11-4** and **11-5**, respectively.

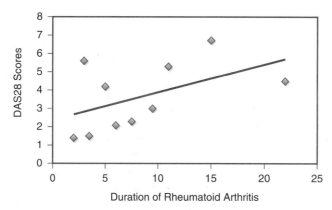

**FIGURE 11-3** Scatterplot of rheumatoid arthritis duration and disease activity scores (DAS28).

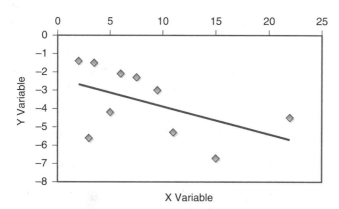

**FIGURE 11-4** Scatterplot showing an inverse or negative correlation with a calculated $r = -0.5$. The negative correlation value indicates that as the value of $x$ increases, the value of $y$ decreases.

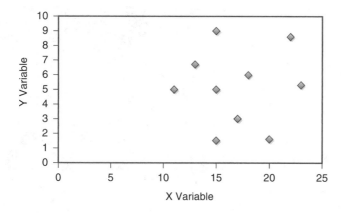

**FIGURE 11-5** A scatterplot with no clear linear relationship ($r = 0.032$).

## REGRESSION

Although correlation provides valuable information on the strength of a relationship between two variables, it provides little other information, such as the true nature of the relationship (e.g., a predictor-and-response relationship). This is where regression, essentially an extension of correlation, is used. Regression allows for the prediction of the magnitude of change in one variable based on the change in another variable by use of an equation. Because of the predictive nature of regression, a dependent, or response, variable and one or more independent, or predictor, variables need to be identified.[2,5,7,8,11] For the purposes of regression, independent variables are generally considered to be those variables that are known, whereas the dependent variables are undetermined and follow the independent variable.[2] Returning to the arthritis example described earlier, correlation was used to determine if there was a relationship between duration of disease and disease severity, and a strong correlation was found between the two variables. Regression can now be used as the next step in the analysis of this relationship, with a mathematical equation or model developed that will allow the prediction of disease severity based on the duration of arthritis.[12] Disease duration can be used as the predictor (independent) variable ($x$) and severity (as DAS28) as the response (dependent) variable ($y$).

### Types of Regression

A number of types of regression are possible, based on both the type and number of variables involved in the analysis (see **Box 11-3**).[13,14] The focus of this chapter will be linear regression, where the outcome variable is continuous.[15]

### Linear Regression

The predictive model used in linear regression is based on the equation for a straight line, $y = a + bx$, where $a$ is the **$y$-intercept** (the value of $y$ when $x = 0$) and $b$ is the slope of the line (the increase in $y$ for each unit change in $x$).[5,13] In linear regression, this model (referred to as the **regression model**) is given as $y = b_0 + b_1x$, where $y$ is the response variable, $b_0$ is the $y$-intercept (the theoretical value of $y$ when $x = 0$), $b_1$ is the **regression coefficient** (indicating the change in $y$ for a unit change in $x$), and $x$ is the predictor

---

**BOX 11-3** | TYPES OF REGRESSION ANALYSIS

- *Simple or univariable regression*: A single predictor variable and a single response variable.
- *Multiple or multivariable regression*:[a] Two or more predictor variables and a single response variable.
- *Linear regression*:[b] A continuous predictor variable and a continuous response variable.
- *Logistic regression*: A continuous or categorical predictor variable and a categorical response variable.

---

[a] The term *multivariate regression* has occasionally been used to describe multiple regression. However, multivariate regression describes regression analyses with more than one response variable and differs from multiple or multivariable regression, which considers only a single response variable. A discussion of multivariate regression is beyond the scope of this chapter.
[b] In multiple linear regression, the predictor variables may be continuous as well as categorical.
Data from Indrayan A. *Medical Biostatistics*. 3rd ed. New York, NY: CRC Press; 2013; Lang TA, Secic M. *How to Report Statistics in Medicine*. 2nd ed. Philadelphia, PA: American College of Physicians; 2006 and Schneider A, Hommel G, Blettner M. Linear regression analysis. *Dtsch Arztbl Int*. 2010;107(44):776-782.

variable. For population data ($X$ and $Y$), the Greek letter beta ($\beta$) is used; for samples ($x$ and $y$), the intercept and coefficient are represented by the letter $b$.

### Assumptions of Linear Regression

Several assumptions are made with the use of linear regression.[5-7,11,12] First, a linear relationship needs to exist between the predictor and response variables. The variables for linear regression need to be continuous (or categorical for multiple linear regression) for the predictor variable and continuous for the response variable. The populations from which the response variables are drawn (for each value of $x$) should follow a normal distribution, and the $y$ values need to be independent. There should also be a constant variance among the predictor variables (referred to as *homoscedasticity*). Lastly, for multiple linear regression where there is more than a single predictor, there should be no perfect correlation between any of the predictor variables (referred to as *multicollinearity*). This would result in similar regression coefficients for these variables, making it difficult to identify the effects of the predictors on the response variable.

### Developing the Linear Regression Model

The intercept and coefficient of the regression model are determined by the method of least squares.[5,6,13] Although a detailed explanation of this method is beyond the scope of this chapter, the method of least squares essentially looks at the vertical differences (called *residuals*) between each observed data point and the line of the proposed model. These residuals represent how far off the value predicted by the proposed regression model is from the actual observed value. The least squares method is then used to determine the regression coefficients that describe the model with the "best fit" to the data (i.e., the least differences between the data points and the line, essentially the line with the smallest residuals). Once the model is established, the correlation coefficient and the coefficient of determination (usually as $R^2$ in regression rather than $r^2$) can both be used to describe just how well the model fits the data, with $R^2$ representing the variability of the response variable accounted for by the predictor variables or by the regression model.[6,8,9] When there is only one predictor variable, as in simple linear regression, $R^2$ is equal to $r^2$.

For a simple linear regression, the regression coefficients and the correlation values can be determined using one of several statistical software programs or a spreadsheet program with a data analysis option. Using the same data on the duration of rheumatoid arthritis and DAS28, the intercept and regression coefficient were calculated to develop a model for predicting DAS28 based on the duration of rheumatoid arthritis. With these intercept and regression coefficient values, the general regression model $y = b_0 + b_1x$ can be rewritten as shown in **Box 11-4**.

In Box 11-4, the positive regression coefficient (0.401878271) for $x$ indicates that as the duration (in years) of rheumatoid arthritis increases, so does the severity of the disease (with an increase in DAS28 score of approximately 0.4 for each unit change in duration).[13] The large correlation coefficient (0.97) and coefficient of determination

**BOX 11-4     LINEAR REGRESSION MODEL**

DAS28 = −0.005871389 + 0.401878271 (duration in years)

**TABLE 11-3**  Sample Data for Duration of Arthritis, Age, and Severity

| Observations | Duration of Rheumatoid Arthritis (years) | Patient Age (years) | DAS28 |
|:---:|:---:|:---:|:---:|
| 1 | 5 | 35 | 1.6 |
| 2 | 7.5 | 26 | 2.3 |
| 3 | 3 | 45 | 1.4 |
| 4 | 2 | 52 | 1.4 |
| 5 | 15 | 70 | 6.7 |
| 6 | 6 | 37 | 2.1 |
| 7 | 9.5 | 42 | 3.0 |
| 8 | 11 | 54 | 5.3 |
| 9 | 3.5 | 40 | 1.5 |
| 10 | 22 | 67 | 8.6 |

(0.94) calculated earlier both suggest that the model is a good fit for the data. Now this model can be used to predict DAS28 based on disease duration. For example, a patient who has had rheumatoid arthritis for 8 years can be expected to have a DAS28 of about 3.2. For a patient with rheumatoid arthritis for 26 years, a DAS28 of approximately 10.44 can be estimated.

### Multiple Linear Regression

As with any disease state, many factors can influence an outcome. To improve the predictive value of the regression model, additional predictors can be added to the model, expanding the equation to: $y = b_0 + bx_1 + b_2x_2 + \cdots + b_kx_k$.[9,16] In the example for rheumatoid arthritis, other variables that might influence the disease can now be added to the model, such as patient age (see **Table 11–3**), and the intercept and regression coefficients can be recalculated.

The new regression model with this additional predictor is shown in **Box 11–5**.

Now, for a 40-year-old patient with rheumatoid arthritis for 8 years, the DAS28 is estimated to be approximately 2.9. Similarly, a 76-year-old patient with a 26-year disease duration is estimated to have a DAS28 of 10.55. The addition of age resulted in an $R^2$ value of 0.98, indicating that the variables in the model account for nearly all of the variability in the response variable. Therefore, the model including disease duration and age is a better predictor than the model including only disease duration. Adding more predictors can usually increase the predictive value of the regression model, providing a better fit for the data.[2] However, adding a large number of predictors does not always result in a good regression model. A good model is considered to be one where a large $R^2$ value can be achieved with only a few predictors. In addition, for multiple regression,

---

**BOX 11-5**    MULTIPLE LINEAR REGRESSION MODEL

DAS28 = −1.64013 + 0.328086 (duration in years) + 0.048244 (age)

only predictors that are considered statistically significant are included in the model; those that contribute little to the predictive value of the model usually have a very small regression coefficient and a nonsignificant *p*-value. Most statistical software programs apply an algorithm to determine which predictors should be kept in the model.

### Standardized Regression Coefficients

When using multiple linear regression, where there are several predictors in the model, it may be of interest to compare the relative contribution of each predictor on the value of the response variable.[2,9] If each predictor is in the same unit of measure, this is not a problem. However, most often the predictors are measured on different scales, making comparison difficult. To account for this, a **standardized regression coefficient** may be used. These standardized regression coefficients are analogous to correlation coefficients, in that the regression coefficients have been rescaled or standardized through the use of the standard deviations of both the response and predictor variables. After standardization, the change in the response variable per increase or decrease in the predictor can now be considered as a change in standard deviation units for both the response and predictor variables (i.e., number of standard deviation unit changes in the response variable for each 1-unit standard deviation change in the predictor), allowing for a comparison of the contributions to the model between the predictors. This standardization is done prior to developing the regression model and is applicable only to predictor variables that are measured on a continuous scale.

## Logistic Regression

A brief mention of logistic regression is important in the discussion of regression because it is frequently encountered in the medical literature. The main difference between linear regression and logistic regression is the type of outcome assessed in the model. In contrast to linear regression, the outcome or response variable in logistic regression is categorical rather than continuous and is often binary (i.e., a yes/no or response/no response).[13,17] Logistic regression is primarily used to predict the probability of an outcome given a single predictor (simple logistic regression) or a set of predictors (multiple logistic regression), with the calculation of an odds ratio. Both an intercept and regression coefficients are calculated with logistic regression.

Using the example of disease duration and rheumatoid arthritis severity, changing the response variable from a numeric value on the DAS28 to a categorical outcome of a DAS28 $\geq 5.0$ can allow for the use of logistic regression. Now with a continuous predictor (disease duration) and a categorical response (DAS28 $\geq 5.0$), logistic regression can be used to determine an odds ratio of achieving this outcome in comparison to a DAS28 of $< 5.0$.

## SUMMARY

Both correlation and regression are important statistical techniques to help describe and assess the nature of a relationship between two or more variables. With correlation, the strength and direction of a relationship can be assessed to determine how these variables "covary" from their respective means. Although not able to determine causality, correlation can help to determine if two variables have a direct or inverse relationship as well as the strength of that relationship. Regression, considered the next step after correlation, can provide information on the predictive strength of an independent or predictor variable for a given dependent or response variable. With linear regression, one or more independent variables (or predictors) can be used to develop a mathematical equation or model, which can then be used to estimate the value of a continuous response variable. For categorical response variables, logistic regression can be used to provide an estimate of the odds of the event occurring using continuous and categorical predictors.

# REFERENCES

1. Tuuli MG, Odibo AO. Statistical analysis and interpretation of prenatal diagnostic imaging studies, part 2. *J Ultrasound Med.* 2011;30(8):1129-1137.
2. Indrayan A. *Medical Biostatistics.* 3rd ed. New York, NY: CRC Press; 2013.
3. Sistrom CL, Garvan CW. Proportions, odds and risk. *Radiology.* 2004;230(1):12-19.
4. DeMuth JE. Overview of biostatistics used in clinical research. *Am J Health-Syst Pharm.* 2009;66(1):70-81.
5. Logan M. *Biostatistical Design and Analysis Using R: A Practical Guide.* Hoboken, NJ: Wiley-Blackwell; 2010.
6. Field A. *Discovering Statistics Using SPSS.* 3rd ed. Thousand Oaks, CA: SAGE Publications; 2009.
7. Vogt WP, Johnson RB. *Dictionary of Statistics and Methodology.* 4th ed. Thousand Oaks, CA: SAGE Publications; 2011.
8. Riffenburgh RH. *Statistics in Medicine.* 2nd ed. Boston, MA: Elsevier; 2006.
9. Vittinghoff E, Glidden DV, Shiboski SC, McCulloch CE. *Regression Methods in Biostatistics.* 2nd ed. New York, NY: Springer Science and Business Media; 2012.
10. Freedman D, Pisani R, Purves R. *Statistics.* New York, NY: WW Norton and Company; 1978.
11. Daniel WW. *Biostatistics: A Foundation for Analysis in the Health Sciences.* 5th ed. New York, NY: John Wiley & Sons; 1991.
12. Eberly LE. Correlation and simple linear regression. In: Ambrosius WT, ed. *Methods in Molecular Biology, vol. 404: Topics in Biostatistics.* Totowa, NJ: Humana Press; 2010;143-164.
13. Tripepi G, Jager KJ, Dekker FW, Zoccali C. Linear and logistic regression analysis. *Kidney Int.* 2008;73(7):806-810.
14. Lang TA, Secic M. *How to Report Statistics in Medicine.* 2nd ed. Philadelphia, PA: American College of Physicians; 2006.
15. Schneider A, Hommel G, Blettner M. Linear regression analysis. *Dtsch Arztbl Int.* 2010; 107(44):776-782.
16. Eberly LE. Multiple linear regression. In: Ambrosius WT, ed. *Methods in Molecular Biology, vol. 404: Topics in Biostatistics.* Totowa, NJ: Humana Press; 2010;165-187.
17. Nick TG, Campbell KM. Logistic regression. In: Ambrosius WT, ed. *Methods in Molecular Biology, vol. 404: Topics in Biostatistics.* Totowa, NJ: Humana Press; 2010;273-301.

# 12

# ANALYSIS AND INTERPRETATION OF NONINFERIORITY TRIALS

Ryan Rodriguez, PharmD, BCPS

## CHAPTER OBJECTIVES

▸ List reasons for selecting a noninferiority design for a clinical trial.

▸ Compare statistical testing methods between superiority and noninferiority trials.

▸ Analyze the establishment of a noninferiority margin for appropriateness.

▸ Appropriately interpret the results of a noninferiority trial.

▸ Identify characteristics of trial design that introduce bias in noninferiority trials and describe their effect on results and conclusions.

## CHAPTER OUTLINE

## KEY TERMS

# INTRODUCTION

Conventional clinical trials compare an investigational treatment to an inactive placebo, no treatment, or an **active control**.[1] This trial design is often intended to prove superiority of an investigational drug to a comparator, and is commonly known as a *superiority design*. In contrast, some trials compare an investigational treatment to an active control, but do not intend to prove it superior. Instead, the intent may be to prove the investigational treatment not "unacceptably worse" than the comparator. Because the efficacy of the investigational treatment may be compromised up to a predefined extent, these trials are known as *noninferiority trials*.

Noninferiority trials are being conducted more frequently due to unique characteristics that make them more favorable than superiority trials.[1] In spite of these benefits to investigators, interpretation of results can be troubling for readers. The use of "double-negative" terminology and counterintuitive language contributes to the confusion.

This chapter details the interpretation of results from noninferiority trials through the consideration of important design aspects and by envisioning important concepts from superiority trials "in reverse." Interpretation of results from noninferiority trials follows the same principles as with superiority trials, but with some nuances that make analysis seem reversed because of differences in the null hypotheses between trial designs.

# CONCEPTS IN NONINFERIORITY TRIAL DESIGN

## NULL AND ALTERNATIVE HYPOTHESES OF NONINFERIORITY TRIALS ARE "REVERSED" FROM SUPERIORITY TRIALS

Traditional superiority trials have a **null hypothesis** that an investigational drug is no different from a comparator, which is often placebo, no treatment, or an active control.[2]

When results disprove the null hypothesis, authors conclude that the drugs are different. The direction of difference may either favor or disfavor the investigational drug.

In contrast, the null and alternative hypotheses in noninferiority trials are in some ways reversed because the intent is not to demonstrate difference, but similarity.[2] More specifically, the null hypothesis is that the difference between an active control and an investigational drug is more extreme than an established margin of compromised efficacy. This margin determines how much is "too worse" and is known as the **noninferiority margin**. In other words, the null hypothesis is that the investigational drug is unacceptably worse ("not noninferior") than the comparator. Thus the **alternative hypothesis** is that the investigational drug is not unacceptably inferior (**noninferior**) to the active control. Investigators prespecify the noninferiority margin to be one that allows an acceptable loss of effect with the investigational drug, while still preserving enough benefit to be considered a viable treatment option.

## REASONS FOR NONINFERIORITY TRIAL DESIGN

If noninferiority trials only support a conclusion that a new drug is "good enough" to be utilized but not better than a comparator, why should they be conducted instead of superiority trials? The answer is that something is gained, either by patients or by investigators, in exchange for a treatment that may be less efficacious.[3] For this reason, it is important to consider whether the advantages offered by a drug being proved noninferior are worth the potentially decreased efficacy or safety. Specific examples of benefits from noninferiority trials that justify such a trade-off follow.

Some favorable pharmacologic or pharmacokinetic property may justify use of a drug that is potentially less efficacious.[3] For example, the pharmacokinetics of a new drug may allow it to be administered by a more convenient route, less frequently, or without monitoring requirements. Indeed, roughly one quarter of the proposed benefit of drugs studied in recent noninferiority trials included reduced duration of treatment and reduced pill burden.[1] Patients and clinicians may be willing to accept compromised efficacy for such convenience.

### Example 1: Justification of Noninferiority Trial Design

Examples of noninferiority trials that justified potentially compromised efficacy as a trade-off for beneficial drug properties include the new oral anticoagulants dabigatran and rivaroxaban.[4,5] Both drugs were studied in noninferiority trials that assessed their efficacy in preventing embolism in patients with atrial fibrillation. Neither drug requires routine laboratory tests, which improved upon the frequent monitoring of international normalized ratio (INR) required by warfarin, the long-used gold standard.[6,7] Noninferiority trials of dabigatran and rivaroxaban were designed to accept slightly worse treatment outcomes with these drugs than with warfarin because their simpler administration and monitoring may justify their use despite a potential for decreased efficacy in preventing embolism.

Additionally, the required sample size for noninferiority trials is often smaller than that for active-controlled superiority trials, making their conduct more feasible in the face of difficulties such as limited time or patient recruitment.[2] However, this is not without exception. Because an investigational drug is often compared to an active control in noninferiority trials, their treatment effects are likely similar. This contrasts the usually large difference between an investigational drug and placebo, which is easier to detect and thus requires comparatively smaller sample sizes.[8,9] Because there is a smaller difference in effects between the investigational and comparator drugs in noninferiority trials, the required sample size may increase.[9] These factors may influence the decision of investigators on the selection of noninferiority trial design.

Furthermore, noninferiority trial design allows for the conclusion of reasonable similarity when an unreasonable trial design would otherwise be required.[2] It is virtually impossible to prove two treatments statistically equivalent. For this reason, equivalence trials establish upper and lower margins that define a range of clinically acceptable similarity. This occurs in bioequivalence trials, which allow generic drugs to have slightly higher and lower average pharmacokinetic measures than brand drugs. This is permissible because slight variations in pharmacokinetic parameters do not cause significant variations in clinical outcomes.[10] Thus, generic drugs could be considered clinically equivalent. Although equivalency trials consider both directions of the investigational drug's effect in comparison to a control, noninferiority trials only consider whether a drug loses more than a defined amount of efficacy. This will permit the conclusion that the drug is acceptably similar to an active control (as with equivalency trials), but there is no limit on the amount of additional benefit it may have.

Lastly, noninferiority trial design is utilized when inclusion of a placebo arm in a traditional placebo-controlled trial would be unethical.[11,12] A new drug may be tested in a disease for which a known effective treatment already exists, in which case patients should not be denied beneficial care.

### Example 2: Use of Noninferiority Design When Placebo Is Unethical

The use of noninferiority trials for ethical reasons is frequently the case with new antimicrobials. Withholding effective treatment from patients who would likely benefit from available antimicrobial treatment would be unethical, so placebo arms are not included.

Ethical justification for noninferiority trials is evident in the trial that evaluated the new antimicrobial fidaxomicin in the treatment of *Clostridium difficile*–associated diarrhea (CDAD) in comparison to vancomycin, a gold standard treatment for severe CDAD.[13,14] In place of exposing patients to undue risk by receiving placebo, vancomycin was instead chosen with the willingness to accept that fidaxomicin may be slightly less efficacious.

## CONFIDENCE INTERVALS AND REFERENCE POINTS

To fully appreciate the statistical and clinical implications of noninferiority trial results, a review of confidence interval interpretation in different trial designs is warranted. Clinical trials report results for differences in treatment effects with a point estimate and confidence interval, which may be expressed in relative or absolute terms and plotted on a forest plot (**Figure 12-1**).[2] Relative comparisons express risk differences as a ratio (one event rate divided by another). Therefore, two treatments with equal risk would produce a quotient (called the **relative risk**, RR) of 1. Any treatment that protects against a negative outcome would have an RR less than 1, indicating a lower chance of the event occurring. In contrast, absolute comparisons subtract a measure of effect of one treatment from another. Therefore, two treatments conferring equal risk of an outcome would have an arithmetic difference of 0. Thus, any treatment with a protective effect against a negative outcome would have a negative **absolute risk difference** (ARD). Confidence intervals for statistically significant results do not cross a **reference point** (Figure 12-1, confidence intervals A and B); if they did, it would

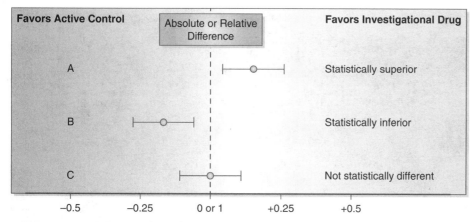

**FIGURE 12-1** Interpretation of confidence intervals using a Forest Plot. Confidence intervals represent results that are (A) statistically superior, (B) statistically inferior, and (C) not statistically different.

indicate the possibility that there is no difference between treatments (Figure 12-1, confidence interval C).

Evaluation of the confidence interval for these results allows determination of the presence of **statistically significant differences**.[2] Confidence intervals estimate the possible range of treatment effects; either bound of the confidence interval represents the least or most beneficial estimate of effect. These are often called the *lower* and *upper* **confidence interval bounds**, respectively. However, depending on the type of outcome, beneficial measures of risk can be above or below the reference point; this is the case for treatments that promote positive or negative outcomes, respectively. Therefore, the terms *lower* and *upper* bounds may be inconsistent in their indication of beneficial effects. Referring to these as the *least effective* and *most effective* bounds may be more intuitive and will be utilized in this chapter.

## ESTABLISHING MARGINS OF CLINICALLY SIGNIFICANT DIFFERENCES

Even when results show that treatments are statistically different, the magnitude of the difference may not warrant changes in practice. For this reason, margins are established that represent a **clinically significant difference** that would warrant such a change (**Figures 12-2, 12-3**, and **12-4**).[2] The establishment of these margins varies based on the type of clinical trial and is especially important in noninferiority trial design.

Because superiority trials intend to demonstrate that an investigational drug is better than a control, a margin for the clinically significant difference is established on the side of the reference point that favors investigational treatment (Figure 12-2). Although it is not traditionally described as such, this margin could be considered the *superiority margin*. The least effective bound of confidence interval A lies completely to the right of the reference point, allowing conclusion of statistical superiority. However, this is not the case with the superiority margin; thus, confidence interval A indicates statistical, but not clinical, superiority. Similarly, confidence interval B indicates statistical superiority, although there is uncertainty regarding clinical superiority because it crosses the margin of clinical significance. Finally, confidence interval C indicates statistical superiority and, because its least effective bound lies completely to the right of the margin of clinical

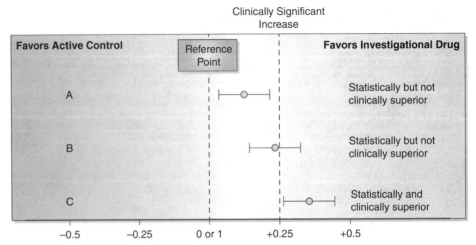

**FIGURE 12-2** Interpretation of confidence intervals in superiority trials. Confidence intervals represent treatments that are (A, B) statistically but not clinically superior, and (C) both statistically and clinically superior.

significance, also indicates definite clinical superiority. To support statistical and clinical superiority, the confidence interval must not cross either the reference point or margin of clinical significance and be on the side that favors the investigational drug.

Sometimes it is necessary for a drug to be simultaneously no worse than and no better than a comparator.[2] This is not frequent, but it occurs in bioequivalency trials. To be bioequivalent to a control (brand) drug, an investigational (generic) drug is not permitted to have therapeutic effects that are too high (toxic) or too low (subtherapeutic) than the control. Therefore, two margins are established—one on either side of the reference point—to define the furthest permissible extents of gain and loss of effect (Figure 12-3). Confidence intervals A, B, and C show that results must lie entirely

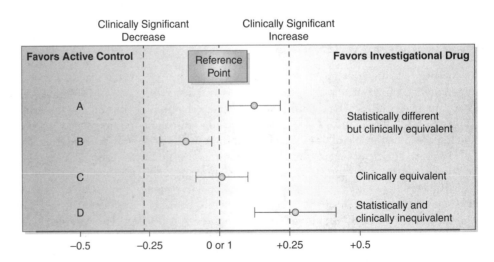

**FIGURE 12-3** Interpretation of confidence intervals in equivalency trials. Confidence intervals represent results that are (A) statistically better than control but not clinically different, (B) statistically worse than control but not clinically different, (C) neither statistically nor clinically different, and (D) statistically and clinically inequivalent.

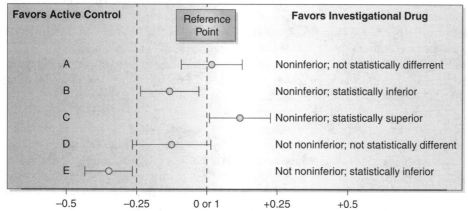

FIGURE 12-4 Interpreting confidence intervals for noninferiority trials. Confidence intervals represent results that are (A) noninferior but not statistically different, (B) noninferior but statistically inferior, (C) noninferior and statistically superior, (D) not noninferior and not statistically different, and (E) not noninferior and statistically inferior.

between both margins to permit the conclusion of clinical equivalence. Confidence intervals may cross the reference point in equivalency trials (confidence interval C), because the intent is to prove similarity, not difference. Inequivalent results would be those with a confidence interval that crosses either margin of clinical difference, as with confidence interval D.

Noninferiority trials, like equivalency trials, establish a noninferiority margin representing the lowest acceptable treatment effect from the investigational drug (Figure 12-4).[3,8,9] This margin is similar to a mirror image of a superiority trial's superiority margin. However, there is no upper limit on how much benefit the investigational drug may have; thus, no other clinically significant margin is required. The least effective bound of a confidence interval cannot cross the noninferiority margin and must lie to the side of the forest plot favoring the investigational drug (confidence intervals A, B, and C). Note that confidence intervals may cross 0 or 1 (confidence interval A), because, like equivalency trials, similarity is permissible and desired.

## INTERPRETATION OF RESULTS IN NONINFERIORITY TRIALS

A unique aspect of noninferiority trials is their analysis using essentially two levels of results interpretation. One level includes the null hypothesis—whether the investigational drug is or is not noninferior. This comparison is based on the noninferiority margin, as described earlier. The second level determines whether the investigational treatment is statistically superior or inferior; this comparison focuses on the traditional reference point of 0 or 1. The combinations of possible results often cause dismay and erroneous interpretation. The following examples of analyses of noninferiority trials highlight considerations readers should give first to the attainment of clinical noninferiority and, subsequently, to the attainment of statistical superiority or inferiority.

Consider the null hypothesis that an investigational treatment is not noninferior to a control and the alternative hypothesis that it is noninferior. In order to reject this null hypothesis and conclude that the investigational treatment is noninferior, the entire confidence interval must lie to the side of the noninferiority margin that favors the investigational drug (Figure 12-4, confidence intervals A, B, and C). Importantly, the least effective bound of the confidence interval cannot cross the noninferiority margin, and the most effective bound is not considered in accepting or rejecting the null hypothesis. In fact, because increased benefit is desirable, the most effective bound could stretch far into benefit and would not affect the conclusion of noninferiority.

In contrast, if the confidence interval crossed the noninferiority margin (Figure 12-4, confidence interval D), the conclusion represents one of the "double negatives" of noninferiority trials. A confidence interval that crosses the noninferiority margin demonstrates the possibility for the true result to be on either side. In this case, the confidence interval does not lie completely to the side of the noninferiority margin favoring the investigational drug. Therefore, the null hypothesis cannot be rejected, leading to the conclusion that the investigational drug is "not noninferior." Readers who encounter this result will often interpret this phrase as suggesting that the investigational drug is inferior; however, this is erroneous. The conclusion of inferiority is based on the finding of statistically significant differences between treatments.

After analyzing a confidence interval to accept or reject noninferiority, analysis proceeds to identifying any statistical superiority or inferiority. Consider that the confidence interval lies entirely to the left of the noninferiority margin (Figure 12-4, confidence interval E). The least effective bound of the confidence interval may lie to the side of the noninferiority margin favoring the active control, thus we must conclude that the investigational treatment is not noninferior. Moreover, the most effective bound also lies to the left of the noninferiority margin, excluding the statistical probability that the true result could be noninferior. Because the confidence interval does not cross the 0 or 1 reference point, we also know that the treatments are statistically different. Therefore, these results would describe a treatment that is not noninferior and also statistically inferior.

Confidence intervals for noninferior treatments may also fit entirely between the noninferiority margin and a reference point (Figure 12-4, confidence interval B). Noninferiority is supported because the least effective bound lies to the side of the noninferiority margin, favoring the investigational drug. Furthermore, because the most effective bound does not cross the reference point, the treatments are statistically different. Oddly, the investigational treatment is statistically worse than the control because the most effective bound lies completely to the left of the reference point. This situation represents another counterintuitive conclusion—the treatment is noninferior and statistically inferior. This is possible because the treatment is statistically worse than its comparator (because the confidence interval does not cross 0 or 1), but not so much worse that it would be clinically noninferior. This reinforces the point that selection of the noninferiority margin is somewhat arbitrary, which is important in differentiating statistical from clinical inferiority.

Confidence intervals supporting noninferiority may not support superiority or inferiority. If the confidence interval crosses the reference point (Figure 12-4, confidence interval A), it is uncertain whether the true effect is statistically inferior or superior. Although this supports noninferiority, no conclusion is possible regarding inferiority or superiority, because either could statistically be possible.

Lastly, a confidence interval may support both noninferiority and superiority. This occurs when a confidence interval lies entirely to the side of both the noninferiority margin and the reference point favoring the investigational drug (Figure 12-4, confidence interval C). Because the least effective bound lies to the right of the non-inferiority margin, the treatment is noninferior to the comparator. Additionally, the least effective bound lies to the right of the reference point, excluding the statistical probability that the true effect could be worse. It is therefore noninferior and statistically superior.

## SUPERIORITY TESTING IN NONINFERIORITY TRIALS

Investigators often perform **superiority testing** after noninferiority testing; this protocol is wholly possible and appropriate.[2,8] The hypothesis that the investigational treatment is superior to the active control is inherent within the hypothesis that the investigational treatment is noninferior.[2] The level of type I error is controlled with this testing procedure, which is termed *closed testing*. Correction for multiple testing is not required when investigators test for superiority after noninferiority.

Proceeding in the opposite order is not as statistically sound or advisable, as this is not always a closed procedure.[2] Furthermore, the selection of the noninferiority margin is somewhat arbitrary and can be placed in such a fashion that noninferiority could always be concluded given a certain set of results.[8] Therefore, authors who fail to show superiority and later perform a post hoc noninferiority test with known results may have knowingly established the margin to favor a conclusion of noninferiority. Thus, if noninferiority testing is planned, it should be predefined and performed before superiority testing. This avoids problems with testing procedures and also provides an a priori estimation of the required sample size for superiority testing, which is typically greater than that required for noninferiority testing.

# DESIGNING AND EVALUATING THE NONINFERIORITY HYPOTHESIS

The most straightforward method to establish or evaluate the design of noninferiority trials is called the **95%–95% confidence interval approach**.[2,15,16] This method uses the 95% confidence interval describing the historical effect of the active control to select the noninferiority margin and the 95% confidence interval of the results achieved in the noninferiority trial.

## WHAT IS THE EFFECT OF THE ACTIVE CONTROL TREATMENT?

The first 95% in the 95%-95% method is used to determine the expected treatment effect from the active control that will be used in the noninferiority trial.[2] Historical data describing the effect of the active control versus placebo are used to base this estimate in statistical reasoning. Often results are available from multiple controlled trials, which may have been pooled into a meta-analysis to provide a robust estimate of the active control's effect. However, when meta-analyses or clinical trials are unavailable, clinical judgment is required to make reasonable assumptions in extrapolating results from few or heterogeneous trials to the planned noninferiority trial.

Regardless of the extent of available historical data, the estimation of the treatment effect of the active control should be conservative.[15] This is why the least effective bound of the confidence interval for the estimated treatment effect is chosen as the expected effect in the noninferiority trial (**Figure 12-5**).[2,12] Because the estimate is low, it is

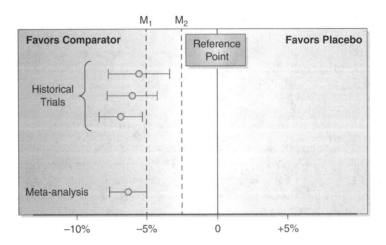

**FIGURE 12-5** Conservative selection of $M_1$ (the least expected effect from active control) and $M_2$ (the noninferiority margin) based on historical trials.

conservative and also likely to be achieved. The expected effect of the active control is an important margin and is often termed $M_1$ in methods sections.[12] Figure 12-5 demonstrates the selection of $M_1$ in this situation.

## HOW MUCH WORSE CAN THE INVESTIGATIONAL DRUG BE?

If an investigational drug demonstrated no more than the conservative effect estimated by the first step in the 95%-95% method ($M_1$), many clinicians may be reluctant to accept its value. If noninferiority were concluded based on this margin, it would essentially prove that the investigational drug has at least the lowest estimated effect as its comparator—any worse of an effect would be akin to taking placebo.[15] Realistically, a majority of patients taking the active control will derive more benefit than this. As predicted by the normal distribution, most patients will receive a benefit that approximates the point estimate of the confidence interval rather than its least effective bound. Consequently, investigators will aim to prove that an investigational drug has roughly this magnitude of treatment effect in the noninferiority trial.

In this case, a new margin is determined that reflects the desired level of treatment effect retained by the investigational drug (Figure 12-5). Using this clinical reasoning, the margin $M_1$ no longer represents a reasonable treatment effect for the investigational drug. This would be considered unacceptably worse; thus, a margin that would require more beneficial effect from the investigational drug must be established. This margin is termed $M_2$ and is the noninferiority margin upon which conclusions are based. In many trials, and as suggested by the FDA, the investigational treatment often must preserve 50% of the active control's effect.[9,15,17] In fact, some trials establish a noninferiority margin that requires the investigational drug to preserve more effect, such as 66%.[18] In addition to regulatory requirements, clinical judgment is a factor in determining the level of acceptable difference in treatment effects. Investigators may consider how much compromised efficacy they would be willing to accept in exchange for a unique benefit, or how much efficacy could be compromised without affecting routine practice. Although the establishment of $M_2$ should be based in reason and objective data, it may be based on expert opinion.

There is no universal rule for establishing noninferiority margins, which underscores the reader's responsibility in analyzing them before adopting results into practice. Guidance from the International Conference on Harmonisation recommends that the determination should be specified a priori, incorporate statistical and clinical reasoning, and be adequately conservative to protect against variability in data.[19] It is important that readers of noninferiority trials closely scrutinize the rationale behind the establishment of the noninferiority margin and compare it to their own judgment of where this margin should be established; this will help assess the applicability of trial results to the reader's unique practice.

## IS THE INVESTIGATIONAL DRUG NONINFERIOR?

Results from the noninferiority trial itself are used to calculate a confidence interval representing the treatment difference between the investigational drug and the active control. The least effective bound can be used to determine if noninferiority can be concluded and represents the second 95% in the 95%-95% method. Noninferiority is concluded based on this confidence interval, as described previously.

Bear in mind that investigators may choose to report results at levels of confidence other than 95%, such as 97.5% or 90%. This is done at the investigators' discretion depending on their acceptable level of type I error, and the analysis using the method described here will not change.

## DETERMINING NONINFERIORITY MARGINS IN TRIALS THAT REPORT ABSOLUTE AND RELATIVE RISK DIFFERENCES

Consider two example trials that illustrate the selection of noninferiority margins for absolute and relative comparisons of risk. Although the decision-making process in establishing a noninferiority margin may differ based on varied rationale, the following examples highlight frequent methodology in important publications.

### Example 3: Establishing Noninferiority Margins in Absolute Comparisons

In a trial that compared absolute risk differences, the antimicrobial fidaxomicin was compared to vancomycin for the treatment of CDAD.[13] Its potential benefit was a convenient oral tablet rather than a compounded liquid solution, which may have justified potentially compromised efficacy. The authors reviewed a Cochrane meta-analysis of published studies of CDAD treatment to determine the historical treatment effect of vancomycin versus placebo.[20] Several small trials suggested a cure rate with placebo of 10–20%. Therefore, the authors conservatively estimated that a 10% absolute difference in cure rates between fidaxomicin and vancomycin would not be clinically detrimental.[21] The noninferiority margin was thus established at a 10% difference in cure rates, allowing a cure rate 10% lower with fidaxomicin compared with vancomycin. In the noninferiority trial, cure rates were 88.2% for fidaxomicin and 85.8% for vancomycin. The confidence interval for the difference in cure rates crossed the reference point (0), with a least effective bound of −3.1%. Therefore, fidaxomicin did not cure worse than 10% fewer patients than vancomycin and met the authors' criteria for noninferiority.

## Example 4: Establishing Noninferiority Margins in Relative Comparisons

A large cardiovascular trial, the Randomized Evaluation of Long-Term Anticoagulation Therapy (RE-LY), compared the relative risk for stroke or systemic embolism with the new oral anticoagulant dabigatran versus warfarin in atrial fibrillation.[17] The determination of the noninferiority margin in this trial is complicated but important because of the frequency of such trial designs.[1] To estimate the expected treatment effect of warfarin in the RE-LY trial, investigators evaluated a meta-analysis of placebo-controlled trials of warfarin used in atrial fibrillation.[22] The meta-analysis found that, versus placebo, warfarin prevented vascular events in patients with atrial fibrillation with an RR of 0.36 (95% CI: 0.248 to 0.527). The upper bound represents the least effective bound in this case. Therefore, in the RE-LY trial, the authors expected warfarin to show an RR for vascular events of at worst 0.527.

Here, the mirror-image concept elicited by noninferiority trials becomes important. Because noninferiority trials allow a new drug to be worse than an active control, this estimate of benefit from the active control (warfarin) must be converted into one of harm.[15] This allows determination of how much worse a new drug may be compared to the active control. Before conducting RE-LY, only the effect of warfarin versus placebo was known. The meta-analysis calculated this as RR—the event rate with warfarin divided by the event rate with placebo. Performing a similar trial with dabigatran may have compared it to placebo, in which case an RR would be similarly calculated. This hypothetical placebo-controlled trial would calculate this as the event rate with dabigatran divided by the event rate with placebo. This would allow for an easy comparison of risk estimates between placebo-controlled trials of both warfarin and dabigatran, because both RRs would be normalized to a denominator using placebo rates.

However, the RE-LY investigators could not compare dabigatran to placebo for ethical reasons; they instead compared it with warfarin and ensured that it did not lose considerable benefit. Therefore, they needed to estimate how much additional risk would be conferred to patients that did not take warfarin; this is done by using the upper bound of the 95% CI from the meta-analysis (0.527). Thus, the inverse of the RR of warfarin versus placebo is calculated. This risk estimate now depicts event rates with placebo divided by event rates with warfarin and shows that patients not taking warfarin experienced an RR for vascular events of 1.898. If dabigatran showed an RR any worse (numerically higher) than 1.898, it would be akin to taking placebo; in other words, dabigatran would not meet the lowest estimate of warfarin's effect. If the RR were better (numerically lower), it would prove that dabigatran preserved at least the lowest, most conservative estimate of warfarin's effect. As discussed, achieving this level of benefit is sometimes not sufficient. The RE-LY investigators, consistent with FDA recommendations, determined that dabigatran should preserve at least 50% of the beneficial effect of warfarin.[17] Using a log-odds method of calculation, the noninferiority margin was reset at 1.46, which required dabigatran to preserve considerably more effect than the initial, conservative estimate of warfarin's effect.

In the RE-LY trial, embolic events occurred at 1.69% and 1.53% per year with dose-adjusted warfarin and 150 mg dabigatran twice daily, respectively, representing an RR of 0.66 (95% CI: 0.53 to 0.82).[17] The least effective bound (0.82) of this confidence interval did not cross the established noninferiority margin of 1.46, so dabigatran was concluded to be noninferior. Additionally, it did not cross the reference point (1), demonstrating that dabigatran was statistically different (more effective) than warfarin; thus superiority was concluded.

# SYSTEMATIC BIASES IN NONINFERIORITY TRIALS

Analysis of noninferiority trials should consider aspects of design that could affect the results and conclusion. Given the nature of noninferiority trials and the mirror-image concepts that are elicited, some biases that are detrimental to the conclusion of superiority may promote the conclusion of noninferiority.[23] For this reason, readers should consider whether investigators sufficiently protected against an inappropriate conclusion of noninferiority.

Whereas placebo-controlled trials can establish that a drug is effective, noninferiority trials cannot directly determine if two treatments are effective or ineffective—only that they are similar.[12] In other words, a drug found to be noninferior to another could be similarly effective or similarly ineffective. Noninferiority trials therefore rely on historical data, which must support that the active control in a noninferiority trial is superior to placebo.[11] This assumption that both the active control and investigational drugs would be superior to placebo (had placebo been included) is termed **assay sensitivity**. Attaining assay sensitivity is important in trials that assess subjective outcomes, such as achievement of analgesia or remission of depressive symptoms. Because trials of drugs in these classes have inconsistently shown superiority to placebo, it is possible that proving an investigational drug to be noninferior to them may not be proving efficacy at all. Therefore, including a placebo control in a noninferiority trial assessing subjective outcomes would ensure that assay sensitivity is present and that conclusions of noninferiority are clinically meaningful. Readers of noninferiority trials where a placebo arm is not included should consider if the active control provides a clinically meaningful benefit over placebo, and whether it would have been reliably superior to placebo.

Historical data are used to estimate the active control's treatment effect, which is assumed to be present in the noninferiority trial. This is known as the **constancy assumption**.[9] However, the treatment difference between active control and placebo may not be the same at the time of the noninferiority trial as it was in historical trials. This may be due to changes in patient characteristics or medical practices. Changes in this difference in efficacy could affect the ability to conclude noninferiority. For example, if the active control is less effective than it was historically, it may be easier to conclude noninferiority of an investigational drug. For this reason, readers should consider if changes in the treatment effect of the active control would make it easier or more difficult to conclude noninferiority of the investigational drug.

**Intention-to-treat (ITT) analysis** is often used in clinical trials as a way to deal with patients who drop out or violate protocol while maintaining the benefits of randomization. In ITT analysis, early data from patients before they drop out or violate protocol are often analyzed as if they were final values. These data may not represent the full benefit of treatment; therefore, ITT analysis makes treatment groups appear more similar.[23] The detection of differences between treatments thus becomes more difficult. Because ITT analysis decreases the chances of a type I error, it is considered conservative in superiority trials. However, because noninferiority trials aim to prove similarity rather than difference, ITT analysis promotes the conclusion of noninferiority and is considered anticonservative in these trials. Analysis by ITT is contrasted with **per-protocol analysis**, which does not include data from patients who drop out or violate protocol. Readers should always compare results from per-protocol and ITT analyses to determine how much of an effect the type of analysis has on the conclusion. If conclusions are consistent with both ITT and per-protocol analyses, the analytic method should not be overly concerning; if they are inconsistent, however, this suggests that ITT analysis may have unjustifiably promoted the conclusion of noninferiority.

### Example 5: Exanta (Ximelagatran) Sets a Precedent for Cardiovascular Noninferiority Trials

A case study that highlights nearly every important consideration in the design and analysis of noninferiority trials is that of ximelagatran (Exanta). This drug was developed to be one of the pioneer oral anticoagulants that did not require the frequent monitoring associated with warfarin, the gold standard oral anticoagulant. In a randomized, double-blind, placebo-controlled trial, Stroke Prevention Using Oral Thrombin Inhibitor in Atrial Fibrillation (SPORTIF V), patients with chronic non-valvular atrial fibrillation were randomized to ximelagatran or dose-adjusted warfarin.[24] The primary endpoint was the proportion of patients who experienced the composite outcome of systemic embolism, ischemic stroke, or hemorrhagic stroke. Although the authors claimed ximelagatran was noninferior based on their definition, the FDA review of the manufacturer's New Drug Application (NDA) highlighted pitfalls in the trial design and subsequently set an example for the regulatory future of new oral anticoagulants.

The SPORTIF V trial can be analyzed using the framework described earlier. The rationale for conducting the noninferiority trial was based in ethical reasons; warfarin was long regarded as an effective treatment for stroke prevention in atrial fibrillation. Additionally, the convenience of no monitoring requirements with ximelagatran outweighed a potential loss in effect.

The design and results of SPORTIF V can be analyzed using the 95%-95% method. Similar to RE-LY, the SPORTIF investigators first considered the effect of warfarin versus placebo in six historical studies.[22] In a **fixed-effects meta-analysis** of these studies, warfarin provided a relative risk reduction for stroke of 62% (95% CI: 48% to 72%). The annual rate of stroke was 1.4% with dose-adjusted warfarin, compared with 4.5% in untreated patients. The SPORTIF V trial was designed assuming an event rate of 3.1% per year in both treatment groups. The authors determined that an absolute difference in yearly event rates any greater than 2% (ximelagatran minus warfarin) would be unacceptable.[24,25] Therefore, the least effective bound of the confidence interval for the difference in event rates would not be permitted to cross 2% in order to conclude noninferiority of ximelagatran (**Figure 12-6a**).

Results from SPORTIF V showed event rates of 1.2% and 1.6% per year with warfarin and ximelagatran, respectively, rates that were considerably lower than the expected 3.1%. The absolute difference in event rates was 0.45% (95% CI: −0.13% to 1.03%) per year. Although the results numerically favored warfarin, the least effective bound of this confidence interval (1.03%) did not indicate a loss of efficacy more than the noninferiority margin of a 2% absolute difference. The authors were thus able to conclude ximelagatran to be noninferior to and statistically no different from warfarin (Figure 12-6a).

Analysis by the FDA critiqued these findings at each point.[15] The authors expected a 3.1% event rate, but the observed rates were much smaller in SPORTIF V. Several reasons could contribute to this; for example, the fixed-effects meta-analysis performed by the SPORTIF V investigators did not factor in heterogeneity among trials, which individually had varying event rates for the warfarin versus placebo effect. Thus, the noninferiority margin of a 2% absolute difference is not valid if event rates substantially differ from expected values.

Despite variability within historical trials in absolute rates and differences, relative differences could be expected to remain constant throughout time (e.g., consider that

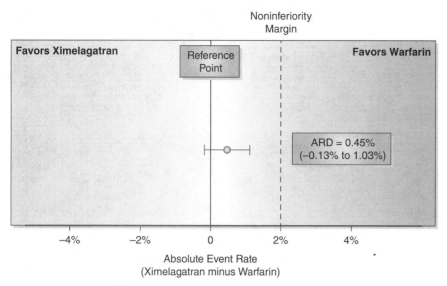

**FIGURE 12-6A** Findings of noninferiority by SPORTIF V investigators using an absolute comparison. ARD = absolute risk difference.

pairs of event rates of 20% versus 30% and 10% versus 15% have unique absolute risk differences [10% and 5%, respectively], but identical RRs [0.66]). For this reason, the FDA combined the results of the six historical trials in a more conservative **random effects meta-analysis**, which considers heterogeneity among trials, to produce a relative risk estimate. With this analysis, warfarin conferred an RR compared with placebo of 0.361 (95% CI: 0.248 to 0.527). Using the conservative 95%-95% method, the inverse of the least effective bound of the confidence interval produces a noninferiority margin of 1.898, just as in RE-LY. However, the FDA decided that a 50% preservation of the warfarin effect was desired, which would produce a noninferiority margin ($M_2$) of 1.378 using the log hazard risk ratio.

Next, the FDA reanalyzed the SPORTIF V data to produce a relative risk estimate. The point estimate for the RR of ximelagatran versus warfarin was 1.39 (95% CI: 0.91 to 2.12; **Figure 12-6b**). The least effective bound of this confidence interval (2.12) shows that the RR of the primary outcome with ximelagatran may have been up to 2.12 times greater than that with warfarin. Because this bound crossed the FDA's noninferiority margin of 1.378, they concluded that ximelagatran was not noninferior. In fact, this bound also crossed 1.898, indicating that ximelagatran could have been less efficacious than the lowest estimated effect of warfarin.

Concern was raised by the FDA, which stated that the investigators did not thoroughly justify the selection of the noninferiority margin of 2%. Furthermore, use of the absolute risk difference was unfounded, because the investigators based their assumptions on a meta-analysis that estimated relative risk difference.[22] Even if the FDA considered absolute risk difference (as the manufacturer initially did), the results still would not have favored ximelagatran. Using the 95%-95% method to define an absolute risk difference, the noninferiority margin would have allowed at most a difference of 0.76% more events with ximelagatran—more conservative than the 2% defined by the investigators.[15] Indeed, SPORTIF V results would not have supported noninferiority in this case either. Thus, no matter what analysis was used, the authors allowed ximelagatran to be worse than what the FDA was comfortable with.

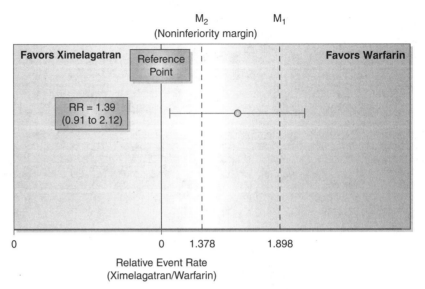

**FIGURE 12-6B**  Inconclusive findings by FDA using a relative comparison. RR = relative risk.

The case study of ximelagatran illustrates the importance of a thorough critique of noninferiority trials. Although the noninferiority design was appropriate because of ethical concerns with a placebo-controlled trial, hepatotoxicity associated with ximelagatran attenuated any theoretical benefit from convenient dosing.[26] Furthermore, although the investigators justified their rationale for establishment of the noninferiority margin, it was not sufficiently conservative according to the FDA—the effect of the active control was not consistent with historical results and the amount of preserved effect was not sufficient. Given the varying event rates in historical studies, the FDA favored analysis using relative, rather than absolute, measures of risk. With either of these analyses, ximelagatran did not provide enough benefit to receive FDA approval. Similarly, readers of noninferiority trials should consider their own interpretations of what constitutes an appropriately determined noninferiority margin before applying results in practice.

## SUMMARY

Noninferiority trials comprise a growing portion of the medical literature and present challenges in interpretation due to complicated statistical testing and terminology. Noninferiority trials are preferable to superiority trials when placebo controls are not feasible or ethical or when a beneficial characteristic of a drug outweighs its potentially decreased efficacy compared with another. Interpretation of results from noninferiority trials may be facilitated by envisioning important concepts "in reverse," including hypothesis testing and confidence interval interpretation. Noninferiority margins represent the furthest acceptable extent of compromised effect from an investigational drug; this margin should be analyzed for its appropriateness before applying results to practice. Results of noninferiority trials can be effectively interpreted by first analyzing whether they indicate noninferiority, then whether they indicate statistical superiority or inferiority. Characteristics of trial design that conservatively protect against type I error in superiority trials may do the opposite in noninferiority trials.

# REFERENCES

1. Suda KJ, Hurley AM, Mckibbin T, Motl Moroney SE. Publication of noninferiority clinical trials: changes over a 20-year interval. *Pharmacotherapy*. 2011;31(9):833-839.
2. Schumi J, Wittes JT. Through the looking glass: understanding non-inferiority. *Trials*. 2011;12:106.
3. Kaul S, Diamond GA. Good enough: a primer on the analysis and interpretation of noninferiority trials. *Ann Intern Med*. 2006;145(1):62-69.
4. Connolly SJ, Ezekowitz MD, Yusuf S, et al. Dabigatran versus warfarin in patients with atrial fibrillation. *N Engl J Med*. 2009; 361(12):1139-1151.
5. Patel MR, Mahaffey KW, Garg J, et al. Rivaroxaban versus warfarin in nonvalvular atrial fibrillation. *N Engl J Med*. 2011;365(10):883-891.
6. Pradaxa (dabigatran) package insert. Ridgefield, CT: Boehringer Ingelheim Pharmaceuticals, Inc; 2012.
7. Xarelto (rivaroxaban) package insert. Titusville, NJ: Janssen Pharmaceuticals, Inc; 2012.
8. Snapinn SM. Noninferiority trials. *Curr Control Trials Cardiovasc Med*. 2000;1(1):19-21.
9. Kaul S, Diamond GA. Making sense of noninferiority: a clinical and statistical perspective on its application to cardiovascular clinical trials. *Prog Cardiovasc Dis*. 2007;49(4):284-299.
10. Davit BM, Nwakama PE, Buehler GJ, et al. Comparing generic and innovator drugs: a review of 12 years of bioequivalence data from the United States Food and Drug Administration. *Ann Pharmacother*. 2009;43(10):1583-1597.
11. D'agostino RB, Massaro JM, Sullivan LM. Non-inferiority trials: design concepts and issues—the encounters of academic consultants in statistics. *Stat Med*. 2003;22(2):169-186.
12. Kaul S, Diamond GA, Weintraub WS. Trials and tribulations of non-inferiority: the ximelagatran experience. *J Am Coll Cardiol*. 2005;46(11):1986-1995.
13. Crook DW, Walker AS, Kean Y, et al. Fidaxomicin versus vancomycin for Clostridium difficile infection: meta-analysis of pivotal randomized controlled trials. *Clin Infect Dis*. 2012;55 Suppl 2:S93-103.
14. Cohen SH, Gerding DN, Johnson S, et al. Clinical practice guidelines for Clostridium difficile infection in adults: 2010 update by the society for healthcare epidemiology of America (SHEA) and the infectious diseases society of America (IDSA). *Infect Control Hosp Epidemiol*. 2010;31(5):431-455.
15. Statistical Review and Evaluation, NDA/Serial Number 21-686. United States Food and Drug Administration website. http://www.fda.gov/ohrms/dockets/ac/04/briefing/2004-4069B1_07_FDA-Backgrounder-C-R-stat%20Review.pdf. Accessed July 21, 2014.
16. Guidance for industry: Non-inferiority trials. United States Food and Drug Administration website. http://www.fda.gov/downloads/Drugs/GuidanceComplianceRegulatoryInformation/Guidances/UCM202140.pdf. Accessed July 21, 2014.
17. Connolly SJ, Ezekowitz MD, Yusuf S, et al. Dabigatran versus warfarin in patients with atrial fibrillation. *N Engl J Med*. 2009;361(12):1139-1151.
18. Oral direct factor Xa inhibitor rivaroxaban in patients with acute symptomatic deep-vein thrombosis or pulmonary embolism. New England Journal of Medicine website. http://www.nejm.org/doi/suppl/10.1056/NEJMoa1007903/suppl_file/nejmoa1007903_protocol.pdf. Accessed July 21, 2014.
19. ICH Harmonised Tripartite Guideline. Statistical principles for clinical trials. International Conference on Harmonisation E9 Expert Working Group. *Stat Med*. 1999;18(15):1905-1942.
20. Bricker E, Garg R, Nelson R, Loza A, Novak T, Hansen J. Antibiotic treatment for Clostridium difficile-associated diarrhea in adults. *Cochrane Database Syst Rev*. 2005;(1):CD004610.
21. Protocol for: Louie TJ, Miller MA, Mullane KM, et al. Fidaxomicin versus vancomycin for Clostridium difficile infection. New England Journal of Medicine website. http://www.nejm.org/doi/suppl/10.1056/NEJMoa0910812/suppl_file/nejmoa0910812_protocol.pdf. Accessed July 21, 2014.
22. Hart RG, Benavente O, Mcbride R, Pearce LA. Antithrombotic therapy to prevent stroke in patients with atrial fibrillation: a meta-analysis. *Ann Intern Med*. 1999;131(7):492-501.
23. Mulla SM, Scott IA, Jackevicius CA, You JJ, Guyatt GH. How to use a noninferiority trial: users' guides to the medical literature. *JAMA*. 2012;308(24):2605-2611.

24. Albers GW, Diener HC, Frison L, et al. Ximelagatran vs warfarin for stroke prevention in patients with nonvalvular atrial fibrillation: a randomized trial. *JAMA*. 2005;293(6):690-698.
25. Halperin JL. Ximelagatran compared with warfarin for prevention of thromboembolism in patients with nonvalvular atrial fibrillation: rationale, objectives, and design of a pair of clinical studies and baseline patient characteristics (SPORTIF III and V). *Am Heart J*. 2003;146(3):431-438.
26. Stewart RA. Clinical trials of direct thrombin and factor Xa inhibitors in atrial fibrillation. *Curr Opin Cardiol*. 2011;26(4):294-299.

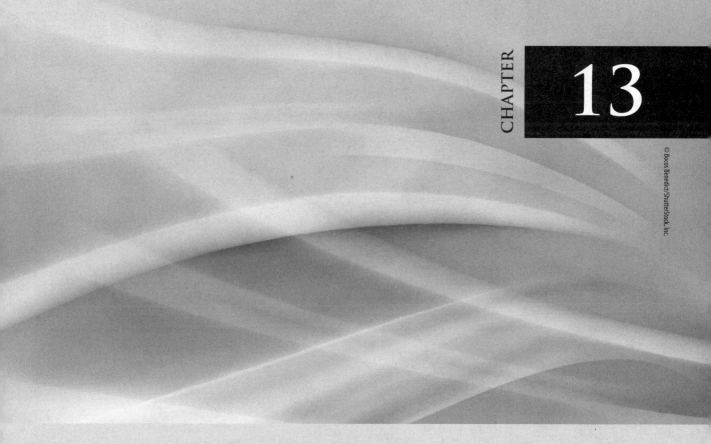

## CHAPTER 13

© Bocos Benedict/ShutterStock, Inc.

# ERRORS RELATED TO CLINICAL RESEARCH

Joshua L. Conrad, PharmD

## CHAPTER OBJECTIVES

▸ Define errors in clinical research and differentiate between type I and type II errors.

▸ Compare and contrast biases, confounders, and chance with regard to clinical research.

▸ Identify and differentiate between various selection and information biases in clinical research.

▸ Describe the relationships between alpha, power, sample size, and effect size in hypothesis testing.

# CHAPTER OUTLINE

# KEY TERMS

# INTRODUCTION

The purpose of clinical research is to answer clinical questions about phenomena in a population by studying samples of that population, with the intention of using the results to inform health and medical decisions for the greater population. Unfortunately, there is always a risk that the observations made and conclusions drawn from clinical research conducted in a sample may not actually apply to the greater population, either on the whole or to the extent demonstrated in the research. For example, a hypothetical clinical study conducted in a sample of subjects with elevated plasma low-density lipoprotein cholesterol (LDL-c) levels demonstrates that a lipid-lowering drug reduces cardiovascular-related death compared to placebo, when in reality the drug does not reduce cardiovascular-related death in the population. Such situations do occur and can be the result of a number of variables, not the least of which is sheer randomness.

When an answer to a clinical question that is obtained through clinical research does not accurately reflect what occurs or would occur in the greater population, an **error** has occurred. In the context of clinical research, therefore, we can define error as a deviation between the truth about a phenomenon in a population and what is observed in a clinical study about that phenomenon that is significant enough in magnitude to result in a false conclusion being drawn. The latter portion of this definition is important because miniscule mistakes and happenstances will frequently occur in clinical studies that cause the observations made therein to be slightly different from the real circumstances in the greater population. However, when such minor incidences are not significant enough to cause major changes in the results or conclusions of the study, they would not be considered true study errors.

For instance, a study nurse accidentally records the blood pressure of a single subject at a single visit as 130/85 mm Hg instead of 120/85 mm Hg, as it was actually measured. This is a mistake, to be sure, but it is unlikely to change the conclusions of the entire study. As another example, study researchers accidentally state in the published article that hyperkalemia was observed in 3% of subjects taking the study drug, when these subjects actually experienced hypokalemia. While this could affect the manner in which and patients in whom the drug is subsequently used, the typographical discrepancy is likely to be noticed and corrected in a future issue of the journal and the electronic version of the original article revised. This, also, would not be considered a true error in the clinical study, because it actually occurred after the completion of the study and would be unlikely to result in significant clinical misinterpretation in the long run. With acknowledgment that minor human mistakes can occur in the course of clinical research, the discussion of clinical research errors in this chapter will be limited to those discrepancies from the truth that can lead to significantly misguided conclusions.

For obvious reasons, it is important to avoid errors in clinical research whenever possible and to clearly identify, quantify, and report factors that could contribute to such occurrences when they have manifested or cannot be avoided. This chapter will examine types of errors that can occur in clinical studies, their causes, and ways in which they can be avoided or mitigated.

## TYPES OF ERROR IN CLINICAL RESEARCH

To begin our examination of the types of errors that can occur in clinical research, let us reflect on the aforementioned hypothetical clinical study in which was observed a reduced incidence of cardiovascular-related death with administration of a drug compared to the incidence observed with placebo, when in truth the drug does not have this effect in the larger population. When such a scenario exists, the result is called a type I error. A **type I error** is an error in which a meaningful difference between groups is observed for an outcome when that difference actually does not or would not exist in the population. In statistical terms, a type I error occurs when we reject the null hypothesis when we should have failed to reject it. Thus, a type I error can only occur when we have rejected the null hypothesis—that is, when a statistically significant difference has been demonstrated. Correspondingly, a type I error cannot occur when we have failed to reject the null hypothesis—that is, when a statistically significant difference has not been demonstrated. The term *positive* is often used to designate the circumstance of rejecting the null hypothesis, indicating that a statistical difference between groups has been demonstrated. Using this terminology, a type I error is a **false positive**—*positive* because a difference in the outcome was observed and *false* because the observation in the sample does not reflect the actual circumstance in the population.

The term **positive study** has also been used conventionally to describe a study that demonstrates what the researchers intended it to demonstrate for an outcome of clinical importance, usually the primary outcome. Thus, a positive superiority study would be one in which was demonstrated a difference between groups in a major outcome. Conversely, a positive equivalency study would be one in which equivalence was demonstrated in all important outcomes. The term *positive* in this context, however, should not be inferred to mean that the study has identified a desirable circumstance. For instance, a study demonstrates that children of lower socioeconomic status are more likely to suffer from obesity than children of higher socioeconomic status. Although this study shows a difference between groups and might therefore be referred to as a positive study, the circumstance of higher obesity rates in lower socioeconomic status children is not likely to be considered desirable. It will be important not to confuse a positive outcome, meaning that a statistically significant difference was demonstrated for that outcome, with a positive study, meaning that the overall study demonstrated what was intended, which could very well have been equivalence.

In contrast to the type I error, a **type II error** is an error in which no meaningful difference between groups is observed for an outcome when a meaningful difference actually does or would exist in the population. In statistical terms, a type II error occurs when we fail to reject the null hypothesis when we should have rejected it. Thus, a type II error can only occur when we have failed to reject the null hypothesis—that is, when a statistically significant difference has not been demonstrated. Correspondingly, a type II error cannot occur when we have rejected the null hypothesis—that is, when a statistically significant difference has been demonstrated. If rejecting the null hypothesis can be termed a positive result for an outcome, failing to reject the null hypothesis, and thus concluding that a statistically significant difference does not exist, can be termed a *negative* result for an outcome. Using this terminology, a type II error is a **false negative**—*negative* because no difference in the outcome was observed and *false* because the observation in the sample does not reflect the actual circumstance in the population. As with the term *positive* for studies demonstrating what was intended, the term **negative study** has been used conventionally to describe studies in which the results are not as intended, and the same discretion should be applied with the implications of the term in this context. The relationships between observations made in clinical studies and truth in the populations to which they apply are presented in **Table 13-1**.

| **TABLE 13-1** | Relationships Between Study Observations and Reality | | |
|---|---|---|---|
| | | **Reality** | |
| | | **Difference Exists** | **No Difference Exists** |
| **Clinical Study Outcome** | **Difference Observed** | True positive* | False positive (type I error) |
| | **No Difference Observed** | False negative (type II error) | True negative |

* A type III error is possible, but usually highly unlikely.

It can be argued that in any given situation in which a difference could theoretically exist, a difference probably does exist, and that if we were able to examine enough samples and could measure with nearly infinite precision, we would detect that difference. In other words, it can be argued that the circumstance of no difference existing is impossible. Think about a factory that makes yardsticks. If we compared the yardsticks that are produced by one machine with the yardsticks that are produced by another, we would likely find that there is no difference. But what if we measured the yardsticks down to the angstrom and then compared? It is likely that they are actually different lengths. In fact, it is likely that the yardsticks produced by a single machine are different from one another at that level. The same can be said about clinical research. If we compare enough subjects taking drug A to enough subjects taking drug B, both believed to have the same effect on blood pressure, and we could measure blood pressure down to the μm Hg, then we would likely find a statistically significant difference. However, this is not pragmatic or meaningful in real life. Therefore, when we discuss the circumstance of no difference existing, we must be practical about how that circumstance is interpreted.

In addition to types I and II errors, a third type of error, the **type III error**, has been described in the literature.[1] Type III error refers to a circumstance that can occur in a two-sided superiority study, in which a statistical difference between two groups is observed for an outcome when the opposite difference actually does or would exist in the population. For instance, it is observed in a clinical study that drug A increases the QT interval to a significantly greater extent than drug B does. However, in reality, drug B increases the QT interval more than drug A does. This is a type III error. Obviously, a type III error cannot occur when we have failed to reject the null hypothesis—that is, when a statistically significant difference has not been demonstrated. The actual risk of committing a type III error in most clinical studies is so minute that we typically do not consider it unless there are major flaws in the study design or execution. However, it is presented here for completeness.

In nearly all instances, it is impossible to definitively determine if any type of error that is possible to occur has, indeed, occurred. This is because it is impossible to know what the true circumstance in the greater population is or would be. If we somehow did have omniscient knowledge of the true circumstance in the population, there would be little need to conduct clinical research on that phenomenon. Practically speaking, therefore, we can merely attempt to identify and quantify the risks that such errors have occurred in a given study or for a given study outcome.

# BIASES IN CLINICAL RESEARCH

A number of circumstances can lead to errors in clinical studies, and these circumstances can be divided into three types. The first to be discussed is bias. Recall that an error in clinical research can be defined as a deviation between the truth about a phenomenon in a population and what is observed in a clinical study about that phenomenon that is significant enough in magnitude to result in a false conclusion being drawn. Given this definition of error, **biases** in clinical studies are identifiable and sometimes quantifiable circumstances that are systematically, or nonrandomly, introduced consciously or unconsciously by actions or decisions made by persons connected to the research and that lead to errors in the interpretation of study results. Because biases are introduced by individuals conducting, participating in, or publishing clinical research, they are theoretically avoidable.

In a seminal article, Sackett catalogued 35 types of bias that can occur in clinical research and divided these into seven categories.[2] Other types of clinical research biases exist as well. The scope of this chapter is insufficient to describe every type of bias that can occur in clinical research, and doing so would likely be of limited value, because their differences are often relatively minor and some of them are not as applicable to or prevalent in studies using more contemporary clinical research methods. Therefore, this chapter will focus only on a select number of biases that are the most relevant at present. Clinical research biases can be divided into two broad categories: selection biases and information biases.

A **selection bias** is any type of bias that causes a systematic difference between the probability of choosing or assigning one individual from the target population and the probability of choosing or assigning another individual from the same population. In general, selection biases occur in the study period up to and including the point of enrollment of subjects in a study and assignment of those subjects to groups. An **information bias** is any type of bias that causes a systematic error in the measurement, analysis, interpretation, or reporting of data in a clinical study. In general, information biases occur after subjects have been enrolled in a study and assigned to groups. In the following sections are presented a number of important selection and information biases and ways in which many of them can be avoided or mitigated. Table 13-3 summarizes the causes of selected selection biases and Table 13-4 summarizes the causes of selected information biases.

## PARTICIPATION (NONRESPONSE) BIAS AND THE VOLUNTEER EFFECT

A hypothetical clinical study was conducted to examine the effects of ultraviolet (UV) phototherapy in patients with psoriasis. Subjects were required to undergo 20 minutes of phototherapy in a clinical setting three times weekly for 3 months. Subjects in the experimental group received UV phototherapy. Subjects in the control group underwent a similar procedure, but with a dummy lamp that did not emit UV light. The treatment location was a community health clinic in a downtown metropolitan area, situated so that it was easily accessible via public transportation. In addition, study subjects were offered an incentive of $20 per treatment to offset their time and expense of participation. Ultimately, the study did not demonstrate efficacy of the UV phototherapy for reducing symptoms of psoriasis, despite sufficient subject enrollment.

A significant difference between the two groups in this study may not have been detected for a number of reasons. Of course, it could be that this type of UV phototherapy simply is ineffective for treating psoriasis. But what if there was something about the study design that resulted in certain individuals from the population, consisting of all patients with psoriasis, being more willing to enroll in the study than others? And, what if those individuals who were more willing to enroll in the study were also more likely to possess some other characteristic that made them less likely to respond to UV phototherapy than those less willing to enroll? This type of bias is referred to as participation bias.

**Participation bias** is a type of selection bias that can occur when the subjects who are willing to participate in a study have different characteristics than those who are unwilling to participate in the study, and those characteristics have an impact on an outcome of interest. The propensity for systematic differences to exist between individuals more open to participating in research and those less willing to participate in research has also been called the **volunteer effect**. Another form of participation bias can occur when the willingness of subjects with a condition of interest to participate in a study differs from the willingness of subjects without the condition of interest to participate in the study, and that difference alters the results. Participation bias has sometimes been referred to as **nonresponse bias**, especially in the context of survey research. Nonresponse bias and participation bias are essentially the same insofar as they both refer to a circumstance in which systematic differences exist in subjects' willingness to engage in research based on characteristics of importance or conditions of interest.

In the hypothetical study above, it is reasonable to suspect that individuals of lower socioeconomic status might be more willing to participate. The location of the treatment clinic may be less convenient for individuals of higher means, who might not routinely use public transportation and might not wish to drive to and park in an inner city location on a frequent basis. In addition, the amount of remuneration offered may be more enticing to those with lower incomes than to those with higher incomes. Finally, the time commitment may be less practical for those of higher socioeconomic status. It might also be reasonable to suspect that individuals of higher socioeconomic status have some characteristics that would have predisposed them to better response to UV phototherapy, such as generally better hygiene and fewer skin infections. Therefore, this study could have been subject to participation bias.

To minimize the risk of participation bias, the researcher should attempt to identify individual characteristics that could result in differences in responses to the exposure or intervention being studied, and then incorporate sampling techniques that encourage equal participation of individuals with and without those characteristics. In the example study, including another treatment location in an area more convenient to those of higher socioeconomic status or offering the option of UV phototherapy equipment that can be used properly in one's home, if possible, could have mitigated some of the risk of participation bias.

## ADMISSION RATE (BERKSON) BIAS

A hypothetical case-control study was conducted to determine whether an association exists between herpes simplex virus (HSV) infection and human immunodeficiency virus (HIV) infection. A retrospective review of the past 10 years of hospital admissions of patients with a diagnosis of HIV and a diagnostic test for HSV was undertaken and compared with control subjects without HIV who were admitted for other chronic diseases and who also had a diagnostic test for HSV. Care was taken to match control subjects to case subjects on numerous factors, including age, sex, race, date of admission, prognosis, etc. The study found that significantly fewer subjects admitted with a diagnosis of HIV had a positive test for HSV than subjects admitted with other chronic diseases. These data were unexpected, given that HSV and HIV can both be transmitted through sexual contact, and led to a conclusion that presence of HSV may suppress HIV transmission.

If the conclusion drawn from this hypothetical study is false, it could be the result of a type of bias known as admission rate bias. **Admission rate bias** is a type of selection bias in which the rates of exposed and unexposed individuals enrolled in a study systematically differ from the rates of exposed and unexposed individuals not enrolled in the study as a result of the setting in which the subjects are selected. This results in study data that are divergent from the data in the greater population. The most common instances of admission rate bias occur when subjects are drawn from those seeking care in acute care settings. Berkson described this type of bias in the context of a case-control study demonstrating a correlation between cholecystitis and diabetes among hospitalized patients.[3] For this reason, admission rate bias is sometimes referred to as **Berkson bias** or **Berkson's paradox**.

In this hypothetical study examining the correlation between HSV and HIV, it is possible that individuals with concurrent HSV and HIV were systematically underrepresented by limiting the sample to those admitted to the hospital. For instance, what if more individuals with concurrent HSV and HIV die faster when they have complications than individuals with HIV without HSV do? Many of those individuals with both viruses in the greater population may not have had time to seek acute care, which likely would have resulted in a smaller incidence of HSV in the hospital-admitted HIV sample. In contrast, it is possible that individuals with concurrent HSV and chronic non-HIV diseases were systematically overrepresented by taking the sample from those admitted to the hospital. For instance, what if more individuals with concurrent HSV and chronic non-HIV diseases develop complications requiring acute care than individuals with chronic non-HIV diseases without HSV do? The incidence of HSV in individuals with chronic non-HIV diseases would be higher among those seeking acute care than those in the entire chronic non-HIV disease population.

Admission rate bias can be avoided by ensuring that samples are representative of their entire respective populations. A common way to do this is to include only subjects who are identified at the time of diagnosis, regardless of the setting in which this occurs. For instance, the risk of admission rate bias could have been mitigated in the example study if the researchers had examined the presence or absence of HSV in individuals with HIV versus other chronic disease at the time that the diagnosis of HIV or other chronic disease was made, whether in a primary care or acute care setting, rather than looking only at those individuals who were admitted to the hospital at some point thereafter.

## Prevalence-Incidence (Neyman) Bias

A hypothetical study was conducted to assess whether a particular class of lipid-lowering agents (class A drugs) is associated with an increased risk of QT prolongation when compared with another class of lipid-lowering agents (class B drugs). The study examined a group of 1,000 subjects with coronary artery disease (CAD), each of whom had been taking a class A drug for at least 5 years, and another group of 1,000 similar subjects with CAD, each of whom had been taking a class B for at least 5 years. All subjects had QT interval measurements on file. In the class A drug group, 22 subjects were found to have had at least one documentation of QT prolongation, a 2.2% prevalence. In the class B drug group, 23 subjects were found to have had at least one documentation of QT prolongation, a 2.3% prevalence. The conclusion drawn from the study was that class A drugs do not increase the risk of developing QT prolongation compared to class B drugs.

Another hypothetical study was conducted to compare the same effects in subjects with CAD. The researchers followed 1,000 subjects who were prescribed class A drugs and 1,000 similar subjects who were prescribed class B drugs. None of the subjects had baseline QT prolongation at study entry, and each subject was observed for 5 years, with QT measurements taken at regular intervals. In the class A drug group, 100 subjects developed QT prolongation, and 78 of these subjects died from sudden death associated with this condition within the 5 years of the study. In the class B drug group, 25 subjects developed QT prolongation, and 2 of these subjects died from sudden death associated with this condition within the 5 years of the study. Thus, the incidence rates of QT prolongation were demonstrated as 10% for class A drugs and 2.5% for class B drugs. The conclusion drawn from the study was that class A drugs do increase the risk of developing QT prolongation compared to class B drugs.

Is it possible that the results of both of these hypothetical studies can be adequately extrapolated to the general population? Or, is it more likely that one of them is less valid? Of course, many factors may have contributed to misleading results in one of the studies. However, there is a high likelihood that the first study suffered from a type of bias known as prevalence-incidence bias. **Prevalence-incidence bias** is a type of selection bias that can occur in studies in which cases that are mild and self-resolving and those that are rapidly fatal are not captured, resulting in a systematic failure to include these cases. This type of bias is named *prevalence-incidence bias* because it is introduced when prevalence is mistaken for or inappropriately used instead of incidence. **Prevalence** is the proportion of individuals with a given condition of interest at a specific point in time. Prevalence answers the question, "What proportion of the sampled population has the condition right now?" In contrast, **incidence** is the rate with which individuals develop a condition of interest in a specific period of time. Incidence answers the question, "What proportion of the sampled population will develop the condition in the specific period of time?" One of the earliest descriptions of prevalence-incidence bias was published by Jerzy Neyman in 1955.[4] For this reason, it is often called **Neyman bias**.

Prevalence-incidence bias is similar in many respects to admission rate bias, except that admission rate bias is associated with the setting from which the subjects are selected and prevalence-incidence bias is associated with the ability to detect the condition being studied within the parameters of the study. In the hypothetical study involving HSV and HIV, it was not the inability to detect the presence or absence of these conditions that led to the biased results; rather, it was the setting from which the subjects were selected that misrepresented the population. In the two hypothetical CAD studies, the subjects could have been drawn from the exact same pool. Yet, the design of the first study was insufficient to detect cases before they became fatal. Another way to look at this is to examine the actual populations being sampled in the two studies to see if they are truly identical. The second study sampled from the population of all individuals with CAD who were starting treatment with a class A or class B drug. In contrast, the first study sampled from the population of all living individuals who had CAD and who had been taking a class A or class B drug for 5 years. In this case, these are two very different populations. To illustrate this point, let us examine what would have happened if we had applied the first CAD study's design to the second CAD study's population. **Table 13-2** shows the data collected in the second CAD study.

At the end of 5 years of taking class A drugs, 922 subjects were alive, and 22 of these subjects have had documented QT prolongation. Now, if we use the methods from the first CAD study and apply them to the second study sample, we would only be looking at individuals who are alive and have been taking class A drugs for at least 5 years. Those 78 individuals who died of QT-related sudden death within the study period are not even considered in this analysis. Thus, the prevalence of QT prolongation in the class A drug group appears to be approximately 2.4% [(22 ÷ 922) × 100%]. Among the 998 living subjects who had been taking class B drugs for at least 5 years, 23 have had documented QT prolongation, resulting in an apparent prevalence of about 2.3% [(23 ÷ 998) × 100%]. When examined using the methods employed in the first study, the subjects from the second study appear to have much different rates of QT prolongation (2.4% and 2.3%) than was observed using the methods of the second study (10% and 2.5%), even though it is the exact same pool of subjects.

| **TABLE 13-2** | Data from Second Example CAD Study | | |
|---|---|---|---|
| | **Subject Disposition at 5 Years** | | |
| **Subject Group** | **Dead from QT Prolongation** | **Alive with QT Prolongation** | **Alive without QT Prolongation** |
| Class A drugs | 78 | 22 | 900 |
| Class B drugs | 2 | 23 | 975 |

How might the data have looked in the two CAD studies if there had been no physical symptoms or other manifestations to warrant investigation of the QT interval? The first study relied on QT interval data that were already collected. Therefore, most individuals who experienced nonsymptomatic QT prolongation would likely not have been identified. In contrast, the second study called for routine measurement of the QT interval in all subjects, regardless of the presence or absence of a clinical reason, which certainly would have captured more instances of nonsymptomatic QT prolongation.

It should be apparent that prevalence-incidence bias can be avoided by identifying subjects as they are first exposed to the element of interest (i.e., measuring incidence), rather than picking them up at some point thereafter (i.e., measuring prevalence). For some conditions, this requires routine data collection on the outcome of interest from all subjects, regardless of a clinical indication.

## MEDICAL SURVEILLANCE BIAS

A hypothetical study was conducted to assess whether a particular class of lipid-lowering agents (class A drugs) is associated with an increased risk of QT prolongation when compared with another class of lipid-lowering agents (class B drugs). Included subjects were those who had a record of receiving a class A or class B drug for at least 1 year, had a normal QT interval documented within 1 year prior to starting the drug, and had at least one QT interval measurement documented while taking the drug. Subjects who had also received a nonstudy drug known to cause QT prolongation at any time between the pretreatment QT interval measurement and the last on-treatment QT interval measurement were excluded from the analysis. The researchers observed documented QT prolongation in 2.4% of subjects taking class A drugs and 2.1% of subjects taking class B drugs, a difference that was not statistically significant. The conclusion drawn from the study was that class A drugs do not significantly increase the risk of developing QT prolongation compared to class B drugs.

In this hypothetical study, subjects in both groups were required to have documented normal pretreatment QT intervals, minimizing the risk that QT prolongation was present in subjects when they started on the study drugs. In addition, all subjects were followed from the start of treatment so as to mitigate the risk of prevalence-incidence bias. Yet, there is still a potential bias in this study, that being medical surveillance bias.

**Medical surveillance bias** is a type of selection bias that can occur in retrospective studies when the inclusion of subjects is limited to those who have received a certain nonroutine screening or diagnostic test. Most individuals, even those with elevated plasma cholesterol, do not undergo routine QT interval measurement unless they have had some precipitating event. When only individuals with documentation of a particular nonroutine test are enrolled in a study, it may create a circumstance in which individuals already at higher risk for developing the condition that the test detects are overrepresented in the study. There was some reason why these individuals underwent screening in the first place. If the overrepresentation of individuals at risk for the condition causes a systematic inflation of the incidence of that condition in one group more than in the other or a systematic dilution of the incidence of that condition in one group more than in the other, medical surveillance bias has occurred.

In this hypothetical QT interval study, it is possible that most of the subjects who developed QT prolongation in both groups would have developed it anyway, given that they were probably already at some risk. Otherwise, why would they have had QT interval screenings in the first place? For illustrative purposes, let us say that class A drugs actually do cause QT prolongation and class B drugs actually do not. If the pool of subjects receiving class A drugs who would develop QT prolongation significantly overlaps with the pool of subjects in that group who would have developed it anyway, without receiving the drug, then the incidence would appear to be similar with and without the drug.

Avoiding medical surveillance bias is difficult in observational studies when the screening for the condition of interest is not routine in all individuals. For this reason, it is best to conduct interventional studies for detecting these types of conditions. For instance, if the example study had been conducted as a clinical trial and subjects were randomly selected from the entire population of patients with high cholesterol, not just those who had already undergone QT interval screening, the subject pool would be less likely to be overwhelmed with individuals already at higher risk for QT prolongation, and drug-induced QT prolongation would be more easily identifiable.

## DETECTION BIAS

A hypothetical clinical study was conducted to determine if a promising new antineoplastic agent increases the survival time of patients with peritoneal cancer when compared to traditional chemotherapies for this condition. Because the condition is so rare, the potential subject pool was limited. Therefore, the researchers used the survival data from patients who had already been treated with traditional chemotherapies as a control and used the new agent in all subjects agreeing to participate in the study, thus increasing the total potential sample size of the experimental group. All subjects used as controls were required to have well-documented dates of diagnoses, treatment courses, and deaths. All experimental group subjects were matched to control subjects with regard to clinically important factors such as age at diagnosis, race, sex, and coexisting conditions, and all were followed until death. When compared with traditional chemotherapies, the new agent increased survival time by an average of 6 months.

Can we be confident in the results of this study? If the experimental group subjects and historical controls were well matched, it could seem so. But what if some of the control subjects had been diagnosed at a time when techniques for identifying peritoneal cancer were not as sensitive as when the study was conducted? It is likely that many of the control subjects would have been diagnosed further into the course of their disease than those in the experimental group. If this was the case, it would give the false impression that the increased survival time in the experimental group was attributable to the new antineoplastic agent, when it was actually due to earlier detection of the condition in these subjects. This case demonstrates detection bias.

**Detection bias** is a type of selection bias that can occur when the methods of screening for the condition of interest differ between the control group and the experimental group. This often occurs when the control group is historical, but it can also occur in case-control studies if the difference occurs between the cases and controls. It is also important that the same definitions of the condition are used, because these can change over time. For instance, the definition of hypertension was a blood pressure of at least 160/96 mm Hg in the early 1980s, but had changed to at least 140/90 mm Hg by the mid-1990s, thereby making it difficult to compare outcomes in patients with diagnoses of hypertension between these two periods.[5]

Specific subtypes of detection bias, referred to as **noncontemporaneous control bias** and **starting time bias**, have also been described in the literature.[2] However, these refer to the same basic concept as detection bias. These types of bias can be avoided by ensuring that the techniques used for all potential subjects in all groups are identical and that the timing of subjects' assignment to groups is relatively similar. When subject enrollment must extend for a long period of time, such as when the condition being studied is rare or when the timing of subject enrollment can have a significant impact on the outcomes, such as with seasonal conditions, using a blocked randomization technique can help prevent detection bias, particularly starting time bias. However, if this cannot be avoided, cases and controls can be matched based on diagnostic techniques and timing.

## PROCEDURE SELECTION BIAS

A hypothetical clinical study was conducted to compare thrombolytic drug therapy versus embolectomy via arterial catheter for the emergent treatment of pulmonary embolism (PE). Both interventions had previously been established as effective for treatment of PE through prior clinical studies, and the risks of these interventions had also been previously well documented. Because of the potential morbidity of the condition and severity of the complications from either intervention, the treating clinicians were allowed to assign each subject to the intervention of the clinician's choice based on the clinical presentation and an evaluation of relative risks and benefits for the individual subject. At the conclusion of the study, it was demonstrated that performing embolectomy resulted in fewer deaths than treatment with thrombolytic drugs.

In the course of routine practice, clinicians make decisions about treatments every day that are based on assessments of potential risks and benefits. So, it can be instinctual to treat such practices in the context of a clinical study as allowable. In fact, such practices can even be seen as desirable if they make the study more like "real life." However, we must remember that clinical studies are not real life. They exist to answer questions about real life that would otherwise be less convincing if certain aspects remained uncontrolled.

In the context of the hypothetical clinical study of PE treatment, the clinicians deciding on treatments for the individual subjects may approach them differently in a systematic manner, such that a bias is created. For instance, the clinicians may routinely assign generally healthier subjects (PE notwithstanding) to receive the more invasive treatment, embolectomy, and generally less healthy subjects to receive the less invasive treatment, thrombolytics. If this occurs and causes the results to be spurious, a bias has been committed. This type of bias is referred to as procedure selection bias.

**Procedure selection bias** most commonly occurs when individual subjects are decidedly assigned to groups based on clinical judgment instead of being randomly assigned. Thus, the easiest way to avoid this type of bias is to randomize subjects to groups. In cases when this is deemed potentially inappropriate, one should question the appropriateness of conducting the study altogether. For instance, if assigning subjects to treatment groups randomly is considered potentially inappropriate because prior evidence suggests that certain individuals will benefit more from one intervention and other individuals will benefit more from another, one should ask whether this prior evidence is sufficient enough to accept as truth. If so, there is little reason to conduct another clinical study on the matter. However, if the prior evidence is still insufficient to accept as truth, the researcher should not be apprehensive about using random assignments. If there is only compelling prior evidence that one subset of the population would benefit more or less with one of the interventions, consideration should be given to excluding those individuals from the study and only including subjects for which there is yet insufficient evidence supporting one of the interventions over the other.

## MEMBERSHIP BIAS

A hypothetical large cohort study was conducted to determine if regular exposure to secondhand cigarette smoke (SCS) is a risk factor for recurrent community-acquired pneumonia (CAP) in children. Children with a new diagnosis of CAP who participated in the study were assigned to groups based on presence (SCS-exposed group) or absence (SCS-unexposed group) of exposure to a habitual cigarette smoker in the home. Children with a chronic condition significantly affecting the cardiovascular, pulmonary, or immune system, such as congenital heart disease, cystic fibrosis, asthma, or HIV infection, were excluded from the study. Diagnosis of CAP was made with a standard combination of chest x-ray, clinical evaluation, and microbiologic evidence. Subjects were followed for 18 months from initial CAP diagnosis to observe recurrence. Baseline demographics of study subjects were similar between groups with regard to sex, age, race, and initial CAP pathogen. At the conclusion of the study, 8% of subjects in the SCS-exposed group and 4% of subjects in the SCS-unexposed group had suffered recurrent CAP. This difference was determined to be statistically significant, and the researchers concluded that exposure to household SCS is a positive risk factor for recurrent CAP in children.

It is not difficult to believe that regular SCS exposure might be a risk factor for recurrent CAP in children. But can we be sure from this hypothetical study that SCS was solely responsible for the observed difference in recurrent CAP between the two groups? What if children who live in households with cigarette smokers are more likely to have other characteristics that also predispose them to recurrent CAP than do children who live in smoke-free homes? If this is the case, the study may suffer from membership bias.

**Membership bias** is a type of selection bias that can occur when subjects in one group have a higher prevalence of a characteristic that may alter their outcomes than subjects in another group have, and that characteristic is systematically tied to another characteristic upon which group assignments are based. For clarity, we can use the term *assigning characteristic* to mean a characteristic upon which assignment to a study group is based and the term *biasing characteristic* to mean a characteristic that can alter a subject's disposition relative to a study outcome. In these terms, membership bias can occur when subjects with a particular biasing characteristic are systematically assigned to one group more than to another group because the biasing characteristic is somehow linked to an assigning characteristic. To be membership bias, the link between the assigning characteristic and the biasing characteristic cannot be random. The link must also exist in the greater population. In other words, subjects in one study group are more likely to be members of a group with a biasing characteristic than are subjects in another study group because that is the way they exist in the population. The natural link between the biasing characteristic and the assigning characteristic is emphasized here because a later discussion of causes for errors in clinical studies in this chapter will examine a similar circumstance, but one in which the characteristic causing the error is not naturally linked to an assigning characteristic.

Because membership bias and participation bias can both involve higher prevalence of a biasing characteristic in one group than in another, it is important to be clear about the cause of this circumstance in order to differentiate between these two types of bias. Recall that with participation bias it is subjects' willingness or unwillingness to participate in the research that introduces the bias. With membership bias, however, the cause is a natural link between the biasing characteristic and an assigning characteristic, not a difference in subjects' willingness to participate.

In the context of the hypothetical CAP study, membership bias is possible if some biasing characteristic that predisposes a child to recurrent CAP is more prevalent in the SCS-exposed group than in the SCS-unexposed group because that biasing characteristic is generally more prevalent in SCS-exposed children than in SCS-unexposed children in the greater population. For instance, what if children who live with smokers are more likely to come from a lower socioeconomic status than children who live in smoke-free homes? Families of lower socioeconomic status are typically larger and suffer from more crowding than those of higher socioeconomic status, and these characteristics have been previously identified as increasing the risk of recurrent CAP. If more subjects in the SCS-exposed group than in the SCS-unexposed group had these characteristics because of their link to households with smokers, it may have been these characteristics, and not the actual SCS exposure, that resulted in the observed difference in recurrent CAP rates between groups.

Membership bias is sometimes difficult to avoid because we are often unaware of all the possible causes of a given outcome. Researchers should perform due diligence in identifying the known and probable biasing characteristics that could alter the results. When these have been systematically linked to a characteristic upon which subjects will be assigned to groups, care should be taken to ensure that the biasing characteristics are also balanced between groups. This may require use of special randomization techniques, such as stratified randomization. If the biasing and assigning characteristics are too closely linked, it may be impossible to balance the biasing characteristic between groups. When this is the case, there are complex statistical methods that can be applied to identify and adjust for the contributions of the biasing characteristic to the outcome measurements.

## RESPONSE BIAS

A hypothetical randomized, double-dummy, superiority clinical trial was conducted to compare the relative efficacy of oral nicotinic receptor blocker tablets (active tablets) and transdermal nicotine patches (active patches) for smoking cessation. Subjects

| TABLE 13-3    Causes of Selected Selection Biases in Clinical Research | |
| --- | --- |
| **Bias** | **Cause** |
| Admission rate (Berkson) bias | Rates of exposed and unexposed individuals enrolled in a study systematically differ from rates of exposed and unexposed individuals not enrolled in the study as a result of the setting in which the subjects are selected (e.g., hospital admissions). |
| Detection bias | The definition or screening method for the condition of interest differs between groups, usually due to a difference in study entry time between groups. |
| Medical surveillance bias | Inclusion of subjects in a retrospective study is limited to those who have received a certain nonroutine screening or diagnostic test. |
| Membership bias | Subjects in one group have a higher prevalence of a characteristic that alters their outcomes than subjects in another group have, and that characteristic is systematically tied to another characteristic upon which group assignments are based. |
| Participation (nonresponse) bias | Subjects who are willing to participate in a study have different impactful characteristics than those who are unwilling to participate in the study or the willingness of subjects with a condition of interest to participate in a study differs from the willingness of subjects without the condition of interest to participate in the study. |
| Prevalence-incidence (Neyman) bias | Cases that are mild and self-resolving and those that are rapidly fatal are not captured; prevalence is mistaken for or inappropriately used as incidence for an outcome measurement. |
| Procedure selection bias | Decisions about treatment group assignments for individual subjects are based on characteristics that cause unintended changes in results. |

were randomly assigned to receive active tablets plus placebo patches or active patches plus placebo tablets for 10 weeks. All subjects received smoking cessation counseling, which included discussion of the risks of smoking, the benefits of quitting smoking, and how to take the tablets and use the patches properly. Efficacy was assessed by subject self-reported smoking status at 3 months after treatment. At the 3-month post-treatment assessment, 64% of subjects in the active tablet group and 60% of subjects in the active patch group reported successful abstention from smoking. The relative benefit of treatment with active tablets compared to active patches was calculated to be 6.3% $[(0.64 - 0.60) \div 0.64]$, which was not determined to be statistically significant. The researchers concluded that neither treatment is more efficacious than the other for smoking cessation.

Is there anything about this hypothetical study that might cause us to question the validity of the results? Self-reported responses can lead to imprecise measurements. They can also lead to outright inaccurate measurements when subjects introduce response bias. **Response bias** is a type of information bias that can occur when subjects respond to questions in a way that they believe the researcher wishes them to answer, rather than in a truthful way. (It should be noted that response bias is not the opposite of nonresponse bias, the latter of which is another term for participation bias, described earlier in this chapter.) Response bias can lead to data inaccuracies that can significantly affect the results of a study.

To illustrate this, let us think about what the data would be if, say, a third of the subjects in both groups who reported quitting smoking actually had not quit because they knew that this was the response desired by the researchers. This would mean that instead of 36% of subjects in the active tablet group having not quit smoking, 57% actually had not quit. Likewise, in the active patch group, 60% would not have quit smoking instead of the 40% reported. In other terms, 43% of subjects in the active tablet group and 40% of subjects in the active patch group were actually successful at quitting smoking, for a relative benefit of 13% $[(0.46 - 0.40) \div 0.46]$, as opposed to 6.3%. This new value might have been determined to be statistically significant.

The best way to avoid response bias is to use objective measurements. When this is not feasible, the researcher should take precautions not to lead subjects in a particular direction with regard to self-reported responses and to instill confidence in subjects that getting truthful responses is preferable to getting responses that the subject thinks are "correct" or "desired." The risk of response bias is especially high when subjects feel that giving certain responses will result in them being chastised, penalized, or stigmatized. Therefore, extra care should be paid to situations in which sensitive questions are asked, such as about intimate matters (e.g., sexual history), illegal activities (e.g., illicit drug use), or potentially sensitive or inflammatory topics (e.g., suicidal or homicidal ideations). Where possible, the researcher should reinforce the compact of privacy and that no retribution will occur as the result of any admissions.

## RECALL BIAS

A hypothetical clinical study was conducted to determine the risk of sudden infant death syndrome (SIDS) in infants who are breastfed by mothers taking over-the-counter (OTC) analgesics for acute pain. Women who had breastfed an infant who had died from SIDS (case mothers) were asked about OTC analgesic use during the time of breastfeeding. Each case mother was matched with a control mother who had breastfed an infant who had not died from SIDS, but who was otherwise similar in numerous regards, such as date of delivery, maternal age at delivery, infant gestational age at delivery, method of delivery, complications of delivery, maternal and household member smoking status before and during breastfeeding, use of pacifiers, infant sleeping position, socioeconomic status, and amount of postpartum pain. The control mothers were asked the same questions about OTC analgesic use during the time of breastfeeding. To mitigate the risk of response bias, the researchers were careful to assure all respondents that their answers would be kept anonymous and confidential, that completely honest responses were desired, and that there would be no negative consequences for any response given. Subjects were also reassured that no study to that date had established a link between SIDS and OTC analgesic use in breastfeeding mothers. In the case mothers, the incidence of OTC analgesic use was reported to be 22%, while the incidence in control mothers was reported to be 8%. The difference was found to be statistically significant, and the researchers concluded that OTC analgesic use in breastfeeding mothers is associated with SIDS in their infants.

The concept of response bias has already been discussed, and this type of bias could, indeed, be present in this hypothetical study. However, it is probably safe to assume that the typical subject in this study would believe that the response associated with fewer repercussions would be that she did not use OTC analgesics during breastfeeding. Thus, response bias in this study would only have minimized the apparent difference between the two groups, leading to a type II error, as we observed in the example smoking cessation study. In the SIDS study, a statistically significant difference was observed between the groups, so a type II error is impossible. There does exist, however, another possible type of bias in the SIDS study—recall bias.

**Recall bias** is a type of information bias that can occur when subjects are asked to remember events from the past. If subjects in one group are systematically more likely to remember events of interest than are subjects in another group, this can lead to recall bias. In the example SIDS study, is there a reason to suspect that mothers who experienced the loss of a child to SIDS might remember events surrounding that experience more or less vividly or accurately than mothers whose children did not die? A mother whose child dies of SIDS may frequently reflect on what she might have done that caused this to happen or what she might have done differently to prevent it. This might include whether she took medications while breastfeeding. Therefore, it is possible that more mothers of infants who died of SIDS accurately remember that they took OTC analgesics while breastfeeding than do mothers of infants who did not die from SIDS. Thus, the reporting of this act could be higher in the case mothers than in the control mothers, even if the actual truth is that the incidence of OTC analgesic use in both groups was the same.

Of course, recall bias can be avoided by conducting studies that do not rely as heavily on subject memory, such as prospective cohort studies. This might not be feasible or ethical in some cases. If relying on subject memory is unavoidable, the researcher should attempt to enroll subjects as quickly as possible following the event of interest in order to increase the chance that all subjects' memories are fresh.

## ATTENTION BIAS, THE HAWTHORNE EFFECT, AND THE PLACEBO EFFECT

A hypothetical clinical trial was conducted to evaluate the efficacy of a gastrointestinal lipase inhibitor for adjunct treatment of metabolic syndrome. Study subjects were randomized in a 2:1:1 ratio to receive lifestyle modification counseling plus study drug (group 1), lifestyle modification counseling plus active control drug (group 2), or lifestyle modification counseling plus placebo (group 3). The active control drug was another drug previously demonstrated in several studies to be effective for adjunct treatment of metabolic syndrome, but was generally considered an optional part of the standard of care. The study duration was 1 year. At the beginning of the study and at monthly intervals throughout, subjects were evaluated by a composite endpoint composed of relevant dichotomous clinical parameters, including normalization of fasting plasma glucose, normalization of glucose tolerance, decrease in body mass index (BMI), decrease in waist circumference, normalization of plasma LDL-c levels, increase in high-density lipoprotein cholesterol (HDL-c) levels, normalization of plasma triglyceride levels, and normalization of blood pressure. Subjects were also interviewed at these same intervals about relevant lifestyle and social habits, such as diet, exercise, smoking, and alcohol use. The researchers planned to compare results between groups 1 and 2 via noninferiority analysis and between groups 1 and 3 via superiority analysis. To avoid increasing the risk of errors, groups 2 and 3 were not directly compared, because the active control drug had already been established as effective for metabolic syndrome. At the conclusion of the study, the composite endpoint results from group 1 were determined to be noninferior to those from group 2. However, the composite endpoint results from group 1 were not statistically superior to those from group 3. The researchers were confused by these results, given that the study drug was demonstrated to be noninferior to a drug that had been previously shown in several studies to be superior to placebo for metabolic syndrome. The researchers did note that group 3 subjects appeared to have improved their diets, increased their exercise, and stopped smoking to a greater extent than typically occurs in patients receiving only lifestyle modification counseling, based on a recent large cross-sectional study. These subjects' clinical parameters of metabolic syndrome also improved more than typical patients who receive only lifestyle modification counseling.

If this hypothetical study was conducted well, as it appears to have been, does it seem odd that the study drug would be found to be not superior to placebo, but not inferior to another drug that was previously found to be superior to placebo? What might have accounted for this situation? The fact that subjects in group 3 appeared to have fared better than they normally would have outside the study may offer a clue that attention bias has occurred in the study.

**Attention bias** is a type of information bias that can occur when subjects change their behavior because they know that their actions are being observed. Attention bias has sometimes been referred to as **observation bias**, but this term can be misleading, because it can seem to imply that this type of bias is only possible in observational studies. In contrast to response bias, in which subjects respond untruthfully to questions, and recall bias, in which subjects cannot remember events accurately, attention bias results from subjects actually doing things differently than they otherwise would if they were not in the clinical study. This can obviously cause a difference between what happens in a clinical study and what might happen under the same circumstances outside the study.

One of the first modern observations of what we can refer to as attention bias was published by Henry Landsberger in 1958.[6] In reviewing productivity studies conducted at a company named Hawthorne Works, Landsberger noted that workers were more productive when being observed as part of studies, but returned to prior levels of productivity after the studies had concluded. The term **Hawthorne effect** has been used to describe this circumstance. The Hawthorne effect, and indeed attention bias, can be the result of conscious or unconscious motivation. Another term, the **placebo effect**, has been used when subjects receiving a placebo exhibit changes in the course of a condition of interest, despite the lack of a true intervention. The Hawthorne effect and the placebo effect differ in that the Hawthorne effect describes observable behaviors in a clinical study that differ from what would be observed outside the study, whereas the placebo effect describes observable outcomes in a clinical study that differ from what would occur outside the study, despite the lack of observable behavior changes in subjects. In other words, subjects experiencing the placebo effect do nothing differently, yet have changes in outcomes. When study subjects are all exposed to the same degree of scrutiny, the Hawthorne effect will typically affect all groups of subjects to a similar degree. Thus, the Hawthorne effect will have fewer propensities to cause biased differences between groups than to cause differences between observations in the study versus those circumstances outside the study. In contrast, the placebo effect is more likely to result in decreased differences between groups within a study. Although the placebo effect has been observed more frequently in studies with more subjective outcomes, such as in the areas of psychiatry and pain management, studies with more objective outcomes are not free from potential bias from placebo effects.[7-9]

In the hypothetical study on metabolic syndrome, it appears that attention bias may have resulted in more group 3 subjects improving their diet, exercise, and smoking habits than they might have if they were not enrolled in the study. Although this may have also been the case in the other study groups, it also may not have. Consider, for instance, if the drugs used in groups 1 and 2 were effective in helping subjects improve their clinical parameters of metabolic syndrome. Those subjects may have had less motivation to improve their lifestyle and social habits. If this was the case, the Hawthorne effect in group 3 subjects could have contributed to attention bias. Adding to this, a placebo effect could also have contributed to group 3 subjects' improvement in clinical parameters of metabolic syndrome.

Attention bias is difficult to avoid in clinical research involving subjects who are aware that they are enrolled in a study. Because it is generally unethical to expose individuals to prospective clinical study observation without their knowledge and consent, this is one of the few advantages that retrospective studies have over prospective studies. Subjects included in retrospective studies were generally not aware that their data would later be used for clinical research when their information was being collected. In prospective studies, it is important to balance the intrusion of study observation and frequent data collection with the desire to create a scenario that resembles "real life." In the example study on metabolic syndrome, by performing analyses and interviews of subjects every month, the researchers placed the subjects under much closer scrutiny than they likely would have experienced outside the study. Such a scenario can contribute to attention bias.

## EXPOSURE SUSPICION BIAS

A hypothetical randomized, double-blind clinical trial was conducted to determine the efficacy of a new antihistamine in treating seasonal allergic rhinitis (SAR). Individuals with clinically diagnosed SAR were eligible for the study. Because prior clinical studies with similar antihistamines had been associated with hematologic laboratory abnormalities, potential subjects were screened via complete blood count (CBC), and those found to have anemia, leukopenia, or thrombocytopenia were excluded from study entry. Potential subjects wishing to enroll in the study were required to give consent to participation after being informed of the potential risks and benefits, to the extent that they could be anticipated. Enrolled subjects were randomly assigned to receive the antihistamine or matching placebo for the duration of the allergy season. At the conclusion of the study, 82% of subjects in the antihistamine group and 28% of subjects in the placebo group had reported a decrease in allergy symptoms, the primary outcome of the study; 56% of subjects in the antihistamine group and 12% of subjects in the placebo group had reported experiencing anticholinergic effects, such as dry mouth, constipation, and blurry vision; and 7% of subjects in the antihistamine group and 0.5% of subjects in the placebo group were reported to have developed hematologic laboratory abnormalities, including anemia, leukopenia, and thrombocytopenia. All of these differences were determined to be statistically significant.

This hypothetical study appears to be relatively straightforward, with little risk of bias. However, what if the fact that a significantly greater number of subjects in the antihistamine group experienced drowsiness, a well-known adverse effect of many antihistamines, led researchers to follow more of these subjects more closely because they believed that subjects reporting drowsiness were likely to be receiving the study drug and not the placebo? And, what if this closer monitoring led to a disproportionate number of CBC investigations in the absence of more compelling clinical manifestations of hematologic abnormalities in the antihistamine group than in the placebo group because the researchers knew that the antihistamine might cause such effects? If this was the case, it is possible that some or all of the difference that was observed in the incidence rates of hematologic abnormalities between groups could have been attributable to the simple fact that more investigations were conducted in subjects in the antihistamine group than in the placebo group. This is an example of exposure suspicion bias.

**Exposure suspicion bias** is a type of information bias that can occur when subjects in one group are systematically exposed to diagnostic procedures or investigations that subjects in another group are not as a result of the researchers' knowledge or beliefs about the group to which individual subjects have been assigned—in other words, because they are suspicious about those individuals' specific exposures. This scenario can increase the chances that conditions will be identified to a greater extent in one group than another, even if the incidence rates are actually the same in both groups. Exposure suspicion bias is not limited to clinical trials; it can occur in other types of clinical research as well. For instance, if the researcher is suspicious of subjects' assigned groups in a case-control or cohort study, she may consciously or unconsciously dig deeper for evidence of certain circumstances in one group more than in the other.

Obviously, exposure suspicion bias can occur in studies in which the researchers are not blinded to the subjects' assigned groups. (In this case, the researchers need not be suspicious of a subject's disposition in the study; it is already known to them.) Alternatively, the researcher or subject may become effectively unblinded to the subject's group assignment, as might have occurred in our example study, due to circumstances such as obvious and expected adverse effects (e.g., anticholinergic effects). Using appropriate blinding and dummying techniques can minimize the risk of exposure suspicion bias. Indeed, this is one of the main reasons that these methods are employed in clinical research. In addition, and especially when the potential for significant unblinding can occur, ensuring that all subjects in all groups are routinely screened at regular intervals for effects that are anticipated to possibly occur in any given group can mitigate the risk of exposure suspicion bias.

## UNMASKING BIAS AND MIMICRY BIAS

A hypothetical randomized, double-blind, noninferiority clinical trial was conducted to compare the relative efficacy of a new sulfonamide antibiotic with a beta-lactam antibiotic previously established as a standard treatment of care for uncomplicated urinary tract infection (UTI) in women. Eligible women were randomly assigned to receive treatment with either agent. The study demonstrated noninferiority of the new sulfonamide compared to the established beta-lactam for efficacy in treating uncomplicated UTI in this population. However, there was also noted a small number of subjects in the sulfonamide group who were diagnosed with systemic lupus erythematosus (SLE) while or shortly after taking the drug. Although the cases of SLE in the sulfonamide group were few, there were no such cases reported in the beta-lactam group, and the difference was found to be statistically significant. No other serious adverse effects were reported in either group. Mild diarrhea and mild nausea were more common in subjects in the beta-lactam group, while mild rash and mild photosensitivity were more common in subjects in the sulfonamide group. The researchers concluded that the sulfonamide was not inferior to standard treatment with the beta-lactam, but that there was an increased risk of SLE with the sulfonamide.

Given these hypothetical results, there would seem to be little reason to use the new sulfonamide instead of the established beta-lactam in most women with uncomplicated UTI, provided that the beta-lactam had previously been established relatively free from causing serious adverse effects. But is there a reason to be suspicious that this clinical study is biased where the diagnoses of SLE are concerned? What if every subject who experienced any adverse effect underwent a thorough diagnostic evaluation of the possible causes, regardless of treatment group, in order to mitigate the risk for exposure suspicion bias and to assess whether the effect was deemed to be related to the drug? Would this make us more or less confident that the sulfonamide caused SLE? In this hypothetical study, it is possible that the increased incidence of SLE in the sulfonamide group is the result of unmasking bias, rather than because the drug causes SLE.

**Unmasking bias** is a type of information bias that can occur when an inciting condition that is unrelated to a condition of interest creates a situation in which the condition of interest is more likely to be discovered. The inciting condition does not have to look like the condition of interest. It merely has to create a circumstance in which the condition of interest is more likely to be discovered if it does exist. When it happens that the inciting condition does present similarly to the condition of interest, unmasking bias has sometimes been referred to as **mimicry bias**. In either case, the condition of interest is detected to a systematically greater extent in one group than in another group, but not necessarily because the actual prevalence rates between the groups differ.

When SLE manifests itself, hallmark symptoms include rash and photosensitivity. However, many cases of SLE are asymptomatic for long periods of time. In this hypothetical UTI study, more subjects in the sulfonamide group experienced rash and photosensitivity than in the beta-lactam group. This resulted in more thorough evaluations into possible causes of these effects in the sulfonamide group than in the beta-lactam group, which could have resulted in detecting more instances of SLE in the sulfonamide group, even if this condition actually existed at the same prevalence in both groups. Rash and photosensitivity (caused by the sulfonamide) would be the inciting conditions and SLE would be the unmasked condition. It could be that the sulfonamide does not cause SLE at all, or that it merely exacerbates the condition when it already exists. In other words, the subjects in the beta-lactam group could have the exact same prevalence of SLE, but without identifiable manifestations yet and no other reason to investigate for the condition.

It is important to distinguish between exposure suspicion bias and unmasking bias. Although both types of bias can result in inflated differences in observed effects between groups because of disproportionate discovery of cases that might otherwise go undetected, they are caused by different circumstances. Whereas exposure suspicion bias is the result of a belief about the treatment group to which a subject is assigned and can be mitigated by proper blinding and purposefully planned screening, unmasking bias is the result of warranted investigation into unexpected effects when they actually occur, without any knowledge or assumption about the subject's assigned group. Unmasking bias is not mitigated by blinding and is sometimes quite difficult to avoid, because it is important to investigate adverse effects in clinical studies. When there is suspicion that unmasking bias has occurred, it may be necessary to conduct new studies specifically designed to determine the risk of the unmasked condition with the intervention.

## Sample Size Bias

A hypothetical clinical trial was conducted to determine the efficacy of a new drug in preventing cardiovascular-related death. A total of 100 subjects were enrolled and randomized to receive either the drug or matching placebo. At the conclusion of the study, the incidence rates of cardiovascular-related death in the drug and placebo groups were 10% and 14%, respectively. The superiority analysis determined that this difference was not statistically significant, and the researchers concluded that the drug does not significantly reduce the risk of cardiovascular death compared to placebo.

Another hypothetical clinical trial was conducted, sampling from the exact same population and using the exact same interventions and primary outcome. This study enrolled 10,000 subjects. The incidence rates of cardiovascular-related death in this study's drug and placebo groups were 11% and 13%, respectively. In contrast to the first study, this difference was determined to be statistically significant, and the researchers concluded that the drug was superior to placebo in preventing cardiovascular-related death in the sampled population.

To be compelling, clinical studies must enroll the correct number of subjects. If they do not, they may suffer from a type of information bias known as sample size bias. **Sample size bias** is a systematic error that occurs because too few or too many subjects than are appropriate are included in the study. With too few subjects, as in the first hypothetical study, the statistical analyses may have insufficient power to definitively demonstrate a difference when one truly exists in the population. (Statistical power will be discussed in more detail later in this chapter.) With too many subjects, as in the second hypothetical study, the analyses may be oversensitive and therefore detect statistically significant differences that are misleading in that they do not represent clinically significant differences. Although sample size bias concerns the number of subjects enrolled in a clinical study, and as such would appear to be a type of selection bias, sample size bias is truly a type of information bias because it affects the statistical analyses and interpretation of the study data, not whether subjects between groups or between the sample and the population are similar.

In addition to being insufficient or misleading, conducting clinical trials with an inappropriate number of subjects can be unethical, because the researcher is exposing subjects to interventions that are potentially less effective or more dangerous than what those individuals might have received otherwise. It is obvious why we would not wish to conduct clinical trials of unproven agents with too many subjects. However, enrolling too few subjects can be just as unethical, because their participation and exposure will be meaningless should the low statistical power of the study lead to a type II error. Sample size biases are avoided by determining a priori how many subjects are necessary to detect statistically significant differences when a clinically significant difference has been achieved, and enrolling a number of subjects close to that figure.

## Missing Data Bias and Withdrawal Bias

A hypothetical randomized clinical trial was conducted to compare the long-term efficacy of two established outpatient programs for treating alcohol dependence. Subjects were randomly assigned to one of the two programs and were followed for a period of 2 years. Program A consisted of oral drug treatment taken once daily for 3 months and attendance of twice-weekly meetings for 2 years. Program B consisted of intramuscular drug treatment given once monthly for 6 months and attendance of once-weekly meetings for 2 years. During the 2-year study period, subjects also made weekly visits to a research clinic, where they were evaluated for relapse via breath analysis and questionnaire and received their study drug. Subjects were also requested to proactively inform researchers by phone if they experienced a relapse as soon as possible after the relapse. If subjects were discovered to have experienced a relapse by breath analysis or self-report or if they stopped making clinic visits and could not be contacted after multiple attempts, they were considered treatment failures. Of subjects who were present at their last scheduled clinic visit and who had not suffered a relapse during the duration of the study, 75% were counted as treatment successes and 25% were counted as treatment failures in the final analysis. This was supported by multiple previous studies that had demonstrated that 70-80% of patients with alcohol dependence who do not suffer a relapse in the first 2 years after initial treatment have similar life outcomes compared to non-alcohol-dependent individuals. At the conclusion of the study, the success rates of programs A and B were determined to be 52% and 66%, respectively. This difference was found to be statistically significant, and the researchers concluded that program B was superior to program A with regard to success rate.

Avoiding participation and response biases would be important factors in designing and executing this study. But assuming adequate measures were taken to minimize the risk of these biases, are there other potential problems in this study? What about the way in which the data from subjects lost to follow-up or from those who were determined to have not relapsed were handled? This could raise concerns of missing data bias. **Missing data bias** occurs as the result of a disproportionate number of subjects between groups or high numbers of subjects in all groups discontinuing their participation in a study. Missing data bias has sometimes been referred to as **withdrawal bias**.

Missing data bias is a type of information bias that can occur when data that are absent are omitted, assumed, imputed, or otherwise treated. Most clinical studies, and certainly most clinical trials, will have missing data. Some subjects will voluntarily drop out of a study before the researcher has an opportunity to collect all the intended data on them. Other subjects will miss study visits in the middle of the study or be lost to follow-up with unknown outcomes. Laboratory specimens for some subjects may get lost. Certain items on questionnaires will be left unanswered. Retrospective study subjects will simply have certain desired data missing from their records. These are common occurrences, and there a number of accepted methods for properly dealing with such missing data. However, when a difference exists between study groups that systematically causes absent information from one group to be different than that from another group, this missing data can lead to biased results.

Let us examine the concept of missing data bias in the context of the hypothetical study on alcohol dependence. There are two primary places in this study where data are absent—from subjects who were lost to follow-up and from subjects who did not relapse by the end of the study. Assuming that the post-2-year treatment failure rate is similar in both groups, and that those rates are close to the 25% estimated in the study, applying a 75% treatment success rate to both groups for subjects completing the study without relapse is probably fine, albeit not as optimal as following them for a longer period. But is it appropriate to assign all subjects lost to follow-up as treatment failures? It might seem so, because we are applying the same parameter to both groups equally. But what if there were significantly more dropouts in one group than in the other, or if the dropout rate in both groups was approximately equal but high? If the dropout rates were different enough between groups or high enough in both groups, counting them all as treatment failures could bias the results, even if only a small and equal proportion of the total dropouts in both groups were actually treatment successes. Furthermore, it is possible that more dropout subjects in one group than in the other had successful treatment but dropped out because they found the burden of continuing to participate in the study for the full 2 years too great. One could easily see how subjects in program A might drop out earlier than those in program B, because program A subjects completed their drug therapy component in half the time. In addition, subjects in program A were required to appear at designated appointments three times per week (twice for meetings and once for clinic visits), whereas subjects in program B were only required to be present two times per week (once for meetings and once for clinic visits). This could also have led to more successfully treated subjects dropping out, and thus being counted as treatment failures, from program A than from program B.

Missing data are nearly ubiquitous in clinical studies, and a number of valid methods for dealing with this issue appropriately are available. No single method exists for optimally handling all types of missing data. The best technique for handling a given set of missing data must be predicated on its type and context in the study. When assumptions about missing data must be made, they should tend toward conservatism. That is, in a superiority study, any assumptions that are made about missing data should be more likely to push the result toward the line of equivalence instead of away from it. Conversely, in an equivalency study, any assumptions that are made about missing data should be more likely to push the result away from the line of equivalence instead of toward it. In a noninferiority study, any assumptions that are made about missing data should be more likely to push the result in favor of the control group instead of in favor of the experimental group.

Given the complexity of dealing with missing data, it can be tempting to simply exclude subjects with significant amounts of missing data from the final study analysis. However, this can create a circumstance in which the data do not accurately reflect what happened in the entire study. For this reason, it is preferred to determine a priori how missing data will be handled and include the data (real or assumed) for all subjects in the final analysis. This also ensures that the correct sample size will be maintained. Analyses that use data from all subjects who were enrolled in the study, even if some of those subjects' data must be assumed, are called **intention-to-treat (ITT) analyses**. ITT analyses are the accepted standard for most clinical studies. Another accepted method is commonly referred to as **modified intention-to-treat** (mITT). Although this term can be appropriately applied to almost any analysis that deviates only slightly from a true ITT analysis, in most mITT analyses all subjects who were enrolled in the study and continued to a prespecified point that is very early in the study, such as having received the first dose of a study drug, are included in the analysis. This method allows for exclusion of subjects who enrolled and then immediately withdrew, were lost, or died without actually having received any study maneuvers.

Sometimes, researchers may wish to analyze the data from only those subjects who completed the study properly, with minimal or no missing data and few or no deviations from the study procedures. Such analyses are referred to as **per-protocol analyses**. Care should be taken when extrapolating conclusions drawn from per-protocol analyses to a general population, especially when the results of these analyses significantly differ from the results of ITT or mITT analyses. However, when the results from per-protocol analyses are relatively similar to the results of ITT or mITT analyses, this can serve as an indicator that missing data were handled appropriately in the latter analyses.

## MIGRATION (CONTAMINATION) BIAS

A hypothetical prospective cohort study was conducted to compare long-term cardiovascular outcomes between adults aged 50–60 years who primarily participate in aerobic exercise and those who primarily participate in strength training exercise. Volunteer subjects who had identified spending at least 2.5 hours/week exercising and at least 80% of their total exercise time exclusively devoted to either aerobic exercise or strength training exercise were assigned to respective groups and followed for 10 years. Subjects attended annual research clinic visits, where they received blood pressure and plasma lipid monitoring and were administered a questionnaire about new cardiovascular events and diagnoses over the previous year. Pertinent baseline demographics, such as age, sex, race, blood pressure, plasma lipid levels, smoking status, presence of diabetes, renal function, and family history of cardiovascular disease, were similar between groups. Mean BMI was slightly higher at baseline in the strength training exercise group than in the aerobic exercise group, which was expected. Body fat percentage and waist circumference were similar between groups. A low and equal number of subjects withdrew or were lost to follow-up during the 10-year study period. Appropriate measures were taken to estimate missing data. At study conclusion, it was determined from multiple metrics, including serious cardiovascular-related events, blood pressure, and plasma lipid levels, that neither aerobic exercise nor strength training exercise was superior to the other with regard to cardiovascular outcomes.

Ten years is a long time. What would happen if subjects changed their exercise habits over the 10 years of the study? This hypothetical study raises the issue of **migration bias**, which is also sometimes referred to as **contamination bias**. Migration bias is a type of information bias that can occur when subjects unintentionally "migrate" from one group to another during the course of the study, but whose outcome data are not missing and are treated as still belonging to their assigned group. In reality, these subjects do not actually change groups. Rather, they start following a protocol that is more similar to a group to which they are not assigned than to the group to which they are assigned, but are still counted as being in their assigned group. The group to which a given subject migrates may be another group within the study, or it may be to a group that is not actually included in the study. Thus, the term **migration** refers to the circumstance in which a subject assigned to a group associated with a specific course transitions to a course that is more associated with a different group, but is still counted as if he were following the course associated with his original group. For instance, a subject is assigned to the group of subjects receiving drug A in a clinical trial comparing drug A to drug B. At some point during the study, that subject unintentionally stops receiving drug A and starts receiving drug B. Despite this, the subject is still counted as being in the drug A group. This describes a subject who has migrated. The subject would also have migrated if he had stopped receiving drug A and started receiving drug C or no drug at all, even if no such groups existed in the study, as long as he is still counted as being in the drug A group. Yet another instance of migration could be if a subject in the drug A group started taking a second drug for the condition of interest, drug D, in addition to continuing drug A. This would represent migration to a nonstudy group, the drug A/drug D combination group. The point is that the subject is now following the protocol of another study or nonstudy group, but is still being counted as if he were following the protocol of his assigned group.

In cases where a subject migrates to the protocol of another study group, migration bias results in a simple decrease in the magnitude of observed differences in outcomes between groups. As more subjects migrate to other groups within the study, these groups become more similar to one another. Thus, the risk of committing a type II error increases. In some cases, however, differences can exist between groups that systematically cause more subjects in one group to migrate out of their assigned group than subjects in another group. When this occurs, the consequences of migration bias can be less predictable and the result can be an error in any direction. The consequences of migration bias can also be less predictable when many subjects migrate to nonstudy groups.

Let us examine how migration bias might have affected the hypothetical study of different types of exercise. It is relatively obvious that some subjects in each of the groups might decide during the course of the study that the other type of exercise is more to their liking and change their habits. Because the researchers assigned subjects to groups based on baseline exercise habits and did not account for changes in such habits throughout the study, the groups may be more similar to each other by the end of the study than at the outset of the study, making observed differences in the study outcomes less prominent. But what if aerobic exercisers and strength training exercisers inherently differ in some systematic way that causes them to change exercise habits disproportionately? For instance, what if aerobic exercise is associated with more injury and aerobic exercisers are more likely to stop exercising altogether when they get injured? This could lead to a greater increase in incidence of cardiovascular outcomes in the aerobic exercise group than in the strength training exercise group. What if, in addition, the general trend as people age is for them to reduce their strength training exercise in favor of aerobic exercise? From baseline, individuals assigned to the aerobic exercise group could only increase the proportion of their total exercise devoted to aerobic exercise by a maximum of 20%, because aerobic exercise already accounted for at least 80% of their baseline total exercise. In contrast, individuals in the strength training exercise group could increase their proportion of aerobic exercise 80% or more, because their baseline proportion of aerobic exercise was only 20% or less. So, if aerobic exercise is actually more beneficial on cardiovascular outcomes than is strength training exercise, migration bias might have been the cause for this effect to have not been observed in the hypothetical clinical study.

Like missing data, data from subjects who have migrated (assuming such migration is captured by the researcher) can be handled appropriately by a variety of methods. Also like with missing data, the optimal method for a given set of data from migratory subjects must be determined by the data type and context. In addition, measures should be implemented to minimize subject migration, when appropriate, and to proactively discover when migration has occurred. Comparing per-protocol analyses of data from subjects who did not migrate to the ITT or mITT analysis can also help to quantify the effect of migration on study outcomes.

## COMPLIANCE (ADHERENCE) BIAS

A hypothetical randomized, double-blind, double-dummy, superiority clinical trial was conducted to compare two regimens of an oral antibiotic for treatment of acute bacterial sinusitis (ABS) caused by susceptible organisms in adult outpatients. Potential subjects were required to be adults with a suspected or confirmed diagnosis of uncomplicated ABS to be eligible. Eligible subjects with a history of persistent cough, recent prior ABS, chronic sinusitis, seasonal or persistent allergies, chronic pain, or sinus surgery were excluded. Study subjects were randomized to receive either regimen 1 or regimen 2. Regimen 1 consisted of one high-dose tablet taken twice daily for 3 days. Regimen 2 consisted of one low-dose tablet taken twice daily for 10 days. To ensure blinding, subjects in the regimen 1 group also took placebo tablets appearing to be low-dose tablets twice daily for 10 days. Likewise, subjects in the regimen 2 group took placebo tablets appearing to be high-dose tablets twice daily for the first 3 days. Subjects were requested to only take medications for symptoms of ABS, such as decongestants, as needed (i.e., not routinely). All enrolled subjects underwent sinus culture and sensitivity at the time of enrollment. The efficacy data from subjects determined to have nonbacterial sinusitis or ABS caused by an organism resistant to the antibiotic were reported, but were excluded from the primary efficacy analysis because the study was intended only to assess the relative efficacy of the two regimens in ABS caused by susceptible organisms. Subjects with resistant-organism ABS were transitioned to appropriate alternate treatment. The primary outcome was time to patient-reported symptom resolution, which was counted as the first full day that the subject experienced complete absence of nasal congestion, sinus headache, sore throat, persistent cough, and fever. Each subject was contacted every day by automated telephone response system to determine if the previous day had been symptom-free. At the conclusion of the study, the mean times to patient-reported symptom resolution in the regimen 1 and 2 groups were 5.7 days and 7.4 days, respectively, a difference determined to be statistically significant. The incidence of absolute treatment failure was slightly, but not statistically significantly, higher in the regimen 2 group. The researchers concluded that regimen 1 was faster than regimen 2 at relieving symptoms of uncomplicated ABS caused by susceptible organisms in adults.

It would appear from the results of this hypothetical study that the researchers' conclusion about the difference in speed of symptom resolution between the two antibiotic regimens is well founded. But is there anything about the design of this study that calls into question the validity of the results? It is certainly reasonable to think that a higher dose of antibiotic could lead to faster symptom resolution. But what if similar numbers of subjects in both groups started to feel better within the first few days? Even if these subjects had not yet achieved complete symptom resolution according to the definition used in the study, some of them may have decided that the burden of continuing to take the medication as directed was unnecessary and, therefore, stopped taking the medication. Other subjects may have been very compliant at the start, when their symptoms were most severe, and then less compliant as their symptoms diminished but had not completely resolved. By day 3, subjects in the regimen 1 group had already received their entire course of active drug, while subjects in the regimen 2 group had only received 30% of theirs. Even if equal numbers of subjects in both groups stopped early, it is clear to see how subjects in the regimen 1 group would fare better. This is an example of compliance bias.

**Compliance bias**, also referred to as **adherence bias**, is a type of information bias that occurs when more subjects in one group systematically fail to properly follow study protocols than subjects in another group do because of inconvenience of or intolerance to their assigned intervention, or when equal amounts of noncompliance between groups exists, but the noncompliance affects the outcomes of one group more than it affects the outcomes of another. Compliance bias most commonly occurs when one intervention is more burdensome than another. One medication must be taken twice daily, whereas the other need only be taken once daily. One medication is taken orally, whereas the other must be administered by painful injection. One medication causes significant nausea, whereas the other is relatively free from bothersome side effects. One procedure is invasive, whereas the other is mundane. These are all differences that can lead to subjects in one group adhering to study protocols more than subjects in another group. It is important to note that compliance does not only refer to completing the entire course of treatment. Compliance also refers to completing the course of treatment in the manner intended. For instance, if a drug is prescribed to be taken every morning, but a subject takes it every evening instead, this is a form of noncompliance, even if she took the entire course of treatment.

In the hypothetical ABS study, subjects in both groups received the same number of tablets. This might be fine if the courses of active treatment were the same in duration, leading to equal numbers of incomplete regimens in both groups. However, the fact that one group's active regimen was complete at day 3 and the other group's active regimen required 10 days created a situation in which noncompliance was more likely to affect one group more than another. In fact, dummying in this study created a falsely inflated pill burden in both groups and may have led to even more noncompliance than if dummying had not been used. Even when treatment courses are identical, compliance bias can be introduced when one intervention has more bothersome adverse effects than the other. Such cases may also lead to missing data bias if too many subjects withdraw from the study and the resultant absent data are not properly handled.

Dummying can assist in maintaining study blinding. Under many circumstances, this can reduce the risk of certain types of bias. However, in some instances, dummying can also increase the risk of introducing bias, as demonstrated by the hypothetical ABS study. Therefore, the potential risks and benefits of dummying in a clinical trial must be weighed. In some instances, it may actually be more desirable to create a research scenario that more resembles "real life." For instance, if one antibiotic regimen requires only 3 days to complete and another requires 10 days, it may be desirable to simply give one group the 3-day treatment and the other group the 10-day treatment and compare the results unblinded. If the 10-day treatment is too burdensome for some subjects in the clinical trial, and they have worse outcomes because of this, then it may be appropriate to assume the same thing might happen outside the study. But at least those subjects whose symptoms start resolving early will not stop taking their medication after 3 days because they think they have received the 3-day regimen.

Noncompliance can be minimized by frequent follow-up and protocol reinforcement. However, like missing data, noncompliance of some degree is nearly unavoidable in clinical studies. Therefore, steps should be taken to accurately quantify noncompliance. Such steps might include pill counts, plasma drug-level monitoring, subject questionnaires, etc. In addition, statistical comparisons can be conducted between subjects identified as relatively compliant (i.e., per-protocol subjects) versus subjects identified as less compliant (i.e., ITT or mITT subjects) to help quantify the impact of noncompliance.

## SCALE DEGRADATION BIAS

A hypothetical clinical trial was conducted to compare the effects of two drugs given as part of a standard regimen for graft-versus-host disease (GVHD) prophylaxis on renal function. Both drugs had been demonstrated in previous studies to be effective as part of the regimen for GVHD prophylaxis following hematopoietic cell transplantation (HCT), and both had previously been implicated in causing nephrotoxicity. Subjects who had undergone HCT were randomly assigned to receive prophylaxis for GVHD with the standard regimen backbone plus either drug A or drug B. Except for the two study drugs, the regimens were identical. No drugs in the standard regimen backbone had been previously implicated as potentially nephrotoxic. The primary outcome was degree of renal function worsening at the end of 6 months of treatment or at study drug discontinuation, if the latter occurred before completing 6 months of treatment. Renal function was determined by calculating estimated glomerular filtration rate (eGFR) using the Modification of Diet in Renal Disease equation at baseline, at weekly intervals for the first month, and at monthly intervals for the remainder of treatment duration. Renal function worsening was categorized as absent (decrease in eGFR < 10 mL/min), mild-moderate (decrease in eGFR = 10-50 mL/min), or severe (decrease in eGFR > 50 mL/min). If severe renal function worsening was observed in a subject prior to 6 months of treatment, the study drug was automatically discontinued. At the conclusion of the study, the differences in renal function worsening between groups were not determined to be statistically significant, and the researchers concluded that neither drug is more nephrotoxic than the other when used for 6 months following HCT.

Without even knowing the numbers of subjects in each group who fell into each of the renal function worsening categories, we can see how using such a system can introduce bias into the results. When data that are measured on numeric scales are collapsed into categories, the result can be scale degradation bias. **Scale degradation bias** is a type of information bias that can occur when data are not analyzed in the most specific and precise manner possible. Although it may be desirable in some contexts to group data ranges into distinct categories for descriptive purposes or clinical decision making, applying statistical analyses to categorical data when the data could be analyzed in their original continuous numeric state is generally unacceptable because this could lead to biased results.

In the hypothetical GVHD study, it is fairly clear to see how significant differences in actual eGFR values could be categorized together, making them indistinguishable from one another. This is especially problematic in the mild-moderate renal function worsening category, wherein the range is quite wide and includes values that represent major clinical differences from one another (e.g., eGFR decreases of 15 mL/min vs. 45 mL/min).

Think of scale degradation as an extreme form of rounding. The bias is introduced when the rounding creates a circumstance in which sufficient precision is lost. Think about rounding the value 15.8 mL/min. If we round to the nearest ones place, we get 16 mL/min. Not much precision is lost here. What if we round 15.8 mL/min to the nearest tens place? The result is 20 mL/min. This is quite a bit less precise, because the rounded value 20 mL/min encompasses all values from 15.0 mL/min to 24.9 mL/min, a range of about 10 mL/min. Now, take that one step further to place the value 15.8 mL/min in the category of "mild-moderate worsening," and it is even more obvious how much precision is lost, because the category encompasses a 30 mL/min range of values.

When categories have been clinically established for data that are measured on numeric scales, it is often appropriate to present the data in terms of those clinical categories. However, this type of presentation should be in addition to presenting the data in their original form. For instance, hypertriglyceridemia can be defined as a fasting plasma triglyceride level of 150 mg/dL or greater.[10] In a clinical study, it may be desirable to report the number of new cases of hypertriglyceridemia, based on this value. The categories would be hypertriglyceridemia and no hypertriglyceridemia. However, it would also be important to present the fasting plasma triglyceride level data in their original continuous numeric form, in order to see the magnitude of triglyceride levels.

## REFERENCE BIAS

A hypothetical clinical trial was conducted to compare two drugs for the treatment of acne vulgaris. The well-conducted study demonstrated superiority of drug A over drug B in reducing both noninflammatory and inflammatory acne lesions. In the discussion section of the study article, the researchers cited three previous articles about studies comparing these two drugs for acne vulgaris treatment that showed similar results. The researchers went on to state that the four studies, together, provided sufficient evidence to support use of drug A over drug B in most patients.

Does anything about this scenario seem odd? If three previous studies all showed superiority of drug A over drug B for the treatment of acne vulgaris, does it seem redundant that the researchers conducted yet another study about this same topic? Is it possible that the results of other studies have conflicted with the results of this and the three cited studies? The absence of any mention of whether refuting evidence exists is a red flag that indicates possible reference bias.

**Reference bias** is a type of information bias that can actually occur after the completion of a study. For this reason, reference bias does not technically cause study errors, but rather reporting errors. When a published article cites only references that do not accurately represent the entire body of knowledge on the topic, reference bias has occurred. Although this is often intentional, it can also represent an unconscious bias toward a particular belief or even a deficiency in literature retrieval skills on the part of the authors. For obvious reasons, researchers should make every attempt to present their research in the context of all previous evidence. This is not to suggest that every article ever published on a given topic needs to be cited in every new original research article. Rather, the cited previous works should be a fair representation of all the previous evidence. Readers of the literature should use caution when relying on authors to provide a complete picture of evidence from related research. When research bias is suspected, it is prudent to conduct one's own literature search and evaluation before making clinical decisions.

## RHETORICAL BIAS

A hypothetical superiority clinical study is conducted to compare two drugs for the treatment of early-stage Alzheimer's disease. The well-conducted study failed to demonstrate superiority of either drug. In the results section of the study article, the researchers identify that, although the difference between mean standardized mental status assessment scores was not determined to be statistically significant, there was a trend toward superiority of drug A over drug B in these scores. In the discussion section of the article, the researchers describe the individual assessment items that led to the higher scores in drug A subjects than in drug B subjects. In the conclusion, the researchers state that in the absence of other clinical study evidence, it may be prudent to use drug A in early-stage Alzheimer's disease patients unless compelling clinical reasons exist for using drug B in a given patient.

Clearly, the researchers in this study favor drug A over drug B. But is this because they truly believe it to be better? Even if they do, the evidence from this study is insufficient to make such a claim, and the language they choose to use in the study article suggests rhetorical bias.

**Rhetorical bias** is a type of information bias that can occur when authors of scientific literature use language and innuendo to lead the reader to a conclusion that is not supported by evidence. Like reference bias, rhetorical bias does not occur during a study, but after it. The hypothetical study on Alzheimer's disease included language that was fairly obviously biased. However, rhetorical bias can be much more subtle. Authors of scientific literature should limit their statements to what can be supported by the evidence and avoid making assumptions or connections that are not fully substantiated. Readers of the literature should be aware of language suggestive of rhetorical bias. If authors appear to focus on minutia, use ambiguous terms (e.g., "trend"), or use criteria that are subjective or undefined (e.g., "compelling clinical reasons"), these are warning signs that one may be facing rhetorical bias.

## PUBLICATION BIAS

A hypothetical clinical trial was conducted to compare the relative efficacy of two topical treatments for seborrheic dermatitis of the scalp. The well-conducted study demonstrated that neither treatment was superior to the other for this condition. The researchers submitted a manuscript describing the study and its results to an appropriate medical journal, but it was not accepted for publication. Subsequent submissions to other appropriate journal resulted in the same outcome.

Sometimes researchers are not the best writers, and this might have been the reason that this article was not published. Another reason for the lack of interest could be that sufficient literature already existed in support of the same results demonstrated in this study and there had been no studies published to refute these findings. Yet another reason could be publication bias.

**Publication bias** is a type of information bias that can occur as a result of the propensity against researchers submitting articles to biomedical journals describing studies that do not demonstrate what the researchers intended to demonstrate (i.e., negative studies) for publication and the propensity for biomedical journal publishers to pass over such articles that are submitted in favor of publishing those studies that do demonstrate what the researchers intended to demonstrate (i.e., positive studies). Like reference and rhetorical biases, publication bias occurs after a study has been completed. Publication bias can result in an underrepresentation of negative study results being available to the scientific community, even when such studies exist and have been well conducted. Not only can publication bias lead to imbalanced literature, it can result in the execution of redundant studies, putting more subjects at risk and costing more resources than necessary. For these reasons, researchers are encouraged to submit articles describing well-conducted negative studies, and publishers of scientific journals should consider them as having the same merit as articles about positive studies.

**TABLE 13-4    Causes of Selected Information Biases in Clinical Research**

| Bias | Cause |
|---|---|
| Attention bias | Subjects change their behavior because they know that their actions are being observed. |
| Compliance (adherence) bias | More subjects in one group systematically fail to properly follow study protocols than subjects in another group do because of inconvenience of or intolerance to their assigned intervention or equal noncompliance between groups affects outcomes of one group more than another. |
| Exposure suspicion bias | Subjects in one group are systematically exposed to diagnostic procedures or investigations that subjects in another group are not exposed to as a result of the researchers' knowledge or beliefs about the group to which individual subjects have been assigned. |
| Migration (contamination) bias | Subjects unintentionally follow a protocol more closely resembling that of a group to which they are not assigned, but are still counted as members of their original group. |
| Missing data bias/withdrawal bias | Data that are absent are omitted or inappropriately assumed, imputed, or otherwise treated; considered withdrawal bias when this is the result of subjects being removed from the study. |
| Publication bias | Negative studies are not submitted or accepted for publication in favor of positive studies. |
| Recall bias | Subjects in one group are systematically more likely to accurately remember events of interest than are subjects in another group. |
| Reference bias | A published article cites studies that do not accurately or fairly represent the entire body of knowledge on a topic. |
| Response bias | Subjects respond to questions in a way that they believe the researcher wishes them to answer, rather than in a truthful way. |
| Rhetorical bias | Authors of scientific literature use language and innuendo to lead the reader to a conclusion that is not supported by evidence. |
| Sample size bias | Too few or too many subjects than are appropriate are included in the study. |
| Scale degradation bias | Data scales are collapsed such that the data are not analyzed in the most specific and precise manner possible. |
| Unmasking bias/mimicry bias | An inciting condition that is unrelated to a condition of interest creates a situation in which the condition of interest is more likely to be discovered; considered mimicry bias when the inciting condition presents similarly to the condition of interest. |

# CONFOUNDERS IN CLINICAL RESEARCH

This chapter has taken an extensive look at various ways that clinical study researchers, subjects, and publishers can introduce systematic, or nonrandom, errors in the results of clinical research and in the conclusions about populations drawn thereon. Furthermore, it has been described how these are theoretically avoidable, because they are introduced into studies by individuals who are somehow connected with the research. Now the focus will turn to examining clinical study circumstances that can also result in errors and that are also avoidable, but that are introduced into clinical research randomly, rather than systematically. Such circumstances are called confounders. In the context of clinical research, a **confounder** is an identifiable and usually quantifiable circumstance that is randomly introduced into a clinical study and that causes an error in the interpretation of the results of the study. The important distinction between biases and confounders is that the former are introduced nonrandomly by individuals connected to a clinical study, whereas the latter are introduced into a study randomly. To illustrate this, let us look at an example of a clinical study in which confounding has occurred.

A hypothetical noninferiority clinical trial was conducted to demonstrate the efficacy of a new oral antibiotic for empiric treatment of uncomplicated skin and soft tissue infection (SSTI). The control was another oral antibiotic drug previously established as the standard of care for empiric treatment of this condition. Eligible subjects were randomly assigned to treatment groups, and treatment outcomes were assessed appropriately. Treatment success was considered to be resolution of signs and symptoms of infection without addition of or transition to other treatment modalities and without recurrence within 3 months. Any other result was deemed a treatment failure. At the conclusion of the study, the new antibiotic was not determined to be noninferior to the standard treatment. It was noticed, however, that a significantly greater number of subjects in the study drug group were taking chronic oral corticosteroids, a treatment that can suppress the immune system. When these subjects were removed from the analysis, the results supported statistical noninferiority.

In this hypothetical study, we can see how a random, yet identifiable and avoidable, circumstance caused the results to differ from what they were when the circumstance was removed. The greater prevalence of oral corticosteroid treatment in the study group compared to the control group could clearly have resulted in fewer treatment successes in the former group than in the latter. Thus, oral corticosteroid use in this study was a confounder. Fortunately, this confounder was noticed and adjusted for. However, this is not always the case. Even when discovered and accounted for properly, the presence of confounders can call into question the validity of a study.

When groups within a study intentionally differ, we can see how they can be subject to membership bias. Recall that membership biases are the result of natural links that exist between characteristics of interest that are used to assign subjects to groups and characteristics that can alter the outcomes being studied. However, in the hypothetical SSTI study, it is clear to see that oral corticosteroid use is not naturally linked to one group or the other, because the subjects were not assigned to different groups based on any characteristics. They all had uncomplicated SSTI. The fact that more subjects in one group than the other were taking oral corticosteroids was the result of pure randomness. Thus, this is considered confounding rather than bias. Membership bias cannot occur in studies in which subjects are randomly assigned to groups that are intended to be similar in all regards. In studies in which subjects are assigned to groups based on a particular characteristic, however, both membership biases and confounders are possible, and it is sometimes difficult to distinguish between the two. Indeed, what appears to be a random confounder may actually be a membership bias for which the link between the assigning characteristic and the biasing characteristic has not been previously recognized.

Like membership bias, confounding is sometimes difficult to avoid because we are often unaware of all the possible causes of a given outcome. Researchers should perform due diligence in identifying the known and probable confounding characteristics that could alter the results a priori and ensure that these are equally distributed to all groups. This may require use of special randomization techniques, such as stratified randomization. When confounders are found to be unequally distributed between groups a posteriori, statistical methods to adjust for their contributions to outcome measurements may be employed.

# CHANCE IN CLINICAL RESEARCH

In addition to biases and confounders, there is a third phenomenon that can lead to errors in clinical research, that phenomenon being chance. Recall that an error in clinical research can be defined as a deviation between the truth about a phenomenon in a population and what is observed in a clinical study about that phenomenon that is significant enough in magnitude to result in a false conclusion being drawn. In this context, **chance** is an unidentifiable circumstance that is randomly introduced into a clinical study and that causes an error in the interpretation of the results of the study. The key characteristic that differentiates chance from biases and confounders is that chance is unidentifiable, and thus unavoidable.

Because errors due to chance are unavoidable in clinical research, it is commonplace in most clinical studies to include inferential statistical analyses that estimate the probabilities that chance errors in study observations have occurred. We will not go into detail about these statistical analyses here; however, we will present some basic concepts about these analyses that are germane to the discussion of errors in clinical research.

## ALPHA AND *P*-VALUE

Recall that a type I error is a false positive—that is, observing a statistically significant difference in a study outcome when that difference does not or would not truly exist in the population. But what constitutes a statistically significant difference? A **statistically significant** difference is a difference between groups that has a relatively low probability of being observed in error. In statistical hypothesis testing, an estimate of the probability of type I error is expressed as a *p*-value, with *p* representing "probability." When comparing a measureable aspect between groups, the ***p*-value** is the estimated probability of observing a given difference or a more extreme difference in that aspect between groups if no difference truly exists. For instance, if a study reported that the difference in mean plasma LDL-c levels between two groups was 10 mg/dL ($p = 0.04$), this could be interpreted as a 4% probability of observing a difference of at least 10 mg/dL if the true difference is actually 0 mg/dL. In more practical terms, one can think of the *p*-value as the probability that the observed difference is due to chance.

As previously mentioned, chance errors are unavoidable in clinical research. Therefore, we must decide a priori the threshold for the *p*-value to claim that a difference observed is statistically significant and, therefore, sufficiently compelling. In statistics, we call this threshold the alpha value, or simply the **alpha** ($\alpha$). By convention, most clinical studies will set the alpha value for the primary outcome at 0.05; however, it may be acceptable to use a more or less stringent alpha value in certain circumstances. Recall that most superiority studies should be two sided—that is to say that superiority can be demonstrated in either direction. In such studies, there is a risk of committing a type I error in either direction. Therefore, the alpha value is often split between these two directions, allotting half (e.g., 0.025) to one side and half to the other. Whatever the alpha value is set to be, the *p*-value must be equal to or lower than the alpha value to claim that the observed difference is statistically significant.

The term *statistically significant* has been used repeatedly throughout this chapter, and it is a term that you will encounter frequently in the literature. It is important, however, not to overvalue this term when interpreting the literature. Just as scale degradation can introduce bias into clinical study results, reducing probability of chance errors to dichotomous categories of statistically significant versus not statistically significant, when probability is actually measured on a numeric scale, can lead to a lack of true understanding of the risk of error. For instance, if the alpha value is set at 0.05, *p*-values of 0.04 and 0.0004 are both statistically significant. However, it is not difficult to see that an estimated probability of chance error of 4% is rather different than an estimated probability of chance error of 0.04%. In older literature, you may encounter *p*-values that are simply reported as less than some value, for example, < 0.05. This is because complex statistical calculations were much more difficult to perform before modern computer programs capable of accomplishing these tasks were widely available, so calculated *p*-values were less precise. However, this is no longer the case, and suspicion is warranted if contemporary studies do not report more exact *p*-values.

It is becoming more common in larger clinical studies having greater numbers of measured outcomes to apply a predetermined alpha value to the entire study, rather than to each single measured outcome. For instance, instead of allowing a 5% risk of type I error in the primary outcome, and another 5% risk for the first secondary outcome, and another 5% risk for the second secondary outcome, and so on, the overall study is given a cumulative 5% type I error risk. In a simplified example of a study with an overall alpha value of 0.05, if the *p*-value for the primary outcome was 0.001, then there would be approximately 0.049 of the cumulative alpha value left for the remainder of the outcomes. If the *p*-value for the first secondary outcome was 0.03, then there would be approximately 0.019 of the cumulative alpha value left for the next outcome. If the *p*-value for the second secondary outcome was 0.04, then there would not be enough of the cumulative alpha value left to claim statistical significance in the second secondary outcome, even though its individual *p*-value was < 0.05. You can see how allowing a 5% risk of type I error for each individual outcome can result in claiming statistically significant differences in multiple outcomes when the cumulative probability that an error has occurred somewhere across all of these outcomes is well over 5%. Allotting an overall study alpha value of 0.05 prevents such inflated statements of significance and allows more appropriate conclusions to be drawn on the entirety of the study, rather than solely on the primary outcome.

## BETA AND POWER

In addition to error due to chance when a difference between groups is observed in a clinical study, there is also the possibility of error due to chance when a difference between groups is not observed in a clinical study. You will recall that these latter types of errors are type II errors, or false negatives. Whereas alpha represents the risk we are willing to accept for committing a type I error, **beta** (β) represents the risk we are willing to accept for committing a type II error. For a number of reasons, medical science is generally accepting of a greater risk of type II errors than type I errors. In other words, we are generally more willing to accept a claim that two things are the same when they are truly different than we are to accept a claim that two things are different when they

| **TABLE 13-5** | Relationships Between Study Observations and Reality | | |
|---|---|---|---|
| | | Reality | |
| | | **Difference Exists** | **No Difference Exists** |
| **Probability** | **Difference Will Be Observed** | Power (1 – Beta) | Alpha (type I error) |
| | **No Difference Will Be Observed** | Beta (type II error) | (1 – Alpha) |

are truly the same. This is probably because there are few situations in which two different circumstance lead to exactly the same outcome, even though the outcomes may be similar. So, the tendency toward dissimilarity already exists in nature. But for whatever reasons, beta is often allowed to be set higher than alpha. In a 1988 publication, Jacob Cohen, a prolific psychologist and statistician at New York University, suggested that a beta of 0.2 is probably adequate for clinical studies in the behavioral sciences.[11] In contemporary clinical studies, the maximum acceptable beta is typically 0.2; however, it is frequently set at a lower threshold.

Avoiding type II errors in clinical research is important. However, in most clinical studies we are more concerned with being able to detect a difference if one truly exists. The astute observer will intuitively notice that the concepts of avoiding a type II error and of ensuring that a difference is detected if one truly exists are closely linked. In fact, they are essentially the same concept. The probability to detect a statistically significant difference in a study if a difference truly exists is called **statistical power**, or simply *power*. Power is equal to 1 – beta. Thus, if the beta of a study is 0.2, then the power is 0.8, or 80%. In other words, if there is a 20% chance of not detecting a difference when a difference truly exists (a false negative), there is an 80% chance of detecting a difference if a difference truly exists (a true positive). For some people, it helps to think about it from the perspective of reality. If a difference truly exists in reality, there are only two options for how it might be perceived through a clinical study—either the difference is detected (true positive) or the difference is not detected (false negative). No other options exist. Thus, the sum of the chances of the difference being detected (true positive) and of it not being detected (false negative) must equal 100%. **Table 13-5** shows how alpha and beta values represent the probability of observing a difference in a clinical study relative to the existence or absence of a difference in reality.

When we discuss beta and power in the context of a clinical study, we are typically referring to these concepts as they relate to the primary outcome. However, beta and power can be set for any study outcome, or even for a set of study outcomes, if desired.

## EFFECT SIZE, EFFECT VARIANCE, AND SAMPLE SIZE

If alpha is the level of risk that we are willing to accept of a type I error (i.e., declaring a statistically significant difference where one does not exist) and power is the probability that we will detect a difference if one exists, then it is easy to see how making the alpha value more stringent will make achieving power more difficult. So, how do we maintain an acceptable power given a specifically stringent alpha? The answer lies in three other variables that have not yet been discussed—the magnitude of the difference observed, the variability of the observations, and the number of subjects included in the study.

If the observed difference between two groups in a clinical study is relatively large, then it stands to reason that we can be more confident that a true difference exists between the two groups, even if the magnitude of the difference is not quite as large in the population as was observed in the study. In contrast, if the observed difference between these groups is relatively small, we would naturally be less confident that a true difference exists in the population. Thus, the magnitude of the difference observed plays a role in determining whether a statistically significant difference can be declared—that is, whether the calculated *p*-value is equal to or less than the designated alpha. The magnitude of difference is called the **effect size**. In addition, some measure of the **variance** in the effect size data is a factor. If the pooled data have large variability, it will be more difficult to be confident that the results reflect what exists in the greater population. Obviously, we cannot know beforehand the magnitude of the difference that we will observe between two groups in a clinical study or its variability, and we certainly cannot artificially create a difference of a specific magnitude and variability. Therefore, the effect size and variance must be estimated. The estimation of effect size and variance may be determined by previous studies with similar interventions or circumstances. In addition, the effect size should be one of **clinical significance**. That is to say that the magnitude of difference between two groups that we hope to see is one that is achievable based on prior evidence and it is one that is sufficiently important enough to affect clinical decisions. In the absence of prior evidence of effect size, researchers must rely more on the clinical significance component for determining the magnitude of difference desired to be observed in the study.

So, if we must have a sufficiently low alpha value and a sufficiently high power, and we cannot control the effect size or variance that we will see, then we must make adjustments to the last variable, the number of subjects included in the study, to maintain the other variables at desired levels. This last variable is called the **sample size** (*n*). There is no single equation for determining the sample size required for a study. It depends on the type of data being collected and the statistical analyses to be applied to that data. Fortunately, the relationships between sample size, alpha, power, and effect size and variance are consistent across all methods. The following general rules apply:

- If all other variables remain constant, assigning a more stringent (i.e., lower) alpha requires a larger sample size.
- If all other variables remain constant, increasing the desired power (i.e., decreasing the beta) requires a larger sample size.
- If all other variables remain constant, expecting a smaller observed effect size will result in the need for a larger sample size.
- If all other variables remain constant, expecting a larger variance in the observed effect will result in the need for a larger sample size.

With these general rules, it is clear how changes to the statistical variables affect the size of the sample that will be required in the study. Because effect size and variance are (or should be) beyond the control of the researcher and acceptable values for alpha and power have been fairly concretely established by the scientific community, the variable that the researcher has the most control over is sample size. Thus, it can be helpful to express the general rules in terms of the effects that adjusting the sample size will have on these variables:

- If all other variables remain constant, increasing the sample size can allow the researcher to apply a more stringent (i.e., lower) alpha.
- If all other variables remain constant, increasing the sample size can allow the researcher to have a higher power (i.e., lower beta).
- If all other variables remain constant, increasing the sample size can allow the researcher to declare a smaller effect size as statistically significant.
- If all other variables remain constant, increasing the sample size can reduce the expected variance in the observed effect.

As discussed in the section of this chapter on biases, sample size bias is a type of information bias related to the number of subjects included in a study. In order to avoid errors due to sample size bias, researchers should conduct a priori sample size calculations that take into account the desired alpha value and power and expected effect size. In the context of errors due to chance, a sufficient sample size is also required to mitigate the risk of type II errors.

In practice, it is not uncommon for a researcher to start by calculating the minimum number of subjects required to enroll in a study to achieve a power of 80%, given an alpha of 0.05 and the expected effect size and variance. If the researcher believes that she can reasonably enroll more subjects than this minimum, she may recalculate what level of power she can achieve with increasingly larger sample sizes, ultimately arriving at a good balance between sample size feasibility and desired power.

## RETROSPECTIVE POWER

In original research reports, we expect to see a *p*-value reported if a difference of any magnitude was observed between groups for any major outcome, even if the *p*-value for that outcome exceeds the alpha value and the result is deemed to be not statistically significant. In the same manner that a *p*-value can be calculated to estimate the probability that a type I error has occurred when a difference is observed, it is also possible to calculate the estimated probability that a type II error has been avoided when a statistically significant difference was not observed. This value is referred to as the **retrospective power**. If power is the a priori probability of avoiding a type II error if a difference truly exists, then the retrospective power is the a posteriori probability that the study had to prevent a type II error, given what was actually observed in the study (i.e., using the actual number of subjects analyzed and the actual effect size observed).

As discussed earlier, the estimated sample size can be calculated given a designated alpha value, desired power, and expected effect size and variance. This same equation can be rearranged algebraically to calculate the retrospective power of the study given the calculated *p*-value (substituting for alpha), the observed effect size and variance (substituting for expected effect size and variance), and the actual sample size used (substituting for estimated sample size). A retrospective power calculation gives some insight into the probability that a type II error has occurred when a study fails to demonstrate a statistically significant difference in a major outcome.

# RELATIONSHIPS BETWEEN BIASES, CONFOUNDERS, AND CHANCE

It may seem as though differentiating between biases, confounders, and chance can sometimes be difficult. Indeed, there can be subtle differences and interdependencies between these three potential causes of research errors. For example, confounders and membership bias can be similar. Increasing sample size can reduce the risk of chance error, but it can also cause sample size bias. Although it is probably advisable to put greater attention toward identifying the potential for errors and mitigating their risk, regardless of their type, classifying a potential cause of error can help in guiding the effort to mitigate or avoid it. To that end, one can ask two questions of any given source of research error to determine its type.

The first question to ask is if the circumstance or its impact on the clinical study is or was potentially avoidable. Recall that errors due to biases and confounders are at least theoretically avoidable, whereas errors due to chance are not. For all practical purposes, anything that can be identified can be avoided, or at least adjusted for. It may sometimes be difficult to determine if a bias occurred or if a confounder was present. But, with enough scrutiny and effort, they can be discovered. However, one can never determine for certain if an error will or did occur in a clinical study simply due to chance. Even the most carefully planned studies are subject to some form of chance error. Furthermore, although most modern statistical methods are very good at estimating the probability of an error due solely to chance, even these methods are inherently imperfect because they do not take into account the size of the sample relative to the size of the population. To illustrate this, imagine a study that enrolled 500 subjects with a given disease. Statistically speaking, it should matter whether the total population of persons with that disease number 1,000 versus 1,000,000. If 50% of all the possible cases are included in the study, the results observed in the study are far more likely to be similar to what can be expected in the entire population than they are if only 0.05% of all the possible cases are included. However, most statistical methods used in clinical studies do not take into account the size of the population. This is because the actual size of the population can never truly be known. In addition, if we wish to extrapolate the study results to future cases, the theoretical population is as infinite as time.

The second question to ask is if the circumstance was introduced into the study systematically, or nonrandomly. Remember that biases are systematically introduced by decisions or actions made by individuals connected to a clinical study. There are discernible patterns to biases. In contrast, confounders and chance result from randomness. Another way to think of this is that the direction that a bias will push the result is usually predictable, whereas the direction that a confounder or chance will push the result is completely unpredictable. To illustrate this, let us once again compare a membership bias with a confounder. With a membership bias, one group is more likely than the other to have a certain characteristic that has been determined to possibly affect the outcome. We know this because the characteristic has been identified to be connected with a characteristic that we are using to designate the groups. So, we already know which group it will favor. With a confounder, in contrast, either group has an equal probability of having more members with the characteristic that will alter the outcome because it is not linked to one group more than another. So, we cannot predict if or how it might affect the outcome.

**Table 13-6** illustrates in a gridlike fashion the relationships between biases, confounders, and chance with respect to whether each is avoidable and/or random. Confounders are both random and avoidable; biases are nonrandom and avoidable; chance is random and unavoidable. Notice that one cell in the grid, the cell associated with circumstances that are both unavoidable and nonrandom, contains a new term that we have not discussed—temporal truth. **Temporal truth** simply refers to reality as it exists in a population at a single instant in time. Because temporal truth represents reality, it is unavoidable, and because it is static at any given instant, it is nonrandom. Hopefully, it is evident what role temporal truth plays in clinical research observations. It represents the conditions that exist in a population that research is attempting to identify and quantify.

| **TABLE 13-6** | Relationships Between Biases, Confounders, and Chance | | |
|---|---|---|---|
| | | **Avoidable** | |
| | | **Yes** | **No** |
| **Random** | **Yes** | Confounder | Chance |
| | **No** | Bias | (Temporal truth) |

So, while we attempt to minimize the impacts of biases, confounders, and chance in clinical studies, it is temporal truth that we wish to elucidate through such research.

## SUMMARY

In the context of clinical research, an error is any deviation between the truth about a phenomenon in a population and what is observed in a clinical study about that phenomenon that is significant enough in magnitude to result in a false conclusion being drawn. For obvious reasons, it is important to avoid errors in clinical research whenever possible and to clearly identify, quantify, and report factors that could contribute to such occurrences when they have manifested or cannot be avoided.

Most errors can be categorized as one of two types: false positive or false negative. A false positive, or type I error, occurs when we reject the null hypothesis when we should have failed to reject it. A false negative, or type II error, occurs when we fail to reject the null hypothesis when we should have rejected it. A number of circumstances can lead to these types of errors in clinical studies. These circumstances can be divided into three categories: biases, confounders, and chance. These categories differ from one another in terms of their ability to be identified (and therefore avoided) and whether they are introduced randomly (as opposed to systematically). Biases are identifiable and introduced systematically. Confounders are identifiable and introduced randomly. Chance is unidentifiable and introduced randomly.

Biases in clinical studies are identifiable and sometimes quantifiable circumstances that are systematically, or nonrandomly, introduced consciously or unconsciously by actions or decisions made by persons connected to the research and that lead to errors in the interpretation of study results. Biases can be further divided into two categories—selection biases and information biases—based on their effects on a study. Selection biases cause systematic differences between the probability of choosing or assigning one individual from the target population and the probability of choosing or assigning another individual from the same population. Some of the more pertinent selection biases are admission rate (Berkson) bias, detection bias, medical surveillance bias, membership bias, participation (nonresponse) bias, prevalence-incidence (Neyman) bias, and procedure selection bias. In contrast, information biases cause systematic errors in the measurement, analysis, interpretation, and reporting of data in clinical studies. Some of the more pertinent information biases are attention bias, compliance (adherence) bias, exposure suspicion bias, migration (contamination) bias, mimicry bias, missing data bias, publication bias, recall bias, reference bias, response bias, rhetorical bias, sample size bias, scale degradation bias, unmasking bias, and withdrawal bias.

Confounders are identifiable and usually quantifiable circumstances that are randomly introduced into clinical studies and that cause errors in the interpretation of study results. The important distinction between biases and confounders is that the former are introduced nonrandomly by individuals connected to a clinical study, whereas the latter are introduced into a study randomly.

Chance is an unidentifiable circumstance that is randomly introduced into a clinical study and that causes an error in the interpretation of the results of the study. The key characteristic that differentiates chance from biases and confounders is that chance is unidentifiable, and thus unavoidable. Because errors due to chance are unavoidable in clinical research, it is commonplace in most clinical studies to include inferential statistical analyses that estimate the probabilities that chance errors in study observations have occurred. Concepts that are important to understand in the context of such analyses are alpha and $p$-value; beta and power; and effect size, effect variance, and sample size. All of these values affect one another in predictable ways, and the most common and generally acceptable value to alter to minimize errors due to chance is sample size.

The ultimate goal of conducting clinical studies is to discover a temporal truth about a phenomenon. The only way to be confident in such discoveries is to minimize the risk of errors introduced through biases, confounders, and chance.

# REFERENCES

1. Leventhal L, Huynh C. Directional decisions for two-tailed tests: power, error rates, and sample size. *Psychol Methods*. 1996;1(3):278-292.
2. Sackett DL. Bias in analytic research. *J Chron Dis*. 1979;32(1-2):51-63.
3. Berkson J. Limitations of the application of fourfold table analysis to hospital data. *Biom Bull*. 1946;2(3):47-53.
4. Neyman J. Statistics—servant of all sciences. *Science*. 1955;122(3166):401-406.
5. Antikainen RL, Moltchanov VA, Chukwuma C Sr, et al; WHO MONICA Project. Trends in the prevalence, awareness, treatment and control of hypertension: the WHO MONICA Project. *Eur J Cardiovasc Prev Rehabil*. 2006;13(1):13-29.
6. Landsberger HA. *Hawthorne Revisited: Management and the Worker, Its Critics, and Developments in Human Relations in Industry*. Ithaca, NY: Cornell University; 1958.
7. Bienenfeld L, Frishman W, Glasser SP. The placebo effect in cardiovascular disease. *Am Heart J*. 1996;132(6):1207-1221.
8. Joyce DP, Jackevicius C, Chapman KR, McIvor RA, Kesten S. The placebo effect in asthma drug therapy trials: a meta-analysis. *J Asthma*. 2000;37(4):303-318.
9. Wang X, Shang D, Ribbing J, et al. Placebo effect model in asthma clinical studies: longitudinal meta-analysis of forced expiratory volume in 1 second. *Eur J Clin Pharmacol*. 2012;68(8):1157-1166.
10. Berglund L, Brunzell JD, Goldberg AC, et al; Endocrine Society. Evaluation and treatment of hypertriglyceridemia: an Endocrine Society clinical practice guideline. *J Clin Endocrinol Metab*. 2012;97(9):2969-2989.
11. Cohen J. *Statistical Power Analysis for the Behavioral Sciences*. 2nd ed. Hillsdale, NJ: Lawrence Erlbaum Associates; 1988.

# EVIDENCE-BASED MEDICINE

Miki Goldwire, PharmD, MSc, BS, BCPS
Jason Babby, PharmD, BCPS

## CHAPTER OBJECTIVES

▸ Define evidence-based medicine (EBM).
▸ List the six steps of applying the evidence-based medicine process.
▸ List the four components of a well-formulated question.
▸ Build a well-formulated question based on a patient case.
▸ Describe databases and search strategies for retrieval of evidence.
▸ Identify factors that determine the validity of a randomized controlled trial.
▸ Identify factors that determine the validity of observational trials.
▸ Calculate relative risk, odds ratio, and number needed to treat.
▸ Identify factors that determine the validity of meta-analyses and systematic reviews.
▸ Identify key factors for assessing clinical practice guidelines.
▸ Describe the positive and negative factors for use of clinical practice guidelines.
▸ Explain the barriers and limitations of evidence-based medicine.
▸ Describe the role of evidence-based medicine in the individualized care of the patient.

# CHAPTER OUTLINE

# KEY TERMS

Absolute risk reduction
AGREE Instrument
Blinding
Boolean operators
Case report
Case series
Case-control study
Clinical practice guidelines
Cochrane Database of Systematic Reviews
Cohort study
Comparative effectiveness research
Confounders
Cross-sectional study
Cumulative Index of Nursing and Allied
    Health Literature (CINAHL)
Database of Abstracts of Reviews of
    Effects (DARE)
Effectiveness
Efficacy
Evidence-based medicine
Experimental study
External validity

GRADE
Hawthorne effect
Hazard ratio
Hierarchy of evidence
Internal validity
MEDLINE
Meta-analysis
Noninferiority margin
Noninferiority study
Number needed to treat
Observational study
Odds ratio
PICO
POEM
Pragmatic trials
Publication bias
Randomized controlled trial
Relative risk
Relative risk reduction
Selection bias
Systematic review

# INTRODUCTION

**Evidence-based medicine** (EBM) places emphasis on the use of literature to guide recommendations in clinical practice. The best-known definition of EBM is "the conscientious, explicit, and judicious use of current best evidence in making clinical decisions about the care of the individual patients. The practice of EBM means integrating individual clinical experience with the best available external clinical evidence from systematic research."[1] Best research includes evidence from randomized controlled trials, observational trials, laboratory experiments, and epidemiological and outcomes

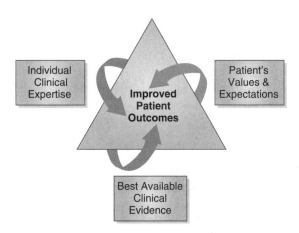

**FIGURE 14-1** Fundamental principles of evidence-based medicine practice.

Reproduced from BMJ, Evidence-based medicine: what it is and what it isn't., Sackett DL, Rosenberg MC, Gray JA, Haynes RB, Richardson WS. 312, pp. 71-72, copyright 1996 with permission from BMJ Publishing Group Ltd.

research. Clinical expertise is knowledge obtained from experiences in clinical practice, including clinical reasoning skills. EBM is not just applying current evidence in practice, but also incorporating two other important aspects—clinical experience and patient values (**Figure 14–1**). Patient values and circumstances are the individualized preferences, concerns, expectations, and financial resources of the patient.[2] Incorporating these three factors will provide the greatest benefit to the patient by ensuring that the best possible clinical decision is made.

Literature by itself is not sufficient to provide a recommendation.[3] It is essential to use clinical expertise, because it is the knowledge gained throughout years of practice. Sackett states, "without clinical expertise, practice risks becoming tyrannized by evidence, for even excellent external evidence may be inapplicable to or inappropriate for an individual patient. Without current best evidence, practice risks becoming rapidly out of date, to the detriment of patients."[1] Discussing the benefits and risks of therapy with patients enhances their role in the decision-making process. The patient's beliefs, values, priorities, preferences, and clinical situation must be taken into consideration in order to successfully practice EBM.[3] Medicine must be individualized; thus, optimal treatment will vary from one patient to another.

Why use EBM? This approach encourages the use of critical-thinking skills by the healthcare practitioner. It causes practitioners to question their recommendations and find support for their reasoning. Practitioners will want to know if there is an intervention with more favorable outcomes in the literature that is suitable for their patient.[4] Healthcare practitioners must learn several skills in order to properly practice EBM. These skills include developing a structured clinical question, formulating a systematic search strategy to obtain the best available evidence, evaluating the literature properly, comprehending the study results, and incorporating evidence into patient care.[5]

EBM has changed clinical practice over the years to focus on the quality of care the patient receives. Studies are now more likely to focus on patient-oriented evidence that matters (**POEM**) rather than focusing exclusively on disease states.[6] Studies focused on disease states do not provide information on long-term patient outcomes, instead focusing on outcomes such as glucose or blood pressure. These intermediate outcomes are not indicators of overall mortality or safety. Basing practice on these types of studies can cause harm to patients, because the long-term effects of interventions are not known. In contrast, studies focusing on POEM evaluate "quality of life, improving function, staying independent, overall mortality, and cost-effectiveness."[6] These types of studies evaluate the overall effectiveness of interventions and long-term patient outcomes.

# PRACTICING EVIDENCE-BASED MEDICINE

The incorporation of EBM into clinical practice guidelines, hospital protocols, and best practices has changed the practice of medicine.[7] Locating evidence is key to successfully incorporating EBM into clinical practice. Without the best available evidence, it is difficult to practice EBM. Technological advances have made literature easily accessible. However, case reports, case series, randomized controlled trials, and systematic reviews are not the only evidence to review when answering a clinical question.[1] External resources, such as results from the patient's history and physical, supplement scientific literature to provide the best evidence. **Table 14-1** lists several EBM resources. These electronic EBM resources help place information at the healthcare professional's fingertips.

| TABLE 14-1 Evidence-Based Medicine Resources | |
|---|---|
| **Resource** | **Description** |
| American College of Physicians (ACP) Journal Club | • Summarizes pertinent literature with commentary<br>• Published monthly<br>• Requires a paid subscription |
| American Family Physician | • Published monthly<br>• Provides review articles on disease states<br>• Free online access |
| Bandolier | • Summarizes articles that "are both interesting and make sense"<br>• Free online access |
| Clinical Evidence | • Summarizes current literature<br>• Requires a paid subscription |
| The Cochrane Database of Systematic Reviews | • Internationally recognized systematic reviews<br>• Requires a paid subscription |
| Database of Abstracts of Review of Effects (DARE) | • Systematic reviews that discuss the effects or impact of interventions<br>• Free access online |
| DynaMed | • A "diagnosis support decision tool"<br>• Summaries of literature on over 3,200 topics<br>• Requires a paid subscription |
| Essential Evidence Plus | • Contains over 1,000 evidence-based summaries of various diseases<br>• Requires a paid subscription |

**TABLE 14-1**   Evidence-Based Medicine Resources *(Continued)*

| Resource | Description |
| --- | --- |
| FIRSTConsult | • Provides current information on diseases from diagnosis to treatment using literature from the well-known databases<br>• Requires a paid subscription |
| Institute for Clinical Systems Improvement (ISCI) | • Offers access to guidelines, order sets, and patient resources<br>• Free access online |
| Journal of Family Practice | • Published monthly<br>• Issues include practice alerts and articles on applied evidence and clinical inquires<br>• Free access online |
| National Guidelines Clearinghouse (NGC) | • Public resource for evidence-based guidelines<br>• Free access online |
| SUMSearch2 | • Searches evidence from MEDLINE, DARE, and the National Guidelines Clearinghouse<br>• Free access online |
| Turning Research Into Practice (TRIP) Database | • Clinical search engine to provide high-quality evidence<br>• Free access online |
| UpToDate | • Clinical decision support providing point-of-care EBM<br>• Requires a paid subscription |
| U.S. Preventive Services Task Force (USPSTF) | • Information on preventive medicine<br>• Free access online |

Once evidence has been located, it must be evaluated before it can be incorporated into daily practice. Applying evidence without properly evaluating it may cause more harm to patients than benefit. Evidence should be evaluated using literature evaluation skills. Some questions to ask when evaluating the evidence include:

- Is this a problem I see in practice?
- Was the patient population studied similar to the one I encounter?
- What was the patient population size studied?
- Was the intervention used standard of care? If not, why was the standard of care not used?
- Would the primary and secondary outcomes affect my patients?
- Did the study meet power?
- Were the results statistically significant?
- Were the results clinically significant?
- What was the number needed to treat?
- What was the number needed to harm?
- Was any type of bias evident?

After the evidence has been deemed to be applicable to current practice, it can then be incorporated. When incorporating evidence into practice, it is important not to forget that medicine is individualized. The patient is a major factor who should be taken into consideration prior to making a recommendation. This is the one step of EBM that is completely "do it yourself."[7] It is essential to integrate all three factors—evidence, clinical expertise, and the patient—when applying EBM to clinical situations.

## A SIX-STEP PROCESS

Pharmacists routinely receive questions about drug therapy. Just as with the systematic approach to answering drug information questions, answering questions using EBM techniques requires a judicious and thorough thought process. The EBM process has six steps:[8-10]

1. Create an answerable clinical question.
2. Find the best evidence.
3. Critically appraise the evidence.
4. Integrate evidence with clinical judgment/expertise and patient preferences.*
5. Implement intervention or apply the evidence.
6. Evaluate the effectiveness of the intervention.

## STEP 1: CREATE AN ANSWERABLE CLINICAL QUESTION

The first step is to formulate an answerable question that is relevant to the clinical situation. In doing so, the question should be phrased to facilitate a search for the best evidence. The result is a well-built, searchable question that is relevant to the patient and specific for the clinical situation. This is not unlike discovering the true, ultimate question the requestor needs answered. For example, a physician asking for an alternative to olanzapine in the treatment of schizophrenia may in fact have a patient receiving olanzapine who is failing or unable to tolerate therapy. To use EBM techniques, the question needs to be relevant to a patient and formulated to facilitate the search for the answer.

## STEP 2: FIND THE BEST EVIDENCE

A key principle to EBM is finding the best evidence, because not all evidence is equal. Evidence can come from several sources, including consensus statements, clinical practice guidelines, expert opinion, primary journal articles, review articles, and numerous online resources. In order to review the *best* evidence, the source should be up-to-date and valid.[14] Textbooks may be out-of-date, consensus statements and clinical practice guidelines may be incomplete, and online sources may be too superficial. The **hierarchy of evidence** attempts to define the best evidence. Study designs susceptible to weak internal validity occupy the bottom, whereas those study designs at the top routinely deliver strong internal validity.[16,17] Coincidentally, study designs susceptible to weak internal validity often have strong external validity, and designs with strong internal validity often have weak external validity. **Internal validity** describes the degree to which the intervention or treatment contributes to the results. **External validity** describes the generalizability of the results to a population (or patient) of interest.

The traditional hierarchy of evidence (**Figure 14–2**) places the meta-analysis of randomized controlled trials (RCTs) at the top of the pyramid. However, depending on the clinical question to be answered (therapy, prevention, harm, prognosis, diagnosis, prevalence), a different study design may provide an appropriate answer.[18]

---

* Some consider clinical judgment/expertise and patient preferences to be step 2;[10] others combine steps 4 and 5.[8,9]

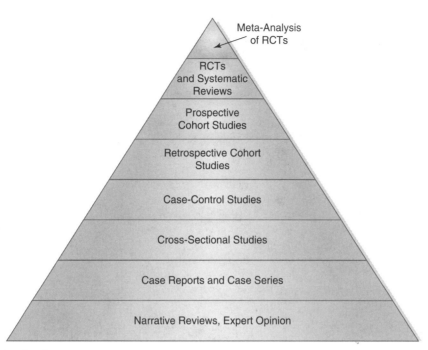

**FIGURE 14-2** Hierarchy of evidence.

| CASE STUDY 14-1 | **Switching Atypical Antipsychotic Therapy** |

A 42-year-old female receiving olanzapine for schizophrenia for the past 3 months returns to the clinic for follow-up. The patient presents with a 20-pound weight gain, amenorrhea, and decreased libido. Recent fasting labs reveal a blood glucose of 164 mg/dL and total cholesterol of 220 mg/dL. Fasting labs drawn 6 months ago indicate a fasting glucose of 83 mg/dL and total cholesterol of 170 mg/dL. The physician would like to change olanzapine to another atypical antipsychotic, either aripiprazole or quetiapine. What therapy should the pharmacist recommend?

Founders of EBM categorized clinical questions as being either foreground or background questions.[11,12] Foreground questions ask specific information relevant to the clinical situation. Four distinct elements devise an answerable question and are often identified by the acronym **PICO**: patient (or problem), intervention, comparison (or control), and outcome (see **Table 14-2**).[13]

For example, using the case scenario, the following PICO search strategy results in a well-built, searchable question that is relevant to the patient and specific for the clinical situation: Which atypical antipsychotic, aripiprazole or quetiapine, is the best choice for treatment of schizophrenia in a 42-year-old woman who experienced increased fasting glucose and serum cholesterol within 3 months of starting olanzapine therapy?

P: Schizophrenia
I: Olanzapine
C: Aripiprazole or quetiapine
O: Hypercholestermia or hyperglycemia

The key to searching for the best evidence is to construct a well-built question. The question needs to address the patient/problem, intervention, comparison/control, and outcome. Parameters relevant to the question also need to be included. For the treatment of schizophrenia, sex of the patient is not relevant to treatment; therefore, the sex of the patient does not need to be included in the patient description.

| TABLE 14-2    Four Elements of the Well-Built Question (PICO) | |
|---|---|
| **Element** | **Description** |
| Patient or problem | What patient population or problem is being treated?<br>Describe the pertinent features of the patient or problem.<br>Examples:<br>• Post–myocardial infarction middle-aged man with risk factors<br>• Geriatric hypertension<br>• Child with influenza A |
| Intervention | What is the desired treatment or therapy?<br>State the desired specific treatment or therapy.<br>Examples:<br>• Warfarin<br>• Ramipril<br>• Oseltamivir |
| Comparison or control | What is the desired comparator treatment or therapy?<br>Examples:<br>• Aspirin<br>• Candesartan<br>• Zanamivir |
| Outcome | What is the desired outcome?<br>State the most important outcome.<br>Examples:<br>• Decreased risk of stroke<br>• Reduced diastolic blood pressure<br>• Treatment of influenza A |

Unfamiliar topics warrant further review. Background questions answer the who, what, where, when, and why of a disease or treatment. For example, the following background questions might aid in understanding the clinical scenario:

- What drugs are recommended for treatment of schizophrenia?
- Who would devise clinical practice guidelines for treatment of schizophrenia?
- What atypical antipsychotics are currently available?
- Which atypical antipsychotics do not affect glucose or cholesterol?
- What is a reasonable duration of treatment for an atypical antipsychotic when used to treat schizophrenia?

Background questions are essential for understanding the clinical condition and devising the best searchable question. Oftentimes, students do not realize the extent of their knowledge gap until searching for the answer. Background questions may arise as searching begins or while in conversation with the requestor. Do not be embarrassed to ask questions, even if those questions reveal knowledge gaps.

Devising a well-built, searchable question that is relevant to the patient and specific for the clinical situation is crucial, because finding the best evidence depends upon the question. Trying to answer unfocused questions may lead to frustration, increased time, and the wrong answer. Strive to devise a well-built question that encompasses what the requestor truly wants answered.

The following are examples of poorly focused questions:

- Does vitamin D decrease the risk for development of diabetes?
- What is recommended for treatment of migraine?
- Does ranitidine cause thrombocytopenia?
- What is an alternative to blood transfusions?
- What is the best proton pump inhibitor to use in pregnancy?

Rephrasing poorly focused questions while conversing with the requestor helps to determine the true question. Taking the poorly focused questions and rephrasing them using PICO elements results in patient-specific, searchable questions:

- Does daily vitamin D decrease the risk for development of type 2 diabetes in a prediabetic patient compliant with diet and exercise?
- What is recommended for treatment of migraine in a prison inmate who has a substance abuse history?
- Is famotidine safe to use for treatment of GERD in a patient who experienced thrombocytopenia with ranitidine?
- How does tranexamic acid compare to blood transfusions for treatment of postpartum hemorrhage?
- Is one proton pump inhibitor more efficacious and safer than another in the treatment of GERD for a 16-week pregnant woman who failed nonpharmacologic therapy?

Clinical questions broadly encompass questions about therapy, harm, prognosis, prevention, and diagnosis.[14] The best evidence to answer questions about these four categories varies.[15]

The medical literature consists of two types of clinical studies: experimental and observational. **Experimental studies** contain at least two groups in which members of one group receive active therapy and members of the other group may receive the standard of care or placebo. Researchers measure effects of therapy on predetermined outcomes. During **observational studies**, participants may be assigned to groups, but are not assigned a treatment or therapy. Researchers observe participants for the desired outcome. Key features of study designs are shown in **Table 14–3**.[19,20]

## EXPERIMENTAL DESIGNS: RANDOMIZED CONTROLLED TRIALS

Considered the gold standard trial design for assessing research questions about therapy, **randomized controlled trials** (RCTs) are designed to test if therapies are beneficial and do more good than harm. Researchers report the mean treatment effect in the specific patient population.[21] The RCT design also controls for known and unknown confounders.[22] Researchers design RCTs to occur under ideal conditions. To create such conditions, researchers employ various techniques to limit systematic error, or the error not due to chance. One such technique is to randomize patients into groups. Randomization increases the chance patients with known and unknown variables distribute evenly into the groups.[23] Every participant in the trial has an equal chance of receiving treatment. The following should be considered when reviewing RCTs:

- Randomization limits **selection bias** and allows for all participants to have an equal chance of being chosen for the treatment group.
- **Blinding** reduces the chance of observation bias from either the researcher or the patient. Blinding also reduces the Hawthorne effect and the placebo effect.[24] In a double-blind study, both patient and researcher are blinded to who is receiving active treatment.
- The **Hawthorne effect** is a type of bias in which patients respond to therapy (either control or treatment) because they are being studied.
- The placebo effect is a type of Hawthorne effect in which patients respond favorably to placebo.

- **Confounders** are independent factors related to both the outcome and treatment.[24,25] To limit potential confounders, such as comorbidities, concomitant medications, or past medical history, researchers develop inclusion and exclusion criteria patients must meet in order to participate in the trial.

Once randomized into groups, one group receives active treatment and the other placebo or the standard of care. Researchers measure the effects of the a priori determined outcome variable in both groups to assess for differences between the groups.

EBM considers the RCT the gold standard trial design for answering questions about therapy.[26] The RCT offers a high degree of internal validity, which is the degree

**TABLE 14-3**    Characteristics of Study Designs

| Study Design | Features | Element Assessed | Outcome Measured |
|---|---|---|---|
| **Experimental/interventional study:** One group receives the intervention and one group does not; analyzes cause and effect; has high internal validity and medium to low external validity. | | | |
| Randomized controlled trial (RCT): special types include crossover, noninferiority | Highly controlled population and environment; groups are randomized to minimize potential differences among subjects. Determines a cause-and-effect relationship between treatment and outcome. | Efficacy | $p$-value, 95% confidence intervals (CI) |
| **Observational study:** Groups are observed; has low internal validity and high external validity. | | | |
| Cohort studies: prospective or longitudinal | Diverse population in which exposure is determined before outcome; establishes relationship between exposure and outcome over time; patients are followed forward in time. | Natural history of disease, prognosis, risk factors | Relative risk (RR) Absolute risk reduction (ARR) Number needed to treat (NNT) Hazard ratio (HR) |
| Cohort studies: retrospective | Diverse population in which exposure is determined before outcome; determines the relationship of exposure to outcome over time; information is gathered after events have occurred; watch for selection and recall bias. | Natural history of disease, prognosis, risk factors | Odds ratio (OR) |
| Case-control studies: retrospective | Cases have the disease (or outcome of interest), controls do not; analyze relationship of disease to exposure; watch for selection and recall bias. | Relationship between disease and exposure; best design for determining causes of rare diseases | Odds ratio (OR) |
| Cross-sectional studies, surveys (prevalence) | Targeted population in which risk or disease prevalence is determined between two groups. | Disease description, diagnosis and staging, disease processes | Group observed at one point in time |

Data from Carlson MDA, Morrison RS. Study design, precision and validity in observational studies. *J Palliat Med.* 2009;12(1):77-82; and DiPietro NA. Methods in epidemiology: observational study designs. *Pharmacotherapy.* 2010;30(10):973-984.

treatment contributes to results. When using an RCT design, the patient's exposure to treatment occurs before assessment of outcome(s), thereby allowing a more definitive cause-and-effect relationship to be established. Researchers rule out other potential causes for the result (confounders), thereby increasing certainty that the treatment was responsible for the outcome.

Although RCTs provide excellent designs for answering questions about drug efficacy, results of RCTs are often limited because of external validity. External validity is the extent to which the results apply to the population of interest.[24] Results established by well-designed RCTs average outcomes and do not represent individual patients but a sample population. In other words, would the results pertain to a specific patient in clinical practice? When determining if results from an RCT apply to an individual patient, critically evaluating the trial for applicability of inclusion criteria, exclusion criteria, duration of therapy, dosage, primary outcome, and use of surrogate outcomes aids in making an informed decision.

## Limited External Validity

Patients enrolled in RCTs designed to assess the treatment of bipolar disease with valproate or the treatment of schizophrenia with the second-generation atypical antipsychotic agents were compared to patients treated at a physician research network. Using inclusion and exclusion criteria set forth in the RCTs, 41 of 92 (45%) practice patients with bipolar disease and 51 of 81 (63%) practice patients with schizophrenia would have qualified to participate in the RCT.[27] The most common cause for ineligibility was comorbid mental illness.

## Comorbidities

Patients with comorbidities are often excluded from RCTs assessing treatment for chronic diseases, such as diabetes, heart failure, chronic obstructive pulmonary disease, and stroke.[28] A review of inclusion and exclusion criteria of patients with comorbidities, the reporting of comorbidities, and whether comorbidities were considered a confounder for data analysis revealed that many researchers excluded patients with comorbidities. Exclusion for comorbid conditions was most common in trials assessing treatment of COPD (0-55%), diabetes (0-44%), heart failure (0-42%), and stroke (0-39%). Only 70 of the 161 (43%) trials reported the prevalence of comorbidities. Of note, 42% of heart failure trials, 38% of diabetes trials, and 77% of COPD trials excluded patients with coronary heart disease. Additionally, 19% of heart failure trials and 44% of diabetes trials excluded patients with renal insufficiency. Of the stroke trials, 30% excluded patients with coronary artery disease and 24% excluded people with heart failure.

## Noninferiority RCTs

Traditionally, researchers design RCTs in which patients received either active drug or placebo. However, in many cases, it is unethical to randomize patients to receive placebo. In such cases, a **noninferiority study** permits researchers to randomize patients to receive active drug or the drug considered as the gold standard.[29] Researchers design the study to show that the new treatment is not inferior to the standard treatment. In doing so, a **noninferiority margin** is established a priori. For example, a recent trial designed to compare aliskiren to ramipril for treatment of hypertension assigned a noninferiority margin of 3.5 mm Hg difference in systolic blood pressure (SBP).[30] By the end of the 36-week trial, aliskiren was considered noninferior to ramipril if the difference in SBP between the patients was no greater than 3.5 mm Hg.

## OBSERVATIONAL STUDIES

Results from observational studies answer questions about treatment, prognosis, and harm and shed light on questions about therapy, specifically under real-world conditions and not ideal conditions, as set forth in the RCT. Results from observational studies only draw associations between therapy and outcome rather than cause and effect between treatment and disease.

### Case Reports

Authors describe events that have not been previously reported in the medical literature through **case reports**. Events may include adverse drug reactions or treatment with a drug and/or dose that has not been associated with the disease. A **case series** is a description of more than one patient with the same event. The association of statins causing rhabdomyolysis was first reported via case reports.[31] Case reports provide information on data not yet reported and should be considered for those questions in which answers are not forthcoming in the other types of studies.

### Case-Control Studies

**Case-control studies** allow researchers to identify risk factors associated with an event or disease and are often chosen when the event to be studied is rare. Cases are those patients who have the disease, and controls are those patients who do not have the disease.[20] To minimize confounders, researchers match cases to controls based on patient characteristics such as age, sex, and comorbidities. Researchers collect data by searching through patients' medical records or by asking patients to recall their own medical history through interview or survey. The differences in the outcome of interest are compared between the groups. Internal validity of case-control studies, which are often conducted retrospectively, is not only influenced by selection bias, but also recall bias.[32]

Researchers employed a case-control study design to assess whether type 2 diabetes (DM) is a risk factor for proton pump inhibitor (PPI) failure for treatment of gastro-esophageal reflux disease (GERD).[33] Medical records from adult patients recently diagnosed with GERD were reviewed during the study period from January 2004 to 2009. Cases were patients newly diagnosed with GERD who experienced PPI therapy failure in which more than once-daily dosing or add-on therapy was required. Controls were patients newly diagnosed with GERD who successfully completed 3 months of once-daily PPI therapy. Of the 285 patients who experienced PPI failure, 122 (42.8%) had a diagnosis of type 2 DM, whereas 157 of the 447 (35.1%) patients who responded to PPI therapy had type 2 DM. The odds of having type 2 DM is 38% higher in patients newly diagnosed with GERD who experienced PPI failure compared to those who responded to PPI therapy (OR = 1.38; 95% CI: 1.02 to 1.86; $p = 0.03$). **Figure 14-3** illustrates a case-study design.

Results of case-control studies are often reported using an **odds ratio** (OR). The OR is the odds of the event occurring in the exposed group divided by the odds of the event occurring in the unexposed group. The odds of an event occurring are the number of persons with the event divided by the number of persons without the event.[34] In this example, the odds of patients failing PPI therapy and having type 2 DM is $122 \div 163$, or 0.748. The odds of PPI responders having type 2 DM is $157 \div 290$, or 0.541. The OR is $0.748 \div 0.541$, or 1.38. An OR of 1.0 means that the odds of having the outcome is the same in each group.

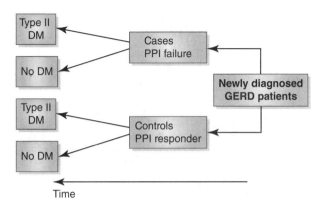

**FIGURE 14-3** Case-control study.

## Cohort Studies

In **cohort studies**, researchers follow a group of people (a cohort), of which some have the exposure of interest and some do not. Patients are followed over time and at the completion of the study the incidence of the outcome in each group is assessed. A cohort is a group of people with a common trait. For example, researchers designed the Framingham Heart Study, which began in 1948, to determine risk factors for cardiovascular disease among a cohort from Framingham, Massachusetts.[35] Researchers make inferences between risk factors and outcomes in both the exposed and unexposed groups.[20]

Cohort studies can be retrospective or prospective. With prospective cohort studies, researchers follow cohort members forward in time; with retrospective cohort studies, researchers collect data by reviewing patients' medical records or by asking patients to recall their own medical history through interview or survey, much like retrospective data collection for a case–control study. However, unlike case–control studies, in which the patient's outcome is known before the study begins, in a cohort study the outcome is not known.

Researchers chose a prospective cohort study to assess the effect of *Clostridium difficile* infection (CDI) in hospitalized patients on the risk of all-cause predischarge death during hospitalization for patients with CDI compared to those without CDI during calendar year 2009.[36] Documented CDI occurred in 185 of 38,644 patients (0.48%). Overall, 24 of the 185 patients (13%) with documented CDI died, and 1,021 of the 38,459 (2.7%) without documented CDI died during their hospital stay. Documented CDI increased the relative risk of predischarge death by 4.89 (95% CI: 3.35 to 7.13); after adjustment for age, sex, and comorbidities, the relative risk of predischarge death was 2.74 (95% CI: 1.82 to 4.10; $p < 0.0001$). Regardless of age, sex, and comorbidities, hospitalized patients with documented CDI were 2.74 times more likely to die during hospitalization than those without documented CDI. **Figure 14-4** illustrates a cohort study design.

Researchers often use **relative risk** (RR) to describe results from cohort studies. Unlike odds, risk is calculated as the number of persons with the outcome divided by the total number of persons in the group.[37] The relative risk or risk ratio compares the risk of the exposure group to the risk of the unexposed group. In the CDI example, the risk of death for patients with documented CDI was 24 ÷ 185, or 0.13. The risk of death for patients without documented CDI was 1,021 ÷ 38,459, or 0.027, so the relative risk was 0.13 ÷ 0.027, or 4.81.

## Cross-Sectional Studies

**Cross-sectional studies** take place in the present time. The outcome of interest, such as the presence or absence of a disease, is determined for each member of the study

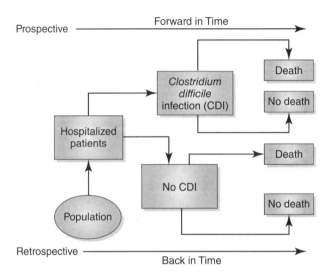

**FIGURE 14-4** Cohort study design.

population at one point in time. These observational studies are inexpensive compared to cohort and case-control studies and measure disease prevalence.[20]

Researchers utilized a cross-sectional study design to determine the prevalence of tobacco use and interest in cessation among active duty soldiers assigned to Fort Riley, Kansas.[38] A total of 6,181 active duty soldiers participated in the study, of which 39% reported using smoked tobacco and 19% smokeless tobacco; 36% reported interest in cessation. Results indicate that active-duty soldiers serving at Fort Riley Army Post represent a high-risk population for tobacco use, of which roughly half are interested in stopping. **Figure 14–5** illustrates a cross-sectional study.

## COMPARATIVE EFFECTIVENESS RESEARCH AND PRAGMATIC TRIALS

In its 2009 report, "Initial National Priorities for Comparative Effectiveness Research," the Institute of Medicine (IOM) defined **comparative effectiveness research** (CER) as:

> the generation and synthesis of evidence that compares the benefits and harms of alternative methods to prevent, diagnose, treat, and monitor a clinical condition or to improve the delivery of care. The purpose of CER is to assist consumers, clinicians, purchasers, and policy makers to make informed decisions that will improve health care at both the individual and population levels.[39]

CER uses results from pragmatic trials to make informed decisions. **Pragmatic trials** measure effectiveness or the benefit of interventions under real-world conditions and are

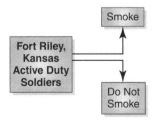

One-Time Assessment

**FIGURE 14-5** Cross-sectional study design.

also referred to as *naturalistic randomized controlled trials*.[40,41] In a pragmatic trial, heterogeneity of the patient population is highly desirable; therefore, exclusion criteria are limited.[42] Patients are still randomized to treatment groups. These trials allow researchers to evaluate therapy despite presence of traditional confounders (e.g., compliance with therapy, use of concomitant therapies, presence of comorbidities, and changing symptoms over time). Because results from pragmatic trials add to the body of evidence, clinicians will be able to make more informed decisions for their patients.

## TRIALS THAT REVIEW OTHER TRIALS

### Systematic Reviews

A **systematic review** summarizes the primary literature and often accompanies a meta-analysis. In a systematic review, authors explicitly state the research question and identify studies in the literature that attempt to answer this question.[43] Explicit methods for identifying studies for inclusion provide scientific rigor. A well-conducted systematic review includes published and unpublished data. **Publication bias** occurs because studies with positive results tend to be published. Unpublished data (data from clinical trials that were never published), incomplete data (data published in abstract form at professional medical meetings), non-English-language data, or data published in books or letters to the editor are considered *grey literature*.[44]

Including grey literature in systematic reviews strengthens conclusions. Sources of grey literature include Food and Drug Administration (FDA) review documents, clinical trial registries, abstracts, editorials, and letters to the editor.

### Meta-Analyses

A **meta-analysis** combines results from different trials through statistical analysis. EBM ranks a meta-analysis of RCTs at the top of the hierarchy of literature. A well-conducted meta-analysis includes published and unpublished data to derive an overall treatment effect. By combining individual studies into one statistical analysis, the power of the sample size increases as well as the precision of the treatment effect.[37] Trials meeting the rigor of systematic review comprise the meta-analysis. The treatment effect, or effect size, is the targeted difference between the groups. It is expressed by the OR, RR, or **hazard ratio** (HR). Researchers first calculate the treatment effect of each individual study along with the 95% CI and then calculate an overall treatment effect from a weighted average from the treatment effect of each individual study. Results displayed graphically in a forest plot provide a summary of effect size from individual trials and an overall summary of all trials. The power of the meta-analysis is the chance of detecting a difference between the groups.

### A Note on Efficacy and Effectiveness

The RCT design is considered the gold standard for determining cause and effect of therapy, or **efficacy**.[21] The rigorous nature of the RCT establishes an average overall benefit and risk of therapy in a select sample population. The FDA requires drug companies to prove the safety and efficacy of a drug before marketing it. Although the results of an RCT establish a cause-and-effect relationship between a treatment and disease under ideal conditions, the same effect may not be seen with the treatment when used in practice.[21,45] Moreover, limited external validity or generalizability of results from RCTs may cause healthcare providers to use therapies for patients in whom the therapies have not been studied. **Effectiveness** describes the effect of therapy under real-world conditions. Observational studies assess effectiveness.[21,45]

## SEARCHING THE LITERATURE

Searching for answers to EBM questions uses many of the same resources as those used in the systematic approach to searching for answers to drug information questions. Secondary sources such as MEDLINE, the Cochrane Library, Embase, and the Cumulative Index of Nursing and Allied Health Literature (CINAHL) aid in locating primary literature as well as tertiary sources that provide summaries of EBM topics. Other important resources in EBM research include Clinical Evidence, DynaMed, Physicians' Information and Education Research (PIER), and UpToDate.

### MEDLINE

**MEDLINE** (www.pubmed.org), a collection of 19 million biomedical journal abstracts and citations from around the world, is one of the most widely used secondary resources for locating primary literature.[46] MEDLINE is available through a variety of services, including PubMed, Ovid, and EBSCO Host. In order to navigate through MEDLINE to find the best evidence, professional indexers assign Medical Subject Headings (MeSH) to individual articles. Searching for articles using MeSH terms rather than keywords results in efficient searches because of the greater likelihood of locating relevant articles.[47,48] Additionally, using Boolean logic operators ensures that relevant articles are returned (**Figure 14-6**). **Boolean operators** (AND, OR, NOT) allow searching with multiple terms by creating relationships between those terms within a search.[49] Use of the Boolean operator AND returns articles containing both search terms. The operator OR returns articles with one or more of the search terms. The operator NOT returns articles that do not contain the search term. Many search engines, including the Cochrane Library and CINAHL, utilize Boolean logic operators.

### *Searching MEDLINE: An Example*

A physician would like to know if adding clopidogrel to aspirin therapy would reduce recurrence of stroke. He is treating a 63-year-old man with a history of hypertension who was admitted for treatment of lacunar stroke. The patient's current blood pressure is 148/78 mm Hg. He is currently taking ramipril 10 mg daily.

A well-designed question would be: Does adding clopidogrel to aspirin reduce recurrence of stroke in patients with recent lacunar stroke?

P: Lacunar stroke
I: Clopidogrel plus aspirin
C: Aspirin
O: Recurrence

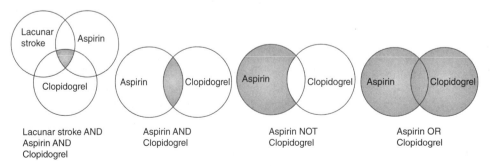

**FIGURE 14-6** Boolean operators.

## Search MEDLINE Through PubMed Using MeSH

**1.** Type in "lacunar stroke," which brings up the MeSH term "Stroke, Lacunar." Notice that this term was added to the MeSH database in 2012. Click the "Add to search builder" bar.

**2.** Type in "clopidogrel," which returns four supplementary concepts: clopidogrel, 2-oxo-clopidogrel, clopidogrel carboxylic acid, and clopidogrel resinate. Click each supplementary term for a complete description. The first term refers to clopidogrel without isomeric designation; additionally, Plavix is listed under Entry Terms. Click the "Add to search builder" bar, making certain that *and* is chosen as the Boolean operator.

**3.** Type "aspirin" into the MeSH search bar, click on the first term, and then click the "Add to search builder" bar, making certain that *and* is chosen as the Boolean operator.

**4.** Click "Search PubMed." Two articles are retrieved. The article "Effects of clopidogrel added to aspirin in patients with recent lacunar stroke" appears to be a reasonable choice.[50]

This article describes a double-blind, multicenter trial of patients with recent lacunar infarct who received aspirin daily plus clopidogrel or placebo.[50] The primary outcome was recurrence of any stroke. According to the hierarchy of evidence, an RCT is an appropriate design to answer questions about therapy. Evaluation of this article should provide an answer to the question.

## The Cochrane Library

The Cochrane Library (www.cochrane.org) is composed of seven databases that include evidence-based information on healthcare interventions. The Cochrane Library aims to make the results of well-conducted trials readily available and routinely incorporates unpublished data. The following is a brief overview of some of the Cochrane Library databases:

- The **Cochrane Database of Systematic Reviews** (Cochrane Reviews) contains rigorous systematic reviews of the primary literature. Each review answers a focused question. Reviews are updated routinely and often include unpublished literature and non-English articles. Explicit methodology, interpretation, and presentation aid in literature appraisal. Results include a summary of conclusive evidence as well as implications for practice.

- The **Database of Abstracts of Reviews of Effects (DARE)** provides summaries of systematic reviews and meta-analyses published in the literature. Each citation includes a summary of the original article and a critical commentary by Cochrane personnel.

- The Cochrane Central Register of Controlled Trials (Clinical Trials, or CENTRAL) includes the title, source of publication, and often the abstract, from bibliographic databases such as MEDLINE and Embase, as well as other published and unpublished sources.

- The Cochrane Methodology Register (CMR) includes bibliographic information of articles that report methodology used when conducting controlled trials and includes journal articles, books, and conference proceedings.

- The Health Technology Assessment Database (HTA) includes information on completed and ongoing health technology assessments (studies of the medical, social, ethical, and economic implications of healthcare interventions) from around the world.

- The NHS Economic Evaluation Database (NHS EED) includes published economic evaluations from around the world. The articles are assessed for quality, including strengths and weaknesses.

### Embase

Embase (www.embase.com) is a database that indexes bibliographic information from over 2,000 medical journals, including those that are not part of MEDLINE. Conference abstracts and conference sessions are also included. It is the largest database of bibliographic information from around the world.

### Cumulative Index of Nursing and Allied Health Literature

The **Cumulative Index of Nursing and Allied Health Literature (CINAHL)** is a database that contains bibliographic information from journals specific to nursing and allied health professionals, such as respiratory therapists, physical therapists, occupational therapists, and pharmacists. Some of the subjects include nursing, biomedicine, health sciences librarianship, alternative and complementary medicine, audiology, bereavement, consumer health, and allied health disciplines.

### Clinical Evidence

Clinical Evidence (clinicalevidence.bmj.com) is a database that contains summaries, based on thorough searches and appraisal of the literature, about prevention and treatment of clinical conditions. Summaries describe the best available evidence from systematic reviews, RCTs, and observational studies, where appropriate, and recommendations for treatment.

### DynaMed

DynaMed is a clinical reference database created by physicians to aid in information retrieval. Individual disease summaries include general information about the disease, causes and risk factors, complications, history and physical presentation, diagnosis, treatment, prognosis, prevention and screening, and patient information. It also lists current medical guidelines and resources for more information about the disease. DynaMed is organized in an outline fashion with bullet points. DynaMed is updated daily.

### Physicians' Information and Education Research

Physicians' Information and Education Research, or PIER, is a clinical decision support tool that provides evidence-based guidance on the diagnosis and treatment of disease as well as links to clinical articles and patient information. Reviews fall into one of five areas: diseases, screening and prevention, complementary and alternative medicine, ethical and legal issues, and procedures.

### UpToDate

UpToDate offers fully referenced expert answers written in paragraph style to clinical questions. Expert authorities write the topical reviews, which synthesize the evidence, summarize key findings, and provide specific recommendations.

**TABLE 14-4**   Questions to Consider During the Critical Appraisal Process

**Step 1: Assess the strengths and weaknesses of the study (internal validity).**

What is the research question?
How were study participants identified and recruited?
For case-control studies, how were cases matched to controls?
Who was included and excluded?
For RCTs, how were patients allocated to treatment and control groups?
For RCTs, how was treatment allocation concealed? Who was blinded?
Was the sample size adequate?
Were the outcomes explicitly stated?

**Step 2: Assess the results.**

Did the study results answer the research question?
How was the statistical analysis done, and was this appropriate?
Were all patients who began the study accounted for in the results? Why did patients leave the study?
Were results calculated according to an intention-to-treat (ITT) analysis or a per-protocol (PP) analysis? How was a modified ITT analysis defined?
Are the authors' conclusions supported by the data presented?

**Step 3: Assess generalizability of the results (external validity).**

Are the patients in the study representative of the patient(s) I am treating?
Would the patient I am treating be included in the study? If not, why not?

Data from Timm DF, Banks DE, McLarty J. Critical appraisal process: step-by-step. *South Med J*. 2012;105(3):144-148; and Akobeng AK. Understanding systematic reviews and meta-analysis. *Arch Dis Child*. 2005;90(8):845-848.

# STEP 3: CRITICALLY APPRAISE THE EVIDENCE

Critically appraising the evidence is crucial to providing proper patient care. Critically appraising an article involves reviewing the article in an objective and structured way.[51] **Table 14-4** provides a list of questions to consider when appraising an article.[11,37] The first step is to decide if the studies provide reliable results or to assess internal validity. The second step is to assess the results for magnitude and precision. The third step is to determine the generalizability of the results or assess external validity.

## STEP 1: ASSESS INTERNAL VALIDITY

When assessing internal validity or potential for bias, knowing the study design assists in determining if results are valid. Different study designs are inherently susceptible to specific types of bias (**Table 14-5**).[18]

## STEP 2: ASSESS THE RESULTS

After assessing internal validity to determine if the study design was appropriate, evaluation of the results is next. When evaluating results, an understanding of statistical methods and measures of treatment effects aids in determining magnitude expected by the intervention (**Table 14-6**).[11,37,52] In study designs in which two groups are compared, such as RCTs and cohort and case-control studies, measures of treatment effect are often expressed as an OR, RR, or HR. A *p*-value or level of statistical significance is the probability that the difference between the groups occurred by chance. *p*-values are often reported along with other measures of treatment effect. Confidence intervals (CI)

**TABLE 14-5**    Potential Bias According to Study Design*

| Bias | Definition | Study Design Affected | How to Minimize |
|---|---|---|---|
| Publication bias | Studies with positive results tend to be published | Meta-analyses, systematic reviews | Include unpublished data, data from presented abstracts, meeting symposia, letters to the editor |
| Selection bias | Groups are not equal with regard to patient demographics or medical history | RCT, case-control | Randomization (RCT), matching (case-control) |
| Information bias | Misclassification of data | Case-control, retrospective cohort | Use more than one person to collect data |
| Recall bias | Patients do not recall all information | Case-control, retrospective cohort | Provide surveys or interviews more often to minimize time between exposure and recall |
| Performance bias | Differences in care provided or exposure to confounders | RCT | Blinding |

* Not all-inclusive.
Data from Morris MJ, Fewell AE, Oleszewski T. Evidence-based medicine: specific skills necessary for developing expertise in critical appraisal. *South Med Assoc.* 2012;105(3):114-119.

**TABLE 14-6**    Measures of Effect Size

| Measures of Effect | Abbreviation | Description | Interpretation |
|---|---|---|---|
| Absolute risk reduction | ARR | Absolute change in risk between control and treatment groups; the risk of the event in the control group minus the risk of the event in the treatment group, expressed as a percentage. | No effect, ARR = 0% |
| Relative risk | RR | The risk of an event in the treatment group divided by the risk of the event in the control and treatment groups; usually expressed as a decimal. | No effect, RR = 1, or 100% |
| Relative risk reduction | RRR | 1 – RR; expressed as a percentage | No effect, RRR = 0% |
| Odds ratio | OR | Odds of an event occurring in the exposed group divided by the odds of the event occurring in the unexposed group; usually expressed as a decimal. | No effect, OR = 1 |
| Hazard ratio | HR | Chance of an event occurring in the treatment arm divided by the chance of the event occurring in the control arm; the event, or hazard, is expressed as a rate or number of events per unit time; written as a decimal. | No effect, HR = 1 |
| Number needed to treat | NNT | The number of patients who need to be treated to prevent one event; reciprocal of the ARR expressed as a decimal proportion; usually rounded to a whole number. | No effect, NNT = infinity |

Data from Davies HT, Crombie IK. What are confidence intervals and p-values? What is …? series. Hayward Medical Communications. 2009.

describe the precision of the data, whereas *p*-values describe statistical significance.[53] A *p*-value of 0.05 means that by chance alone, 1 out of 20 identical trials would have a non-significant result. A 95% CI correlates to a *p*-value of 0.05, where the 95% CI means that if the experiment were repeated 100 times, 95 times the result would fall within the CI range. The CI provides a range for the treatment effect.

For example, researchers designed a multicenter, double-blind, placebo-controlled trial to determine if use of bisphosphonates in men with osteoporosis decreases the rate of fractures.[54] Men aged 50–85 years with primary osteoporosis or secondary osteroporosis due to low testosterone were randomized to receive zoledronic acid 5 mg intravenously or placebo at baseline and again at month 12. Of the 553 men in the treatment group, 9 men (1.6%) suffered a vertebral fracture over the course of 24 months compared to 19 of 575 (4.9%) who received placebo. This represents a reduction in vertebral fractures of 67% in men treated with zoledronic acid compared to placebo (RR = 0.33; 95% CI: 0.16 to 0.70; *p* = 0.002). Zoledronic acid reduced the risk of vertebral fractures in men with osteoporosis.

These results indicate that men treated with zoledronic acid are 67% less likely to suffer a vertebral fracture relative to those treated with placebo and that this difference is statistically significant with a *p*-value of 0.002. This *p*-value means that if zoledronic acid was no different in efficacy than placebo, by chance alone the relative risk of 67% would be higher or lower in 1 out of 500 identical trials. The 95% CI expands this further: men treated with zoledronic acid are 30-84% less likely to suffer a vertebral fracture compared to those treated with placebo. The *p*-value expresses statistical significance, whereas the confidence interval adds precision to the effect size.

Within the same trial, the absolute risk reduction is 3.3%. The absolute risk reduction is always lower than the relative risk reduction. The **absolute risk reduction** (ARR) is the difference in risk between the treatment and control groups, whereas the **relative risk reduction** (RRR) is the difference in risk between the treatment group and the entire sample population (i.e., the treatment group and the control group). The RRR describes the risk eliminated by the treatment. The **number needed to treat** (NNT) is the reciprocal of the ARR (expressed as a decimal proportion), or $1 \div 0.033$, which is equal to 30. Thirty patients need to be treated with zoledronic acid before one patient is less likely to experience a vertebral fracture.

## STEP 3: ASSESS THE GENERALIZABILITY OF THE RESULTS

After determining if the results are valid, assessing if the results are generalizable to the patient in question (i.e., external validity) is the next step.

### Determining Generalizability: An Example

A physician would like to know if his patient with osteoporosis should receive zoledronic acid. He is treating a 78-year-old man with primary osteoporosis. His medical history is unremarkable except for a thyroidectomy secondary to thyroid cancer back in 1972. His medications include levothyroxine 0.25 mg once daily. He does not smoke and tries to eat a healthy, balanced diet. All labs are normal except for his latest bone mineral density (BMD) test, which showed a T score of −2.8.

A well-designed question would be: Would starting zoledronic acid prevent fractures in a 78-year-old man with primary osteoporosis?

P: Man with osteoporosis
I: Zoledronic acid
C:
O: Decrease rate of fractures

Searching MEDLINE with the terms and Boolean operators "Male AND Osteo-porosis AND Zoledronic acid AND fractures" returns several articles. Limiting results to randomized control trial and English returns fewer articles, one of which is an RCT by Boonen and colleagues.[54] To assess generalizability, or external validity, the patient population of the RCT should be examined. This is best accomplished by reviewing the inclusion and exclusion criteria of the trial and asking, "Would my patient be a candidate for this trial?"

The article presented the following inclusion criteria:[54]

> Men, 50 to 85 years, who had primary osteoporosis or osteoporosis associated with low testosterone levels were eligible if they had a bone mineral density T score of –1.5 or less at the total hip or femoral neck and one to three, mild to moderate grade, vertebral fractures. Men without fractures were eligible if they had a bone mineral density T score –2.5 or less at the total hip, femoral neck, or lumbar spine.

The exclusion criteria were as follows:[54]

> Exclusion criteria included ≥ 4 prevalent vertebral fractures; a 25-hydroxyvitamin D level of < 15 ng/mL during screening; baseline renal insufficiency; an alkaline phosphatase level > 1.5 times the upper limit of normal (ULN) or an aspartate aminotransferase or alanine aminotransferase level > 3 times ULN; hypercalcemia or hypocalcemia; and bisphosphonate hypersensitivity. Patients who were receiving bisphosphonates, teriparatide, calcitonin, or glucocorticoids were eligible if the prespecified washout criteria were met before randomization.

Notice the explicit inclusion and exclusion criteria. In order to minimize the chance for bias and provide conditions in which the result may be definitively attributed to the treatment, researchers design RCTs with explicit inclusion and exclusion criteria. The patient is 78 years old and has primary osteoporosis, which meets the inclusion criteria. His history of Graves disease requiring a thyroidectomy and daily thyroid supplementation is not listed as an exclusion criterion. He appears to be a candidate for zoledronic acid.

Critical appraisal of experimental and observational studies involves asking different questions (Table 14-4). Several critical appraisal worksheets are available to help in this process. The Critical Appraisal Skills Programme, developed in Oxford in 1993, publishes several appraisal checklists for each type of study: RCT, systematic reviews, cohort studies, case-control studies, economic evaluations, and diagnostic studies. The Centre for Evidence-Based Medicine, under EBM Tools, lists several critical appraisal forms, including ones for RCTs, systematic reviews, diagnosis, and prognosis.

# STEP 4: INTEGRATE EVIDENCE WITH CLINICAL JUDGMENT/EXPERTISE AND PATIENT PREFERENCES

In addition to determining efficacy and effectiveness of a therapy, risk of adverse events and patient preferences, including cost of therapy, need to be considered. When integrating the evidence with clinical judgment, one should ask if the therapy makes sense. Returning to the example about zoledronic acid, the efficacy of zoledronic acid for treatment of osteoporosis in men resulted in a 67% decrease in vertebral fractures compared to patients who received placebo. Although the CI was wide, thus resulting in a potential decrease in vertebral fractures of 30-84%, the benefit of zoledronic acid is apparent. However, consideration of potential adverse drug events and whether the benefits of therapy outweigh the risks is essential. Zoledronic acid, a bisphosphonate, may cause renal insufficiency, requiring dialysis in some patients.[55] Bisphosphonates may also cause osteonecrosis of the jaw. Only after a discussion with the patient's physician will an appropriate decision on starting therapy with zoledronic acid be made.

In addition to clinical expertise, EBM takes into account patient preferences. Zoledronic acid is administered as an intravenous infusion over at least 15 minutes once a year. This means the patient will be required to come to the hospital or clinic to receive the drug. Additionally, determining if the drug is covered by the patient's medical insurance will help drive the decision of whether to implement therapy. The drug will not benefit the patient if it is not taken. Asking the patient about his preferences will result in the best therapy.

# STEPS 5 AND 6: IMPLEMENT INTERVENTION AND EVALUATE EFFECTIVENESS

The remaining two steps are to implement the intervention and evaluate its effectiveness. After implementation of the therapy, following the patient's progress ensures that the intervention or therapy accomplishes the desired outcome. Individual patients may or may not react to the therapy as patients treated during clinical trials. Results reported from clinical trials represent the average patient for which the clinical trial enrolled. In addition, the treatment effect may be decreased under real-world conditions. The strict methodology of RCTs enforces a high rate of compliance.

# CLINICAL PRACTICE GUIDELINES

In 2011, the Institute of Medicine defined **clinical practice guidelines** as "statements that include recommendations intended to optimize patient care that are informed by a systematic review of evidence and an assessment of the benefits and harms of alternative care options."[56] Clinical practice guidelines assist healthcare practitioners in making informed decisions to treat patients. Guidelines may provide information on epidemiology, screening, diagnosis, and nonpharmacologic and pharmacologic treatment. Guidelines are essential in clinical practice because they provide a standard of care and ultimately improve the quality of health care.[57]

Guidelines are decision-making tools providing treatment algorithms. It is important to note that guidelines are not a "cookbook" to medicine. All decisions should not be made solely based on guidelines, because each patient is unique. While taking clinical practice guidelines into consideration, it is also important to rely on one's own clinical judgment and the values of the patient in making therapeutic recommendations.

## TYPES OF GUIDELINES AND GUIDELINE DEVELOPMENT

The three types of clinical practice guidelines are informal consensus panel, formal consensus panel, and evidence-based guidelines. Each guideline is unique in the way it is developed.

Informal consensus guidelines are developed during a meeting of experts. These guidelines may be based solely on expert opinion and provide recommendations. The quality of such guidelines are questionable because they usually do not explain how recommendations are supported by clinical evidence. When reading informal consensus guidelines, it is important to be aware of bias. During a meeting of experts, some individuals may not have been as assertive as others in presenting their opinions; thus, their views may not become a part of the guidelines. In addition, there may also be a conflict of interest if the full methodology for developing the recommendations is not clearly stated within the guidelines. Another possible bias in these types of guidelines occurs if experts have recommended certain diagnostics tests or medications in which they have a financial interest.[58] Expert opinions are not necessarily substantiated by literature or considered best practice. An evaluation of additional literature may be needed in order to determine if expert opinion guidelines are appropriate to apply to a clinical situation.

Formal consensus panels are developed in a more structured 2.5-day meeting by expert thought leaders. Similar to the informal consensus panel, there is a discussion on recommendations; however, experts may work through the night to reach a consensus. On the third day, the guidelines are unveiled to an audience. Some of the flaws with formal consensus panel guidelines may be inconsistent levels of evidence for recommendations and variable referencing of recommendations.[58]

Evidence-based guidelines have the most rigorous development, which includes extensive documentation of methodology and appropriate levels of evidence for recommendations.[58] The development of these types of guidelines does not occur in a few days; rather, it occurs over months to years and is an expensive process.[59] Evidence-based guidelines are considered to be superior to both informal and formal consensus-based guidelines because the recommendations are supported by literature. Today, these types of guidelines are used by several organizations, such as the American Heart Association and the American College of Cardiology.

In general, evidence-based clinical practice guideline development consists of four phases: preparing for the creation of guidelines, evaluating the literature, drafting guidelines, and reviewing guidelines.[60] The first phase involves determining the topic and scope of the guidelines, the audience to whom the guidelines are directed, and selecting members of the guideline development group. During the second phase, the focused clinical question will be determined, a literature search will be conducted, and the evidence will be evaluated.[61] The drafting of the clinical practice guidelines consists of the development of the recommendations, categorization of recommendations based on levels of evidence, creating a strategy to implement the guidelines, and drafting the executive summary.[61,62] The last phase of clinical guideline development focuses on the updating and implementation of the guidelines.[62]

The goal of the Grading of Recommendations, Assessment, Development, and Evaluation (**GRADE**) working group is to create a standardized process to rate the quality of literature and determine the appropriate level of evidence of a recommendation.[62] Based on GRADE, literature is categorized on the overall quality (study design, inconsistent results, indirectness of evidence, and bias) as high, moderate, low, or very low.[63] In addition, recommendations are classified as strong or weak depending on evidence supporting its use. The strength of each recommendation is based upon the risk of benefit versus harm, quality of evidence, values and preferences, and cost. Strong recommendations propose that "most informed patients would choose the recommended management and that clinicians can structure their interactions with patients accordingly," whereas weak recommendations suggest that "patients' choices will vary according to their values and preferences, and clinicians must ensure that patients' care is in keeping with their values and preferences."[64] Explanations of the advantages of the GRADE approach are described in **Table 14-7**. Many organizations, including the American College of Chest Physicians (ACCP), the World Health Organization (WHO), the Agency for Healthcare Research and Quality (AHRQ), and the Centers for Disease Control (CDC), have adopted the GRADE approach.[61,62]

**TABLE 14-7**    Comparison of GRADE and Other Systems

| Factor | Other Systems | GRADE | Advantages of GRADE System* |
|---|---|---|---|
| Definitions | Implicit definitions of quality (level) of evidence and strength of recommendation. | Explicit definitions. | Makes clear what grades indicate and what should be considered in making these judgments. |
| Judgments | Implicit judgments regarding which outcomes are important, quality of evidence for each important outcome, overall quality of evidence, balance between benefits and harms, and value of incremental benefits. | Sequential, explicit judgments. | Clarifies each of these judgments and reduces risks of introducing errors or bias that can arise when they are made implicitly. |
| Key components of quality of evidence | Not considered for each important outcome. Judgments about quality of evidence are often based on study design alone. | Systematic and explicit consideration of study design, study quality, consistency, and directness of evidence in judgments about quality of evidence. | Ensures that these factors are considered appropriately. |
| Other factors that can affect quality of evidence | Not explicitly taken into account. | Explicit consideration of imprecise or sparse data, reporting bias, strength of association, evidence of a dose-response gradient, and plausible confounding. | Ensures consideration of other factors. |
| Overall quality of evidence | Implicitly based on the quality of evidence for benefits. | Based on the lowest quality of evidence for any of the outcomes that are critical to making a decision. | Reduces likelihood of mislabeling overall quality of evidence when evidence for a critical outcome is lacking. |
| Relative importance of outcomes | Considered implicitly. | Explicit judgments about which outcomes are critical, which ones are important but not critical, and which ones are unimportant and can be ignored. | Ensures appropriate consideration of each outcome when grading overall quality of evidence and strength of recommendations. |
| Balance between health benefits and harms | Not explicitly considered. | Explicit consideration of trade-offs between important benefits and harms, the quality of evidence for these, translation of evidence into specific circumstances, and certainty of baseline risks. | Clarifies and improves transparency of judgments on harms and benefits. |
| Whether incremental health benefits are worth the costs | Not explicitly considered. | Explicit consideration after first considering whether there are net health benefits. | Ensures that judgments about value of net health benefits are transparent. |
| Summaries of evidence and findings | Inconsistent presentation. | Consistent GRADE evidence profiles, including quality assessment and summary of findings. | Ensures that all panel members base their judgments on the same information and that this information is available to others. |
| Extent of use | Seldom used by more than one organization and little, if any, empirical evaluation. | International collaboration across wide range of organizations in development and evaluation. | Builds on previous experience to achieve a system that is more sensible, reliable, and widely applicable. |

*Most other approaches do not include any of these advantages, although some may incorporate some of these advantages.
Reproduced from *BMJ*, GRADE Working Group. Grading quality of evidence and strength of recommendations., Atkins D, Best D, Briss PA, et al., 328, p. 1490, copyright 2004 with permission from BMJ Publishing Group Ltd.

**TABLE 14-8**    Institute of Medicine Standards for Developing Trustworthy Clinical Practice Guidelines

| Standard | Select Inclusions to Meet Standards |
|---|---|
| 1. Establishing transparency | Explain methodology of guideline development. |
| 2. Management of conflict of interest | Individuals being considered to be selected in the Guideline Development Group must provide full disclosures (i.e. intellectual, institutional, or financial involvement). |
| 3. Guideline group composition | A multidisciplinary group who will be directly affected by the guideline's development. |
| 4. Clinical practice guideline–systematic review intersection | Systematic reviews included in development should meet standards of the Institute of Medicine Committee on Standards for Systematic Reviews of Comparative Effectiveness Research. |
| 5. Establishing evidence foundations for and rating strength of recommendations | Recommendations should have information on benefits and risks and where the information for the recommendation was obtained (i.e., literature, expert opinion, etc.). In addition, the recommendation should be rated based on evidence supporting the recommendation. |
| 6. Articulation of recommendation | Recommendations should be presented in a standard format stating the situation in which the recommendation should be applied to practice. |
| 7. External review | Peer review group should consist of clinicians, health organizations, federal agencies, and public. |
| 8. Updating | Guidelines should be updated regularly based on new literature available. |

Data from Graham R, Macher M, Wolman DM, et al, eds. *Clinical Practice Guidelines We Can Trust*. Washington, DC: National Academies Press; 2011.

## EVALUATING GUIDELINES

The Institute of Medicine evaluated the best practices for the development of guidelines due to various methods being used by organizations and published a consensus report in 2011 discussing all aspects of clinical practice guidelines.[63] In the consensus report, eight standards are described to develop trustworthy guidelines. **Table 14–8** lists each standard and summarizes select inclusion criteria for each. Many guidelines follow the standards set forth by the Institute of Medicine; however, it is still essential to evaluate the trustworthiness of each guideline.

In order to assess and evaluate the quality of clinical practice guidelines, the Appraisal of Guidelines Research and Evaluation (AGREE) Instrument was created. The **AGREE Instrument** can be used by policy makers, guideline developers, health-care professionals, and educators to assist in the evaluation of clinical practice guidelines. The original AGREE Instrument, published in 2001, contained six domains with 23 key items.[65] AGREE II was published in 2009 with revised key items to include public health considerations (www.agreetrust.org).[66] Each domain focuses on part of the guideline development process through a series of questions that determine if the guideline and recommendations are truly evidence based.[67] "The AGREE Instrument assesses both the quality of the reporting, and the quality of some aspects of recommendations," which can be used on new, current, and updated clinical guidelines.[66]

The introduction and/or methodology sections of clinical practice guidelines should always be read prior to reviewing recommendations. These sections explain development of the guideline as well as the rating system used. Moreover, the entire process for guideline development is stated, from the focused question to the formation of the clinical recommendations. The methodology section also contains a description of how the panel of individuals reviewed the literature considered for guideline inclusion.

**TABLE 14-9**   Strength of Recommendations from CHEST Guidelines

| Grade of Recommendation | Benefit vs. Risk and Burdens | Methodologic Strength of Supporting Evidence | Implications |
|---|---|---|---|
| Strong recommendation, high-quality evidence (1A) | Benefits clearly outweigh risk and burdens or vice versa. | Consistent evidence from randomized controlled trials without important limitations or exceptionally strong evidence from observational studies. | Recommendation can apply to most patients in most circumstances. Further research is very unlikely to change our confidence in the estimate of effect. |
| Strong recommendation, moderate-quality evidence (1B) | Benefits clearly outweigh risk and burdens or vice versa. | Evidence from randomized controlled trials with important limitations (inconsistent results, methodologic flaws, indirect or imprecise) or very strong evidence from observational studies. | Recommendation can apply to most patients in most circumstances. Higher-quality research may well have an important impact on our confidence in the estimate of effect and may change the estimate. |
| Strong recommendation, low- or very-low-quality evidence (1C) | Benefits clearly outweigh risk and burdens or vice versa. | Evidence for at least one critical outcome from observational studies, case series, or randomized controlled trials, with serious flaws or indirect evidence. | Recommendation can apply to most patients in many circumstances. Higher-quality research is likely to have an important impact on our confidence in the estimate of effect and may well change the estimate. |
| Weak recommendation, high-quality evidence (2A) | Benefits closely balanced with risks and burden. | Consistent evidence from randomized controlled trials without important limitations or exceptionally strong evidence from observational studies. | The best action may differ depending on circumstances or patient or societal values. Further research is very unlikely to change our confidence in the estimate of effect. |
| Weak recommendation, moderate-quality evidence (2B) | Benefits closely balanced with risks and burden. | Evidence from randomized controlled trials with important limitations (inconsistent results, methodologic flaws, indirect or imprecise) or very strong evidence from observational studies. | Best action may differ depending on circumstances or patient or societal values. Higher-quality research may well have an important impact on our confidence in the estimate of effect and may change the estimate. |

Data from Guyatt GH, Norris SL, Schulman S, et al. American College of Chest Physicians Antithrombotic and thrombolytic therapy: American College of Chest Physicians Evidence-Based Clinical Practice Guidelines (9th edition). *CHEST*. 2012;141(2 suppl):53S-70S.

Subsequently, rating the strengths and recommendations of the guideline differs between individual guidelines. Some authors use the GRADE system for rating the guidelines, whereas others may use their own criteria. For example, the CHEST Guidelines and the Use of Antiretroviral Agents in HIV-1–Infected Adults and Adolescents both have adapted the GRADE system (**Tables 14–9** and **14–10**).[68,69] Because different guidelines use different rating systems, it is crucial to review the methodology section accurately to consider the criteria used for the strength of each recommendation. The strength of recommendation is listed after each recommendation provided. Knowing the rating

**TABLE 14-10**    Rating Scheme of Recommendations from the Guidelines for the Use of Antiretroviral Agents in HIV-1-Infected Adults and Adolescents

| Strength of Recommendation | Quality of Evidence for a Recommendation |
|---|---|
| A: Strong recommendation for this statement<br>B: Moderate recommendation for this statement<br>C: Optional recommendation for this statement | I: One or more randomized trials with clinical outcomes and/or validated laboratory endpoints<br>II: One or more well-designed, nonrandomized trials or observational cohort studies with long-term clinical outcomes<br>III: Expert opinion |

Data from Panel on Antiretroviral Guidelines for Adults and Adolescents. Guidelines for the use of antiretroviral agents in HIV-1-infected adults and adolescents. Department of Health and Human Services. Available at http://aidsinfo.nih.gov/ContentFiles/AdultandAdolescentGL.pdf.

scheme for the recommendations before reading the recommendation puts into perspective the strength of the recommendation.

## INCORPORATING GUIDELINES INTO PRACTICE

Once clinical practice guidelines are developed and published, the question becomes how to incorporate the guidelines into practice. Incorporating guidelines involves communication of recommendations, education to other healthcare professionals, and overcoming barriers to change.[70] Pharmacists can reinforce new guidelines while rounding on a team and making recommendations for clinical interventions, thereby reinforcing guideline recommendations to other healthcare professionals. Keeping abreast of current or new guideline recommendations is essential. Several forms of education are available to disseminate information from new guidelines to healthcare professionals, such as continuing education programs, national conferences, mailed letters or handouts, and academic detailing.[71] Academic detailing involves a trained healthcare professional speaking one-to-one with a physician in the physician's practice setting. In order to disseminate the clinical guidelines information appropriately, multiple educational approaches must be aimed at physicians.[72]

Factors that may increase the probability of incorporating guidelines into everyday practice include the practice setting itself, incentives, and regulations. The hospital environment can affect the opinions and practices of others such that physicians not accepting of guidelines may feel pressured by those who accept the guidelines.[72] However, this may not be an issue in an institution where healthcare professionals have guideline-driven practices. Insurance companies may not provide adequate reimbursement for services for physicians who do not follow guidelines. Thus, reimbursement by insurance companies may provide an incentive for physicians to increase the use of guideline recommendations in practice. Regulatory bodies such as The Joint Commission may require institutions to adapt guideline standards in order to receive accreditation. The Centers for Medicare and Medicaid Services (CMS) is another regulatory body that has recommended core measures for both pediatric and adult patients. Examples of CMS core measures include heart failure, pneumonia, and immunizations.

An effective method to incorporate guidelines into practice is through the use of informatics. Clinical decision support (CDS) allows the incorporation of guidelines into order sets or the creation of guideline-enhanced electronic medical records.[73] Although recommendations may appear for a patient, a practitioner may have several options available, such as selecting a treatment option from a generated list, rejecting the recommendation and stating why, or choosing an alternative treatment option that was not included in the guideline-enhanced medical record.[74] An institution that incorporates guidelines into electronic medical records can evaluate the use of clinical decision support. Adherence to the guideline can be reviewed to determine if the patient truly received optimal therapy. Additionally, physicians who consistently do not follow guideline recommendations can be identified and educated.

## BARRIERS TO GUIDELINE USE

Clinical practice guidelines assist in the standardization and improvement of patient care. Guidelines provide the necessary information for healthcare practitioners to screen, prevent, diagnose, and treat diseases in a consistent and efficient manner. Using evidence-based guidelines in practice or within institutions may reduce healthcare costs and promote an image of excellence.[75] Using clinical practice guidelines provides several benefits; however, there are also barriers to its use. The following limitations should be taken into consideration when integrating information to practice.

Published guidelines may not be updated regularly and may become outdated. As a result, using this information when additional evidence is available may be detrimental to the patient when there are newer therapies for treatment or a new gold standard for diagnosis. Recommendations made based on outdated guidelines may be ineffective or harmful to the patient.[75] Additional literature should be evaluated in a timely manner in order to keep up with changes to treatments for a particular disease state. Another

---

**CASE STUDY 14-2**     **Treatment of Crohn's Disease**

PF is a 35-year-old female with a past medical history of Crohn's disease. She has been receiving infliximab for maintenance therapy. In July, she developed CDI and was subsequently treated with oral metronidazole, which was switched to oral vancomycin due to intolerance. One month passed and she tested negative for *C. difficile* prior to her scheduled infliximab infusion. She is currently due for this infusion; however, she now has a recurrence of CDI. The team is not sure how to proceed. The medical resident asks the pharmacy student on rounds to check the guidelines for Crohn's disease.

After a literature search, the pharmacy student finds a few guidelines for Crohn's disease. The pharmacy student then verifies the trustworthiness of the guidelines by asking several questions. Using the AGREE Instrument found at agreetrust.org, the pharmacy student asks himself the following questions:

- Who developed the guidelines? What type of guideline is it?
- How recent are the guidelines? What is the most current literature that was included in the review? Was the literature search method described?
- Are the recommendations stated in the guidelines valid? Was the GRADE approach used? Are the guidelines peer reviewed?
- Were outcomes relevant to the disease state considered (i.e., quality of life)?
- Do the guidelines account for recent clinical developments?
- Are the guidelines applicable to this patient?

If the answer to just one of these questions is "no," it does not mean that the guideline is completely untrustworthy. An answer of "no" to one or more of the questions, however, means that the student's recommendation based on the guideline may be limited. After determining the trustworthiness of the guidelines, the pharmacy student then searches for the evidence to answer the clinical question that is specific to the patient.

limitation is that guidelines for a disease state that are published by different organizations may have conflicting information. If guidelines conflict, health professionals may be confused with what recommendation to follow.[76] When presented with conflicting guidelines, it is essential to evaluate each guideline for development, literature used, and if expert opinion was incorporated.

When applying guidelines to practice, it is essential to consider the individual patient. Clinical practice guidelines standardize care for the general population; however, it is important to remember that care should be individualized per patient.[77] In other words, the same recommendation may not be appropriate for all patients.

Public policy may be affected by changes in clinical practice guidelines. Insurance coverage of diagnostic tests or therapeutic options can be limited based on the recommendations of guidelines.[77] For instance, if a medication is expensive and not a first-line agent for a disease state, the insurance company may decide to decrease coverage, thereby restricting it. However, as stated earlier, it is important to incorporate the patient into the decision. If a patient has a contraindication or is allergic to a medication, then a first- or second-line agent may not be a suitable option. A higher copayment for another medication (not first or second line) may deter the patient from obtaining the medication, thus affecting patient care.

Guidelines may be an influencing factor for future clinical studies. It may cause harm if a guideline states that an intervention is not appropriate without adequate evidence or literature. Future studies may not be funded for this specific intervention due to a negative statement in a guideline.[77] The intervention may have been proven useful if studied in a certain population of patients.

## LOCATING GUIDELINES

Clinical practice guidelines can be accessed from the organizations that developed the guidelines, from secondary resources (e.g., MEDLINE), and from tertiary resources (e.g., DrugDex Drug Consults from Micromedex, Lexicomp drug monographs, DynaMed disease state monograph, etc.). **Table 14–11** provides a list of select national organizations from which to obtain guidelines. The websites of a number of organizations, such as the National Guideline Clearinghouse (www.guideline.gov), Turning Research Into Practice (TRIP) Database (www.tripdatabase.com), and the Guidelines International Network (www.g-i-n.net), provide access to guidelines and additional EBM resources.

# BARRIERS TO EVIDENCE-BASED MEDICINE

Incorporation of EBM in practice is growing due to the number of benefits seen by applying this information. It promotes recommendations that have been thoroughly evaluated, decreases use of ineffective recommendations, and ultimately has the ability to improve the quality of patient care.[63,78] Although there are many benefits to EBM, a number of barriers are preventing its use in clinical practice.

Barriers to practicing EBM range from lack of confidence in literature evaluation to lack of resources. In one study, conflicting results from studies followed by not having a skilled individual evaluating the evidence were the main reasons practitioners did not fully implement EBM into their practice.[79] In a study that evaluated EBM barriers for Australian practitioners, the primary barrier identified was "patient demand for treatment despite highly rated barriers related to lack of time."[80] Lack of time in general was cited as a barrier due to constraints for searching for literature, evaluating the literature,

| TABLE 14-11 | Select Resources to Obtain Guidelines |
|---|---|
| **Therapeutic Area** | **Organization** |
| Cardiology | American College of Cardiology (ACC)<br>American Heart Association (AHA)<br>American College of Chest Physicians (ACCP)<br>National Heart, Lung, and Blood Institute (NHLBI) |
| Endocrinology | American Association of Clinical Endocrinologists (AACE)<br>American Diabetes Association (ADA)<br>National Osteoporosis Foundation (NOF) |
| Gastroenterology | American College of Gastroenterology (ACG) |
| Infectious diseases | Infectious Disease Society of America (IDSA) |
| Nephrology | Kidney Disease: Improving Global Outcomes (KDIGO)<br>Kidney Disease Outcomes Quality Initiative (KDOQI) |
| Neurology | American Academy of Neurology (AAN) |
| Obstetrics | American Congress of Obstetricians and Gynecologists (ACOG) |
| Oncology | National Comprehensive Cancer Network (NCCN) |
| Pediatrics | American Academy of Pediatrics (AAP) |
| Psychiatry | American Psychiatric Association (APA)<br>American Academy of Child and Adolescent Psychiatry (AACAP) |
| Pulmonary | National Heart, Lung, and Blood Institute (NHLBI)<br>Global Initiative for Chronic Obstructive Lung Disease (GOLD) |

and discussing the recommendations with patients. Lack of EBM resources was an obstacle cited; however, the studies that published these results were from the 1990s.[81] Currently, the use of mobile technology and online resources has reduced several of these barriers. Systematic reviews, clinical practice guidelines, and electronic databases that summarize the evidence are available for practitioners to use for quick reference, thus providing point-of-care use.

Barriers may also be a result of patient preference. General practitioners (GPs) stated that when patient preferences do not match EBM, it prevented them from incorporating it into practice in order to please the patient: "As concluded in a qualitative study, the quality of the relationship with a patient is considered a barrier to using evidence. Especially when GPs know their patients well, they find it hard to translate the evidence to their patients because they felt that deviating from guidelines based on experience or patient preferences is not evidenced-based behavior."[82] It is important to remember that the definition of EBM is to incorporate evidence, expertise, and patient values in order to make the most appropriate clinical intervention. Each patient is unique; some may have allergies or contraindications to medications. Clinical expertise is essential in applying EBM to practice, because this is a skill that allows practitioners to evaluate the patient and determine whether the evidence applies to them.

Some barriers to practice cannot be altered. This is applying EBM "at the right time, in the right place, and in the right way."[83] Practitioners cannot control the clinical situations of their patients (i.e., if they have a stroke and it is not recognized in time for proper treatment). EBM is difficult to implement in cases such as these, because there is a specific time frame for the most effective treatment options. Sometimes a practitioner may come across a problem in that there is no high-quality evidence available. In this situation, the practitioner relies on tertiary resources, expert opinion, or his or her own expertise. As more EBM is available to guide decisions, this barrier to practice will be reduced.[84]

Financial and organizational barriers are a concern with EBM practice.[84] Patients may insist against an intervention due to cost, because their insurance may not fully cover the expense. Aiding patients in finding financial assistance programs for medications may provide patients the ability to accept an intervention. Organizational barriers could exist, which may hinder physicians who want to provide EBM to their patients. For instance, say that an internal medicine physician wants to prescribe fidaxomicin for a patient who failed therapy with metronidazole for CDI; however, in this hospital, the antibiotic is restricted to infectious diseases. The physician will need to request a consult or obtain approval from the infectious disease team, thus delaying therapy. As a practitioner, it is essential to understand the logistical issues in an organization and the potential for changes.[84]

# LIMITATIONS OF EVIDENCE-BASED MEDICINE

EBM has a number of limitations that may be based on the evidence itself. These limitations are related to publication bias, the tendency toward a "one-size-fits-all" approach when using RCTs, and the nature of medicine.

## PUBLICATION BIAS

EBM developed, in part, because of variation in medical practice. Relying on the best available evidence, physicians benefit patients while improving variation in medical practice.[85] Finding the best available evidence, however, is not always achievable. Publication bias is a well-founded concern that impedes availability of evidence. In a recent review of 546 drug trials registered with ClinicalTrials.gov, 346 (63%) were primarily funded by industry.[86] Of the 362 (66.3%) trials with published results, positive outcomes occurred in 85.4% of industry-sponsored trials, 50.0% of government-funded trials, and 71.9% of those trials funded by nonfederal organizations ($p < 0.001$). Additionally, 50% of non–federally funded trials received contributions from industry. These trials were more likely to report positive outcomes compared to those without industry contributions (85.0% vs. 61.2%; $p = 0.013$). Targeted trials included those involving anticholesteremics, antidepressants, antipsychotics, PPIs, and vasodilators.

ClinicalTrials.gov is a registry developed by the National Institute of Health for tracking clinical trial data. As a result of the Food and Drug Administration Amendments Act of 2007 (FDAAA), sponsors and investigators are required to enter clinical trial data, including results, into the ClinicalTrials.gov registry.[87] Despite legal requirements, compliance is poor.[88] This registry could provide a mechanism for easy retrieval of unpublished trial results. However, lack of compliance limits availability of unpublished trial results.

Selective publication of antidepressant premarketing clinical trials provided only a partial picture of drug efficacy. Researchers identified publication of trials in which results were stated in the package inserts for 12 commonly used antidepressants.[89] Of the 74 trials identified, 40 (54%) were published with results consistent with the FDA reviewer's critique of the data; 37 of these yielded positive results and 3 questionable results. Eleven (15%) trials were published with positive results when the FDA reviewers deemed the results to be negative, and the remaining 23 (31%) were not published, of which 22 had negative results. Selective reporting of clinical trial results defeats the purpose of EBM and limits the clinician's ability to find the best available evidence.

## RANDOMIZED CONTROLLED TRIALS AND DOSING RECOMMENDATIONS

EBM places results from RCTs as the highest level of evidence for clinician-based treatment decisions. Likewise, regulatory agencies base proof of safety and efficacy on results from RCTs. Subsequently, recommended dosages are based on results from the average patient in an RCT, a type of "one-size-fits-all" dosing.[90] This population-based medicine provided a backdrop for unexpected adverse drug events, including myocardial infarction (MI) associated with rofecoxib (Vioxx®), MI and increased cardiovascular risk with rosiglitazone (Avandia®), and increased cardiovascular risk with sibutramine (Meridia®).[90]

Real-effectiveness medicine attempts to improve EBM by considering the best evidence for effectiveness of therapies in a real-world setting.[91] Extrapolation of results from RCTs to populations outside inclusion and exclusion criteria may result in undesirable effects. Patients with more severe disease, multiple comorbidities, older and younger age, and rare diseases are often excluded from participation in RCTs. RCTs designed to include elderly patients generally restrict inclusion criteria to the relatively healthy patient.

## NATURE OF MEDICINE

Medicine itself does not provide consistent, readily definable, adequately measurable patient outcomes for all conditions.[92] For example, patients tolerate different levels of pain and define quality of life according to personal beliefs. Principals of EBM place patient individuality under patient preferences and clinical expertise, which in some cases may require anecdotal or empiric evidence. As one researcher stated, "Medicine is complex, messy, difficult and constantly requires normative judgment."[92] The actual practice of medicine is complex. Unfortunately, adequate controlled clinical trials that enroll complex patients are often lacking.

## THE FUTURE OF EVIDENCE-BASED MEDICINE

Making sound medical recommendations and decisions requires not only knowing the best evidence and having that evidence available but also caring for and treating a person, a unique individual. EBM is more than a simple guide to decision making. True EBM practice includes caring for the individual patient and taking into account patient preferences. A redesign of EBM to evaluate and consider the goals of evidence in medicine as well as the goals of medicine has been suggested.[92] Questions to continually ask include:

- What is the evidence being used for?
- What counts as evidence and what evidence counts?
- What is the evidence we have, or seek, evidence of?
- What weight are we giving to each type of evidence?
- How are we to incorporate these different types/pieces of evidence into our decisions?

The best evidence depends upon the question asked as well as the individual patient case. Patients often require more than clinical expertise, "but care and respect at a time of great vulnerability."[92] Clinicians should weigh the evidence against the patient's individual goals and preferences. Ultimately, judgment of the patient's individual case informs the best therapy.

Clinicians still use personalized or individualized medicine in which specific medical needs of the individual patient such as delivering the right drug at the right dose at the right time are met.[93] Testing to determine which patients respond to what therapies is well established in the treatment of hormone-positive or hormone-negative breast cancer.[91] Individualized care through genomic testing identifies patients with abnormalities in proteins and enzymes, such as those patients who are slow or fast metabolizers of medications that rely on the P-450 enzyme system for metabolism.[94]

# SUMMARY

Providing the best possible care for patients is a worthy charge for any healthcare professional. EBM promotes the use of scientific literature in clinical decision actions. Along with incorporating patient preferences and circumstances and clinician expertise, EBM serves to promote the well-being of individual patients. Practicing EBM through use of a systematic method provides healthcare professionals a road map. Developing an answerable question, systematically searching the best available evidence, critically evaluating the evidence, incorporating evidence with patient preferences, implementing evidence into patient care, and evaluating the intervention devise the road map. What starts with population-based evidence through review of results from clinical trials becomes individualized for the patient through incorporating patient preferences and clinical judgment.

Study design with the RCT occupying the top of the literature evidence provides the basis for proving efficacy of a therapy. However, applying data from an RCT to individual patients may be difficult because of limited generalizability or external validity. In such cases, results from observational trials may augment findings from RCTs and provide a better picture of the best available evidence. Finding all available evidence may be limited by publication bias. Despite possible limitations, practice guidelines devised from the best available evidence provide the healthcare professional further guidance. Incorporating EBM into medical practice provides a mechanism for healthcare professionals to stay abreast of current therapies and treatments. Incorporating EBM principles into individualized patient care provides the best possible therapy for each individual patient.

# REFERENCES

1. Sackett D, Rosenberg WM, Gray JA, et al. Evidence-based medicine: what it is and what it isn't. *BMJ*. 1996;312(7023):71-72.
2. National Research Council. *Health Professions Education: A Bridge to Quality*. Washington, DC: The National Academies Press; 2003.
3. Guyatt G. Evidence-based medicine: past, present, future. *MUMJ*. 2003;1(1):27-32.
4. Salmond S. Finding the evidence to support evidence-based practice. *Orthop Nurs*. 2013;32(1):16-22.
5. Guyatt G, Rennie D, eds. *Users' Guides to the Medical Literature: A Manual for Evidence-Based Clinical Practice*. Chicago, IL: AMA Press; 2002.
6. Miser W. An introduction to evidence-based medicine. *Prim Care*. 2006;33(4):811-829.
7. Brandi W. Making evidence-based medicine doable in everyday practice. *Fam Pract Manag*. 2004;11(2):51-58.
8. Sackett DL. Evidence-based medicine. *Semin Perinatol*. 1997;21(1):3-5.
9. Slawson DC, Shaughnessy AF. Teaching evidence-based medicine: should we be teaching information management instead? *Acad Med*. 2005;80(7):685-689.

10. Porzsolt F, Ohletz A, Thim A, et al. Evidence-based decision making—the 6-step approach. *ACP J Club*. 2003;139(3):A11-A12.

11. Timm DF, Banks DE, McLarty J. Critical appraisal process: step-by-step. *South Med J*. 2012;105(3):144-148.

12. Kelly AM. Evidence based practice: an introduction and overview. *Seminars Roentgenol*. 2009;44(3):131-139.

13. Richardson WS, Wilson MC, Nishikawa J, et al. The well-built clinical question: a key to evidence-based decisions. *ACP J Club*. 1995;123(3):A12-A13.

14. Wilton NK, Slim AM. Application of the principles of evidence-based medicine to patient care. *South Med J*. 2012;105(3):136-143.

15. Webster AC, Cross NB, Mitchell R, et al. How to get the most from the medical literature: searching the medical literature effectively. *Nephrology*. 2010;15(1):12-19.

16. Worrall J. Evidence in medicine and evidence-based medicine. *Philosophy Compass*. 2007;2(6):981-1022.

17. Burns PB, Rohrich RJ, Chung KC. The levels of evidence and their role in evidence-based medicine. *Plast Reconstr Surg*. 2011 Jul;128(1):305-310.

18. Morris MJ, Fewell AE, Oleszewski T. Evidence-based medicine: specific skills necessary for developing expertise in critical appraisal. *South Med Assoc*. 2012;105(3):114-119.

19. Carlson MDA, Morrison RS. Study design, precision and validity in observational studies. *J Palliat Med*. 2009;12(1):77-82.

20. DiPietro NA. Methods in epidemiology: observational study designs. *Pharmacotherapy*. 2010;30(10):973-984.

21. Nallamothu BK, Hayward RA, Bates ER. Beyond the randomized clinical trial: the role of effectiveness studies in evaluating cardiovascular therapies. *Circulation*. 2008;118(12):1294-1303.

22. Berbano EP, Baxi N. Impact of patient selection in various study designs: identifying potential bias in clinical results. *South Med J*. 2012;105(3):149-155.

23. Slack MK, Draugalis JR. Establishing the internal and external validity of experimental studies. *Am J Health Syst Pharm*. 2001;58(22):2173-2181.

24. Hartung DM, Touchette D. Overview of clinical research design. *Am J Health Syst Pharm*. 2009;66(4):398-408.

25. Coleman CI, Talati R, White CM. A clinician's perspective on rating the strength of evidence in a systematic review. *Pharmacotherapy*. 2009;29(9):1017-1029.

26. Facchiano L, Snyder CH. Evidence-based practice for the busy nurse practitioner: part two: searching for the best evidence to clinical inquiries. *J Am Acad Nurse Pract*. 2012;24(11):640-648.

27. Zarin DA, Young JL, Wes JC. Challenges to evidence-based medicine: a comparison of patients and treatments in randomized controlled trials with patients and treatments in a practice research network. *Soc Psychiatry Psychiatr Epidemiol*. 2005;40(1):27-35.

28. Boyd CM, Vollenweider D, Puhan MA. Informing evidence-based decision-making for patients with comorbidity: availability of necessary information in clinical trials for chronic diseases. *PLoS ONE*. 2012;7(8):e41601.

29. Wellek S, Blettner M: Establishing equivalence or noninferiority in clinical trials—part 20 of a series on evaluation of scientific publications. *Dtsch Arztebl Int*. 2012;109(41):674-679.

30. Duprez DA, Munger MA, Botha J, et al. Aliskiren for geriatric lowering of systolic hypertension: a randomized controlled trial. *J Hum Hypertens*. 2010;24(9):600-608.

31. Omar MA, Wilson JP. FDA adverse event reports on statin-associated rhabdomyolysis. *Ann Pharmacother*. 2002;36(2):288-295.

32. Song JW, Chung KC. Observational studies: cohort and case-control studies. *Plast Reconstr Surg*. 2010;126(6):2234-2242.

33. Hershcovici T, Jha LK, Gadam R, et al. The relationship between type 2 diabetes mellitus and failure to proton pump inhibitor treatment in gastroesophageal reflux disease. *J Clin Gastroenterol*. 2012;46(8):662-668.

34. Szumilas M. Explaining odds ratios. *J Can Acad Child Adolesc Psychiatry*. 2010;19(3):227-229.

35. History of the Framingham Heart Study. Framingham Heart Study website. www.framingham heartstudy.org/about-fhs/history.php. Accessed July 22, 2014.

36. Wenisch JM, Schmid D, Tucek G, et al. A prospective cohort study on hospital mortality due to Clostridium difficile infection. *Infection*. 2012;40(5):479-484.

37. Akobeng AK. Understanding systematic reviews and meta-analysis. *Arch Dis Child*. 2005;90(8):845-848.

38. Ornelas S. Benne PD, Rosenkranz RR. Tobacco use at Fort Riley: a study of the prevalence of tobacco use among active duty soldiers assigned to Fort Riley, Kansas. *Mil Med*. 2012;177(7):780-785.

39. The Institute of Medicine. Initial national priorities for comparative effectiveness research. Institute of Medicine. 2009. http://www.iom.edu/Reports/2009/ComparativeEffectivenessResearch Priorities.aspx. Accessed July 22, 2014.

40. Roland M, Torgerson DT. What are pragmatic trials? *BMJ*. 1998;316(7127):285.

41. Tunis SR, Stryer DB, Clancy CM. Practical clinical trials: increasing the value of clinical research for decision making in clinical and health policy. *JAMA*. 2003;290(12):1624-1632.

42. Price D, Chisholm A, van der Molen, et al. Reassessing the evidence hierarchy in asthma: evaluating comparative effectiveness. *Curr Allergy Asthma Rep*. 2011;11(6):526-538.

43. Greenhalgh T. How to read a paper. Papers that summarise other papers (systematic reviews and meta-analyses). *BMJ*. 1997;315(7109):672-675.

44. Ahmed I, Sutton AJ, Riley RD. Assessment of publication bias, selection bias, and unavailable data in meta-analyses using individual participant data: a database survey. *BMJ*. 2012;344:d7762. doi: 10.1136/bmj.d7762.

45. Eichler H, Abadie E, Breckenridge A, et al. Bridging the efficacy–effectiveness gap: a regulator's perspective on addressing variability of drug response. *Nat Rev Drug Discov*. 2011;10(7):495-506.

46. US National Library of Medicine National Institute of Health. Medline/PubMed Resources Guide. www.nlm.nih.gov/bsd/pmresources.html. Accessed July 22, 2014.

47. Young S, Duffull SB. A learning-based approach for performing an in-depth literature search using Medline. *J Clin Pharm Ther*. 2011;36(4):504-512.

48. Richter RR, Austin TM. Using MeSH (medical subject headings) to enhance PubMed search strategies for evidence-based practice in physical therapy. *Phys Ther*. 2012;92(1):124-132.

49. Aoki NJ, Enticott JC, Phillips LE. Searching the literature: four simple steps. *Transfusion*. 2013;53(1):14-17.

50. SPS3 Investigators, Benavente OR, Hart RG, McClure LA, Szychowski JM, Coffey CS, Pearce LA. Effects of clopidogrel added to aspirin in patients with recent lacunar stroke. *N Engl J Med*. 2012;367(9):817-825.

51. Abalos E, Carroli G, Mackey ME. The tools and techniques of evidence-based medicine. *Best Pract Res Clin Obstet Gynaecol*. 2005;19(1)15-26.

52. Davies HT, Crombie IK. What are confidence intervals and p-values? What is …? series. Hayward Medical Communications. 2009.

53. Mansi IA. Statistics for the nonstatistician: a premier for reading clinical studies. *South Med J*. 2012;105(3):120-125.

54. Boonen S, Reginster J Y, Kaufman JM, et al. Fracture risk and zoledronic acid therapy in men with osteoporosis. *N Eng J Med*. 2012;367(18):1714-1723.

55. Zoledronic acid. In DynaMed [database online]. EBSCO Publishing. http://web.ebscohost.com .dml.regis.edu/dynamed. Updated March 6, 2013. Accessed April 13, 2013.

56. Graham R, Macher M, Wolman DM, et al, eds. *Clinical Practice Guidelines We Can Trust*. Washington, DC: National Academies Press; 2011.

57. Wollersheim H, Burgers J, Grol R. Clinical guidelines to improve patient care. *Neth J Med*. 2005;63(6):188-192.

58. Woolf S. Practice guidelines, a new reality in medicine. II. Methods of developing guidelines. *Arch Intern Med*. 1992;152(5):946-952.

59. Cruse H, Winiarek M, Marshburn J, et al. Quality and methods of developing practice guidelines. *BMC Health Serv Res*. 2002;2:1.

60. Turner T, Misso M, Harris C, et al. Development of evidence-based clinical practice guidelines (CPGs): comparing approaches. *Implement Sci*. 2008;3:45. doi: 10.1186/1748-5908-3-45.

61. Jaeschke R, Jankowski M, Brozek J, et al. How to develop guidelines for clinical practice. *Minerva Anestesiol*. 2009;75(9):504-508.

62. GRADE Working Group. GRADE Working Group website. http://gradeworkinggroup.org /index.htm. Accessed July 22, 2014.

63. Guyatt G, Oxman A, Vist GE, et al. GRADE: what is "quality of evidence" and why is it important to clinicians? *BMJ*. 2008;336(7651):995-998.

64. Guyatt G, Oxman A, Kunz R, et al. GRADE: going from evidence to recommendations. *BMJ*. 2008;336(7652):1049-1051.

65. The AGREE Collaboration. *The Appraisal of Guidelines for Research & Evaluation (AGREE) Instrument, 2001*. London: The AGREE Research Trust; 2001.

66. The AGREE Collaboration. *The Appraisal of Guidelines for Research and Evaluation (AGREE II) Instrument, 2009*. London: The AGREE Research Trust; 2009.

67. Graham I, Harrison M. Evaluation and adaptation of clinical practice guidelines. *Evid Based Nurs*. 2005;8(3):68-72.

68. Guyatt GH, Norris SL, Schulman S, et al. Methodology for the development of antithrombotic therapy and prevention of thrombosis guidelines: antithrombotic therapy and prevention of thrombosis, 9th ed: American College of Chest Physicians Evidence-Based Clinical Practice Guidelines. *Chest.* 2012;141(2 suppl):53S-70S.

69. Panel on Antiretroviral Guidelines for Adults and Adolescents. Guidelines for the use of antiretroviral agents in HIV-1-infected adults and adolescents. Department of Health and Human Services. http://aidsinfo.nih.gov/ContentFiles/AdultandAdolescentGL.pdf. Accessed July 22, 2014.

70. Davis D, Vaisey AL. Translating guidelines into practice. A systematic review of theoretic concepts, practical experience and research evidence in the adoption of clinical practice guidelines. *CMAJ.* 1997;157(4):408-416.

71. Ishii LE. Closing the clinical gap: translating best practice knowledge to performance with guideline implementation. *Otolaryngol Head Neck Surg.* 2013;148(6):898-901.

72. Browman GP, Levine MN, Mohide EA, et al. The practice guidelines development cycle: a conceptual tool for practice guidelines development and implementation. *J Clin Oncol.* 1995;13(2):502-512.

73. Eytan T, Goldberg H. How effective is the computer-based clinical practice guideline? *Eff Clin Prac.* 2001;4(1):24-33.

74. Fox J, Patkar V, Chronakis I, et al. From practice guidelines to clinical decision support: closing the loop. *J R Soc Med.* 2009;102(11):464-473.

75. Woolf S, Grol R, Hutchinson A, et al. Clinical guidelines. Potential benefits, limitations, and harms of clinical guidelines. *BMJ.* 1999;318(7182):527-530.

76. Feder G. Management of mild hypertension: which guidelines to follow? *BMJ.* 1994;308(6926):470-471.

77. Woolf SH. Shared decision-making: the case for letting patients decide which choice is best. *J Fam Pract.* 1997;45(3):205-208.

78. Hasnain-Wynia R. Is evidence-based medicine patient-centered and is patient-centered care evidence-based? *Health Serv Res.* 2006;41(1):1-8.

79. McKenna H, Ashton S, Keeney S. Barriers to evidence-based practice in primary care. *J Adv Nurs.* 2004;45(2):178-189.

80. Young J, Ward J. Evidence-based medicine in general practice: beliefs and barriers amount Australian GPs. *J Eval Clin Pract.* 2001;7(2):201-210.

81. McKenna H, Ashton S, Keeney S. Barriers to evidence-based practice in primary care: a review of the literature. *Int J Nurs Stud.* 2004;41(4):369-378.

82. Zwolsman SE, Pas E, Waard MW, et al. Barrier to GPs' use of evidence-based medicine: a systematic review. *Br J Gen Pract.* 2012;62(600):e511-e521.

83. Haynes B, Haines A. Barriers and bridges to evidence based clinical practice. *BMJ.* 1998;317(7153):273-276.

84. Vogel E. Challenges to using evidence-based medicine in daily clinical practice. *Sem Med Pract.* 1999;2(3):21-24.

85. Timmermans A, Ou H. The continued social transformation of the medical profession. *J Health Soc Behav.* 2010;51(suppl):S94-S106.

86. Bourgeois FT, Murthy S, Mandl KD. Outcome reporting among drug trials registered in ClinicalTrials.gov. *Ann Intern Med.* 2010;153(3):158-166.

87. Lester M, Godlew B. ClinicalTrials.gov registration and results reporting updates and recent activities. *J Clin Res Best Pract.* 2011;7(2):1-2.

88. Prayle AP, Hurley MN, Smyth AR. Compliance with mandatory reporting of clinical trial results on ClinicalTrials.gov: cross sectional study. *BMJ.* 2012;344:d7373. doi: 10.1136/bmj.d7373.

89. Turner EH, Matthews AM, Linardatos E, et al. Selective publication of antidepressant trials and its influence on apparent efficacy. *N Engl J Med.* 2008;358(3):252-260.

90. Lesko LJ, Schmidt S. Individualization of drug therapy: history, present state, and opportunities for the future. *Clin Pharmacol Ther.* 2012;92(4):458-466.

91. Malmivaara A. Real-effectiveness medicine—pursuing the best effectiveness in the ordinary care of patients. *Ann Med.* 2013;45(2):103-106.

92. Kerridge I. Ethics and EBM: acknowledging bias, accepting difference and embracing politics. *J Eval Clin Prac.* 2010;16(2):365-373.

93. Nardini C, Annoni M, Schiavone G. Mechanistic understanding in clinical practice: complementing evidence-based medicine with personalized medicine. *J Eval Clin Prac.* 2012;18(5):1000-1005.

94. Tremblay J, Hamet P. Role of genomics on the path to personalized medicine. *Metabolism.* 2013;62(suppl 1):S2-S5.

# HOW TO PREPARE AN EFFECTIVE JOURNAL CLUB

Dianne May, PharmD, BCPS
Jacquelyn Bryant, PharmD

## CHAPTER OBJECTIVES

▸ Define the specific goals and target audiences for a journal club.

▸ Describe the various settings in which to hold a journal club.

▸ Differentiate between the various formats and styles of journal clubs.

▸ Identify important critical appraisal skills that should be used when evaluating articles for a journal club.

▸ Apply strategies for assessing and evaluating a journal club.

# CHAPTER OUTLINE

# KEY TERMS

Content expert
Continuing professional development
Critical appraisal

Journal club coordinator
Virtual journal club

# INTRODUCTION

A journal club has been described as "a group of individuals who meet regularly to discuss critically the clinical applicability of articles in the current medical journals."[1,2] Journal clubs date back to the 1800s when physicians, such as Sir James Paget and Sir William Osler, met with their students to disseminate and discuss the latest medical literature.[2,3] This was considered an effective way to provide important educational concepts in an interactive, informal setting. Since that time, medical professionals have used journal clubs as a forum to evaluate and discuss the impact of published research on their clinical practice, promote evidence-based practice, develop drug literature evaluation skills, teach **critical appraisal** skills, and keep up with the medical literature.[4]

As an educational tool, journal clubs offer students learning opportunities aimed at improving their ability to retrieve, analyze, and interpret the literature and apply this information when making evidence-based decisions, as outlined by the Center for the Advancement of Pharmaceutical Education (CAPE) recommendations.[5,6] With the high bar set by educational accrediting committees and the underlying need for high-quality, patient-centered care, many colleges and medical centers have begun incorporating journal clubs into their classroom lectures, small group discussions, and advanced experiential clinical practice experiences.[5] The skills learners develop from journal clubs can easily be applied to the clinical practice setting for decision-making purposes and as an avenue for continuing professional development (CPD).

Several steps can be taken to increase the level of success seen with journal clubs. These include (1) defining the audience and the specific goals, (2) identifying a designated leader, (3) choosing an appropriate location, (4) selecting an article with clinical impact (e.g., landmark trials), (5) choosing the best format for reviewing the article, and (6) evaluating the quality of the journal club.[3,7] Journal clubs should strive to stimulate interest, attendance, and participation.[2] This can be accomplished by knowing the target audience and setting clear goals for the journal club. One novel approach involves offering continuing education credit to attendees as a means to increase participation.[8] **Table 15-1** lists some of the keys points to conducting a successful journal club.[3,7,9-11]

| **TABLE 15-1** Key Points for Ensuring a Successful Journal Club |
| --- |

- Have clear, concise goals.
- Use a trained leader/facilitator.
- Expect invitees to attend.
- Meet at regular, predictable intervals (e.g., monthly).
- Communicate the article citation in advance; electronic communication is preferred (~ 1 week).
- Set a discussion time limit (~ 1 hour); stop and start on time.
- Relate the teaching component to critical appraisal skills.
- Engage in a structured, organized discussion using established critical appraisal processes.
- Discuss the article in the context of how it fits in clinical practice.
- Evaluate relevant articles with clinical impact to generate interest.
- Include a content expert and drug literature evaluation/statistics expert.

Data from Alguire PC. A review of journal clubs in postgraduate medical education. *J Gen Intern Med*. 1998;13(5):347-353; Swift G. How to make journal clubs interesting. *Adv Psychiatr Treat*. 2004;10:67-72; Moberg-Wolff EA, Kosasih JB. Journal clubs. Prevalence, format, and efficacy in PM&R. *Am J Phys Med Rehabil*. 1995; 74(3):224-229; Deenadayalan Y, Grimmer-Somers K, Prior M, Kumar S. How to run an effective journal club: a systematic review. *J Eval Clin Pract*. 2008;14(5):898-911; and Valentini RP, Daniels SR. The journal club. *Postgrad Med J*. 1997;73(856):81-85.

# DEFINE THE AUDIENCE AND GOALS FOR THE JOURNAL CLUB

A variety of audiences may participate in journal clubs. The goals and most appropriate format may vary depending on the skill level of the audience as well as the objective. Some common goals of journal clubs include teaching critical appraisal skills, affecting clinical practice, promoting evidence-based practice, staying up-to-date with the literature, and providing a means for **continuing professional development** (CPD).[3] The Accreditation Council for Pharmacy Education (ACPE) defines CPD as "the life-long process of active participation in learning activities that assists individuals in developing and maintaining continuing competence, enhancing their professional practice, and supporting achievement of their career goals."[12] A journal club may also meet a more social goal by gathering colleagues together on a regular basis.[7]

## PROFESSIONAL YEAR 2 AND 3 STUDENTS

Professional year 2 (P2) and year 3 (P3) students generally are beginning to learn drug literature evaluation skills in their didactic drug information courses. They tend to have limited clinical experience from which to draw upon. The goal for this group is to teach critical appraisal skills, assessing not only clinical content and applicability, but also drug literature evaluation skills and statistical knowledge. For this level, using a checklist is very helpful in guiding the students in evaluating the literature. By answering guided questions, the learner becomes more skilled and efficient at critiquing important aspects of an article. A checklist is a useful memory tool when organizing and highlighting key points during evaluation, ensuring that the learners stay organized and focused in their evaluation. An example of important features of a checklist for randomized controlled trials is found in **Table 15-2**. Other examples of checklists are available through the *Pharmacist's Letter* and the Cochrane Library. Although these checklists are good for evaluating randomized controlled trials, they may not be ideal for other types of studies, such as non-inferiority studies or systematic reviews. Checklists are available that may be valuable for these types of studies. For example, the Consolidated Standards of Reporting Trials

**TABLE 15-2**    Components of a Checklist to Evaluate Journal Articles

| Parameter | Common Questions to Ask |
|---|---|
| Journal | • Is the journal reputable?<br>• What is the peer-review process?<br>• What is the impact factor and scope of the journal? |
| Title | • Is the title brief and nonbiased?<br>• Does the title represent what was studied? |
| Authors | • Do the authors have expertise in the field of study?<br>• Was a statistician involved in the analysis of the data?<br>• Do any of the authors work for or have financial ties with the pharmaceutical manufacturer? |
| General | • Was the research site appropriate in both location and resources to conduct the study?<br>• Was a statistician involved in the analysis of the data?<br>• What was the funding source for the research?<br>• Do any of the authors work for or have financial ties with the pharmaceutical manufacturer?<br>• Is the abstract clearly written and consistent with the text?<br>• Does the abstract contain information about the purpose, methods, results, and conclusions of the study? |
| Introduction | • Is appropriate background provided in the introduction?<br>• Does it help you understand why this particular study was needed?<br>• Does it highlight results from previous studies?<br>• Is the objective specific and clearly stated?<br>• Was the protocol reviewed by the institutional review board or ethics committee for the institution?<br>• Was informed consent obtained from subjects or their guardians? |
| Methods | • What was the study design? |
| *Study design* | • Are randomization and blinding methods discussed?<br>• Were inclusion and exclusion criteria discussed? |
| *Patients/subjects* | • Are the subjects representative of the general population to which the results are intended to be generalized?<br>• Were any diagnostic criteria for disease states clearly defined?<br>• Were demographic data compared for the treatment and control groups? |
| *Treatment intervention/ control intervention* | • Is the intervention being evaluated and the control intervention clearly stated?<br>• Are the doses, frequencies, and durations appropriate for the indication for which the medication is being used?<br>• Were other interventions between the groups the same?<br>• Was compliance monitored?<br>• Were the variables measured appropriately? |
| *Outcomes* | • What was the primary outcome for the study?<br>• What were the secondary outcomes for the study?<br>• Is there one primary outcome being evaluated? |
| *Data handling* | • Were any subgroup analyses determined a priori?<br>• Were dropouts reconciled with the number randomized? |
| *Statistical analysis* | • Did the author describe how sample size was calculated and report the number needed for stated power?<br>• Did the number of patients who completed the study equal the initial sample size calculated?<br>• Was the sample size large enough to detect a difference?<br>• Was the appropriate statistical test used to report the results?<br>• Was a pharmaceutical sponsor involved in the statistical analysis? |

| TABLE 15-2 | Components of a Checklist to Evaluate Journal Articles (*Continued*) |
|---|---|
| **Parameter** | **Common Questions to Ask** |
| Results | • Are the data presented in a clear and understandable format?<br>• Are adverse reactions and dropouts described?<br>• Are data in charts, figures, and text described consistently?<br>• Is visual presentation of data accurate (e.g., drawn to scale, no missing data, etc.)?<br>• Were primary and secondary outcome results reported for each group?<br>• Were *p*-values and/or confidence intervals reported? |
| Conclusions/ discussion | • Are the conclusions consistent with the results?<br>• Do the conclusions answer the original study question?<br>• Were limitations of the study discussed?<br>• Were recommendations for use in clinical practice made?<br>• Is the therapy cost-effective? |
| References | • Are the references current and representative of current knowledge?<br>• Are the references reputable? |
| Clinical significance to practice | • What are the implications of this study in clinical practice?<br>• Is it generalizable to other patient populations?<br>• Does this represent new knowledge on the subject? |

(CONSORT) Group has additional guidance for reporting on randomized controlled trials and other types of studies, such as cluster trials, noninferiority and equivalence trials, and pragmatic trials.[13-16] Additionally, the Preferred Reporting Items for Systematic Reviews and Meta-Analyses (PRISMA) group provide an evidence-based minimum set of items for reporting in systematic reviews and meta-analyses.[17]

The classroom or a small group discussion setting may be the best environment to incorporate journal clubs for this group of learners. The principles they have learned in class can easily be demonstrated through participation in an in-class journal club. An example of how this can work involves the educator choosing what is considered to be a "good" article with a sound study design and the students using the checklist to evaluate the merits of the trial. This is compared to a "bad" article with many study design flaws, enabling the students to clearly see the differences. A student can choose an article using the same checklist after obtaining approval of the facilitator. This active learning process conducted as a journal club during class affords the students the opportunity to apply the skills and knowledge learned during their drug information course(s).

## PROFESSIONAL YEAR 4 STUDENTS

Students in their final professional year (P4) have completed all of their didactic training in drug information and should be more competent to evaluate the literature. At this level, however, students still have limited clinical experience from which to draw upon. The goal for this group is to build on their didactic training, incorporating patient care and applicability. This can be done through journal clubs held on advanced experiential practice experiences. A checklist may still be helpful, but the aim is to learn how to apply the information from the article to a patient population that they follow. Students should learn how to apply the evidence to their specific patients. The best setting for this group may be small group discussions with preceptors, residents, peers, and the multidisciplinary team.

## RESIDENTS AND PRACTITIONERS

Residents and practitioners have more experience and expertise in evaluating the literature. For this group, a checklist may be less important; however, a structured, guided discussion is still helpful. The goals for this group may be to promote evidence-based practice, answer a specific clinical question, keep up-to-date with the most cutting-edge therapies in order to better care for their patients, or use the journal club as a means of providing CPD. Journal club meetings provide unique opportunities to accomplish this; the discussions can be turned into new or improved clinical skills for the clinician or academician. Subscribing to a "journal watch" pertaining to a specific area of practice may be one approach to managing the efficiency of journal article review. The journal watch provides summaries of the most recently published articles in a specific practice area.

Moving away from traditional classroom lectures with structured learning environments can be intimidating. Journal clubs provide a way to gather information from many areas of practice and incorporate ideas from evidence-based medicine into recommendations communicated to healthcare teams. For residents, leading a journal club may satisfy a requirement related to obtaining a teaching certificate where small group discussions with evaluations are necessary. As a practitioner, one of the most important aspects of clinical practice is staying up-to-date on current treatment guidelines and new therapeutic agents released into the market. With so many articles being published each year, journal clubs also provide an efficient method for reviewing "hot topics" and controversial practices. A debate format or reviewing classic articles compared to newer articles may be preferred for those with more advanced practice. This promotes discussion and sharing of ideas among peers.

Another innovative approach is to use journal clubs as a means to develop writing skills and teach critical appraisal through subsequent letter writing to the editor generated from the group discussion.[4,7,18]

## DRUG INFORMATION PHARMACISTS AND EDUCATORS

This group is among the most experienced in evaluating the literature. Journal clubs may be used as an active learning technique to teach drug literature evaluation principles in a didactic setting or as part of an advanced experiential practice experience. Journal clubs may also be an effective way for faculty to provide additional elective courses without a major increase in their workload. Elective courses are often needed on satellite campuses where students may not have access to electives on the main campus due to distance. This novel approach involves incorporating P3 students in once-weekly journal club discussions centered around evaluating the evidence related to actual patient cases presented by P4 students and/or residents already on rotation with that faculty member. The workload impact is minimal because the patient case discussions with P4 students were occurring anyway. These introductory encounters for P3 students give the less experienced learner an opportunity to apply knowledge and learn from those with more experience. This will assist in their ability to provide evidence-based recommendations during clinical seminars and advanced experiential practice experiences throughout their fourth professional year.

Possibly the most advanced model is using a form of journal club as a means to make formulary decisions, promote evidence-based practice, and change clinical practice recommendations. This might be where a group of decision makers, such as a subgroup of the pharmacy and therapeutics (P&T) committee, debates the pros and cons of a particular therapy prior to forming recommendations to the full committee.

# CHOOSE A DESIGNATED JOURNAL CLUB COORDINATOR AND DEFINE OTHER ROLES

Journal clubs may be more successful when one person takes responsibility and provides consistent oversight.[7] This person is designated the journal club leader or coordinator. Other roles associated with journal clubs include the facilitator (if not the journal club coordinator), presenter, content expert, and participants. Understanding the expectations of each of these roles can help improve the quality of the journal club and increase participation.

## JOURNAL CLUB COORDINATOR

In general, the **journal club coordinator** should be someone who is enthusiastic about, and understands the importance of, using the journal club as an educational or decision-making tool. This can be an educator/faculty member, preceptor, or practitioner, and it does not necessarily always have to be the same person. However, it is preferred that one person take responsibility for the programmatic aspects of the journal club to ensure consistency. The role of the journal club coordinator includes (1) selecting or approving the article chosen, (2) ensuring that the article citations and meeting dates are communicated in advance, (3) selecting the appropriate environment for the journal club, (4) inviting content experts, (5) facilitating journal club discussions, (6) evaluating learners, and (7) obtaining periodic evaluations of journal club from participants for quality improvement purposes.

## FACILITATOR OR PRESENTER

The role of facilitator may be filled by the journal club coordinator or a different person could be designated as the presenter each time the journal club meets. Oftentimes, the facilitator is a resident or student. After a brief description of the article under review, the facilitator should help guide the discussion by keeping it on track and on time. One person should not be allowed to dominate the discussion, and the presenter should strive not to answer his or her own questions. Asking open-ended questions and soliciting opinions from the group can help facilitate the discussion format. Sidebar conversations that are distracting and off topic should be prevented. The facilitator should also encourage participation and discussion within the group; this stimulates critical thinking and verbalization of thoughts. After concluding the session, the facilitator should follow up with any questions asked of the group that were not able to be answered during the discussion.

When not filled by the facilitator, the role of presenter is often filled by a learner, such as a student or resident. In peer-to-peer journal clubs, the role of presenter may rotate between practitioners or colleagues. The presenter responsibilities may include (1) choosing the article, (2) communicating the article citation to participants, (3) preparing a written synopsis of the study for ease of discussion when required (see **Box 15-1**), (4) verifying and communicating the place and time, and (5) leading the discussion. This means that the presenter should not just read the article summary to the group but spend the majority of time discussing salient points. As a learner, the presenter may also be responsible for providing evaluation forms to participants and preparing and presenting a "clinical pearl" topic pertinent to the discussion.

# EXAMPLE SYNOPSIS OF A JOURNAL CLUB ARTICLE PREPARED BY A STUDENT OR RESIDENT

The ACCESS Study: Evaluation of Acute Candesartan Cilexetil Therapy in Stroke Survivors. Schrader J, Luders S, Kulschewski A, et al. *Stroke*. 2003;34(7):1699-1703.
    By: Kaleigh Marx, PharmD Candidate

**Background:** Current recommendations regarding acute hypertension in cerebral ischemia do not support aggressive lowering of hypertensive states in the acute ischemic period. Although theoretical evidence supports this recommendation, evidence-based data are lacking. Past studies have shown rapid hypotensive action of certain blood pressure–lowering agents have led to a risk of neurological deterioration. This study was countered, however, by another that tested the cautious reduction of blood pressure resulting in an improvement in prognoses. Those involved with this study hypothesized that specific antihypertensives may be more appropriate for the application of blood pressure lowering in the acute stroke period. Antihypertensives such as those that exert their action by $AT_1$ receptor blockade are hypothesized to be protective against stroke. The authors cite convincing data supporting beneficial effects of neurohormonal inhibition as a basis for specifically studying $AT_1$ receptor blockade in this setting.

**Objective:** To assess the safety of modest blood pressure reduction by candesartan cilexetil in the early treatment of stroke, as well as to provide an estimate of the number of cases required to perform a larger phase III efficacy study.

**Design:** Prospective, double-blind, placebo-controlled, randomized multicenter phase II study.

**Patients:** 500 patients, 250 patients per treatment group, provided a sample size large enough to detect a reduction in event rate by 6% to 12% compared with the placebo group with a power of 80% and $\alpha = 0.05$.

**Inclusions:** Motor deficit, cerebral CT scan excluding intracranial hemorrhage, necessity to treat hypertension according to current recommendations (the mean of two blood pressure measurements was ≥ 200 mm Hg systolic and/or ≥ 110 mm Hg diastolic 6-24 hours after admission or ≥ 180 mm Hg systolic and/or ≥ 105mm Hg diastolic 24-36 hours after admission).

**Exclusions:** Age > 85 years, disorders in consciousness potentially preventing acquisition of consent, occlusion or > 70% stenosis of the internal carotid artery, malignant hypertension, manifest cardiac failure (NYHA class III and IV), high-grade aortic or mitral stenosis, unstable angina pectoris, or contraindications against candesartan cilexetil.

**Treatment:**

**Treatment group:** Day 1: 4 mg candesartan cilexetil. Day 2: Dose increase to 8 or 16 mg candesartan cilexetil daily if blood pressure exceeded 160 mm Hg systolic or 100 mm Hg diastolic to a targeted 10-15% blood pressure reduction within 24 hours. Day 7: 24-hour blood pressure profile obtained. If mean daytime blood pressure exceeded 135/85 mm Hg, the dose of candesartan cilexetil was increased or an additional antihypertensive drug was added (hydrochlorothiazide, felodipine, metoprolol).

**Control group:** Same as above with placebo days 1-6. Day 7: If patients showed a hypertensive profile, candesartan cilexetil was started and adjusted to lower blood pressure goals of < 140/90 mm Hg (office blood pressure) or < 135/85 mm Hg (mean daytime blood pressure, automatic blood pressure monitoring).

**Assessments:**

**Baseline:** Carotid ultrasound prior to randomization, vital status, neurologic examination, laboratory values, blood pressure (prior to and during first 3 days of treatment).

**Follow-up visits:** Blood pressure, neurological index/status, adverse events, and medication at 3, 6, and 12 months.

**Efficacy endpoints:**

- **Primary:** Case fatality and disability, measured as functional status with the use of the Barthel Index (BI) 3 months after the end of a placebo-controlled 7-day phase (later shown to be an inappropriate outcome measure for this sample size as well as not useful for assessing minor deficits at a high functional level). BI is a measure of the patient's functioning as it relates to activities of daily living and mobility.
- **Combined secondary endpoints:** Overall mortality and cerebrovascular and cardiovascular events occurring within the study period (assessed 12 months after discharge).

| BOX 15-1 | EXAMPLE SYNOPSIS OF A JOURNAL CLUB ARTICLE PREPARED BY A STUDENT OR RESIDENT (CONTINUED) |
|---|---|

**Statistical analysis:** The Fisher exact test was used for frequency comparisons, whereas the Mantel-Haenszel test was used to calculate odds ratios and 95% confidence intervals. The Mann-Whitney U test was used for mean comparisons. Kaplan-Meier curves were used to present cumulative event rates and were compared with the log-rank test. The *p*-value was set at 0.05.

**Results/Conclusions:**
**Efficacy:**

- The original primary outcome, BI, revealed no significant differences on day 0 and after 3 months (candesartan day 0, 60.0 [SD 30.24] and 3 months, 87.0 [SD 22.91] vs. placebo day 0, 64.1 [SD 27.53] and 3 months, 88.9 [SD 88.9]).
- Cumulative 12-month mortality and number of vascular events, however, did differ significantly in favor of the candesartan cilexetil treatment group.
- The odds ratio was 0.475 (95% CI: 0.252 to 0.895).

| | 12-Month Mortality | Vascular Events (total number) | Cardiovascular Events (fatal and nonfatal) | Cerebrovascular Events (fatal and nonfatal) | Noncardiovascular Mortality | Pulmonary Embolism |
|---|---|---|---|---|---|---|
| **Candesartan cilexetil** | 5 (2.9%) | 17 (9.8%) | 2 | 13 | 1 | 1 |
| **Placebo** | 12 (7.2%) | 31 (18.7%) | 10 | 19 | 1 | 1 |
| *P* | 0.07 | 0.026 | | | | |

**Investigator's conclusion:** When there is need for or no contraindication against early antihypertensive therapy, candesartan cilexetil is a safe therapeutic option. Additionally, the data reveal that a 7-day course of candesartan after an acute ischemic stroke significantly improves cardiovascular morbidity and mortality. Lastly, the same favorable effect is not achieved when candesartan is started 7 days after an acute stroke has occurred.

**Summary:** The results of this study indicate that treatment with $AT_1$ receptor blockers during the acute stroke period may prove to be beneficial. Data collected throughout this trial indicate a lack of significant difference in blood pressure readings between the treatment group and placebo group, as well as a lack of differences in blood pressure throughout the subsequent 12 months of follow-up. The beneficial effects, therefore, are not due to blood pressure lowering but by perhaps other neuroprotective effects of these pharmacologic agents that are currently being investigated. Additionally, the favorable effects displayed in this trial were due to a lower incidence of myocardial ischemic events and not a difference in cerebral ischemic events. The investigators hypothesize that this difference may be supported by evidence that impaired central autonomic regulation has shown to be associated with increased mortality from myocardial infarction. Further studies should be designed to test the effect of local angiotensin II effects on early as well as long-term autonomic function.

**Impact factor for journal:** 6.158

## CONTENT EXPERT

The presence of a **content expert** adds depth to a journal club discussion. With P2 and P3 students, the faculty member most often fills the role of content expert and facilitator. Even when the participants are all practitioners, they may not be comfortable or confident when topics are discussed outside their area of expertise. The content expert is someone who has expertise in the area being discussed during journal club who can provide insight into implications for practice. The presence of experts who are well-versed in drug literature evaluation and statistics is also helpful. These experts can help clarify and elaborate on unclear points during the discussion. Because the topic for the journal club is picked in advance, the coordinator should proactively arrange the date around the schedules of key content experts so they can be in attendance.

## PARTICIPANTS

The journal club participants also play an important role. A successful journal club is dependent on an in-depth discussion where all participants contribute to the conversation. Participants should not take a passive role whereby observation is the primary focus. The participants should read the article in advance and come prepared to share their thoughts and opinions. They may be asked to evaluate the presenter and provide feedback on the quality and effectiveness of the journal club.

# CONSIDER THE BEST LOCATION AND SETTING FOR THE JOURNAL CLUB

Consideration should be given to time and location for journal clubs because convenience may improve participation. A calendar with established dates and times can help participants plan ahead. Starting and stopping the journal club on time provides participants with clear expectations on a set time commitment. The best location for a journal club can vary depending on the audience and the objective. The setting may be formal or informal. It can be held in the classroom setting, small group setting, patient care rounds, at a restaurant, or at someone's home. Virtual journal clubs offer an innovative approach to getting groups together with common interests when face-to-face interaction may not be practical. Regardless of the location, the journal club is more productive when held at a location with the fewest distractions.

## CLASSROOM SETTING

Although ideally done in smaller groups where everyone can participate, a journal club can be an effective teaching tool in the classroom. Teaching drug literature evaluation skills by actually performing a journal club in class helps learners apply their didactic drug literature evaluation knowledge directly and provides them with active learning opportunities. As an educator, the ability to impact a large number of learners at one time is a benefit. This setting is advantageous when the goal is to evaluate a learner's skill set or knowledge base. One potential barrier to the classroom setting is making the journal club a discussion versus a lecture or presentation. This is especially true if teaching from a distant site via technology. As a teaching tool, journal clubs should be different from other types of training sessions, such as grand rounds or didactic lectures. Several things can be done to make a journal club within the classroom more conducive for discussion and active participation.[7] First, the chairs should be arranged in a circle or horseshoe shape to encourage interaction and to make it less comfortable for the learner to be passive at the back row of the room.[7] The article citation should be communicated to the group at least a week in advance to give the learners an opportunity to prepare ahead of time. The learners should be instructed to number their paragraphs in order to keep everyone oriented and focused for the discussion. During the discussion, off-shoot discussions and side conversations should be prevented to keep everyone on task. A checklist should be provided to ensure consistent and thorough review of the article (see Table 15-2). It is sometimes easier to mandate attendance by learners, which has been shown to affect success.[19]

## SMALL GROUP DISCUSSION IN A CONFERENCE ROOM OR OFFICE SETTING

Small group discussions are more intimate and less intimidating than the classroom setting. There are generally fewer distractions, and all participants can sit within close proximity of each other. This is a good environment for P4 students on their advanced experiential practice experience or resident experience. Because the group is smaller, participation may be better. This type of environment facilitates discussion and sharing of ideas and also teaches learners an alternative presentation style. A different skill set is used to facilitate a discussion compared to giving a presentation. This setting also teaches the learner to critically evaluate the literature in an interactive manner. Involving various levels of learners is beneficial. Residents can serve as facilitators, and students can learn from their modeling. As previously stated, a small group discussion may also be ideal when using a journal club format for elective courses. At the other end of the spectrum is a more advanced model where some variation of "journal club" is used by practitioners and policy makers where medication decisions are made, such as when a subgroup of the P&T committee debates the pros and cons of a particular therapy prior to making recommendations to the full committee.

## PATIENT CARE ROUNDS SETTING

Making patient care decisions during multidisciplinary rounds or at point of care is an effective way to affect clinical practice and promote evidence-based recommendations. Residents and practitioners can use a more informal, highly condensed version of a journal club when making patient care recommendations to their multidisciplinary patient care teams. A review of the benefits and limitations of an article can be easily summarized in a concise time period by those with clinical experience and more advanced drug literature evaluation skills. One report suggests that journal club on rounds can be presented in 5-10 minutes, not unlike a complicated patient case presentation. For example, the "chief complaint" of an article is the research question, and it builds from there.[20] The point is that the journal club does not necessarily need to be a formal discussion that lasts an hour. It can be done in a much condensed time and format when used to make patient care decisions on rounds or at point of care.

## PRIVATE HOME, RESTAURANT, OR OTHER CASUAL SETTING

Participants may enjoy a relaxed, nonintimidating environment with group involvement and open discussion. Tips for optimizing the learning environment and interest level include holding a "Bring Your Lunch" journal club, giving attendees a midday break; conducting the journal club outdoors; or hosting a journal club dinner party at a colleague's home following work. Providing food may increase participation in the journal club if attendance is not mandatory.[7,19] Obviously, this may not be feasible in many situations, such as in the classroom. However, if the journal club is held out of the hospital or school setting, such as in the preceptor's home or at a restaurant, providing food may be more practical. This may also increase the social aspect of the journal club, making it more fun, collegial, and attractive to the participants. However, food may be seen as a distraction by some attendees, thus diverting the proper focus of the journal club. The advantages and disadvantages of having food at the journal club should be considered. Outside the classroom setting, it may be preferable to have a core group that attends the journal club regularly, with others attending based on interest or expertise. This ensures an adequate numbers of participants while keeping the journal club fun and pertinent. Attempts should be made to limit distractions as much as possible, because it may be easier to get off track in a more informal environment.

## VIRTUAL JOURNAL CLUBS

A **virtual journal club** conducted online offers an innovative, self-directed approach to allow groups of individuals with common interests, but in different locations, the opportunity to discuss published research in real time as well as asynchronous discussions.[21,22] Interested individuals can participate in evidence-based discussions at a time and place of convenience.[23] Whereas a face-to-face, moderated journal club may be a more effective approach for learners, an online journal club offers an option for more advanced practitioners who are trying to keep up with hot topics in their area of practice.[24] Important considerations for the development of an online journal club include creation of a server site and development of content.[23] Ideally, the site would contain sections describing the goals and rules associated with site use as well as clinical content and subsections directing groups to areas of interest. A moderator is helpful to enforce the rules and facilitate the discussion. The use of a blog format to post research articles and critiques has also been described.[25] Academic and medical blogging allows commentary from experts with possible links to important news or published literature. These novel formats may provide a good forum for individuals with varying expertise to share ideas and to provide a means for CPD among practitioners with busy schedules.[23]

Once the location or setting has been set, the next step is to select an appropriate article and decide the best format for delivering the journal club.

# SELECT AN ARTICLE AND FORMAT FOR THE JOURNAL CLUB

One of the first steps when organizing a journal club is topic selection. Limiting the discussion to one topic is preferable, although more than one article may be discussed. This keeps the discussion focused. Many topics originate from discussions regarding current practice and often stem from clinical questions arising during patient care activities. Formulating a good clinical question will help identify appropriate literature. This may be accomplished by including search terms related to the patient and/or disease population of interest, the intervention being investigated, the comparator intervention, and the outcome of interest. For students, topic selection may be based on the specialty of their advanced experiential practice experience site or on the preceptor's desire to highlight a key drug literature evaluation principle or study design as a learning point. Primary literature related to the chosen topic should be reviewed in search of a specific article of interest. When deciding on a specific topic to discuss, it is also important to know the target audience. Will the journal club be attended by clinicians practicing in a specific area? Is this journal club an advanced experiential practice experience requirement attended by students and residents? Will this journal club constitute a combination of learners without a specific focus area? These questions will guide decision making when choosing between topics that are broad versus those related to a specific practice area. For more experienced practitioners, sharing opinions and expertise may guide article selection.

Learners should consult their preceptor for article suitability before communicating to the group. The article citation should be provided for review well in advance (at least 1 week) so all participants have time to prepare. The journal club coordinator can be instrumental in ensuring that the article chosen for the journal club meets all the goals and objectives. Limiting the time to about 1 hour helps the group prioritize and decreases disinterest due to the time commitment. Regardless of the article chosen, it should (1) be relevant to the clinical practice of the participants, (2) answer a clinical question, and/or (3) provide new knowledge.[26] Not only does the journal club help answer the clinical dilemma, it gives all the participants confidence in dealing with the same issue in the future. Consideration should be given not only to the article chosen, but also the journal. Important aspects include scope, impact factor, target audience, and peer-review process.

Once the journal club topic and article(s) have been chosen, the next step is to decide which journal club format is most appropriate. Several formats are possible that can be used to offer diversity and variety to the journal club, including (1) reviewing a single comparative trial using a checklist (see Table 15-2), (2) debating the pros and cons of a particular intervention, (3) comparing a new article to a classic article, and (4) using various study designs to discuss strengths and weaknesses of that type of design (e.g., prospective, retrospective, case report, meta-analysis).[11]

In addition, providing a brief 3- to 5-minute "clinical pearl" related to a drug literature evaluation principle may be a good way to bring participants up to speed on a concept that is addressed in the article under review.[7]

## CRITICAL APPRAISAL OF A SINGLE ARTICLE

The ability to critically evaluate the literature and determine what impact the published article may have on practice is an important skill set for pharmacists. When the goal of journal club is to teach or improve drug literature evaluation skills, the format most appropriate may be the critical appraisal journal club.[7] For the inexperienced learner, a double-blind, randomized, controlled comparative trial published in the last 1-3 years that answers a specific question may be ideal. It is important for the preceptor to set expectations. The learner can easily evaluate the study design, statistics, results, and important components of the article using a structured checklist. This helps further develop the learner's drug literature evaluation skills and may be helpful to provide the depth and consistency that are desired.

## DEBATE FORMAT

With practitioners, the goal of journal club may be to affect clinical practice, promote evidence-based practice, or keep up with the literature. This may be more extensive than critically evaluating a single article. It may involve a more thorough review of a specific topic where multiple articles are discussed.[7] A debate style where the pros and cons of a particular intervention are demonstrated can be effective in this situation. This format consists of the journal club being presented by "pro" and "con" representatives or teams. It allows for the incorporation of one or more articles with opposite viewpoints to display supporting or refuting evidence.

## HISTORICAL PERSPECTIVE FORMAT

The third type of journal club format is the historical format. This format compares newer published evidence to published evidence supporting the historical gold standard.

In this case, other types of articles may be introduced, including case series or meta-analyses that may help answer a more patient-specific clinical question. Oftentimes, this type of journal club has tremendous implications for changing current standards of practice, making this format another effective style for the more experienced practitioner.

## DISCUSS STRENGTHS AND WEAKNESSES OF A PARTICULAR STUDY DESIGN

Choosing an article based on the type of study design may be an effective format when the goal is to highlight the differences between study designs. An article may be chosen that highlights a particular design, and participants can debate the advantages and disadvantages of that style.[27]

Regardless of the format chosen, all journal clubs should end with a discussion on how the data will affect clinical practice. Where does the information discussed during journal club fit in when you consider the current standard of practice?

Once completed, it is helpful to have some sort of evaluation process associated with the journal club presentation. This may be individual evaluation of the presenter, especially if this was a learner. Equally important is a periodic evaluation of the journal club itself for quality improvement purposes.

# EVALUATE THE JOURNAL CLUB

Several aspects of the journal club should be evaluated. These include preceptor assessment of learners, self-assessments by learners, peer-to-peer assessments, and quality assessment of the journal club process and achievement of goals. If the goal of the journal club is to teach drug literature evaluation skills, then the learner should be evaluated. This may be in the form of an exam or practical if in a didactic classroom setting. For advanced experiential practice experiences and resident experiences, this may be done more with a rubric or self-reflection based on their role as presenter or group leader (see **Table 15-3**).[28,29] A grading rubric is also available in the *Pharmacist's Letter*. For residents, the formative feedback provided can be included in the resident's educational portfolio. If they were the presenter, the evaluations may be used to support teaching certificate requirements. If the goal is to keep up with the literature, answer a specific clinical question, or change practice, as commonly seen with practitioner-oriented journal clubs, then peer-to-peer feedback or assessment may be helpful. One may present an opposing view that was not considered by another, which may influence application of the information at the bedside or in formulary recommendations.

In addition to evaluating the participants associated with the journal club, evaluating the process associated with the journal club is also important. This helps keep the journal club fresh and relevant and identifies areas of improvement involving structure and format. The journal club coordinator should periodically evaluate the journal club process itself to ensure that it is maintaining a high quality and achieving the stated goals. This can be done through surveying participants or asking for feedback by asking specific questions: Is the journal club meeting the stated objectives? Is the location and length of the journal club still appropriate? How many participants attend each journal club? Is there a structured evaluation process? Are there improvements in critical reading skills and knowledge? What is the level of participant satisfaction?

There is limited published data assessing drug literature evaluation skill knowledge and application in learners participating in journal clubs. One study demonstrated that a student's ability to effectively evaluate and communicate pertinent information

**TABLE 15-3**    Rubric for Evaluating Journal Club

**Appendix B**
**Journal Club Presentation – Evaluation Rubric**

Presenter(s):_____    Reviewer:_____

Criteria

| I. STUDY OVERVIEW | 3 Points | 2 Points | 1 Point | 0 Points | Score |
|---|---|---|---|---|---|
| **Introduction**<br>❑ Authors' affiliations/ study support<br>❑ Study objective(s) and rationale<br>**Methods – *Design***<br>❑ Case-control, cohort, controlled exp, etc.<br>❑ Type of design (crossover, parallel, etc.)<br>❑ Type of assignment used<br>❑ Blinding<br>**Methods – *Patients/Subjects***<br>❑ How enrolled/from where?<br>❑ Inclusion/exclusion criteria<br>❑ # enrolled per group | | **Accurately** and **completely** reported ALL relevant introduction, study design, and patient/ subject components | **Accurately** and **completely** reported MOST of the relevant introduction, study design, and patient/subject components | Did not **accurately** and **completely** report most of the relevant introduction, study design, and patient/ subject components | |
| **Methods – *Treatment Regimens***<br>❑ Treatments used<br>❑ Dosages/administration<br>❑ Therapy duration<br>**Methods – *Outcome Measures***<br>❑ Primary measures<br>❑ Secondary measures<br>**Methods – *Data Handling***<br>❑ Intention to treat, per protocol, etc.<br>❑ # lost to follow-up<br>❑ Reasons for dropouts | | **Accurately** and **completely** reported ALL relevant treatment regimens, outcome measures, and data handling components | **Accurately** and **completely** reported MOST relevant treatment regimens, outcome measures, and data handling components | Did not **accurately** and **completely** report MOST relevant treatment regimens, outcome measures, and data handling components | |
| **Methods – *Statistics***<br>❑ Tests used<br>❑ Power of study<br>**Results**<br>❑ Results for each outcome measure<br>❑ Confidence intervals<br>❑ *p*-values<br>❑ Compliance<br>❑ Adverse events<br>**Conclusion**<br>❑ Authors' conclusion(s) | | **Accurately** and **completely** reported ALL relevant statistics, results, and authors' conclusion components | **Accurately** and **completely** reported MOST of the relevant statistics, results, and authors' conclusion components | Did not **accurately** and **completely** report MOST of the relevant statistics, results, and authors' conclusion components | |

**Comments for Study Overview:**

*(continues)*

| TABLE 15-3 | Rubric for Evaluating Journal Club (*Continued*) |
|---|---|

**Appendix B**
**Journal Club Presentation – Evaluation Rubric**

Presenter(s):_____    Reviewer:_____

**Criteria**

| II. STUDY ANALYSIS AND CRITIQUE | 4 Points | 3 Points | 2 Points | 1 Point | 0 Points | Score |
|---|---|---|---|---|---|---|
| Analyzed all parts of study (refer to supplement sheet for guidance) | ALL parts appropriately critiqued, with ALL relevant questions accurately addressed with strengths, weaknesses, and their impact described | Missed only ONE or TWO considerations or relevant questions in critique, with the rest appropriately addressed with strengths, weaknesses, and their impact described | MOST parts appropriately critiqued; some relevant questions with strengths, weaknesses, and their impact overlooked or inaccurate | Only SOME parts appropriately critiqued; most relevant questions with strengths, weaknesses, and their impact overlooked or inaccurate | Failed to appropriately critique any part; all relevant questions with strengths, weaknesses, and their impact overlooked or inaccurate | **Multiply by 2 for this field only** |

**Comments for Study Analysis and Critique:**

| III. STUDY CONCLUSION | 3 Points | 2 Points | 1 Point | 0 Points | Score |
|---|---|---|---|---|---|
| **Clear, Concise Conclusion Stated** | Conclusion summarized accurately and completely all of the following: key points to be taken from study (which reflected study limitations); drug's role in therapy or clinical practice implications; AND need for any further research in area | Conclusion did not summarize accurately and completely one of the following: the key points to be taken from study; the drug's role in therapy or clinical practice implications; or the need for any further research in area | Conclusion did not summarize accurately and completely two of the following: the key points to be taken from study; the drug's role in therapy or clinical practice implications; or the need for any further research in area | Failed to give conclusion OR conclusion completely inaccurate | |

**Comments for Study Conclusion:**

**TABLE 15-3**     Rubric for Evaluating Journal Club (*Continued*)

**Appendix B**
**Journal Club Presentation – Evaluation Rubric**

Presenter(s):_____     Reviewer:_____

| Criteria | | | | | |
|---|---|---|---|---|---|
| **IV. PREPAREDNESS** | **3 Points** | **2 Points** | **1 Point** | **0 Points** | **Score** |
| **Knowledge of Study Details** | | Presenters each well prepared; thoroughly explained ALL details of study | Not all presenters well prepared OR thoroughly explained only some study details | No presenter well prepared OR did not thoroughly explain any study details | |
| **Response to Questions** | Correctly answered ALL questions in a confident manner | Correctly answered ALL questions in a non-confident manner OR correctly answered MOST questions in a confident manner | Conectly answered MOST questions in a non-confident manner OR correctly answered only SOME questions | Incorrectly answered all questions OR handled questions unprofessionally | |

**Comments for Preparedness:**

| **V. PRESENTATION** | **3 Points** | **2 Points** | **1 Point** | **0 Points** | **Score** |
|---|---|---|---|---|---|
| **Speaking Style** | | Spoke clearly; easy to hear and understand | Difficult to hear or understand SOME things spoken | Difficult to hear or understand MOST things spoken | |
| **Timing** | | | Within 12 minutes (+/− 3 minutes) | >15 or <9 minutes | |
| **Distracters (uhs, uhms, etc.) OR Distracting Mannerisms** | | Used few (or no) distracters or distracting mannerisms | Used several distracters or distracting mannerisms | Used distracters or distracting mannerisms throughout | |
| **Eye Contact** | | Maintained eye contact throughout | Occasionally looked at evaluators | Read the presentation | |

**Comments for Presentation:**

Additional Comments: _____     TOTAL SCORE FROM BOTH SIDES
(Maximum = 29 points)

_____

_____

_____

Blommel ML, Abate MA. A rubric to assess critical literature evaluation skills. *Am J of Pharm Educ*. 2007; 71(4):1-8. doi: 10.5688/aj710463 regarding study design, statistics, strength, weaknesses, and application in therapy was improved following advanced experiential practice experiences that incorporated journal clubs.[5] Students' attitudes and confidence improved as they relate to presentation skills and understanding of study design and clinical relevance of a study. In a different study, a systematic review was conducted to identify core processes of a successful journal club.[10] Outcomes that showed improvement included perceived reading habits of journal club members, improved ability to appraise original research articles, critical appraisal knowledge, and overall satisfaction. In another study, reading habits and drug literature evaluation knowledge scores improved following journal club; however, ability to critically appraise the article showed no significant difference.[30]

The following case study highlights the key principles of this chapter, where a postgraduate year 2 (PGY2) critical care pharmacy resident shares her thought process as she prepares for a journal club meeting.

| CASE STUDY 15-1 | PGY2 Critical Care Pharmacy Resident Journal Club Scenario |
|---|---|

The PGY2 critical care pharmacy resident at an academic medical center is assigned the task of facilitating the upcoming journal club. The first task she must complete is the selection of the article to evaluate during the journal club meeting. She recalls an interesting clinical question that surfaced during patient care rounds in the trauma intensive care unit regarding tranexamic acid dosing to inhibit fibrinolysis in a trauma patient. The primary article used to support her evidence-based recommendation would make for a great journal club article evaluation, as it was recently published in a reputable journal and had a positive impact on the patient's therapy management. After deciding on this article, she contacted the journal club coordinator and her residency director for approval of the journal club topic and article selection. Next, she decided that the journal club would be more beneficial for all those involved if there was a content expert present at the meeting who could offer insight and clinical expertise when evaluating the article. She decided the trauma critical care pharmacist would be the perfect content expert for the article. Once she confirmed a date and time that would be suitable for the content expert's schedule, she began to plan the location and decided that a less formal setting at a colleague's residence would provide opportunity for great participation from the group. Two weeks before the journal club's scheduled date, the resident emailed the article citation, date, time, and location to the other pharmacists and residents in the department, inviting them to participate in the meeting. During this time, the resident also began to prepare her evaluation of the journal article by following the format used in Table 15-2. Her final evaluation and summary document resembled the example used in Box 15-1. One day prior to the journal club meeting, she sent out an email as a reminder to those who had signed up to participate. During the journal club meeting, the resident acted as the time-keeper and allowed 30 minutes prior to the group discussion for socialization and refreshments. She then gathered everyone into a quiet room to begin the journal article discussion. During the hour-long discussion, she kept the group on topic and made a point to move along the comments if the group was spending too much time on one section in particular. At the conclusion of the journal club meeting, the resident provided the preceptors and other mentors with evaluation forms that would characterize her success in organizing and leading the meeting.

# SUMMARY

A journal club can be done in a more formal setting, such as a classroom, or a more informal one, such as at a faculty member's home. Even in a more condensed setting, such as on patient care rounds, the discussion should be focused and organized. The format for the journal club may vary depending on its goal. One article may be reviewed from beginning to end using a checklist, or three or four articles may be discussed in a more condensed fashion using a debate format or historical perspective. Evaluation of

**TABLE 15-4**    Barriers to a Successful Journal Club

Lack of an organized method for critical review.
Lack of preparation time.
Poor faculty/content expert attendance.
Evaluating an article with minimal clinical relevance.
Not providing a feedback mechanism.

Modified from Moberg-Wolff EA, Kosasih JB. Journal clubs. Prevalence, format, and efficacy in PM&R. *Am J Phys Med Rehabil.* 1995;74(3):224-229.

learners and the programmatic aspects of the journal club should be routinely performed to ensure quality and to make improvements in both the individuals and the program.

Avoiding potential pitfalls can help ensure success.[9] A list of the most common pitfalls associated with journal club are found in **Table 15-4**.

Innovations continue to evolve that will improve the interest and effectiveness of journal clubs. As demands for interdisciplinary education grows, the journal club offers a practical forum to bring different groups of practitioners together in both training and practice.[30] This can foster multidisciplinary patient care recommendations and develop important relationships.

In summary, journal club should be an enjoyable, educational tool to help learners develop critical appraisal skills and to guide practitioners and educators as they make patient care and formulary decisions or answer patient-specific therapy questions. It is an activity that transcends the boundaries of the classroom to the real world, where continuing professional development is critically important. Even when the lack of "free time" prohibits participation in formal journal clubs, clinicians can use the skills learned and apply them to self-directed reading of journal articles regarding cutting-edge medication therapy or disease state management strategies.

# REFERENCES

1. Linzer M. The journal club and medical education: over one hundred years of unrecorded history. *Br Med J.* 1987;63(740):475-478.
2. Kleinpell RM. Rediscovering the value of the journal club. *Am J Crit Care.* 2002;11(5):412-414.
3. Alguire PC. A review of journal clubs in postgraduate medical education. *J Gen Intern Med.* 1998;13(5):347-353.
4. Stallings A, Borja-Hart N, Fass J. Strategies for reinventing journal club. *Am J Health-Syst Pharm.* 2011;68(1):14-16.
5. Arif SA, Gim S, Nogid A, Shah B. Journal clubs during advanced pharmacy practice experiences to teach literature-evaluation skills. *Am J Pharm Educ.* 2012;76(5):1-8.
6. Center for the Advancement of Pharmacy Education Educational Outcomes 2004, American Association of Colleges of Pharmacy. http://www.aacp.org/resources/education/Documents/PharmacyPracticeDEC006.pdf. Accessed July 23, 2014.
7. Swift G. How to make journal clubs interesting. *Adv Psychiatr Treat.* 2004;10:67-72.
8. Hinkson CR, Kaur N, Sipes MW, Pierson DJ. Impact of offering continuing respiratory care education credit hours on staff participation in a respiratory care journal club. *Respir Care.* 2011;56(3):303-305.
9. Moberg-Wolff EA, Kosasih JB. Journal clubs. Prevalence, format, and efficacy in PM&R. *Am J Phys Med Rehabil.* 1995;74(3):224-229.
10. Deenadayalan Y, Grimmer-Somers K, Prior M, Kumar S. How to run an effective journal club: a systematic review. *J Eval Clin Pract.* 2008;14(5):898-911.
11. Valentini RP, Daniels SR. The journal club. *Postgrad Med J.* 1997;73(856):81-85.
12. Accreditation Council for Pharmacy Education. Guidelines on Continuing Pharmacy Education (CPE) and Continuing Professional Development (CPD). 2014. https://www.acpe-accredit.org/pdf/GuidanceCPE_CPD_June2014.pdf. Accessed December 2, 2014.

13. Schulz KR, Altman DG, Moher D for the CONSORT Group. CONSORT 2010 Statement: updated guidelines for reporting parallel group randomized trials. *Ann Intern Med.* 2010;152(11):726-732.

14. Campbell MK, Elbourn DR, Altman DG; CONSORT Group. CONSORT Statement: extension to cluster randomized trials. *BMJ.* 2004;328(7441):702-708.

15. Piaggio G, Elbourne DR, Altman DG, et al; CONSORT Group. Reporting of noninferiority and equivalence randomized trials: an extension of the CONSORT Statement. *JAMA.* 2006;295(10):1152-1160.

16. Zwarenstein M, Treweek S, Gagnier JJ, et al. CONSORT Group. Improving the reporting of pragmatic trials: an extension of the CONSORT Statement. *BMJ.* 2008;337:a2390.

17. Moher D, Liberati A, Tetzlaff J, et al. PRISMA Group. Preferred reporting items for systematic reviews and meta-analyses: the PRISMA Statement. *Ann Intern Med.* 2009;151(4):264-269.

18. Edwards R, White M, Gray J, Fischbacher. Use of a journal club and letter-writing exercise to teach critical appraisal to medical undergraduates. *Med Educ.* 2001;35(7):691-694.

19. Sidorov J. How are internal medicine journal clubs organized and what makes them successful? *Arch Intern Med.* 1995;155(11):1193-1197.

20. Schwartz MD, Dowell D, Aperi J, Kalet AL. Improving journal club presentations, or, I can present that paper in under 10 minutes. *Evid Based Med.* 2007;12(3):66-68.

21. Berger J, Hardin HK, Topp R. Implementing a virtual journal club in a clinical nursing setting. *J Nurses Staff Dev.* 2011;27(3):116-120.

22. Wombwell E, Murray C, Davis SJ, Palmer K, Nayar M, Konkol J. Leadership journal club. *Am J Health-Syst Pharm.* 2011;68(21):2026-2027.

23. Lizardondo L, Kumar S, Grimmer-Somers K. Online journal clubs: an innovative approach to achieving evidence-based practice. *J Allied Health.* 2010;39(1):e-17-22.

24. McLeod RS, MacRae HM, McKenzie ME. A moderated journal club is more effective than an internet journal club in teaching critical appraisal skills: results of a multicenter randomized controlled trial. *J Am Coll Surg.* 2010;211(6):769-776.

25. Lehna C, Berger J, Truman A, Goldman M, Topp R. Virtual journal club connects evidence to practice. An analysis of participant responses. *J Nurs Adm.* 2010;40(12):522-528.

26. Askew JP. Journal club 101 for the new practitioner: evaluation of a clinical trial. *Am J Health-Syst Pharm.* 2004;61(18):1885-1887.

27. Hartlaub PP. A new approach to the journal club. *Acad Med.* 1999;74(5):607-608.

28. Carpenter CR, Katz E, Char D. Editorial: Journal club and teaching evidence-based medicine. *J Emer Med.* 2006 31(3):306-307.

29. Blommel ML, Abate MA. A rubric to assess critical literature evaluation skills. *Am J Pharm Educ.* 2007;71(4):1-8.

30. Linzer M, Brown JT, Frazier LM, DeLong ER, Siegel WC. Impact of a medical journal club on housestaff reading habits, knowledge and critical appraisal skills: a randomized, controlled trial. *JAMA.* 1988;260(17):2537-2541.

# MEDICATION SAFETY

Sherilyn VanOsdol, PharmD, BCPS

## CHAPTER OBJECTIVES

▸ Compare and contrast definitions of medication errors and adverse drug events.

▸ Describe ways in which human error contributes to adverse drug events.

▸ Compare and contrast medication error detection strategies.

▸ Discuss the role of culture in error reporting and investigation.

▸ Describe root cause analysis and failure modes effects analysis.

▸ Describe populations or processes that may be at higher risk for adverse drug events.

▸ Identify potential sources of error in the medication use process.

▸ Name strategies used to reduce medication errors.

▸ Describe the pharmacist's role in medication safety.

# CHAPTER OUTLINE

# KEY TERMS

Adverse drug event
Adverse drug reaction
Automated dispensing cabinet
Computerized provider order entry
Failure modes and effects analysis
High-alert medication

Incident report
Medication error
Medication safety
Person approach
Root cause analysis
Systems approach

# INTRODUCTION

To understand the importance of medication safety in daily practice, it is important to learn some of the history that has made the medication use system in the United States what it is today. Without context, many of the concepts discussed here may seem intuitive or even unimportant; however, medication use systems and the pharmacist's role in patient safety have changed substantially over time to meet safety needs. Several organizations have been pivotal in restructuring the medical system to make medication safety central to the patient care process. Some of these organizations are focused specifically on medication safety; others focus on patient safety but acknowledge that prevention of adverse drug events (ADEs) is fundamental in the provision of quality patient outcomes.

Betsy Lehman, an acclaimed health columnist for *The Boston Globe*, died from cardiac toxicity after receiving a fourfold overdose of cyclophosphamide at the Dana-Farber Cancer Institute during the fall of 1994.[1] Another patient, on the same experimental protocol, also received an overdose and suffered cardiac toxicity, leaving her with permanent heart damage. Both patients received 16 days' worth of cyclophosphamide over the course of 4 days, and the errors were not detected until data from the protocol were entered into a study document several months later. These cases brought national attention to concerns for the lack of safety systems at a renowned cancer research hospital. They also opened the question: If this could happen at Dana-Farber, could the same thing happen elsewhere?

In 1999, the Institute of Medicine (IOM) published a groundbreaking report titled *To Err Is Human: Building a Safer Health System*, which indicated that an estimated 44,000 to 96,000 Americans die annually as a result of medical errors.[2] Deaths due to medical errors were estimated to exceed those from motor vehicle accidents (43,458), breast cancer (42,297), and AIDS (16,516). The report estimated that medication errors alone account for at least 7,000 deaths annually, and that preventable ADEs occurred in 2 of every 100 hospital admissions.

In 2006, the IOM published *Preventing Medication Errors*, a report focused on medication safety.[3] *Preventing Medication Errors* attempted to define the problem of preventable ADEs across the entire healthcare system, rather than focusing on the inpatient setting. The report estimated that more than 1.5 million preventable ADEs occur each year, with 380,000 to 450,000 occurring in hospitals, 800,000 occurring in long-term care facilities, and 530,000 occurring in ambulatory care. Costs associated with managing preventable ADEs have been estimated to range from $4,700 to $8,700 per ADE in the inpatient setting.[3,4] In 2000, the annual cost of drug-related illness and death in the ambulatory care setting was approximately $177.4 billion.[3]

To emphasize the importance of healthcare quality and patient outcomes, major accreditation bodies have aligned their standards. In 2003, The Joint Commission released its first set of National Patient Safety Goals, which set standards for addressing patient safety issues.[5] The Joint Commission annually revises its National Patient Safety Goals for ambulatory health care, behavioral health care, critical access hospital, home care, and hospital settings—each of which contains a section on medication management.

# MEDICATION SAFETY TERMINOLOGY

Terminology used to describe medication safety and errors is not standardized across medication safety organizations and published literature. In their 1995 *Guidelines on Adverse Drug Reaction Monitoring and Reporting*, the American Society of Health-System Pharmacists (ASHP) called for common definitions of terminology surrounding adverse drug reactions to facilitate reporting, surveillance, and research related to adverse drug reaction trends.[6] The terminology used to define medication safety and ADEs is similarly heterogeneous.[7,8] Commonly used terms with multiple definitions include the following: medication errors, ADEs, adverse drug reactions, drug-related problems, medication misadventures, and drug-related morbidity.

An error is defined as "the failure of a planned action to be completed as intended (error of execution) or the use of a wrong plan to achieve an aim (error of planning)."[3] An error may be an act of commission (doing something wrong) or an act of omission (failing to do the right thing).[3,9] The IOM defines a medication error as any error occurring in the medication use process.[3] The definition used by the National Coordinating Council for Medication Error Reporting and Prevention (NCC MERP) more clearly defines where errors may occur:

> any preventable event that may cause or lead to inappropriate medication use or patient harm while the medication is in the control of the health care professional, patient, or consumer. Such events may be related to professional practice, health care products, procedures, and systems, including prescribing; order communication; product labeling, packaging, and nomenclature; compounding; dispensing; distribution; administration; education; monitoring; and use.[10]

For the purposes of this chapter, an abbreviated form of this definition will be used; a **medication error** is defined as any error in any step of the medication use process. Medication errors often receive a subclassification to indicate in which step of the medication use process the error occurred, such as a prescribing error, dispensing error, or medication administration error. Common medication error prevention strategies in these areas will be discussed in further detail later in the chapter. Following investigation, medication errors may also be categorized by the degree of harm inflicted upon the patient who received the error. Many institutions use the NCC MERP Index for

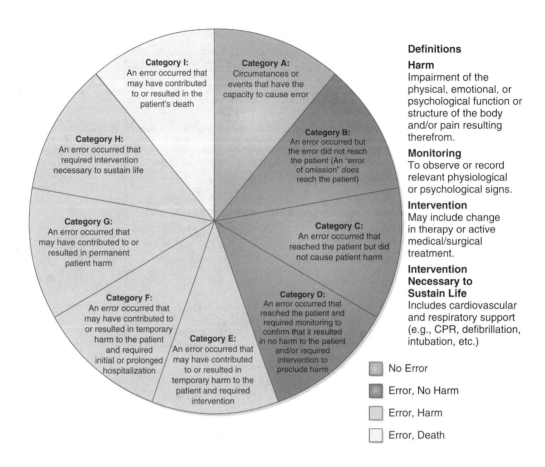

**FIGURE 16-1** NCC MERP index for categorizing medication errors.

Categorizing Medication Errors, or a similar tool, to define the level of harm resulting from a medication error (**Figure 16-1**).

An **adverse drug event** is defined as an adverse event (i.e., injury resulting from medical care) involving medication use.[9] This term encompasses medication errors that cause preventable ADEs and adverse drug reactions (**Figure 16-2**). ADEs are commonly classified by the degree of harm the event causes to the patient. The term significant ADE is used if the event causes symptoms that, although harmful to the patient, pose little or no threat to the patient's life function. These adverse events can include elevated or depressed laboratory test levels. Examples of physical symptoms include dizziness, fatigue, constipation, muscle cramps, insomnia, headaches, and pedal edema.[4] Serious ADEs cause persistent alteration to life function. Serious ADEs can also include elevated or depressed laboratory values that require medical intervention, especially if they suggest organ system dysfunction. Examples of these serious adverse events include clinically significant bleeding, symptoms requiring hospitalization for management (e.g., symptomatic hypoglycemia), and altered mental status. If an ADE causes symptoms that, if left untreated, would put the patient at risk for death, it is called a life-threatening ADE. A life-threatening drug event might have occurred if there are indications of the following: severely altered laboratory values indicating impending failure of a critical

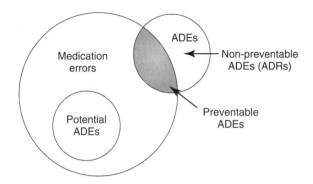

**FIGURE 16-2** Relationships between medication errors, potential adverse drug events, and adverse drug events.

Reproduced from Gandhi TK, Seger DL, Bates DW. Methodology matters identifying drug safety issues: from research to practice. *Int J Qual Health Care.* 2000;12(1):69-76, by permission of Oxford University Press.

physiological system, as well as patient care needs for treating respiratory depression, cardiac arrest, and anaphylaxis.

Although medication errors hold the potential for harm, not all errors cause harm to the patient. Medication errors that have the potential for injury but do not cause harm are called potential ADEs.[7] A potential ADE does not cause harm either because it is intercepted before reaching the patient (also called a near miss) or an error reached the patient but resulted in no patient harm. Medication errors that cause harm, but that could have been avoided with more complete information, are known as preventable ADEs. Examples include a patient receiving and having a reaction to an antibiotic to which she had a known allergic reaction or a patient becoming somnolent following an overdose of a sedating medication.

Not all ADEs are preventable. Nonpreventable ADEs are also called **adverse drug reactions**. Adverse drug reactions occur when a drug is used in the recommended manner and results in an undesired response. An example of an adverse drug reaction would be anaphylaxis after first receipt of penicillin in a patient with no known history of hypersensitivity to the antibiotic. Bear in mind that an adverse drug reaction could occur in the face of a medication error (e.g., a patient unexpectedly has an anaphylactic reaction to penicillin, but never had an order to receive that drug); however, they will retain their separate definitions here.

The terms drug–related problem and medication misadventure are used in the literature as umbrella terms that encompass medication errors, ADEs, adverse drug reactions, and the areas in which they overlap.

**Medication safety** is defined as freedom from accidental injury during the course of medication use. The term encompasses activities to avoid, prevent, or correct ADEs that may result from the use of medications.

## WHY ERRORS OCCUR

In July 2006, a healthy adolescent female was admitted to a hospital to deliver her baby. As part of a standard protocol, her nurse retrieved a bag of penicillin to administer to the patient intravenously.[11] Minutes after the infusion was started, the patient began having seizure activity, respiratory distress, and cardiovascular collapse. The patient's baby was delivered unharmed via emergent cesarean section; however, heroic attempts to resuscitate the mother failed, and she died several hours later. It was later discovered that, rather than penicillin, the nurse mistakenly hung for intravenous infusion a solution of fentanyl and bupivacaine intended for epidural infusion.

## HUMAN ERROR

To understand how to anticipate and minimize harm from human error, it is important to recognize well-characterized sources of human error.[9,12] Similar to the terminology for medication errors, a variety of schema exist for defining causes of human error. The etiological classifications of human causes of medication errors have helped facilitate the design of better prevention methods, and are described here.

Recall that an error may be the failure of a planned action to be completed as intended (error of execution) or the use of a wrong plan to achieve an aim (error of planning).[3,9] Errors of execution are also called skill-based errors; they occur when an action was planned correctly but incorrectly executed, either due to a memory-based error or an action-based error.[13] A memory-based error is also known as a lapse, and may occur if an important piece of information is forgotten during an action (e.g., forgetting a patient had a penicillin allergy and writing her a prescription for Penicillin VK). Action-based errors are also called slips and result when the outcome of an action is different from what was intended (e.g., selecting hydroxyzine rather than hydralazine from a drop-down menu in a pharmacy computer system). Another example of an action-based error is intravenous administration of an epidural infusion to a pregnant woman. Technical errors, such as a miscalculated final concentration of an oral solution, are also considered action-based errors.

An error of planning is also known as a mistake.[13] Mistakes can be caused by incomplete information (knowledge-based errors) or failure to apply a guiding principle (rule-based errors). A knowledge-based error led to the death of Betsy Lehman, as described in the introduction, when an ambiguously written chemotherapy order (i.e., the total dose was indicated, but the time line for administration was missing) was prepared and administered to the patient, rather than clarified.[1,13] Had a standardized process been used for writing chemotherapy orders at the institution, the incorrect order would have been a rule-based error.

### Responding to Human Error

Two schools of thought govern the approach to serious harm caused by human error: the person approach and the systems approach.[12,14]

#### *Person Approach*

In the **person approach**, the individual most directly involved in an error—for example, the nurse administering the epidural infusion via an IV line—is considered at fault for causing the error to occur.[12,14] Performance deficits of the individual, such as inattention, poor motivation, forgetfulness, negligence, and recklessness, are blamed for any harm inflicted upon the patient. Responses to error in the person approach include writing new procedures, disciplinary action, threat of litigation, or firing the responsible individual. A major flaw of the person approach is the assumption that removal of a "problem" person will mitigate the risk for a similar error to occur in the future. In the case of mistakenly giving a pregnant woman epidural medication via IV, the nurse was dismissed from her job and was charged with a felony criminal offense.[11]

## Systems Approach

In the **systems approach**, human errors are anticipated. Errors are considered the result of a culmination of many system weaknesses or failures. The systems approach acknowledges that the conditions in which an individual performs his or her job shape the outcomes; therefore, substituting such a "problem" person with a peer in the same circumstances could very well produce the same results.[12] In health care, safety elements that are removed from direct patient care but that affect how care is delivered exist in what is known as the blunt end of the system.[9] The individual most directly involved in the error is considered to be practicing at the sharp end of the system. The blunt end of the system is responsible for the circumstances in which an error occurs at the sharp end of the system.

## SYSTEMS FAILURES

Several models describe ways in which the blunt end of the system allows errors to occur. James Reason developed the Swiss Cheese model to demonstrate the role of various elements that help prevent, or contribute to, error in highly complex systems (e.g., airline, automotive industries).[12] This model of systems thinking has more recently been adopted in health care, a similarly complex system. In the Swiss Cheese model, each layer of cheese corresponds to defenses and barriers to an error. Technology and equipment, policies and procedures, and highly trained healthcare providers are some examples of these defenses, or slices of cheese, in health care (**Figure 16-3**). No single layer of defense is infallible; each has "holes." Generally, holes in one slice do not lead to a bad outcome. Should enough holes in a system align, an error occurs. If the error is not intercepted before reaching the patient, it holds the potential to cause patient harm or death.

In the Swiss Cheese model, holes are also called latent failures.[9,12] Examples of latent failures include lack of teamwork and communication, poorly designed work schedules or work environments, and variations in the design of equipment. Many latent failures occur in parts of the system that are invisible to frontline healthcare providers (i.e., the blunt end of the system). When an error occurs, it occurs during care provided at the sharp end of the system, and may be due to an active failure (e.g., misprogramming an

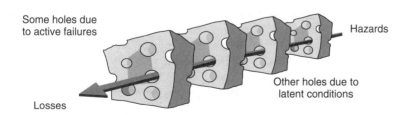

Some holes due to active failures

Hazards

Other holes due to latent conditions

Losses

Successive layers of defenses, barriers, and safeguards

**FIGURE 16-3** Swiss cheese model of accident causation.

infusion pump or administering medication from an oral syringe through an IV catheter) but was most likely caused by many latent failures. Therefore, a key safety strategy is to focus on systems elements and incorporate human factors engineering to make failure difficult. As James Reason notes, "Though we cannot change the human condition, we can change the conditions under which humans work."[12]

## A CULTURE OF SAFETY

Traditionally, healthcare providers were expected to perform all tasks completely error-free. When an error did occur, the person closest to the error was implied as a suboptimal performer, as described in the persons approach.[12] Often called "name, blame, and shame," the healthcare culture deemed error a result of suboptimal provider care, rather than external factors. Following publication of the IOM's *To Err Is Human*, national focus was placed on the fact that humans are, in fact, fallible by nature, and that emphasis should be placed on designing systems to prevent (or reduce the severity of) errors. However, adoption of this approach in institutional settings required a shift in thinking.

Organizational leadership drives much of the attitude that, in turn, drives supervisor and peer response to an error (or near miss). Culture—defined as the shared beliefs, values, norms, and procedures within an organization—shapes provider perceptions of whether a given action, such as reporting an error, is praiseworthy or punishable by hospital leadership, direct supervisors, or peers.

In its 2004 report, *Patient Safety*, the IOM recommended incorporating elements focused on safety into institutional culture.[15] Recommended safety elements included a shared understanding that health care is a high-risk undertaking, an organizational commitment to detecting and analyzing errors and near misses, open communications regarding patient harm, and establishment of a just culture. In a just culture, learning from mistakes is balanced with the need to take disciplinary action in the instance of gross misconduct or blatant disregard to safe practices.[9,15] Importantly, individuals are not held responsible for errors that result from systems failures over which they have no control.[15] This concept is widely embraced as a culture of safety. Adoption of a culture focused on safety has been associated with reductions in adverse events and mortality.[16]

The IOM made further recommendations that healthcare organizations adopt a mind-set of high-reliability organizations, in which error is expected; hence, constant focus is placed on systems improvements to prevent errors.[3] High-reliability organizations acknowledge the high-risk nature of their work. They adopt a culture of safety that focuses on frontline workers and enables frontline management to identify and rapidly respond to threats. They are also resilient when errors occur. These organizations dedicate resources to transparently sharing information learned from analyses of errors and near misses. Such organizations operate with nearly failure-free performance records—examples include air traffic control systems and nuclear power plants.[9]

## HOW ERRORS ARE DETECTED

A key concept of medication safety is that there is no way to detect a true error rate.[17] The estimated incidence of ADEs in various settings helps to define the problem and should be used to focus on quality improvement efforts. Multiple complementary techniques for detecting errors should be used, as no one error detection method is complete.

Many institutions use **incident reports** (voluntary reporting of safety concerns or events by healthcare providers, patients, or parents) to assess their internal ADE incidence.[18] The numbers of reported errors and near misses do not reflect error rates or incidence; evidence has determined that incident reports of errors and ADEs are only the tip of the iceberg, accounting for 2-5% of ADEs.[18,19] The Institute for Safe Medication Practices emphasizes that differences in institutional culture, definitions of errors, patient populations served, and the types of reporting and detection systems used can all lead to significant differences in incident reporting.[20] For these reasons, it is not meaningful to compare the number of incident reports between different healthcare systems. Instead, this information should be used to detect weaknesses in the medication use system and to prevent potential errors from occurring.

Voluntary reporting of system weaknesses can provide rich information for medication safety improvement efforts. However, data gathered from internal incident reporting systems should be supplemented with complementary methods for detecting errors to provide a more comprehensive view of medication safety failures.[2] Other error detection methods include audits of charts or filled prescriptions, detection of ADEs using trigger tools, and direct observation of a step in the medication use process, such as medication administration.

In chart audits (also called chart reviews), a patient's medical records are thoroughly reviewed to search for potential ADEs.[18] Records that might be assessed include medical records, discharge summaries, pharmacy databases, and laboratory data. Chart audits may be conducted when a patient is concurrently admitted or retrospectively; however, this method is very labor-intensive compared to incident reporting or the use of trigger tools. In the trigger tool method, a certain drug used to treat an adverse drug reaction, event, or a laboratory value indicative of a potential ADE is used to "trigger" the review of a patient's medical record. The trigger helps the auditor of the chart determine a time frame and the type of ADE. Well-designed trigger tools can have 100% positive predictive value for detecting ADEs and can be the most efficient method, if well designed.[18] Alerting orders or trigger medications were used to detect the incidence of ADEs in 71.9% of hospitals surveyed in 2009.[21]

Direct observation is another method used for understanding issues in the medication use process.[18] Direct observation refers to a range of methodologies in which real-time observations determine errors or error-prone steps in the medication use process. This is a highly labor-intensive method for detecting ADEs; however, it provides many benefits: it is performed in real-time, can intercept potentially serious medical errors, and focuses on processes and workflows.

# QUALITY IMPROVEMENT IN MEDICATION SAFETY

## ROOT CAUSE ANALYSIS

Once an error or near miss is identified, **root cause analysis** (RCA) identifies active and latent failures that contributed to the event.[14,22] This is a time- and resource-intensive investigation and is often reserved for serious or potentially serious adverse events and near misses. Root cause analysis was originally developed to analyze industrial accidents, such as the Chernobyl nuclear accident and the *Challenger* space shuttle accident. In an RCA, data are collected to reconstruct an event. An interdisciplinary team analyzes all steps of the process leading up to the event, including information obtained from interviewing event participants. Although the term RCA indicates that the goal is to identify a single underlying cause (i.e., "root cause"), this process typically uncovers multiple active and latent failures and may be better described as a systems analysis. Institutions that have adopted a culture of safety share the results from an RCA within their institution, and might even publish the results so that others can learn from the lessons discovered during the RCA process. The Joint Commission and many states require institutions to conduct timely RCA of serious events; in some states, reporting of RCA results is mandatory.

### FAILURE MODES AND EFFECTS ANALYSIS

The medication use process is complex, and each step/process involved could potentially introduce a new source of error. Because of this, it is important to proactively assess risk whenever possible, rather than reactively analyze systems failure. A method to proactively assess risk associated with introduction of a new process, medication, or device into a system is known as a **failure modes and effects analysis** (FMEA).[9] In FMEA, all steps of a process are mapped out, and an interdisciplinary team identifies all possibilities for failures with each step (i.e., failure modes), the probability a failure would occur and that it would be detected, and its severity.[23] This information is fed through a calculation to determine a criticality index; steps with higher criticality index scores become areas of focus for error-proofing before the process is introduced into the system.

### EXTERNAL REPORTING OF DRUG-RELATED PROBLEMS

The IOM and ASHP further emphasize reporting serious errors and ADEs to outside organizations to provide information to other healthcare institutions.[3,24,25] Several organizations in the United States devote resources to promoting medication safety. The Food and Drug Administration (FDA) maintains a database of reported serious adverse events or quality problems associated with FDA-regulated drugs, biologics, dietary supplements, and medical devices.[26] The Institute for Safe Medication Practices (ISMP) is a nonprofit agency focused on medication safety and dissemination of tools and case reports to enhance education in this area. ISMP, in partnership with the United States Pharmacopoeia (USP), maintains the Medication Errors Reporting Program, a voluntary incident reporting system where ADEs can be confidentially reported.[27] Reporting of medication and vaccine errors, preventable ADEs, close calls, and hazardous conditions to this system is encouraged. Field experts then analyze and comment on reported events that are common or severe and provide recommendations for safety measures to minimize the risk of repeated ADEs. The ISMP disseminates these on a regular basis.

The ISMP and USP also partner with the FDA, which maintains the MedWatch program.[26,27] Healthcare providers or consumers can file safety concerns regarding drugs, biologics, medical devices, over-the-counter medications, and special nutritional products to the MedWatch program. ISMP additionally files reports to MedWatch based on voluntary reports submitted to the Medication Errors Reporting Program. Safety issues filed in MedWatch can lead to safety notifications sent to healthcare providers or consumers; new labeling or packaging requirements; increased safety monitoring requirements, such as boxed warnings or risk evaluation mitigation strategies programs; and even recalls.

## RISK FACTORS FOR ADVERSE DRUG EVENTS

Although ADEs may potentially occur in any setting or at any step of the medication use process, certain patient populations and medication use process steps pose a higher risk. Certain patient populations and stages in patient care are more prone to preventable ADEs.

A patient's age, organ function, mental status, and degree of health literacy determine the degree of resilience against harm from, or ability to intercept, an ADE. Transitions of care, high-acuity situations, and polypharmacy also represent risk factors for ADEs.

## HIGH-RISK POPULATIONS

Pediatric patients are uniquely at high risk for preventable ADEs. Some reasons for this include their immature renal and hepatic systems; weight-based dosing, and thus a wide range of possible doses; the risk of 10-fold dosing errors; and potentially limited ability for a pediatric patient to detect and communicate that an error has occurred or is about to occur.[28] Furthermore, most medications used in pediatrics have not been studied for FDA approval in that population and are used off-label.[3]

Elderly patients are also at heightened risk for ADEs. Patients in this population likely have less resilience if a medication error reaches them due to multiple comorbidities, polypharmacy, and variable degrees of drug metabolism and elimination.[29] Patients with multiple comorbidities or impaired renal or hepatic function are usually excluded from the premarketing studies that lead to FDA approval; however, these patients are often prescribed multiple agents to manage their underlying disease state(s).[3] Prior to use of drugs in this rapidly growing population, patients and drug therapy must be assessed to balance the benefits with the risks associated with use of a given agent. The American Geriatrics Society publishes a list of medications considered potentially inappropriate or high risk in the elderly population to help avoid preventable medication-related problems in this population.[30] Multidisciplinary rounding and pharmaceutical care (e.g., thorough drug list reviews) decrease inappropriate prescribing and potential medication-related problems.[29]

## CARE SETTINGS

Transitions of care introduce the potential for inaccurate transfer of information relevant to a patient's current medication regimen. Transitions of care involve movement of a patient between areas of care, such as admission to the hospital from home or a long-term care facility, transfers between units within the hospital, discharge from the hospital, or switching between healthcare systems. Approximately 66% of preventable medication reconciliation errors occur during transitions of care within an institution, 22% at admission, and 12% during the discharge process.[31] At each transition, information related to a patient's drug allergies, prescription drugs and adherence, use of over-the-counter medications and herbals, and recent drug regimen changes is essential. Medication reconciliation is the process of obtaining and maintaining an accurate and detailed list of all prescription and nonprescription drugs a hospital or ambulatory care patient is taking, including dosage and frequency, throughout a healthcare encounter.[32] During transitions of care, physicians, nurses, or pharmacists can perform medication reconciliation. Evidence suggests that pharmacists are the most effective and efficient provider when safely performing medication reconciliation, particularly for patients with risk factors such as polypharmacy, the elderly, or those with multiple comorbidities.[33,34]

## MEDICATION-RELATED FACTORS

The use of certain medications, known as **high-alert medications**, can also pose a high risk. High-alert medications are not necessarily associated with a higher rate of ADEs, but they are associated with an increased risk of significant patient harm when used in error.[35] The ISMP publishes lists of high-alert medications for institutional and inpatient as well as community and ambulatory healthcare settings. Common to both lists are chemotherapeutic agents, oral hypoglycemic agents, all insulin formulations, unfractionated and low-molecular-weight heparin, and opioids. Additionally, in the inpatient setting, anesthetic and sedative agents, intravenous inotropic and antiarrhythmic agents, hypertonic sodium chloride and dextrose, and drugs administered epidurally or intrathecally are considered high alert. In the ambulatory setting, antiretroviral, immunosuppressant, and pregnancy category X medications are considered high alert. Access the ISMP website to find current lists that identify specific high-alert medications.

## MEDICATION USE PROCESS

The medication use process is a highly complex system spanning from formulary management and procurement of drugs to prescribing, administration, and patient monitoring. Each part of the system consists of several steps and may involve input from multiple providers; the ISMP has made recommendations for mitigating safety barriers in what are considered the 10 key elements of the medication use system (**Table 16-1**).

Many strategies have been introduced to minimize risk for ADEs and medication errors. Among these are low-tech strategies such as tools targeted at poor handwriting, identification systems for medications with similar names, and recommendations for safe use of high-alert medications. The following discussion describes some common medication errors and preventive strategies.

### Prescribing Errors

An error due to incorrect selection of a drug, dose, concentration, dosage form, quantity, route, infusion rate, incomplete information, or indication is known as a prescribing error.[24] Poor handwriting or inappropriate abbreviations are also causes of prescribing errors, and serious medication errors can result; for instance, the case described in the introduction was a prescribing error. Methods for minimizing prescribing errors include requirement of complete prescribing information, avoiding use of error-prone abbreviations (**Table 16-2**), access to up-to-date drug information resources, and implementation of computerized prescriber order entry (CPOE).

### Order Communication or Transcribing Errors

Errors associated with order communication include transcribing handwritten or faxed orders into a pharmacy computer system, misheard or misinterpreted verbal orders, and misinterpretation of poor handwriting or error-prone abbreviations. Avoidance of error-prone abbreviations and the use of CPOE systems that interface directly with pharmacy computer systems also help minimize order communication errors. Other strategies to minimize the risk of these errors include policies prohibiting verbal orders or the requirement to read orders back to a provider who calls in a prescription to a community pharmacy. If verbal orders cannot be prohibited, requiring the prescriber to provide an indication can provide an additional mechanism for clarification.

### Product Labeling, Packaging, or Nomenclature Errors

Incorrectly labeling a medication package, use of incorrect auxiliary labels, and ambiguous labeling can lead to a variety of downstream errors. Many drugs have brand and generic names that are both spelled and pronounced similarly. This can lead to many errors with product confusion at any step of the medication use process, particularly during drug product selection during prescribing, compounding, dispensing,

| Element | Description |
| --- | --- |
| **TABLE 16-1**    Ten Key Elements of the Medication Use System | |
| Patient information | Pertinent demographic (age, weight) and clinical (allergies, lab results) information aid in appropriate selection of drug therapy and decreasing preventable adverse drug events. |
| Drug information | Accurate and up-to-date drug information resources should be available to all healthcare providers involved in the medication use process to decrease preventable adverse drug events. Resources should include drug references, formulary information, institutional protocols, and dosing scales. |
| Communication of drug information | Communication barriers between providers should be eliminated to reduce errors associated with miscommunication of drug information. |
| Drug labeling, packaging, and nomenclature | Drugs with confused drug names, confusing labeling, and nondistinct product labeling should be clearly identified and labeled to differentiate between look-alike, sound-alike drug names or similar concentrations to prevent associated errors. |
| Drug storage, stock, standardization, and distribution | Standardization of drug administration times and limiting the number of available concentrations will reduce or mitigate the medication errors associated with their use. |
| Drug device acquisition, use, and monitoring | Appropriate safety assessments should be made at the time of drug delivery device selection and use. A system of double-checks should be employed as appropriate to ensure safe use. |
| Environmental factors | Work environments should be designed to minimize distractions such as noise and interruptions, provide adequate lighting, and ensure that providers have a manageable workload to reduce the risk of error. |
| Staff competency and education | Priority should be placed on staff education regarding new medications, high-risk medications, internal and external medication errors, protocols, policies, and procedures related to medication use to promote medication safety practices. |
| Patient education | Patients should receive education from all healthcare providers regarding appropriate use and indications for all medications they receive. Educating and enabling patients to ask questions allows them to play a key role in medication error prevention. |
| Quality process and risk management | Systems and processes that lead to errors should be redesigned to prevent errors rather than focusing on correcting individuals who make errors. Promoting detection and correction of errors before they occur and creating systems in which it is difficult to make an error are effective strategies for reducing errors. |

Modified from the Institute for Safe Medication Practices. Frequently asked questions #3: What are "ten key elements" of the medication use system? Institute of Safe Medication Practices website. http://www.ismp.org/faq.asp#Question_3. Updated regularly. Accessed April 14, 2013.

or administration. Several strategies have been recommended to minimize the risk for drug product confusion, including the use of Tall Man (mixed case) letters on labeling (e.g., buPROPion vs. busPIRone).[36] The FDA and ISMP maintain a list of commonly confused drug names with recommendations for Tall Man letters (**Table 16-3**). Other recommendations include storing potentially problematic medications out of alphabetical order with "name alert" stickers, using both generic and brand names to provide a second source of identification, requiring order indication, providing patients with drug information that contains both generic and brand names, and assessing risk for look-alike, sound-alike errors when introducing a new medication to a formulary system.[37]

Some medication classes have incorporated standardized colors to help differentiate products, such as in ophthalmic preparations and syringes used during anesthesia.[37]

**TABLE 16-2    The Joint Commission's List of "Do Not Use" Abbreviations**

| Do Not Use | Potential Problem | Use Instead |
|---|---|---|
| U, u (for unit) | Mistaken for "0" (zero), the number "4" (four), or "cc" | Write "unit." |
| IU (for international unit) | Mistaken for "IV" (intravenous) or the number "10" (ten) | Write "international unit." |
| Q.D., QD, q.d., qd (daily) Q.O.D, QOD, q.o.d, qod (every other day) | Mistaken for each other Periods or the "O" mistaken for "I" | Write "daily." Write "every other day." |
| Trailing zero (X.0 mg) Lack of leading zero (.X mg) | Decimal point is missed, can lead to 10-fold errors | Write X mg. Write 0.X mg. |
| MS | Can mean morphine sulfate or magnesium sulfate | Write "morphine sulfate." |
| $MSO_4$ and $MgSO_4$ | Confused for each other | Write "magnesium sulfate." |

Modified from The Joint Commission Official "Do Not Use" List. The Joint Commission. http://www.jointcommission.org /assets/1/18/Do_Not_Use_List.pdf. © The Joint Commission, 2014. Reprinted with permission.

**TABLE 16.3    Use of Tall Man Letters to Differentiate Look-Alike Drug Product Names**

| Established Name | Recommended Name | Established Name | Recommended Name |
|---|---|---|---|
| Acetohexamide Acetazolamide | AcetaHEXAMIDE AcetaZOLAMIDE | Medroxyprogesterone | MedroxyPROGESTERone |
| Bupropion Buspirone | BuPROPion BusPIRone | Methylprednisolone Methyltestosterone | MethylPREDNISolone MethylTESTOSTERone |
| Chlorpromazine Chlorpropamide | ChlorproMAZINE ChlorproPAMIDE | Mitoxantrone | MitoXANTRONE |
| Clomiphene Clomipramine | ClomiPHENE ClomiPRAMINE | Nicardipine Nifedipine | NiCARdipine NIFEdipine |
| Cyclosporine Cycloserine | CycloSPORINE CycloSERINE | Prednisone Prednisolone | PredniSONE PrednisoLONE |
| Daunorubicin Doxorubicin | DAUNOrubicin DOXOrubicin | Risperidone Ropinirole | risperiDONE rOPINIRole |
| Dimenhydrinate Diphenhydramine | DimenhyDRINATE DiphenhydrAMINE | Sulfadiazine Sulfisoxazole | SulfADIAZINE SulfiSOXAZOLE |
| Dobutamine Dopamine | DOBUTamine DOPamine | Tolazamide Tolbutamide | TOLAZamide TOLBUTamide |
| Glipizide Glyburide | GlipiZIDE GlyBURIDE | Vinblastine Vincristine | VinBLAStine VinCRIStine |
| Hydralazine Hydromorphone Hydroxyzine | HydrALAZINE HYDROmorphone HydrOXYzine | | |

Reproduced from the U.S. Food and Drug Administration Name Differentiation Project. United States Food and Drug Administration. http://www.fda.gov/Drugs/ DrugSafety/MedicationErrors/ucm164587.htm. Accessed May 13, 2013.

Drugs with multiple concentrations have also been confused (e.g., heparin flush [1:10] with concentrated heparin [1:10,000]); at the time of this writing, the FDA has distributed for review a draft guidance documentation on Safety Considerations for Product Design to Minimize Medication Errors.[38,39] Incorporation of bar code technology during the drug dispensing and administration phases adds an additional safety layer when working with drugs with commonly confused names.

## Dispensing and Distribution Errors

Dispensing errors include errors with order review, processing or verification, compounding, dispensing, and distribution of medications. These errors may result in preparing the wrong drug for dispensing, dispensing a drug to the wrong patient, delays in delivery, or stocking incorrect medications in medication storage areas. The use of clear labeling using Tall Man letters is one strategy to minimize dispensing errors associated with look-alike, sound-alike drug names.

## Administration Errors

The medication administration process is the last step in which a medication error may be intercepted before reaching the patient; however, it is believed that the majority of the errors at this step are not caught.[4] Medication errors occur in an estimated 11.5-19% of medication administrations; moreover, 3.1-7% of medication administrations might lead to patient harm. Many institutions implement standardized procedures to ensure that nurses follow the "five rights" of medication administration: administering the right drug to the right patient at the right dose via the right route at the right time.

Nurses are commonly distracted by noise and interruptions during medication pass times, compounding the stress of an already high-volume workload.[4] Strategies shown to improve safety during medication administration include forbidding interruptions during a medication pass, quiet medication storage/preparation rooms, nursing double-checks, and implementation of technology such as bar code medication administration and smart IV infusion pumps.

## Monitoring Errors

When a patient is inadequately monitored for response to a drug dose or regimen, a monitoring error occurs. Monitoring may refer to therapeutic drug monitoring; laboratory values indicating undesired response to a drug; other adverse reactions, such as anticipated side effects; or ensuring appropriate response to therapy. Monitoring errors can lead to inappropriate dose adjustments (or no dose adjustment when one would be appropriate), inappropriate duration of therapy, or serious ADEs that could have been mitigated if detected sooner. Failure to document a patient's response and other monitoring parameters is also considered a monitoring error.[37] Medications requiring laboratory monitoring are often ordered concurrently with the appropriate test(s) as part of an order set. Many hospitals have implemented pharmacist-run programs for managing therapeutic drug monitoring and subsequent dose adjustments. Follow-up appointments are commonly scheduled prior to discharge or when laboratory or clinical monitoring for drug response is required in the ambulatory care setting.

## Adherence Errors

More common in the outpatient setting, adherence errors occur when patients do not take a medication regimen as prescribed. Multiple factors can cause adherence errors:

insurance issues preventing patients from obtaining their medications, inadequate education regarding how to take their medications, poor health literacy, and/or cultural factors. Patient and caregiver education is a key component in minimizing adherence errors. Follow-up phone calls are an additional strategy to assess and improve patient adherence following hospital discharge. High-risk patient populations (e.g., those with certain disease states or polypharmacy) may be targeted in these programs to ensure that they have made appropriate changes to their medication regimens and have minimized their risk of medication-related readmissions.

## ROLE OF HEALTH INFORMATION TECHNOLOGY

The IOM recommends that healthcare institutions implement technologies intended to improve safety in the medication use process.[3] These include computerized provider order entry, automated dispensing cabinets, bar code medication administration, electronic medication administration records, and smart infusion pumps. Each form of technology introduces elements of safety to the medication use system, although poorly planned or improper implementation of technology can introduce new sources of error.

### Computerized Provider Order Entry

Prescribing can be a highly error-prone step in the medication use process. **Computerized provider order entry** (CPOE) is a process in which a provider, such as a physician, uses a computer system to directly enter medical orders (e.g., medications, laboratory monitoring, consultation with other providers), thereby avoiding errors associated with handwriting or the transcription process. CPOE offers an additional safety mechanism called clinical decision support (CDS). CDS can include screening for drug–drug interactions, patient allergy cross-reactivity, or alerts that an ordered dose is out of the normal dose range. In addition, many CPOE systems incorporate the use of order sets. An order set related to a medication includes a specific drug and dose order bundled with laboratory monitoring and nurse assessments, thereby eliminating the need for a provider to remember to enter multiple orders. Proposed benefits of CPOE include elimination of illegible or incomplete orders, reduction of incorrect transcription, provision of clinical decision support, and improved communication and tracking of new or changed orders.[28]

### Automated Dispensing Cabinets

**Automated dispensing cabinets** (ADCs) are computerized drug storage and distribution systems that allow medications to be stored securely in patient care areas.[40] These systems allow for control of drug distribution on units or in clinics and are important tools in decentralized drug delivery. ADCs commonly interface with hospital computer systems, allowing pharmacists to control which medications are available for specific patients. This supports pharmacist review of ordered medications prior to administration. Additionally, ADCs improve medication availability to point of care areas, thereby decreasing delays in medication delivery and administration.

### Bar Code Medication Administration

Bar code medication administration (BCMA) involves labeling unit doses of medications with bar codes, which contain unique identifying information about the medication when scanned with an optical scanner.[41] In the inpatient setting, patient wristbands may also have a bar code unique to the patient; this links patient-specific information with the medication administration record and with medications that are scanned for administration. Optimized use of BCMA can lead to decreased medication administration errors by ensuring that the "five rights" are followed, as well as decreasing documentation errors associated with medication administration by interfacing with the electronic medication administration record (where all medication administrations or refusals are documented within a patient's medical record). Use of BCMA is endorsed by the Agency for Healthcare Research and Quality (AHRQ), the IOM, and the ISMP in partnership with the American Hospital Association and Health Research and Educational Trust.[41,42]

## Smart Infusion Pumps

Many medications administered intravenously are classified as high-alert medications.[35] Serious medication administration errors have been attributed to misprogramming of manual infusion pumps, which require calculation of infusion rates based on patient weight and drug concentration. Smart infusion pumps, or smart pumps, are programmed with a library of formulary agents and standardized concentrations and provide appropriate dose infusion rates. Furthermore, the pump will notify the user if an infusion is higher or lower than the defined infusion rate parameters. Some institutions have interfaced BCMA with smart pump technology to introduce additional safety measures in administration of IV infusions.

## Concerns with Technology

The IOM identified three concerns with the introduction of various technologies into patient care. Currently, there is not a standardized set of terms, concepts, or codes to represent drug information, which makes seamless interface between systems impossible.[3] A lack of standardization also exists surrounding how safety alerts are presented to end users of the various technologies. Additionally, alert notifications are often identical, despite varying degrees of clinical importance or different levels of potential severity. Many alerts are not considered to be clinically meaningful and so are overridden; when too many alerts are fired, providers may experience "alert fatigue," which can introduce further safety concerns as providers become less likely to pay attention to a more serious alert. Lastly, systems often lack the intelligence to use patient-specific information in alert-firing logic.

User–technology interfaces should also be engineered to take human factors into account.[3] A poorly designed user interface can contribute to medication errors, as can lack of standardization. When healthcare providers use nonstandardized workflows (i.e., workarounds) when using technology or bypass safety tools built into technologies, they are more likely to introduce new, and likely unanticipated, sources of error.[43]

# PHARMACISTS' ROLES IN PROMOTING MEDICATION SAFETY

## INTERPROFESSIONAL TEAMWORK

Patient care is provided by many providers who must work together and communicate to deliver optimum care. The complexity of medicine is continuously increasing, and knowledge of new disease states and drugs is expanding rapidly. Providers must remain current on best practices in their respective professions and apply this in patient care; however, this should be applied in a team setting, rather than in professional silos. Interprofessional teamwork and communication across disciplines has been identified as a key strategy to improve patient safety and the overall quality of care. In effective interprofessional teamwork, all healthcare team members assume equal status on the team, which fosters collaboration in problem solving and overall better care.[44] Pharmacists play an essential role in the patient care team in both inpatient and outpatient settings. As the medication experts, pharmacists have the ability to assist in safe and effective medication use, including the ability to identify potential drug-related problems and mitigate adverse drug reactions.

## PREVENTING ADVERSE DRUG EVENTS

Pharmacists traditionally have been associated with medication distribution systems within a health system; however, pharmacists play a major role in promoting medication safety. A study evaluating 1,520 significant ADE reports from 1976-1997 concluded that pharmacist intervention could have prevented 50% of those that were preventable.[45] Clinical pharmacists have improved patient care and medication safety in a variety of different practice settings including, but not limited to, the following:[46-48]

- Ambulatory care
- Outpatient/retail setting
- The emergency department
- Inpatient rounds

## MEDICATION SAFETY LEADER

The ASHP takes the position that, although all pharmacists should take responsibility for medication safety, healthcare organizations should further designate a medication safety leader to serve as the authoritative expert in safe medication use.[25] Medication safety should be the major component of a medication safety leader's position. The medical safety leader should provide leadership and medication safety expertise; influence practice change; perform research; and educate healthcare providers, trainees, and patients.

# SUMMARY

There is no way to detect the true incidence of medication errors or ADEs; however, sentinel reports from the IOM indicate that these errors are more prevalent than previously believed and lead to serious patient harm and mortality.

Human error is common and can occur during the planning or execution of an action; however, it is now commonly accepted that latent failures in the blunt end of the situation cause errors that occur at the sharp end. Many new strategies have changed the ways in which medication errors and near misses are approached, including the use of a systems approach, implementation of a just culture and changes in the way that near misses and medication errors are reported, and reducing errors through the use of RCAs and FMEAs.

Incident reporting systems are the most common medication error detection strategy. Data from such systems should be supplemented with other detection strategies, such as chart reviews utilizing trigger tools, to assess near misses and errors that are not reported.

Medication errors can occur in any step of the medication use process (e.g., during prescribing, dispensing, administration, monitoring, or adherence). The use of low-tech strategies such as Tall Man lettering to distinguish between drugs with confused names, avoiding abbreviations known to cause confusion, and changing where drugs are stored have been associated with decreased errors. Appropriately implemented health information technology systems can further improve safety in the medication use system.

Pharmacists play a key role in preventing and mitigating ADEs due to their expertise in medication use. Whether working in drug distribution, rounding with interprofessional teams, educating patients, or serving as the medication safety leader, pharmacists are essential in ensuring safe medication use.

# REFERENCES

1. Roush W. Dana-Farber death sends a warning to research hospitals. *Science*. 1995;269(5222):295-296.
2. Kohn LT, Corrigan JM, Donaldson MS, eds. *To Err Is Human: Building a Safer Health System*. Washington, DC: National Academies Press; 2000.
3. Aspden P, Wolcott J, Bootman JL, Cronenwett LR, eds. *Preventing Medication Errors: Quality Chasm Series*. Washington, DC: National Academies Press; 2007.
4. Kale A, Keohane CA, Maviglia S, Gandhi TK, Poon EG. Adverse drug events caused by serious medication administration errors. *Qual Saf Health Care*. 2012;21(11):933-938.
5. The Joint Commission. Facts about the National Patient Safety Goals. http://www.jointcommission.org/facts_about_the_national_patient_safety_goals. Accessed July 23, 2014.
6. American Society of Health-System Pharmacists. ASHP Guidelines on adverse drug reaction monitoring and reporting. http://www.ashp.org/DocLibrary/BestPractices/MedMisGdlADR.aspx. Accessed July 23, 2014.
7. Gandhi TK, Seger DL, Bates DW. Identifying drug safety issues: from research to practice. *Int J Qual Health Care*. 2000;12(1):69-76.
8. Pintor-Mármol A, Baena MI, Fajardo PC, et al. Terms used in patient safety related to medication: a literature review. *Pharmacoepidemiol Drug Saf*. 2012;21(8):799-809.
9. Agency for Healthcare Research and Quality. AHRQ Patient Safety Network glossary. http://psnet.ahrq.gov/glossary.aspx. Accessed July 23, 2014.
10. The National Coordinating Council for Medication Error Reporting and Prevention (NCC MERP). http://www.nccmerp.org. Accessed July 23, 2014.
11. Smetzer J, Baker C, Byrne FD, Cohen MR. Shaping systems for better behavioral choices: lessons learned from a fatal medication error. *Jt Comm J Qual Patient Saf*. 2010;36(4):152-163.
12. Reason J. Human error: models and management. *BMJ*. 2000;320(7237);768-770.
13. Ferner RE, Aronson JK. Clarification of terminology in medication errors: definitions and classifications. *Drug Saf*. 2006;29(11):1011-1022.
14. Karl R, Karl MC. Adverse events: root causes and latent factors. *Surg Clin North Am*. 2012;92(1):89-100.
15. Aspden P, Corrigan JM, Wolcott J, Erickson SM, eds. *Patient Safety: Achieving a New Standard for Care*. Washington, DC: National Academies Press; 2004.
16. Weaver SJ, Lubomski LJ, Wilson RF, Pfoh ER, Martinez KA, Dy SM. Promoting a culture of safety as a patient safety strategy: a systematic review. *Ann Intern Med*. 2013;158(5 part 2):369-374.
17. Institute for Safe Medication Practices. Benchmarking—when is it dangerous? https://www.ismp.org/Newsletters/acutecare/articles/19980909.asp. Published September 9, 1998. Accessed July 23, 2014.
18. Meyer-Massetti C, Cheng CM, Schwappach DL, et al. Systematic review of medication safety assessment methods. *Am J Health Syst Pharm*. 2011;68(3):227-240.
19. Cullen DJ, Bates DW, Small SD, Cooper JB, Nemeskal AR, Leape LL. The incident reporting system does not detect adverse drug events: a problem for quality improvement. *Jt Comm J Qual Improv*. 1995;21(10):541-548.
20. Institute for Safe Medication Practices. Frequently asked questions. http://www.ismp.org/faq.asp. Accessed July 23, 2014.
21. Pedersen CA, Schneider PJ, Scheckelhoff DJ. ASHP national survey of pharmacy practice in hospital settings: monitoring and patient education—2009. *Am J Health Syst Pharm*. 2010;67(7):542-558.
22. Agency for Healthcare Research and Quality. AHRQ patient safety primers: root cause analysis. Agency for Healthcare Research and Quality Patient Safety Network. http://psnet.ahrq.gov/primer.aspx?primerID=10. Accessed July 23, 2014.
23. Institute for Healthcare Improvement. Failure modes and effects analysis (FMEA) tool. http://www.ihi.org/knowledge/Pages/Tools/FailureModesandEffectsAnalysisTool.aspx. Accessed July 23, 2014.

24. American Society of Health-System Pharmacists. ASHP guidelines on preventing medication errors in hospitals. http://www.ashp.org/DocLibrary/BestPractices/MedMisGdlHosp.aspx. Accessed July 23, 2014.

25. American Society of Health-System Pharmacists. ASHP statement on the role of the medication safety leader. *Am J Health Syst Pharm*. 2013;70(5):448-452.

26. Food and Drug Administration. MedWatch: the FDA safety information and adverse event reporting program. http://www.fda.gov/Safety/MedWatch/default.htm. Accessed July 23, 2014.

27. Institute for Safe Medication Practices. The National Medication Errors Reporting Program (ISMP MERP). https://www.ismp.org/orderforms/reporterrortoismp.asp. Accessed July 23, 2014.

28. Abramson EL, Kaushal R. Computerized provider order entry and patient safety. *Pediatr Clin North Am*. 2012;59(6):1247-1255.

29. Patterson SM, Hughes C, Kerse N, Cardwell CR, Bradley MC. Interventions to improve the appropriate use of polypharmacy for older people. *Cochrane Database Syst Rev*. 2012;(5):CD008165. doi:10.1002/14651858.CD008165.pub2.

30. The American Geriatrics Society. American Geriatrics Society updated Beers Criteria for potentially inappropriate medication use in older adults. *J Am Geriatr Soc*. 2012;60(4):616-631.

31. National Quality Forum, National Priorities Partnership. Preventing medication errors: A $21 billion opportunity. Compact action brief: A roadmap for increasing value in health care. http://www.qualityforum.org/Publications/2010/12/Preventing_Medication_Errors_CAB.aspx. Published December 2010. Accessed July 23, 2014.

32. Institute for Healthcare Improvement. Innovation at its best: medication reconciliation. http://www.ihi.org/knowledge/Pages/ImprovementStories/InnovationatItsBestMedRec.aspx. Accessed July 23, 2014.

33. Mueller SK, Sponsler K, Kripalani S, Schnipper JL. Hospital-based medication reconciliation practices: a systematic review. *Arch Intern Med*. 2012;172(14):1057-1069.

34. Cornu P, Steurbaut S, Leysen T, et al. Effect of medication reconciliation at hospital admission on medication discrepancies during hospitalization and at discharge for geriatric patients. *Ann Pharmacother*. 2012;46(4):484-494.

35. Institute for Safe Medication Practices. ISMP high-alert medications. http://www.ismp.org/Tools/highalertmedicationLists.asp. Accessed July 23, 2014.

36. Food and Drug Administration. Food and Drug Administration Name Differentiation Project. http://www.fda.gov/Drugs/DrugSafety/MedicationErrors/ucm164587.htm. Accessed July 23, 2014.

37. Berman A. Reducing medication errors through naming, labeling, and packaging. *J Med Syst*. 2004;28(1):9-29.

38. Institute for Safe Medication Practices. There's more to the 60 Minutes story on heparin errors. *ISMP Medication Safety Alert!* http://www.ismp.org/newsletters/acutecare/articles/20080327.asp. Published March 27, 2008. Accessed July 23, 2014.

39. Food and Drug Administration Center for Drug Evaluation and Research. Guidance for Industry: Safety considerations for product design to minimize medication errors—draft guidance. http://www.fda.gov/Drugs/GuidanceComplianceRegulatoryInformation/Guidances/ucm331808.htm. Published December 2012. Accessed July 23, 2014.

40. ISMP. Guidance on the interdisciplinary safe use of automated dispensing cabinets. http://www.ismp.org/tools/guidelines/ADC_Guidelines_final.pdf. Published 2008. Accessed July 23, 2014.

41. Cochran GL, Jones KJ, Brockman J, Skinner A, Hicks RW. Errors prevented by and associated with bar-code medication administration systems. *Jt Comm J Qual Patient Saf*. 2007;33(5):293-301,245.

42. American Hospital Association, Health Research and Educational Trust, Institute for Safe Medication Practices. Assessing bedside bar-coding readiness: Pathways for medication safety. http://www.ismp.org/tools/pathwaysection3.pdf. Published 2002. Accessed July 23, 2014.

43. Wulff K, Cummings GG, Marck P, Yurtseven O. Medication administration technologies and patient safety: a mixed-method systematic review. *J Adv Nurs*. 2011;76(10):2080-2095.

44. Hall P. Interprofessional teamwork: professional cultures as barriers. *J Interprof Care*. 2005;19(suppl 1):188-196.

45. Kelly WN. Potential risks and prevention, part 4: reports of significant adverse drug event. *Am J Health Syst Pharm*. 2001;58(15):1406-1412.

46. Kaboli PJ, Hoth AB, McClimon BJ, Schnipper JL. Clinical pharmacists and inpatient medical care: a systematic review. *Arch Intern Med*. 2006;166(9):955-964.

47. Cohen V, Jellinek SP, Hatch A, Motov S. Effect of clinical pharmacists on care in the emergency department: a systematic review. *Am J Health Syst Pharm*. 2009;66(15):1353-1361.

48. Chisholm-Burns MA, Lee JK, Spivey CA, et al. US pharmacists' effect as team members on patient care: Systematic review and meta-analyses. *Med Care*. 2010;48(10):923-933.

# MEDICATION USE POLICY AND PERFORMANCE ASSESSMENT

Keri C. Anderson, PharmD, BCPS
Catherine Brown, PharmD, MSM, BCPS

## CHAPTER OBJECTIVES

▶ Evaluate the purpose of conducting a medication use evaluation.

▶ Analyze the processes involved in preparing and executing a medication use evaluation.

▶ Explain the steps involved in developing and writing a medication policy.

▶ Discuss the major drivers for the development of operational and clinical medication policies and guidelines.

▶ Describe important resources for development of operational and clinical medication policies and guidelines.

▶ Compare methods of assessing performance around medication policy.

## CHAPTER OUTLINE

## KEY TERMS

Benchmarks

Best practice

Clinical practice guideline

Collaborative practice drug therapy
management agreements

Conditions for Coverage

Conditions of Participation

Failure mode and effects analysis

5 Million Lives Campaign

High-alert medications

High-benefit medications

Improvement maps

Institutional review board

Medication error

Medication guideline

Medication management standards

Medication use evaluation

Medication use policy

Medication use process

Metrics

Order set

PDCA cycle

Pharmacy and therapeutics committee

Policy

Position statement

Quality improvement

Root cause analysis

Standards of practice

Tracer methodology

# INTRODUCTION

**Medication use policy** is how **standards of practice** in the profession of pharmacy are defined. In the hospital setting, the primary focus of this chapter, **policy** is how medication use is defined and specified, both operationally and clinically. What is the purpose of defining standards? Standards are defined to outline the operational practices and procedures based on regulatory mandates for safe and legal medication use. They are also defined to outline best practices clinically, and what is known to provide safety and the best outcome for patients given the evidence currently available in the medical literature. These **best practices** are often outlined in institutional **medication guidelines**, a subset of written policies that provide guidance for clinicians in selecting and monitoring appropriate therapy. Drivers for development of medication use policy and guidelines will be discussed later in the chapter.

# HOW MEDICATION POLICIES ARE DEVELOPED AND WRITTEN

It is important to understand how policies are developed and written in the hospital setting. The process of writing and developing medication policies involves a number of key steps:

- Define the policy need.
- Identify key policy stakeholders.
- Obtain stakeholder buy-in and input.

- Write a policy that addresses the identified need in an appropriate format with key elements.
- Obtain approval of stakeholders.
- Obtain institutional approval through the committee process.
- Educate affected staff on the approved policy.
- Implement the approved policy.
- If applicable, monitor the impact of the policy implementation.
- Make any needed changes to the policy based on monitoring.
- Maintain the policy according to system requirements.

A policy will arise from a need to define or clarify an operational or clinical standard of medication use. The *Handbook of Institutional Pharmacy Practice* defines a policy as a written statement that provides guidance on the position and values of an organization.[1] An accompanying procedure will consist of the steps needed to carry out the policy. Alternatively, the organization may choose to develop a guideline. Depending on how the terms *policy* and *guideline* are treated and used in an institution, a choice may be made to develop one or the other based on the need in question. One reasonable standard for choosing whether to develop a policy or a guideline is that a policy can be considered a directive that must always be followed (i.e., deviation is not acceptable), whereas a guideline is a directive that should be followed in most situations, but reasonable deviations are acceptable based on the situation. The latter designation may more reasonably be applied to a clinical directive, where patient-specific factors and clinical situations may warrant an occasional deviation from usual practice.

For example, the institution may want to define how and when herbal medications and dietary supplements may be used in the hospital setting. The point person tasked with policy development will begin by researching this topic. This could include:

- Surveying other hospitals about their supplement policy and obtaining copies for reference.
- Conducting a primary literature search about supplement product standards.
- Researching supplement use in hospitalized patients.
- Researching specific supplements relevant to practice in the region or the institution.
- Reviewing state law.
- Reviewing national guidelines.
- Reviewing medication management standards.

Having defined the need and done considerable research, the next step is to identify the key stakeholders. Those who may have input on this issue include hospital physicians, pharmacists, dieticians, nurses, and risk or quality management hospital staff, who are intimately familiar with regulatory requirements. Although leadership personnel often have clear ideas about policy requirements, it is also important to consider the viewpoint of the bedside staff who must implement and use the policy. This perspective is often a real-world view that is often neglected during policy development. Depending on the organization's culture and size, input and buy-in may be sought individually by the policy writer or it may be obtained in a meeting convened to make decisions about the policy. Once a consensus has been reached, the policy can be drafted.

To draft a policy or guideline, the writer must follow the institution's accepted format. Policy format varies considerably from institution to institution. The Joint Commission (TJC) and other entities do not require a specific format. However, there are some common elements in policies that are reasonable to include, as shown in **Table 17-1**.

It is important to identify the scope of the policy. To what patient population (e.g., adults, pediatrics, neonates) and what treatment setting does the policy apply (e.g., all

| TABLE 17-1    Policy Guideline Elements |
| --- |
| Policy number |
| Scope |
| Policy statement |
| Background/rationale |
| History |
| Inclusion/exclusion criteria |
| Procedure |
| Affected personnel |
| Responsibilities |
| Definitions |
| List of related policies |
| List of related order sets |
| Point person or position |
| Approval dates by various committees |
| Review cycle |

inpatients, critical care patients, patients on telemetry)? For medication guidelines, inclusion and exclusion criteria that describe when the guideline should be used for a specific patient's therapy may be needed. A brief statement of the policy, often with a short background or rationale, is also important. The full document may contain considerable detail, but a brief summary of the policy will clarify the issue for staff who must carry out the policy. For institutions that combine policies and procedures in one document, the policy must also provide a clear outline of any associated procedure and clear definition of who has the responsibility for carrying out the policy. Clear expectations are essential for a successful policy implementation. Sometimes definitions must be included in a policy. If terminology is not immediately clear or staff need a clear definition of a term to understand when to apply the policy, then terms and definitions should be included. For administrative reasons, it may be helpful to include several other elements as well. Identification of related policies, or **order sets**, that are affected by the policy is useful to serve as a reminder of the downstream effects when undergoing policy revisions. Likewise, it may be useful to track approval dates by various hospital committees, identify a point of contact for the policy if there are questions, and specify the review cycle for the policy.

Once a policy has been drafted, the writer should use due diligence and revisit stakeholders to be certain that the final version still represents the original intent of the policy and can be reasonably implemented. Specific word and phrasing choices may be significantly important to provide a final document that staff can follow in the institution and that will fully meet regulatory requirements. Once stakeholders are satisfied, the next hurdle is approval of the policy or guideline through the institution's usual process. This may require presentation at one or more relevant medical staff committees; the **pharmacy and therapeutics committee** (P&T), which has oversight over policies or guidelines involving medications; and the executive policy approval committee or medical executive committee (MEC). Given the steps in the process and the necessary review and oversight for a policy, the time line for approval of a new or revised hospital policy may reasonably take several weeks to months.

Once a new policy, or a policy with significant revisions, is approved, hospital managers or the hospital education department is often tasked with educating staff on the policy in preparation for implementation. Depending on the number and significance of practice changes for bedside staff, this may be a minor or major undertaking. Minor policy changes can often be communicated through staff meetings, tip sheets, memos, or even email. Major changes or policies with a significant impact may require classroom education time or even completion of competencies to document mastery, which can be difficult to schedule for bedside staff.

Once education is completed, a target date is often set for implementation of a policy or guideline. Bedside staff must be made aware that the changes will go into place on the date specified. If improvement in performance is desired for institutional or regulatory purposes, hospital staff may be given specific **metrics** to document during a specified postimplementation period. Metrics may then be analyzed and change in performance documented and communicated. Analysis of performance around medication use—that is, medication use evaluation (MUE)—is discussed in more detail in a later section. This process may also yield information about additional changes to policy or procedure that can be considered when the policy is up for review in the future. As the *Handbook of Institutional Pharmacy Practice* states, "Applying the Deming Plan-Do-Check-Act (PDCA) Cycle to develop and maintain policies and procedures can be helpful."[1] PDCA will be discussed in greater detail later in the chapter. Depending on policy type and regulatory requirements, the review cycle for policies in a hospital typically ranges from every 1 to 3 years.

# DRIVERS FOR DEVELOPMENT OF A MEDICATION USE POLICY

A discussion of the drivers for development of both operational and clinical medication use policy is important for developing a complete understanding of medication use policy. First, the focus will be on drivers for development of operational policy. One significant driver is pharmacy law. Federal and state law both suggest policies that must be developed. In an example from federal law, section 1304.04 of Title 21 (Controlled Substances Act) specifies maintenance and recording of inventories of controlled substances.[2] This section of federal law will prompt institutional policy that outlines how the institution will meet these legal requirements. An institution must also respond to state law. In Washington State law, for example, WAC 246-873-080 states, in part:

> All drug containers in the hospital shall be labeled clearly, legibly and adequately to show the drug's name (generic and/or trade) and strength when applicable. Accessory or cautionary statements and the expiration date shall be applied to containers as appropriate.[3]

This section of state law may prompt the need for specific policy around labeling requirements in the hospital. The law may even explicitly require an institution to write policy. For example, WAC 246-873-080 also states, in part:

> The director [of pharmacy] shall establish, annually review and update when necessary comprehensive written policies and procedures governing the responsibilities and functions of the pharmaceutical service. Policies affecting patient care and treatment involving drug use shall be established by the director of pharmacy with the cooperation and input of the medical staff, nursing service and the administration.[3]

This broad directive not only addresses what policy must encompass, it also offers direction on *how* policy should be developed.

The many requirements from governmental regulatory agencies, such as the Centers for Medicare and Medicaid Services (CMS), also drive policy development. According to the CMS website:

> CMS develops Conditions of Participation (CoPs) and Conditions for Coverage (CfCs) that health care organizations must meet in order to begin and continue participating in the Medicare and Medicaid programs. These health and safety standards are the foundation for improving quality and protecting the health and safety of beneficiaries.[4]

When a hospital undergoes a validation survey by a state agency to ensure adherence to CMS **Conditions of Participation** (CoPs) and **Conditions for Coverage** (CfCs), the agency specifically looks to see if medications are being prepared and administered in line with the law and regulations and with hospital policy. This means that surveyors will observe practice in the hospital, but they will also review hospital policies to be certain that practice is following policy. An example is the need to develop policy around the use of single-dose/single-use medication vials for injection. Single-dose vials, according to CMS, may not be used for multiple patients unless repackaging occurs within USP 797 standards; otherwise it is unacceptable under CMS's infection control regulations.[5] USP 797 is a regulation developed by the US Pharmacopoeia (USP) that applies to any pharmacy that prepares compounded sterile preparations. The Centers for Disease Control (CDC) has also released a guideline and **position statement** on the same topic that reinforces the need for a policy on safe use of single-dose vials.[6] Other governmental agencies that affect the need for policy development include the Food and Drug Administration (FDA) and the National Institute for Occupational Safety and Health (NIOSH).[1]

Hospital accrediting bodies also require policy making. TJC, in its Leadership Standards, requires hospitals to have policies and procedures that support safe medication management.[7] See **Table 17-2** for the list of medication management topics for which TJC requires policies.[8] Although TJC may be familiar to many, other accrediting organizations include the Healthcare Facilities Accreditation Program (HFAP) and Det Norsk Veritas (first approved by CMS to accredit hospitals in 2008). All of these bodies are authorized to survey facilities for CMS's conditions of participation and coverage and must be periodically reauthorized by federal law.

Upon accreditation, institutions are "deemed" to be in compliance with CMS CoPs.[4] Although TJC standards for accreditation are not always exactly the same as CMS CoPs, hospital policy regarding medications relies heavily on TJC's list of required standards specifically regarding medication management. These medication standards guide pharmacists in developing a medication management strategy featuring all stages of medication use, including selection, storage, ordering, dispensing, administration, and monitoring.[9] Policy may be written to outline and refine this strategy. Hospital accrediting bodies, including TJC, also survey to be certain practice is following hospital policy.

Medication policy development or revision may also arise out of the need to improve medication safety. FDA MedWatch alerts can prompt the need for policy change.[10] Safety organizations and institutional needs may push policy development for specific issues. The Institute for Safe Medication Practices (ISMP) is a nonprofit organization dedicated to safe medication use and prevention of **medication errors**.[11] The ISMP provides a variety of tools to help pharmacists and other healthcare providers implement safe practices around medication use, including newsletters, a regular column in *Hospital Pharmacy*, and quarterly action agendas with recommendations about specific medications.[12] It also provides onsite consulting services to evaluate medication use processes at an institution and recommend best practice. The Institute for Healthcare Improvement (IHI) launched the **5 Million Lives Campaign** to reduce morbidity and mortality in health care, including adverse drug events and surgical complications.[13] Out of this, initiatives have emerged to help hospitals improve in core focus areas such as reducing surgical site infections and the incidence of venous thromboembolism. The organization provides **improvement maps** that may trigger policies around a number of medication use issues, such as antibiotic stewardship.[14]

A number of resources are available to access the laws, regulations, accreditation standards, and safety initiatives that will help pharmacists with development of appropriate medication use policy. **Table 17-3** lists some pertinent resources.

**TABLE 17-2** Documentation Specifically Required in Medication Management Standards

| | |
|---|---|
| MM.01.01.01 | The availability of patient information |
| MM.01.01.03 | A list of high-alert and hazardous medications |
| MM.01.02.01 | A list of look-alike and sound-alike medications |
| MM.02.01.01 | Written criteria for formulary agents |
| MM.02.01.01 | A formulary, including medication strength and dosage |
| MM.02.01.01 | Written medication substitution protocols in event of medication shortage or outage |
| MM.03.01.01 | The control of medication between receipt by a healthcare provider and administration of the medication |
| MM.04.01.01 | The types of medication orders deemed acceptable by the organization |
| MM.04.01.01 | Required elements of a complete medication order |
| MM.04.01.01 | Occasions when the indication for use is required on a medication order |
| MM.04.01.01 | Precautions for ordering medications with look-alike or sound-alike names |
| MM.04.01.01 | Actions to take when medication orders are incomplete, illegible, or unclear |
| MM.04.01.01 | The circumstances for which weight-based dosing is required for pediatrics |
| MM.05.01.17 | How medications recalled or discontinued for safety reasons by the manufacturer or FDA will be retrieved and handled |
| MM.06.01.01 | LIPS and clinical staff disciplines who can administer medications |
| MM.06.01.03 | The organization's process for self-administration of medications |
| MM.06.01.05 | The organization's process for investigational medications |
| MM.07.01.03 | Response to actual or potential adverse drug events, significant adverse drug reactions, and medication errors |
| MM.07.01.03 | Notification of the prescriber in the event of an adverse drug event, significant adverse drug reaction, or medication error |

Data from Policies and Procedures Checklist. In Uselton JP, Kienle PC, Murdaugh LB, eds. *Assuring Continuous Compliance with Joint Commission Standards: A Pharmacy Guide.* 8th ed. Washington, DC: ASHP; 2008:203-225.

Finally, institutional needs will also play a role. An institution that has a significant medication error and conducts a **root cause analysis** (RCA) may determine that a policy is needed to prevent a similar error from occurring again. Hospitals may also pursue new policies when they learn about nationally reported medication errors that could potentially occur at their own institution. For example, ISMP reported in the January 12, 2012, issue of the *Medication Safety Alert!* newsletter that multiple instances have occurred where nurses had used the same insulin pen for more than one patient, thinking it was acceptable practice because they had used different needles on the pen for each patient.[30] Due to the risk of cross contamination and infectious disease transmission even with a needle change, ISMP recommends assigning individual pens to patients. For an institution that uses insulin pens, it is important to specify this recommendation in policy.

Likewise, an institution conducting a **failure mode and effects analysis** (FMEA) while reviewing a new drug for its formulary may find that a policy will help prevent an anticipated potential error with a medication. According to the Institute for Healthcare

**TABLE 17-3** Resources for Policy Development

**Federal Drug Law**

Food and Drug Administration: Federal Food, Drug and Cosmetic Act[15]

Drug Enforcement Administration: Title 21 United States Code (USC) Controlled Substances Act[16]

National Institute for Occupational Safety and Health: Preventing Occupational Exposure to Antineoplastic and other Hazardous Drugs in Healthcare Settings[17] and NIOSH List of Antineoplastic and Other Hazardous Drugs in Healthcare Settings[18]

**State Pharmacy Law**

National Association of Boards of Pharmacy[19]

NABPLAW Online: The Source for State Pharmacy Laws and Regulations[20]

**Regulatory Agencies**

Center for Medicare and Medicaid Services: Conditions for Coverage and Conditions of Participations, Hospitals

Food and Drug Administration

Centers for Disease Control[21]

United States Pharmacopeial Convention: Pharmaceutical Compounding—Sterile Preparations <797> (USP 797)[22]

**Accreditation Agencies**

The Joint Commission: National Patient Safety Goals[23]

The Healthcare Facilities Accreditation Program (HFAP)[24]

Det Norsk Veritas: DNV Accreditation Requirements[25]

**Professional Associations**

American Society for Health-System Pharmacists: Guidelines[26]

American Society for Health-System Pharmacists: *Assuring Continuous Compliance with Joint Commission Standards: A Pharmacy Guide, Eighth Edition*[27]

**Safety Organizations**

Institute for Safe Medication Practice: *Medication Safety Alert!* newsletter[28]

Institute for Healthcare Improvement[29]

Improvement, "[FMEA] is a systematic, proactive method for evaluating a process to identify where and how it might fail, and to assess the relative impact of different failures in order to identify the parts of the process that are most in need of change."[31] This assessment can be done with medications to determine what might go wrong with inappropriate use. This could prompt development of a policy or guideline around a medication for safety. One example might be the development of a guideline for fingolimod (Gilenya™), a medication for multiple sclerosis, to be certain that an electrocardiogram (ECG) is performed at appropriate times upon initiation of the medication in an institution.

Operations are not the only realm for policies around medications. To ensure positive outcomes for patients, the institution must also think clinically, and policies or medication guidelines can be an important tool to guide therapy to obtain these outcomes. They help healthcare practitioners make the best decisions about treatment for patients. In this case, the best evidence should guide the institution to outline and follow the best practice. Where are the best evidence and documented best practice found? They are found in national guidelines issued by medical and pharmacy associations, government agencies, and other institutions. See **Table 17-4** for examples of some commonly encountered guidelines and sources. The National Guideline Clearinghouse is also a well-known resource for evidence-based **clinical practice guidelines**.[32]

**TABLE 17-4**    Clinical Practice Guidelines and Sources

**American College of Chest Physicians:** Antithrombotic Therapy and Prevention of Thrombosis[33]

**American Society of Regional Anesthesia and Pain Medicine:** Regional Anesthesia in the Patient Receiving Antithrombotic or Thrombolytic Therapy: Evidence-Based Guidelines[34]

**American College of Chest Physicians/American Heart Association:** Guidelines for the Diagnosis and Management of Heart Failure in Adults[35]

**American College of Cardiology Foundation/American Heart Association Task Force on Practice Guidelines, and the American College of Physicians, American Association for Thoracic Surgery, Preventive Cardiovascular Nurses Association, Society for Cardiovascular Angiography and Interventions, and Society of Thoracic Surgeons:** Guideline for the Diagnosis and Management of Patients With Stable Ischemic Heart Disease: Executive Summary[36]

**National Heart, Lung, and Blood Institute:** The Seventh Report of the Joint National Committee on Prevention, Detection, Evaluation, and Treatment of High Blood Pressure[37]

**National Heart, Lung, and Blood Institute:** Third Report of the Expert Panel on Detection, Evaluation, and Treatment of High Blood Cholesterol in Adults[38]

**National Heart, Lung, and Blood Institute:** Guidelines for the Diagnosis and Management of Asthma[39]

**American Diabetes Association (ADA) and the European Association for the Study of Diabetes (EASD):** Management of Hyperglycemia in Type 2 Diabetes: A Patient-Centered Approach[40]

**Infectious Diseases Society of America:** Immunization of Infants, Children, Adolescents, and Adults: Clinical Practice Guidelines[41]

**American Society of Health-System Pharmacists:** Clinical Practice Guidelines for Antimicrobial Prophylaxis in Surgery[42]

**HHS Panel on Antiretroviral Guidelines for Adults and Adolescents:** Guidelines for the Use of Antiretroviral Agents in HIV-1-Infected Adults and Adolescents[43]

**American Society of Clinical Oncology:** Antiemetics: ASCO Clinical Practice Guideline Update[44]

**American Psychiatric Association:** Practice Guideline for the Treatment of Patients With Major Depressive Disorder[45]

The various national guidelines outline acceptable and approved standards of care that help institutions and providers achieve preferred outcomes. According to the National Library of Medicine:

> Guidelines are statements of principles or procedures that assist professionals in ensuring quality in such areas as clinical practice, biomedical research, and health services. Practice guidelines assist the health care practitioner with patient care decisions about appropriate diagnostic, therapeutic, or other clinical procedures for specific clinical circumstances.[46]

According to the Institute of Medicine's Committee on Standards for Developing Trustworthy Clinical Practice Guidelines:

> Clinical practice guidelines are statements that include recommendations intended to optimize patient care that are informed by a systematic review of evidence and an assessment of the benefits and harms of alternative care options. To be *trustworthy*, guidelines should:

- be based on a systematic review of the existing evidence;
- be developed by a knowledgeable, multidisciplinary panel of experts and representatives from key affected groups;

- consider important patient subgroups and patient preferences, as appropriate;
- be based on an explicit and transparent process that minimizes distortions, biases, and conflicts of interest;
- provide a clear explanation of the logical relationships between alternative care options and health outcomes, and provide ratings of both the quality of evidence and the strength of the recommendations; and
- be reconsidered and revised as appropriate when important new evidence warrants modifications of recommendations.[47]

The nationally accepted guidelines are the building blocks for clinically oriented drug policies in the institution. Some hospital medication guidelines may be written as **collaborative practice drug therapy management agreements**, also commonly referred to as *prescriptive protocols*. Most states allow the pharmacist to manage therapy under the supervision of a physician, and many also allow a pharmacist to initiate therapy under protocol.[48]

In summary, drug policies in the hospital setting are prompted by a variety of needs. **Table 17–5** lists some of the common types of medication use policies that hospitals often develop, many of which are encouraged or required by TJC.[1]

| **TABLE 17-5**  Common Types of Medication Use Policies | |
|---|---|
| Operational | Adverse drug reaction management |
| | Automated dispensing cabinets |
| | Biohazardous medication handling |
| | Controlled substance management |
| | Discharge prescriptions |
| | Drug formulary system |
| | Floor stock medications |
| | Herbal and dietary supplement use |
| | High-alert medications |
| | Investigational drugs |
| | IV admixture services |
| | Look-alike, sound-alike medications |
| | Medication administration and documentation |
| | Medication errors |
| | Medication orders |
| | Medication storage and security |
| | Multiple-dose medication container management |
| | Patient self-administration of medication |
| | Recalled medications |
| | Scope of pharmacy services |
| Clinical | Aminoglycoside and vancomycin dosing |
| | Anticoagulation therapy management |
| | Antiemetic therapy management |
| | IV-to-oral route change |
| | Parenteral nutrition |
| | Potassium administration |
| | Renal dosing |

Data from Tomich DJ, Dydek GJ. The policy and procedure manual. In Brown TR, ed. *Handbook of Institutional Pharmacy Practice.* Washington, DC: ASHP; 2006:297-312.

# ASSESSING PERFORMANCE WITH REGARD TO MEDICATION POLICY

## OPERATIONAL PERFORMANCE ASSESSMENT: LOGS, CHECKLISTS, AND TRACERS

Performance assessment is a critical step to documenting appropriate medication use and adherence to policy in the organization. One significant reason for the assessment is financial. For example, the hospital pharmacy may monitor medication wastage to find ways to minimize associated financial losses. Regulatory reasons for assessing operational performance are also very important. The hospital must ensure that policies that have been written are followed. This will ensure both patient safety and preparation for survey by regulatory agencies.

Operational performance may be assessed in a number of ways. Log sheets and checklists may be used to document that activities and procedures required by hospital medication policies have occurred. Checklists may be used to document that medication storage areas throughout the hospital have been checked on a periodic basis and found to be in compliance with regulations. Temperature logs are used to document that refrigerators and freezers are maintained at appropriate temperatures for vaccines and other temperature-sensitive medications. Regulatory agencies will look for this type of documentation of operational performance during audits. Similarly, they will check that laminar flow hoods in clean rooms have received required periodic maintenance. Hospitals may use log sheets and checklists for safety reasons as well. For example, batch log sheets may be used to document proper preparation and checking of batches of compounded medications. Checklists may also be used to document each step in the preparation of chemotherapy agents to verify that proper procedures were followed, thus ensuring safety.

Operational performance may also be assessed by the tracer methodology. **Tracer methodology** is the survey method favored by TJC. According to TJC:

> Tracer methodology is an evaluation method in which surveyors select a patient, resident, or client and use that individual's record as a roadmap to move through an organization to assess and evaluate the organization's compliance with selected standards and the organization's systems of providing care and services. Surveyors retrace the specific care processes that an individual experienced by observing and talking to staff in areas that the individual received care. As surveyors follow the course of a patient's, resident's, or client's treatment, they assess the healthcare organization's compliance with Joint Commission standards. They conduct this compliance assessment as they review the organization's systems for delivering safe, quality health care.[49]*

TJC also conducts system tracers specifically around medication management. As discussed in TJC's *Survey Activities Guide*, surveyors examine the institution's medication management process from procurement through administration and monitoring. They also look at medication reconciliation as a patient moves from one level of care to the next. Finally, they will review other processes, such as medication error reporting, performance improvement initiatives, education of staff and patients around medications, use of the patient's own medications, information management systems pertaining to medications, and involvement of patients in medication management.[50]

The tracer methodology may also be used by hospital personnel or medication safety teams to monitor their own performance around **medication management standards** and to ensure ongoing survey readiness.

# CLINICAL PERFORMANCE ASSESSMENT: MEDICATION USE EVALUATION

Medication use evaluation is the primary method for clinical performance assessment in the hospital setting. The American Society of Health-System Pharmacists (ASHP) defines a **medication use evaluation** (MUE) as a performance improvement method focused on the evaluation and improvement of medication use processes to optimize patient outcomes.[51] The term medication use evaluation is considered by the Academy of Managed Care Pharmacy to be synonymous with *drug utilization review*, *drug use evaluation*, and *medication use management*.[52] Irrespective of the term utilized, all refer to an observational, systematic evaluation using a **quality improvement** method such as a plan-do-check-act (PDCA) model for improvement.[53] **Table 17-6** provides a description of the steps involved in the model for improvement, which involves defining the purpose of an MUE or performance improvement project and implementing the **PDCA cycle** (also see **Appendix 17-A**).[54,55]

The purpose of conducting an MUE is to identify, resolve, or prevent actual or potential medication problems that could prevent health systems from achieving optimal patient care outcomes.[51] Objectives for MUE have been set forth by ASHP and are as follows:

- Promote optimal medication therapy and evaluate the effectiveness of medication therapy.
- Prevent medication-related problems and improve patient safety.
- Establish interdisciplinary consensus on medication use processes.
- Stimulate improvements and standardization in medication use processes.
- Utilize innovative medication use practices to improve patient outcomes and resource utilization and minimize procedural variations that contribute to suboptimal outcomes.
- Identify areas in which further information and education for healthcare professionals may be needed.
- Minimize costs of medication therapy, including costs of complications and wasted resources.
- Meet or exceed internal and external quality standards (e.g., professional practice standards, accreditation standards, or government laws and regulations).

MUE may focus on the use of one medication, or it can be applied broadly to assess a therapeutic class, disease, condition, outcome, or any step in the **medication use process** (i.e., prescribing, transcribing, dispensing, administering, monitoring).[51] Emphases for MUEs in the hospital may be requested by the P&T committee, medication safety

| TABLE 17-6 | PDCA Model for Improvement | |
|---|---|---|
| Step 1: Purpose | What is the goal? What can be done to improve? How is improvement defined? | |
| Step 2: PDCA cycle | Plan | How will it be done? (who, what, when, where?) |
| | Do | Collect data. |
| | Check (or study) | Summarize what is learned and identify improvements. |
| | Act | Implement improvements. |

Data from American Society of Health-System Pharmacists. The pharmacist's role in quality improvement. http://www
.ashp.org/DocLibrary/Policy/QII/RoleinQI.aspx. Accessed July 23, 2014.

committee, quality improvement committee, multidisciplinary subcommittees, or individuals reporting to these groups. MUEs are commonly conducted on **high-alert medications**, error-prone medications, **high-benefit medications**, or medications that must be utilized properly within a specified time period to achieve a beneficial outcome (e.g., insulin, anticoagulants, antibiotics, alteplase). MUEs may also be conducted following increased reports of adverse events, medication errors, noncompliance with formulary restrictions or criteria for use policies, FDA MedWatch alerts, or TJC indicator updates. **Table 17-7** provides examples of the different emphases of MUEs.

To conduct an MUE, a thorough search of the literature is the first step in determining scope and formulating a proposal. The MUE proposal should include the following elements:

- Objective or purpose of the evaluation
- Background to summarize relevant information on the topic
- Summary of the methods of how the evaluation will be conducted (e.g., retrospective chart review, inclusion criteria, time period assessed)
- Listing of all criteria to be evaluated
- References utilized

The P&T committee, quality improvement committee, or another multidisciplinary committee should review the proposal to provide suggestions for improvement prior to initiation of data collection. An MUE is typically exempt from review by an **institutional review board** (IRB), because it is an observational, internal quality improvement process. An example of an MUE template containing the sections for a proposal is provided in **Appendix 17-B**. The template may vary at each institution,

| **TABLE 17-7** | Medication Use Evaluation Topics | |
|---|---|---|
| **Emphasis** | **Example** | **Description of Evaluation** |
| Medication | Daptomycin | Indications for use, contraindications, dosing, dose adjustments in special populations, duration of therapy, monitoring, infection cure rate, infectious disease service consulted |
| Therapeutic class | Proton pump inhibitors | Discontinuation upon discharge if ordered for stress ulcer prophylaxis |
| Disease state | Acute myocardial infarction | Aspirin administered in patients with chest pain within 24 hours of arrival |
| Condition | Hypoglycemia | Adherence to hospital policy for correction of hypoglycemic events |
| Medication use process | Prescribing | Use of unapproved abbreviations |
| | Transcribing | Accuracy of order entry |
| | Dispensing | Time from order entry to medication administration |
| | Administering | Administrations of medications within 30 minutes of the scheduled administration time |
| | Monitoring | Documentation of pain scores following administration of pain medications |
| Outcome | Length of stay | Use of alvimopan to decrease length of stay following surgery |

and it is important to include sections and follow the formatting for the institution. The U.S. Department of Veterans Affairs published an MUE Toolkit online that includes an MUE template with instructions for completing each section.[56]

Criteria for medication use are defined through internal medication use policies, protocols, guidelines, external standard-setting bodies (e.g., TJC, Medicare), FDA-approved manufacturer labeling, and the primary literature.[51] Criteria are established to assess appropriate use of a medication and may include parameters to assess prescribing, administration, monitoring, safety, effectiveness, timeliness, and many other items. Criteria should be clearly defined in the MUE proposal to avoid variation in the data collection process or misinterpretation of results. For example, criteria to evaluate the appropriate monitoring of warfarin should be described specifically. If monitoring is merely categorized as appropriate or inappropriate, then it is unclear why the monitoring was acceptable or unacceptable, because one can interpret these terms in many different ways. More-specific criteria would include the evaluation of patients with a daily INR ordered while receiving warfarin and those with a baseline INR ordered prior to initiation of warfarin therapy. These criteria assessed individually will provide information of what specifically needs to change to improve the monitoring of warfarin therapy. Additionally, setting **benchmarks**, or acceptable thresholds, for each criterion aids in establishing the goal for the outcome. Benchmarks are typically expressed as a percentage and may be set based on internal standards of the organization, external standard-setting bodies (e.g., TJC, Medicare), by comparison to other hospitals (e.g., www.medicare.gov/hospitalcompare), guidelines, or primary literature articles. Descriptive characteristics should also be predefined to aid in describing the sample; examples include the indication for which the medication was prescribed or the medical service of the ordering physician. Creation of a data collection form (paper or electronic) aids in the data collection process to ensure that all criteria and characteristics are collected and interpreted appropriately. An example of a data collection form is provided in **Appendix 17–C**. Facts and Comparisons eAnswers has published several examples of data collection forms for individual drug products through a subscription to the online Formulary Monograph Service.[57]

Most MUEs are conducted retrospectively; however, data can also be collected prospectively or concurrently.[53] Prospective review occurs prior to dispensing the medication, concurrent review occurs at the time the patient is receiving treatment, and retrospective review is a historical evaluation of medication therapy that occurs after the patient has been administered a medication.[52] Each design has benefits and limitations. Prospective evaluation allows for prescribing trends to be evaluated while still providing the opportunity for interventions to occur prior to the patient receiving therapy. For example, a prospective MUE evaluating the ability of healthcare providers to separate doses of levothyroxine from calcium-, iron-, or aluminum-containing drug products would provide an opportunity to correct the error prior to it ever reaching the patient yet also trend the percentage of prescribed orders that are not separated from these products by at least 4 hours. Concurrent evaluation provides the opportunity for criteria to be evaluated at the time the patient is receiving a medication. For example, if conducting an MUE on postoperative pain management, the evaluation can be designed to ensure that all patients' pain scores are documented at baseline and within an appropriate time frame following medication administration. Qualitative and quantitative measures may be utilized to evaluate the effectiveness of the medication on patient outcomes. Limitations of both prospective and concurrent evaluations include planning for a longer time period for data collection, depending on the sample size needed and frequency of events; reliance on multiple individuals for data collection; and adding more responsibilities to individual healthcare providers. Retrospective review may occur rapidly if software systems with data mining capabilities are utilized for data collection. The time period for retrospective evaluation may be expanded or easily adjusted for seasonal variations in medication use. A significant limitation of retrospective review is the lack of documentation in the medical record for criteria, such as monitoring parameters or adverse events associated with medication use. Missing data may affect the ability to draw complete conclusions or make useful recommendations.

The following are potential sources of data to be evaluated for MUEs:

- The medical record (i.e., orders, progress notes, allergies, labs)
- Clinical decision support system alerts
- Dispensing records or automated dispensing cabinet reports
- Medication administration records
- Bar-coding reports
- Smart-pump alert reports
- Insurance codes or claims

Direct observation of techniques such as compounding or administration of medications may also be evaluated. Data collection is conducted by one individual or a team of trained individuals (e.g., pharmacists, residents, students). The evaluation period may differ depending on the frequency of use or seasonal use of the medication in order to extract an adequate sample size (i.e., 1 month, 6 months, 1 year). **Table 17–8** provides suggested sample sizes for evaluation as provided by the TJC for performance improvement activities.[58] A more sophisticated method for determining sample size has been described and assistance from a statistician may be utilized.[59]

Once collected, the data should be compiled and analyzed. If using a paper data collection form, the information should be transferred into a spreadsheet or database to quantify the results. If the information is initially entered into an electronic form and saved in a database, a more rapid analysis of results can occur. Once the analysis is complete, the information should be represented in the results section of the MUE and expressed as a percentage. Some organizations may request that results are displayed as both a fraction and a percentage. The percentage is calculated by dividing the number of patients meeting the criteria by the total number of patients assessed and then multiplied by 100:

$$\frac{\text{Number of patients meeting the criteria}}{\text{Total number of patients assessed}} \times 100 = \text{Percentage compliant}$$

Tables and graphs provide a visual representation of results and aid in demonstrating trends and should be included in the results section. A notes section embedded in tables with exceptions or variation in outcomes may aid in explanation of results. An explanation for variation in outcomes or limitations of the data collection process may

| TABLE 17-8  Appropriate Sample Sizes for Analysis | |
|---|---|
| **Population** | **Sample** |
| < 30 cases | All cases |
| 30–100 | 30 |
| 101–500 | 50 |
| > 500 | 70 |

be described and included in the discussion section. A multidisciplinary group should analyze the results, identify system improvements, provide insight into formulating a proposed action plan, and propose a time line for implementation. The recommendations from the multidisciplinary group should be included in the conclusion section of the MUE. An example of a completed MUE template is provided in **Appendix 17-D**. Additional examples have been published in the primary literature and online by the World Health Organization.[60]

MUE results and recommendations for improvement should be presented to the organizational body with oversight of the process, which in many institutions is the P&T committee. Recommendations for improvement or corrective action may prompt a combination of the following:

- Creation or revision of medication use policies, processes, or criteria for use.
- Creation or revision of order sets or clinical pathways.
- Formulary changes (i.e., addition, deletion).
- System alerts.
- Departmental education (i.e., medical staff, pharmacy, nursing, lab).

Once the new process is approved, changes should be implemented by a multidisciplinary team. Changes may be tested on a small scale (e.g., one unit, few patients) to identify implementation improvements prior to distribution in the entire organization. Once the processes for implementation are refined, changes should be communicated using multiple means for successful implementation. Communication methods include department meetings, in-services, computer-based learning tools, newsletters, flyers, posters, and e-mail. After implementation, the PDCA model for improvement should be repeated within an appropriate time frame (quarterly, annually) to reassess for continuous quality improvement.

Pharmacists are inherently qualified to conduct and oversee the MUE process given their involvement in medication use. Responsibilities of pharmacists have been previously defined by ASHP and include the following:[61]

- Develop a plan for MUE and identify and plan for evaluation.
- Create policies, processes, and criteria for effective medication use.
- Promote adherence to policies, processes, and criteria.
- Conduct MUEs (plan/collect data/analyze data).
- Work with the multidisciplinary team to develop an action plan based on the MUE results.
- Implement the action plan (education, revising medication use policies).
- Reevaluate after the action plan has been implemented.

MUE should be considered a best practice, because it can substantially improve quality or safety and has a financial return on investment (ROI) of 51-100% of the amount invested.[62,63] MUE has been found to be a moderately complicated element, requiring the investment of 0.5-1.0 full-time employee (FTE) in labor and/or a moderate amount of other direct expenses to implement. Drug information specialists or medication safety officers commonly perform MUE activities and also provide oversight for residents as part of a required component of postgraduate year one (PGY1) residency training.[63-65] All pharmacists should be prepared to participate in the MUE process, because it is conducted in various patient care settings (i.e., health systems, hospitals, ambulatory care clinics, community pharmacies, skilled nursing facilities, managed care organizations) and in both large and small institutions. In 2010, the ASHP national survey of pharmacy practice in hospital settings evaluated the use of drug policy tools by the P&T committee to improve medication use and medication safety and quality

---

**CASE STUDY 17-1**     **Policy Development: Noninjectable Biohazardous Medications**

You are a pharmacist working at a 150-bed community hospital. You have noticed inconsistent practice in the handling of noninjectable biohazardous medications among nursing and pharmacy staff. You are concerned that staff may be at risk from improper handling, and you and bring it up to your supervisor. Your supervisor agrees that there is reason for concern. She assigns you to research further to determine if a policy is needed around proper handling of noninjectable biohazardous medications and, if there is a clear rationale for a policy, that you be the point of contact for getting it approved and implemented in your hospital.

1. Describe how you would define the policy need. (Why is there a policy need? What would the policy accomplish? Should it be developed as a policy or a guideline? How would you determine what needs to be included?)
2. Describe how you would identify key policy stakeholders and obtain their buy-in and input.
3. List some common elements you might include in your policy or guideline.
4. Describe how you would obtain approval of the policy by stakeholders and committees once it is written.
5. Describe how you might educate affected staff on the approved policy or guideline.
6. Describe what steps you might take after implementation.

improvement activities.[66] Of the sample of 1,968 hospitals surveyed, approximately 566, or 29%, responded. To accurately apply results to the population, weights were assigned to responses to adjust for the sampling method used. Results showed that MUEs are conducted by 66.2% ($n = 563$) of hospitals; larger hospitals (> 600 beds, $n = 53$) reported a higher rate of evaluation, at 98.1%, than smaller hospitals (< 50 beds, $n = 93$), which had a rate of 41.9%.

---

**CASE STUDY 17-2**     **Policy Development: Anticoagulation and Neuraxial Procedures**

You are a pharmacist working at a 300-bed community hospital, and you have a strong interest in anticoagulation issues. You have been to a recent national pharmacy conference where updates to national anticoagulation guidelines have been presented and discussed. You speak to two different pharmacists at the talk, and it comes up in conversation that their facilities have a guideline around when neuraxial procedures may be safely performed in patients requiring anticoagulation. You approach your clinical manager when you return with the suggestion that your facility develop one as well. Your clinical manager agrees that it could improve patient care and, because of your interest in this area, she assigns you to develop the guideline, get it approved, and implement it at your facility.

1. Describe how you would define the policy need. (Why is there a policy need? What would the policy accomplish? Should it be developed as a policy or a guideline? How would you determine what needs to be included?)
2. Describe how you would identify key policy stakeholders and obtain their buy-in and input.
3. List some common elements you might include in your policy or guideline.
4. Describe how you would obtain approval of the policy or guideline by stakeholders and committees once it is written.
5. Describe how you might educate affected staff on the approved policy or guideline.
6. Describe what steps you might take after implementation.

**CASE STUDY 17-3     Medication Use Evaluation: Rivaroxaban**

The P&T committee at Seaside Hospital added rivaroxaban to formulary approximately 1 year ago. Medication errors involving rivaroxaban have recently been reported by the medication safety committee. The individual errors were investigated; however, the P&T committee would like more information about the use of the product in the hospital.

1. How would you find out more information about the use of rivaroxaban at Seaside Hospital?
2. What are the potential consequences of inappropriate use of this product?
3. What literature resources would help you find specific information about appropriate use of the product?
4. What specific criteria should be used to assess if rivaroxaban was dosed appropriately in patients with renal dysfunction at Seaside Hospital?
5. How would descriptive information about the service of the prescriber ordering rivaroxaban assist you in evaluating the MUE results?
6. How would you design the MUE (prospective, concurrent, or retrospective) if you are the only individual available to perform data collection?
7. If 15 patients were transitioned from a heparin drip to rivaroxaban therapy for the treatment of deep vein thrombosis and 7 of those patients were started on rivaroxaban at the time of discontinuation of the infusion, what would be the percentage (%) compliance with transition from heparin to rivaroxaban at discontinuation of heparin?
8. What recommendation could be made to improve compliance with initiating rivaroxaban at the time the heparin continuous infusion is discontinued?

# SUMMARY

Medication use policies and guidelines are developed to define and clarify the operational practices and procedures for safe and legal medication use, and to outline best practices clinically. Pharmacists must be prepared to recognize policy need in the context of numerous policy drivers, and be able to research relevant regulatory requirements and best practices. They must also be prepared to collaborate with other healthcare professionals to develop and implement policies and guidelines that meet institutional needs, while assessing their performance.

MUE is a performance improvement method focused on the evaluation and improvement of medication use processes to optimize patient outcomes. The PDCA model for improvement can be utilized to assist in planning and executing the MUE process. All pharmacists should be prepared to conduct MUE in order to promote appropriate medication use in all practice settings.

# REFERENCES

1. Tomich DJ, Dydek GJ. The policy and procedure manual. In Brown TR, ed. *Handbook of Institutional Pharmacy Practice*. Washington, DC: American Society of Health-System Pharmacists; 2006:297-312.
2. Controlled Substances Act. 21 USC § 1304.04.
3. Drug Procurement, Distribution, and Control. WAC 246-873-080.
4. Centers for Medicare and Medicaid Services. Conditions of Participation (CoPs) and Conditions for Coverage (CfCs). http://www.cms.gov/Regulations-and-Guidance/Legislation/CFCsAndCoPs/index.html?redirect=/cfcsandcops/. Accessed July 23, 2014.
5. Centers for Medicare and Medicaid Services. Safe use of single dose/single use medications to prevent healthcare-associated infections. https://www.cms.gov/Medicare/Provider-Enrollment-and-Certification/SurveyCertificationGenInfo/Downloads/Survey-and-Cert-Letter-12-35.pdf. Accessed July 23, 2014.

6. National Center for Emerging and Zoonotic Infectious Diseases, Division of Healthcare Quality Promotion. Single-dose/single-use vial position and messages. Centers for Disease Control website. http://www.cdc.gov/injectionsafety/PDF/CDC-SDV-Position05022012.pdf. Published May 2, 2012. Accessed July 23, 2014.

7. LD 04.01.07. Leadership Standards for Hospitals. The Joint Commission 2010 Comprehensive Accreditation Manual for Hospitals.

8. Policies and procedures checklist. In Uselton JP, Kienle PC, Murdaugh LB, eds. *Assuring Continuous Compliance with Joint Commission Standards: A Pharmacy Guide*. 8th ed. Washington, DC: American Society of Health-System Pharmacists; 2008:203-225.

9. Uselton JP, Kienle PC. Maintaining compliance with Joint Commission medication management standards. *Patient Safety & Quality Healthcare*. July/August 2008.

10. MedWatch: The FDA safety information and adverse event reporting program. U.S. Food and Drug Administration website. http://www.fda.gov/Safety/MedWatch/default.htm. Accessed July 23, 2014.

11. Institute for Safe Medication Practice. http://ismp.org. Accessed July 23, 2014.

12. *Hospital Pharmacy*. Thomas Land Publishers Incorporated. http://www.thomasland.com/hospitalpharmacy.html. Accessed July 23, 2014.

13. Institute for Healthcare Improvement. Protecting 5 Million Lives from Harm. http://www.ihi.org/offerings/Initiatives/PastStrategicInitiatives/5MillionLivesCampaign/Pages/default.aspx. Accessed July 23, 2014.

14. Institute for Healthcare Improvement. The IHI Improvement Map. http://www.ihi.org/offerings/Initiatives/Improvemaphospitals/Pages/default.aspx. Accessed July 23, 2014.

15. Federal Food Drug and Cosmetic Act. Food and Drug Administration website. http://www.fda.gov/regulatoryinformation/legislation/federalfooddrugandcosmeticactfdcact/. Accessed July 23, 2014.

16. Title 21 United States Code (USC) Controlled Substances Act. Drug Enforcement Agency, Office of Diversion Control website. http://www.deadiversion.usdoj.gov/21cfr/21usc/. Accessed July 23, 2014.

17. National Institute for Occupational Safety and Health. Preventing occupational exposure to antineoplastic and other hazardous drugs in healthcare settings. Centers for Disease Control and Prevention website. http://www.cdc.gov/niosh/docs/2004-165/. Accessed July 23, 2014.

18. National Institute for Occupational Safety and Health. NIOSH list of antineoplastic and other hazardous drugs in healthcare settings 2012. Centers for Disease Control and Prevention website. http://www.cdc.gov/niosh/docs/2012-150/. Accessed July 23, 2014.

19. National Association of Boards of Pharmacy. http://www.nabp.net/boards-of-pharmacy. Accessed July 23, 2014.

20. NABP*LAW* Online: The Source for State Pharmacy Laws and Regulations. NABP*LAW* website. http://www.nabp.net/programs/member-services/nabplaw. Accessed July 23, 2014.

21. Centers for Disease Control. http://www.cdc.gov. Accessed July 23, 2014.

22. Pharmaceutical Compounding—Sterile Preparations <797> (USP 797). United States Pharmacopeial Convention website. http://www.usp.org/store/products-services/usp-compounding. Accessed July 23, 2014.

23. The Joint Commission. The National Patient Safety Goals Effective January 1, 2013. http://www.jointcommission.org/assets/1/18/NPSG_Chapter_Jan2013_HAP.pdf. Accessed April 11, 2013.

24. The Healthcare Facilities Accreditation Program (HFAP). http://www.hfap.org. Accessed July 23, 2014.

25. DNV Accreditation Requirements. Det Norsk Veritas. http://dnvaccreditation.com/pr/dnv/downloads.aspx. Accessed July 23, 2014.

26. American Society for Health-System Pharmacists. Policy positions and guidelines. http://www.ashp.org/bestpractices. Accessed July 23, 2014.

27. Uselton JP, Kienle PC, Murdaugh LB, eds. *Assuring Continuous Compliance with Joint Commission Standards: A Pharmacy Guide, Eighth Edition*. Washington, DC: American Society of Health-System Pharmacists; 2008.

28. *Medication Safety Alert!* Institute for Safe Medication Practice website. http://ismp.org/newsletters/default.asp. Accessed July 23, 2014.

29. Institute for Healthcare Improvement. http://www.ihi.org/Pages/default.aspx. Accessed July 23, 2014.

30. *Medication Safety Alert!* January 12, 2012. Institute for Safe Medication Practice website. http://ismp.org/newsletters/acutecare/issue.asp?dt=20120112. Accessed July 23, 2014.

31. Failure Mode and Effects Analysis Tool. Institute for Healthcare Improvement website. http://app.ihi.org/Workspace/tools/fmea/. Accessed July 23, 2014.

32. National Guideline Clearinghouse. http://guideline.gov. Accessed July 23, 2014.

33. Antithrombotic Therapy and Prevention of Thrombosis, 9th ed: American College of Chest Physicians Evidence-Based Clinical Practice Guidelines. *CHEST*. 2012;141(2 suppl).

34. Horlocker TT, Wedel DJ, Rowlingson JC, et al. Regional anesthesia in the patient receiving antithrombotic or thrombolytic therapy: American Society of Regional Anesthesia and Pain Medicine Evidence-Based Guidelines (Third Edition). *Reg Anesth Pain Med*. 2010;35(1):64-101.

35. Jessup M, Abraham WT, Casey DE, et al. 2009 focused update. ACCF/AHA guidelines for the diagnosis and management of heart failure in adults. *J Am Coll Cardiol*. 2009;53(15):1343-1382.

36. Fihn SD, Gardin JM, Abrams J, et al. 2012 ACCF/AHA/ACP/AATS/PCNA/SCAI/STS guideline for the diagnosis and management of patients with stable ischemic heart disease: executive summary. *J Am Coll Cardiol*. 2012;60(24):2564-2603.

37. The Seventh Report of the Joint National Committee on Prevention, Detection, Evaluation, and Treatment of High Blood Pressure (JNC 7). *Hypertension*. 2003;42:1206.

38. Third Report of the Expert Panel on Detection, Evaluation, and Treatment of High Blood Cholesterol in Adults (Adult Treatment Panel III). National Heart, Lung, and Blood Institute website. http://www.nhlbi.nih.gov/guidelines/cholesterol/index.htm. Accessed July 23, 2014.

39. Guidelines for the Diagnosis and Management of Asthma (EPR-3). National Heart, Lung, and Blood Institute website. http://www.nhlbi.nih.gov/guidelines/asthma/index.htm. Accessed July 23, 2014.

40. Inzucchi SE, Bergenstal RM, Buse JB, et al. Management of hyperglycemia in type 2 diabetes: a patient-centered approach: position statement of the American Diabetes Association (ADA) and the European Association for the Study of Diabetes (EAS). *Diabetes Care*. 2012;35(6):1364-1379.

41. Pickering LK, Baker CJ, Freed GL, et al. Immunization of infants, children, adolescents, and adults: clinical practice guidelines by the Infectious Diseases Society of America. *Clin Infect Dis*. 2009;49(6):817-840.

42. Bratzler DW, Dellinger EP, Olsen KM, et al. Clinical practice guidelines for antimicrobial prophylaxis in surgery. *Am J Health Syst Pharm*. 2013;70(3):195-283.

43. Clinical Guidelines Portal. Guidelines for the Use of Antiretroviral Agents in HIV-1-Infected Adults and Adolescents. HHS Panel on Antiretroviral Guidelines for Adults and Adolescents. http://aidsinfo.nih.gov/guidelines/html/1/adult-and-adolescent-arv-guidelines/0/. Accessed July 23, 2014.

44. Basch E, Prestrued AA, Hesketh PJ, et al. Antiemetics: American Society of Clinical Oncology clinical practice guideline update. *J Clin Oncol*. 2011;29(31):4189-4198.

45. American Psychiatric Association. *Practice Guideline for the Treatment of Patients with Major Depressive Disorder*. 3rd ed. Arlington, VA: APA; 2010.

46. *Collection Development Manual*. Standards and guidelines. National Library of Medicine website. http://www.nlm.nih.gov/tsd/acquisitions/cdm/formats46.html. Accessed July 23, 2014.

47. *Clinical Practice Guidelines We Can Trust. Report Brief*. Institute of Medicine. Website http://www.iom.edu/~/media/Files/Report%20Files/2011/Clinical-Practice-Guidelines-We-Can-Trust/Clinical%20Practice%20Guidelines%202011%20Report%20Brief.pdf. Published 2011. Accessed July 23, 2014.

48. Is prescribing the next step in the evolution of pharmacy? *ASHP Intersections*. http://www.ashpintersections.org/2012/05/is-prescribing-the-next-step-in-the-evolution-of-pharmacy/. Published May 15, 2012. Accessed July 23, 2014.

49. Facts About the Tracer Methodology. The Joint Commission website. http://www.jointcommission.org/facts_about_the_tracer_methodology/. Accessed July 23, 2014.

50. Survey Activities Guide for Healthcare Organizations. The Joint Commission website. http://www.jointcommission.org/assets/1/18/2012_Organization_SAG.pdf. Accessed April 11, 2013.

51. Phillips MS, Gayman JE, Todd MW. ASHP guidelines on medication-use evaluation. *Am J Health Syst Pharm*. 1996;53(16):1953-1955.

52. Academy of Managed Care Pharmacy. Drug utilization review. http://amcp.org/WorkArea/DownloadAsset.aspx?id=9296. Accessed July 23, 2014.

53. Tyler LS, Cole SW, May JR, et al. ASHP guidelines on the pharmacy and therapeutics committee and the formulary system. *Am J Health Syst Pharm*. 2008;65(13):1272-1283.

54. American Society of Health-System Pharmacists. The pharmacist's role in quality improvement. http://www.ashp.org/DocLibrary/Policy/QII/RoleinQI.aspx Accessed July 23, 2014.

55. IHI Model for improvement. Institute for Healthcare Improvement website. http://www.ihi.org/knowledge/PulishingImages/ModelforImprovent.gif. Accessed April 12, 2013.

56. U.S. Department of Veteran Affairs. VA Center for Medication Safety. MUE Toolkit. http://www.pbm.va.gov/PBM/vacenterformedicationsafety/tools/MUEToolkit.pdf. Accessed July 23, 2014.

57. Facts and Comparisons eAnswers. Formulary Monograph Service. http://online.factsandcomparisons .com. Accessed April 12, 2013.

58. The Joint Commission. *Comprehensive Accreditation Manual for Hospitals: The Official Handbook*. Oakbrook Terrace, IL: Author; 2010.

59. Durthaler JM, Ernst FR. Evidence-based disease management in medication-use evaluation: application to drotrecogin alfa (activated) in severe sepsis. *Am J Health-Syst Pharm.* 2006;63(15):1453-1460.

60. World Health Organization. Drug and Therapeutics Committees: A Practical Guide. http://apps .who.int/medicinedocs/pdf/s4882e/s4882e.pdf. Accessed July 23, 2014.

61. Vermeulen LC, Rough SS, Thielke TS, et al. Strategic approach for improving the medication-use process in health systems: the high-performance pharmacy practice framework. *Am J Health-Syst Pharm.* 2007;64(16):1699-1710.

62. Vermeulen LC, Beis SJ, Cano SB. Applying outcomes research in improving the medication-use process. *Am J Health-Syst Pharm.* 2000;57(24):2277-2282.

63. ASHP statement on the role of the medication safety leader. *Am J Health-Syst Pharm.* 2013;70(5):448-452.

64. Bernknopf AC, Karpinski JP, McKeever AL, et al. Drug information: from education to practice. *Pharmacotherapy.* 2009;29(3):331-346.

65. ASHP Accreditation Standard for Post-Graduate Year One (PGY1) Residency Programs. http:// www.ashp.org/DocLibrary/Accreditation/ASD-PGY1-Standard.aspx. Accessed July 23, 2014.

66. Pedersen, CA, Schneider PJ, Scheckelhoff DJ. ASHP national survey of pharmacy practice in hospital settings: Prescribing and transcribing - 2010. *Am J Health-Syst Pharm.* 2011;68(8):669-688.

# IHI MODEL FOR IMPROVEMENT

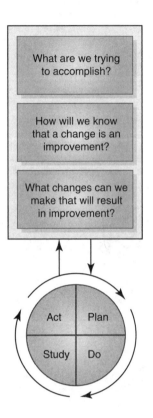

IHI Model for Improvement.

*The Improvement Guide: A Practical Approach to Enhancing Organizational Performance*, 2nd Ed., Langley. Copyright © 2009 Jossey-Bass. Reproduced with permission of John Wiley & Sons Inc.

# EXAMPLE MUE TEMPLATE

**Medication Use Evaluation: Title**

**Objective:** Describe the purpose of the evaluation.

**Background:** Include a description of the medication, therapeutic class, disease, condition, outcome, or any step in the medication use process (i.e., prescribing, transcribing, dispensing, administering, monitoring) that is being evaluated. Include a rationale, or why it is important to evaluate within the organization at this time. Provide information regarding acceptable benchmarks for criteria if available from internal or external resources. List references used for this section in the reference section.

**Methods:** Describe who, what, when, where, and how the evaluation will be conducted.

> **Design:** Describe the overall design or process for collecting data, who will collect the data, what time period will be assessed, what data will be included or excluded, and what will be collected.

> **Criteria:** Describe specifically what criteria will be evaluated and include acceptable benchmarks or thresholds if available.

> **Data collection form:** Include a copy of the data collection form in the proposal if utilized to show what will be collected. The form is not typically included in the final report.

**\*Results:** Provide the total number of charts reviewed or orders assessed for the time period evaluated. Display all outcomes for criteria in various tables and figures as percentages. Also display specific trends that occur with a subset of data.

**\*Discussion:** Provide an interpretation of results. Describe any trends and include limitations of the evaluation.

**\*Conclusion:** Provide a summary of the information that was discovered following the evaluation. Include recommendations for improvement following this evaluation and what actions can be taken to improve outcomes for criteria.

**References:** Include a list of references used.

**Prepared by:** Include names of the individuals who prepared the evaluation or of those who contributed to the project.

---

*\*Section included in final report and not included in the MUE proposal.*

# MUE DATA COLLECTION FORM FOR TAPENTADOL

| Patient Information | | |
|---|---|---|
| Name: | DOB: | Height: |
| MRN: | Gender: | Weight: |
| Prior history of pain?: Y/N | | |
| On pain therapy at home?: Y/N | | |
| Pain medication used at home (including medication regimen): | | |

| Encounter Information | | |
|---|---|---|
| Visit #: | Admitting diagnosis: | Location (unit/room): |
| Admit date: | Admitting physician: | Physician service: |

| Prescribing Information | |
|---|---|
| Tapentadol order: | Ordering physician: |
| | Date/time order written: |

**Dosage**

*Initial dose:*

- 50, 75, or 100 mg with an additional dose allowed within first hour if pain uncontrolled? Y/N
- PO every 4-6 hours? Y/N

*Within max dose limits:*

- 700 mg on day 1 only? Y/N
- 600 mg daily? Y/N

*Dose adjustment:*

- 50 mg every 8 hours in patient with moderate hepatic impairment (Child Pugh grade B)? Y/N

Comments:

**Indication**

- Used for treatment of moderate to severe acute pain in adult patients? Y/N

Comments:

**Restriction for use**

- Utilized for postoperative pain? Y/N
- Prescribed by Ortho Service (restricted to this service)? Y/N

**Contraindications**

*Ordered in patient with:*

- Impaired pulmonary function in an unmonitored setting? Y/N
- Patients with paralytic ileus? Y/N
- Use within 14 days of an MAO inhibitor? Y/N

**Precautions**

*Use avoided in patients with:*

- Head injury or intracranial lesion? Y/N
- History of seizure disorder? Y/N
- Severe hepatic impairment (Child Pugh grade C)? Y/N
- Severe renal impairment (CrCl < 30 ml/min)? Y/N
- Pancreatic or biliary tract disease? Y/N

**Used in patient with medications with duplication or potential interactions:**

- Serotonin Modulators [Monoamine Oxidase inhibitors, Selective Serotonin Reuptake Inhibitors (SSRI), Selective Norepinephrine Reuptake Inhibitors (SNRI), Tricyclic Antidepressants (TCA), Triptans]? Y/N
- CNS Depressants (opiates, anxiolytics, sedatives, hypnotics)? Y/N
- Opiate antagonists (alvimopan, naloxone)? Y/N

### Monitoring/Administration Information

- Monitored control of pain within 2 hours of administration? Y/N        Comments:
- Documented adverse reactions:
  - Nausea? Y/N
  - Vomiting? Y/N
  - Dizziness? Y/N
  - Headache? Y/N
  - Somnolence? Y/N
  - Constipation? Y/N
  - Respiratory depression? Y/N
  - CNS depression? Y/N
  - Serotonin syndrome? Y/N
  - Withdrawal symptoms? Y/N

### Criteria

- Did the patient's pain scores improve with use of the agent? Y/N        Comments:
- Was the patient switched to a different analgesic to control pain? Y/N
- Did the patient require supplemental breakthrough medication? Y/N
- Did the patient need an antiemetic agent to prevent or relieve nausea and vomiting? Y/N
- Did the patient need a laxative to relieve constipation? Y/N

# EXAMPLE OF MUE RESULTS

## MEDICATION USE EVALUATION CONTINUATION OF BETA-BLOCKERS PERIOPERATIVELY

**Purpose:** The objective of this medication use evaluation was to identify areas for improvement with SCIP-Cardiology-2, or the continuation of beta-blocker therapy during the perioperative period.

**Background:** The Surgical Care Improvement Project (SCIP) was created by a steering committee represented by 10 nationally recognized organizations (including the Centers for Medicare and Medicaid Services [CMS] and The Joint Commission) to improve surgical care by reducing the occurrence of surgical complications.[1] A stated goal of the project is to reduce the incidence of preventable surgical complications by 25% nationally by the year 2010. SCIP is composed of process of care measures aimed at reducing infection, venous thromboembolism (VTE), and cardiac events, which have been targeted due to the high incidence and high cost of preventable errors. SCIP's core measures include goals aimed at improving pharmacotherapy and include the appropriate timing and selection of prophylactic antibiotics, controlling serum glucose postoperatively, prophylaxis of venous thromboembolism, and continuation of beta-blockers in the perioperative period.

The continuation of beta-blocker therapy measure (SCIP-Cardiology-2), requires that patients who were receiving a beta-blocker at home prior to arrival receive beta blockade during the perioperative period, which is defined as 24 hours before surgical incision through discharge from the post-anesthesia care unit (PACU) or up to 6 hours after admission to the ICU.[2] This measure stems from a Class I recommendation from the American College of Cardiology Foundation and American Heart Association (ACCF/AHA), which states that beta-blockers should be continued in patients undergoing surgery who are receiving beta-blockers for the treatment of conditions with ACCF/AHA Class I guideline indications for the drugs (e.g., angina, arrhythmia, hypertension).[3] This recommendation is based on clinical trials that have shown that beta-blocker withdrawal in the perioperative period should be avoided due to an increased risk of myocardial infarction and mortality.

The SCIP-Cardiology-2 measure has been defined in the Specifications Manual of National Hospital Inpatient Quality Measures since October 2006; however, CMS recently required reporting of this measure in order for hospitals to receive payment for fiscal year 2010.[4] For the reporting period of January 2009 through June 2009, Seaside Hospital was performing at 81% for this measure, as compared to 89% for all reporting hospitals in the United States and 87% for all hospitals reporting in the state.[5] The top 10% of hospitals nationwide achieved 100% for this measure. The objective of this medication use evaluation is to assess the sample of patients that did not receive beta-blockers during the perioperative period and whose therapy should have been continued for 2009. Data will be evaluated to identify areas for improvement.

**Methods:** The Quality Team was contacted by the multidisciplinary SCIP task force to identify patients that did not meet the SCIP-Cardiology-2 measure from January to December 2009. The following data elements were extracted for each case: surgical procedure, surgeon, anesthesiologist, patient indication for beta-blocker therapy, and regimen.

The following criteria were analyzed by chart review for each patient:

1. Was there documentation in the chart that the patient was on a beta-blocker prior to arrival?
2. Did the patient take their beta-blocker on the morning prior to arrival?
3. Was the beta-blocker taken/administered within 24 hours of anesthesia start time?
4. Was the patient instructed to take their beta-blocker prior to arrival as documented in the preoperative form?
5. Was a beta-blocker ordered?
6. Was a beta-blocker administered on the day of surgery within PACU or < 6 hours in ICU?
7. Was there a contraindication for beta-blocker therapy (bradycardia, hypotension)?
8. Was the reason for not administering a beta-blocker perioperatively documented?
9. Did the patient experience cardiac complications in the perioperative period as a result of not receiving a beta-blocker?

**Results:** The SCIP task force evaluated 48 cases out of 410 assessed that did not meet the SCIP-Cardiology-2 measure from January to December 2009. A summary of criteria results is found in **Table 17D-1**. Monthly and yearly compliance rates can be found in **Figure 17D-1**.

**Discussion:** Average yearly compliance with SCIP-Cardiology-2 for 2009 was 88%. The January to June 2009 period was much lower at 81% and the hospital improved to 92% compliance from July to December 2009. Monthly compliance was lowest in the month of May at 70%, and the drop in compliance for this month was likely caused by the introduction of a revised preoperative record. The new record was designed to improve compliance with the measure; however, it caused confusion among staff. Following education on the new form in June, compliance rose to its highest at 98% in July.

All patients' records contained documentation that they were on a beta-blocker at home prior to surgery, indicating that the medication reconciliation process is being followed at preoperative screening. Thirty-five percent of patients took their beta-blocker on the morning of surgery; however, all of the patients admitted on the day of surgery received instructions to take their beta-blocker prior to arrival, and all charts contained anesthesia orders to take the beta-blocker prior to surgery with the exception of two emergent cases. The

**TABLE 17D-1  Summary of Results**

- Overall, 87% compliance with SCIP-Cardiology-2 for 2009 (Goal 100%).
- Monthly compliance was lowest in the month of May at 70%.
- 100% of patients had documentation that they were on a beta-blocker prior to arrival.
- 35% of patients took their beta-blocker on the morning of surgery prior to arrival.
- 0% of patients received a beta-blocker within 24 hours of anesthesia start.
- 90% of patients had an order for a beta-blocker.
- 50% of patients received a beta-blocker on the day of surgery; however, all received after discharge from PACU, which does not meet the standard for SCIP-Cardiology-2.
- 50% of patients had a reason for not receiving a beta-blocker; however, these patients did not have documentation of the reason.
- 8% of patients experienced complications, and it is unknown if these may have been prevented by administration of the beta-blocker in the perioperative period.

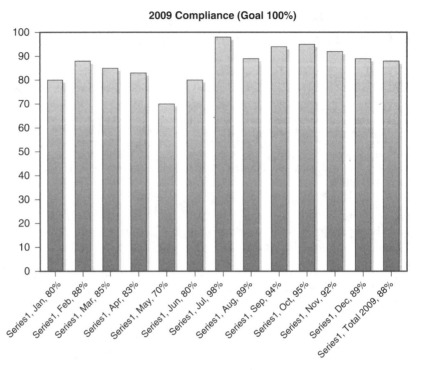

**FIGURE 17D-1** SCIP-Cardiology-2 compliance.

instructions provided to patients do not list the medication specifically but refer to a group of medications (e.g., cardiac, antihypertensives).

No patients received a beta-blocker within 24 hours of anesthesia start time. Thirty-five percent of patients who took their beta-blocker did not have documentation of the time of the last dose to determine if it was within 24 hours of anesthesia start. Ninety percent of patients had an order for a beta-blocker, and approximately 50% of patients received a beta-blocker on the day of surgery. All of these patients receiving a beta-blocker were administered the medication after discharge from the PACU, which does not meet standards. Fifty percent of patients experienced bradycardia or hypotension in the OR; however, the contraindication or reason for not administering a beta-blocker was not documented in the record.

The complications experienced by patients not continuing beta-blockers included the development of atrial fibrillation in 2 patients 48 hours after surgery, which may be unrelated, and hypertension in 2 patients in the PACU.

Limitations of this evaluation include the retrospective chart review in a small number of patients. Electronic copies of handwritten charts were evaluated and not always legible. Many residents and students train at the institution and may affect compliance and the effect of this on outcomes is unknown.

**Conclusion:** Improvements should be made to achieve 100% compliance with SCIP-Cardiology-2. The hospital has improved but is still not at goal.

Improved instructions to patients and orders to include more details regarding what specific medications should be taken prior to surgery may assist with compliance with patients taking their beta-blocker on the morning of surgery. Current educational efforts are focused on what medications to stop, and orders may be unclear to patients about how medications are classified with the terms *beta-blocker, cardiac,* or *antihypertensives* all being used interchangeably by staff. The

SCIP Task Force should formulate a script for nursing staff to use the specific name of the beta-blocker when counseling patients.

Improving documentation of the timing of beta-blocker therapy if taken prior to arrival is an additional area for improvement for reaching compliance with this measure. The most recent updated perioperative record may help prompt for documentation of date and time of the last dose; however, this information at times was inconsistent with the information found in the OR Checklist. More than one individual and more than one area in the chart to document this information may cause confusion. One staff member should be tasked to answer this question on one form. The SCIP Task Force should identify the staff member responsible to answer this question and identify the form to be used.

Prescribers may consider compliance with the measure if the beta-blocker is administered on the day of surgery, but it must be administered prior to discharge from the PACU. The SCIP Task Force should educate prescribers on the definition of the measure. The PACU order set should be modified to include the option to administer a beta-blocker prior to PACU discharge. Additionally, the PACU order set may need revision to document a contraindication or reason for not receiving a beta-blocker. Documentation for not continuing a beta-blocker with clinical data to support the reason could improve measure compliance and should be assigned to a staff member in the PACU and recorded prior to PACU discharge. There were minimal complications experienced by patients in which the beta-blocker was not continued.

The following recommendations (**Table 17D-2**) are provided to improve future compliance with SCIP-Cardiology-2. A multidisciplinary team will meet to discuss action plans for implementation.

**TABLE 17D-2**  Recommendations

- SCIP Task Force to create scripted instructions for nurses to provide to patients prior to surgery. The instructions will specify the name of the beta-blocker that the patient should take on the morning of surgery.
- SCIP Task Force to evaluate duplication of questions on forms and determine whose responsibility it is to document the date and time of receiving a beta-blocker at home. This will aid in determining if a beta-blocker was received 24 hours prior to anesthesia start.
- SCIP Task Force to educate anesthesiologists, physicians, and nurses on compliance with SCIP-Cardiology-2.
- SCIP Task Force to modify the PACU order set to include the option to administer a beta-blocker prior to PACU discharge and include a section for a reason for not continuing a beta-blocker perioperatively with clinical data to support the reason.
- Reevaluate process at 6 months.

# REFERENCES

1. Chen CL, Shapiro ML, Angood PB, Makary MA. Patient safety. In: Brunicardi FC, ed. *Schwartz's Principles of Surgery*. 9th ed. New York, NY: McGraw-Hill; 2009.
2. QualityNet. http://www.qualitynet.org. Accessed February 5, 2010.
3. Fleishmann KE, Beckman JA, Buller CE, et al. 2009 ACCF/AHA focused update on peioperative beta blockade: a report of the American College of Cardiology Foundation/American Heart Association Task Force on Practice Guidelines. *Circulation*. 2009;120:2123-2151.
4. Centers for Medicare and Medicaid Services. http://www.cms.hhs.gov/HospitalQualityInits. Accessed February 1, 2010.
5. Hospital Quality Compare. http://www.hospitalcompare.hhs.gov. Accessed February 1, 2010.

## CHAPTER 18

# FORMULARY MANAGEMENT

Sabrina W. Cole, PharmD, BCPS
Kelli Garrison, PharmD, BCPS
Conor Hanrahan, PharmD, BCPS

## CHAPTER OBJECTIVES

- Differentiate between a formulary and a formulary system.
- Describe the governance of a formulary system and the functions of the governance structure.
- List the components of a formulary system that supports optimal use of medications in an organization.
- Describe the effective strategies for formulary maintenance.
- Apply literature evaluation skills and formulary concepts to determine appropriate therapeutic alternatives in response to a drug shortage.

# CHAPTER OUTLINE

# KEY TERMS

Closed formulary
Formulary
Formulary system
Nonformulary medications

Off-label use
Open formulary
Pharmacy and Therapeutics Committee
Therapeutic alternative

# INTRODUCTION

The drug market is expanding rapidly, with an average of 88 new drugs, 25 new molecular entities (NMEs), and 100 generic products approved by the Food and Drug Administration (FDA) each year.[1-5] The number of NMEs continues to increase, with 39 NMEs approved in 2012, the highest number in over a decade.[2] The availability of these new products often means novel treatments for patients and further advances in health care. However, to make these agents available for patients, the FDA must allow some through the expedited process, via priority review, accelerated approval, and fast-track mechanisms. This shortened review typically means that less data are available for assessment of efficacy and safety.[2]

In addition, the cost of health care has risen dramatically over the past several decades, with pharmacy operations accounting for approximately 20% of the overall operating budget of the average U.S. hospital.[6] As a result, healthcare organizations utilize drug formularies as a means of promoting evidence-based practice, improving patient safety, and containing costs in today's ever-changing economic environment.[7,8] This chapter will serve as a resource regarding formulary management and provide tools to help ensure efficacious, safe, and cost-effective care for patients.

# WHAT IS A FORMULARY?

In simple terms, a **formulary** is a list of medications that are deemed appropriate for use by an organization, whether that organization is a large academic medical center, community hospital, or pharmacy benefit manager (PBM).[9-12] However, this definition is perhaps too simple, because a formulary is much more than just a list of medications. A formulary also includes medication use policies, medication guidelines, and other decision-support tools surrounding medication use (e.g., dosing charts, medication selection algorithms, substitution protocols). This concept is emphasized by the

American Society of Health-System Pharmacists (ASHP), which defines a formulary as a "continually updated list of medications and related information, representing the clinical judgment of physicians, pharmacists, and other experts in the diagnosis, prophylaxis, or treatment of disease and promotion of health."[11] Thus, formularies are dynamic tools used to guide medication use within an organization.

The ongoing process by which changes are made to the formulary is known as a **formulary system**. As one might expect, formularies must be continually updated based on new drug approvals, changes in drug cost, and after-market therapeutic efficacy and safety evaluations. Therefore, organizations must have a formulary system in place to ensure proper formulary maintenance. Such systems are also the means by which organizations evaluate, appraise, and select drug entities for formulary addition; create policies and guidelines regarding drug use; and ultimately promote rational, clinically appropriate, safe, and cost-effective medicine.[11-13] As will be discussed later in this chapter, both formularies and formulary systems exist in a variety of settings, including hospital practice, managed care, long-term care, ambulatory care, and governmental programs (e.g., Medicare, Medicaid, and the U.S. Department of Defense).

Formularies can be categorized as either open or closed and may include a tiered system or a set of restrictions (**Figure 18-1**). Most health systems, for example, maintain a formulary as open or closed with some restrictions in place, whereas the U.S. Department of Defense and managed care plans typically use a preferred list or tiered system to classify inclusion on the formulary.[12,14] Although the characterization of the formulary is slightly different in these settings, the core principles are similar. Section details will

**Open Formulary**

- Includes all medications and dosage forms currently marketed
- Does not distinguish between products for efficacy and safety
- Leads to inefficient inventory management and difficulties in controlling costs
- Challenging to maintain an electronic health record (EHR)
- May be most appropriate for outpatient (retail) settings

**Closed Formulary**

- Only includes medications selected for use
- Involves an evaluation of efficacy, safety, and cost
- Helps promote efficient inventory management and cost containment
- Streamlines build and maintenance of an EHR

**Positive Formulary**

- Start with a "blank" list and require requests from providers to add
- Time intensive process for a new organization since every medication would need to be considered at the beginning

**Negative Formulary**

- Start with all medications in stock then evaluate each therapeutic class to eliminate agents that would be consider duplicate therapy
- May result in a larger formulary

**FIGURE 18-1** Types of formularies.

focus on these core principles and will distinguish between health system pharmacies and PBMs where necessary.

As the name implies, an **open formulary** is unrestrictive and places no limitations on which medications can be used by an organization (i.e., any drug on the market is available for use). This type of formulary can become difficult to manage over time for health systems, because organizations would have to keep large drug inventories on hand. Similarly, open formularies may be cost prohibitive because any drug, regardless of price, would be available for use.

In contrast, a **closed formulary** limits the number of available medications to a select list of agents that have been deemed appropriate by the organization. This strategy is usually preferred because it allows an organization to contain costs while promoting the safest, most efficacious drug therapies. Nevertheless, the organization should have an exception process by which **nonformulary medications** can be given (e.g., when there is therapeutic failure of a formulary medication).[11]

Closed formularies can be further described as positive or negative, depending on how the organization chooses to add medications to its drug library. In a positive formulary, the organization would essentially start with a "blank slate" and wait for specific medications to be requested for formulary addition. Conversely, in a negative formulary, medications already in use are initially added to the formulary, and then drugs are reviewed and removed as necessary over time. Such designations are more relevant to organizations just starting a formulary and are less important for those that are well established. For example, PBMs utilize positive and negative strategies when developing preferred drug list formularies for clients.

Given the benefits of a closed formulary, it is not surprising that most institutions have adopted this strategy. In 2010, a national survey of nonprofit academic medical centers found that the majority of respondents used a closed (restricted) formulary process for their inpatient pharmacies, whereas most outpatient pharmacies used an open formulary structure. In addition, some institutions have adopted a "mixed" model in which nonformulary items can be added via a request process or only certain drug classes are restricted, so that only part of the formulary is considered closed.[7]

Tiered systems were created to help control the costs to managed care organizations or within the Department of Defense. These systems usually involve a preferred list of medications that differentiate between generic and brand classifications. The decision to include a medication on the list is based on the therapeutic equivalence or superiority of medications within each therapeutic class. The different tiers usually have copayments that increase with each tier.[12,15] An example of a tier system is shown in **Figure 18–2**. For the Department of Defense, the formulary process evolved

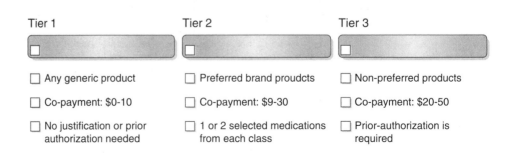

**FIGURE 18-2** Example of a tiered formulary system.

rapidly after the institution of the three-tier Uniform Formulary in 2005. This process is based on the following:[12]

- Evidence-based clinical evaluation and assessment of relative cost-effectiveness (i.e., pharmacoeconomic and budget impact modeling).
- Open competition for manufacturers to have a medication on the formulary, which should lead to better contract pricing.
- Comments from providers and beneficiaries on any potential change to the formulary via a public forum.

The example of the Department of Defense formulary process is unique compared with that of health systems and managed care organizations. Formulary changes to the Department of Defense formulary require congressional approval.

# THE HISTORY AND EVOLUTION OF FORMULARIES

Similar to most novel concepts in health care, formulary systems have evolved over time (**Figure 18-3**). The concept of a formulary can be traced back to 15th-century England, with the creation of the *Edinburgh Pharmacopeia* by the Royal College of Physicians in 1699.[16] The first American formulary, known as the *Lititz Pharmacopeia*, was created in 1778 by Continental Army officers in Lititz, Pennsylvania, during the American Revolution. Other early American formularies included the *Pharmacopeia of the Massachusetts Medical Society* in 1808, the *Pharmacopeia of the New York Hospital* in 1816, and *The United States Pharmacopeia* in 1820.[17]

Despite this early foundation, the major push toward modern-day formularies did not occur until after World War II, when advances in manufacturing practices allowed prescribers to write for "brand-name" medications instead of compounded products. At the same time, thousands of new and duplicate drugs were being introduced into the market, which further added to the complexity and cost of health care.[17]

Recognizing the need for standardization and the rational use of medications, in 1950 the Joint Commission on Accreditation of Hospitals (now known as The Joint Commission [TJC]) began promoting the idea of hospital formularies. Although basic, these formularies attempted to provide inventory control, ensure product consistency, and maintain an adequate supply of medication. However, such efforts were initially met with resistance by groups such as the National Pharmaceutical Council and the American Medical Association (AMA), who tried to prevent pharmacists from performing therapeutic interchanges with generic equivalent drugs.[11,17] Nevertheless, hospitals continued to grow formulary systems and, in 1958, ASHP added formularies to its minimum standards for hospital pharmacies.[11,18]

By the 1960s, organizations started to realize the economic value of formularies and began using them to manage product safety and efficacy. A number of associations, including many that were initially opposed to formulary implementation, also began to promote formulary policies and standards.[11] However, it was not until 1965 that TJC actually required hospitals to establish a formulary system in order to receive accreditation. Simultaneously, Medicare listed formularies as a requirement for reimbursement, which also provided a strong financial incentive for formulary implementation.[11,17]

The adoption of formulary systems continued to grow during the 1980s and 1990s as new literature on their clinical and economic benefits emerged.[11] During this time,

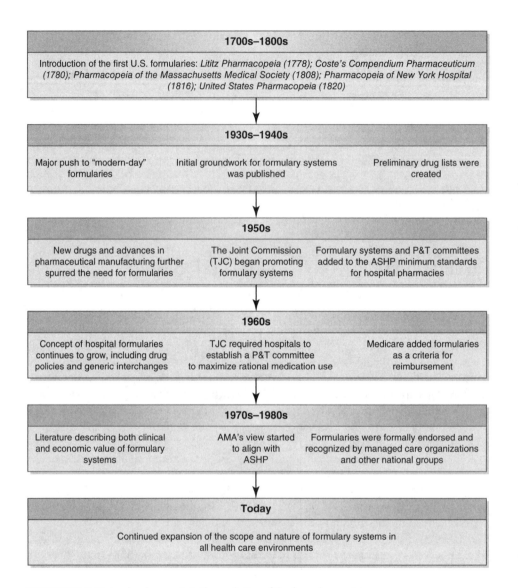

**FIGURE 18-3** Major developments in the evolution of the formulary system.

the Pharmaceutical Research and Manufacturers Association (PhRMA) and the AMA formally recognized drug formularies and therapeutic interchange.[11,19] Similarly, as managed care organizations continued to grow during the 1970s and 1980s, they, too, began using formularies as a means to manage increasing drug costs. Today, formularies have become an essential part of cost-effective, evidence-based health care.

# GOVERNANCE OF A FORMULARY SYSTEM

As mentioned earlier in this chapter, a formulary system is the process by which organizations evaluate, appraise, and select drug entities and drug-related products that are considered most useful in patient care. The responsibility is usually given to a specific committee or group with representatives from within the organization. In the hospital environment, this responsibility is given to the **Pharmacy and Therapeutics (P&T) Committee**, which oversees medication management in the health system. The ultimate goal of the P&T Committee is to promote rational, clinically appropriate, safe, and cost-effective drug therapy.[20] Specific responsibilities of the Committee will vary by institution, but may include the following:[10,12,20,21]

- Develop and maintain the drug formulary.
- Monitor adherence to the formulary (i.e., restrictions, nonformulary use).
- Develop policies and procedures related to medication use (e.g., order set, protocols, practice guidelines).
- Review adverse drug events.
- Conduct medication use evaluations.
- Educate staff on the optimal use of medications.

## MEMBERSHIP

Medication use affects nearly every discipline; therefore, P&T Committees should be multidisciplinary, including physicians, pharmacists, nurses, dietitians, hospital administrators, and other personnel that the institution deems necessary (e.g., risk or quality improvement managers, pharmacoeconomic specialists) (**Figure 18-4**).[11,13] The size of the Committee will vary by institution, but the group will typically have 12-17 voting members who are selected with guidance from the medical staff.[20,22] Members meet an average of seven times per year, although larger hospitals will often hold meetings on a monthly basis.[21]

Although pharmacists will play an important role in the Committee, the majority of voting members are typically physicians, because they are considered the leaders of the healthcare team and are responsible for prescribing medications. Nevertheless, pharmacists still have many responsibilities for supporting the Committee, such as creating

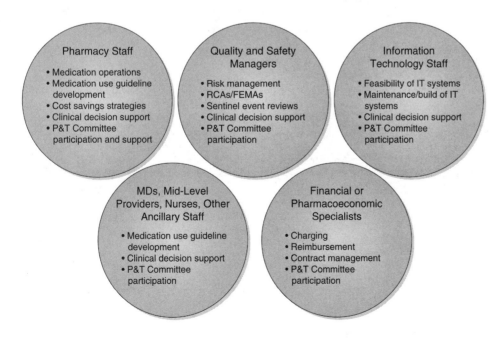

**FIGURE 18-4** Example of P&T Committee membership and general responsibilities.

drug monographs; evaluating medications for formulary addition/deletion; conducting quality assurance reviews; creating policies, procedures, and guidelines; assisting with educational initiatives; and maintaining the formulary publication (e.g., website, hard copy, information system).

## ORGANIZATION AND STRUCTURE

At most hospitals, the P&T Committee is one of several other committees that report directly to the Medical Executive Committee (MEC), which is the group responsible for managing most clinical services within the hospital (**Figure 18-5**). Members of the MEC are elected by the medical staff and work with the hospital management team (e.g., chief executive officer [CEO], chief financial officer [CFO], chief nursing officer [CNO], director of pharmacy) to achieve the organization's mission and vision. Thus, the P&T Committee serves in an advisory capacity to the institution in matters related to medication use. It is important to note that P&T Committees do not exist exclusively in the hospital setting. P&T Committees are also instrumental in the formulary decision process for pharmacy benefits managers for outpatient formulary decisions.

Depending on the size of the institution or organization, the P&T Committee may also have several subcommittees, also known as *ad hoc committees* or *expert panels* (Figure 18-5). These committees are composed of specialists who focus on a particular therapeutic areas important to the institution. For example, due to the complexity and prevalence of antibiotic use within the hospital, some institutions will create an anti-infective subcommittee to review new antibiotics, antiretrovirals, and other matters related to anti-infective policy (e.g., protocols, order sets). Due to its specialized nature, the group would include physicians, pharmacists, and nurses who specialize in

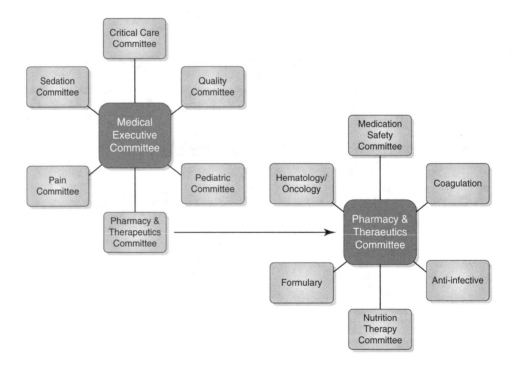

**FIGURE 18-5** Example organization and structure of the P&T Committee and related committees.

infectious diseases. Thus, these subcommittees are able to provide more time, resources, and expertise in a particular area compared with the larger P&T body. However, it is important to remember that these subcommittees are simply advisors to the P&T Committee, and their recommendations cannot be implemented without approval from the main body. The number and type of subcommittees is dependent on the organization and the specialized care that is provided.

# STRATEGIES FOR FORMULARY DEVELOPMENT

## PRODUCT SELECTION/REQUEST PROCESS

The P&T Committee should have a formalized, systematic, and evidence-based review process for the evaluation of products to be considered for formulary addition (**Figure 18-6**).[11] The review process is often initiated by the request for a single medication to be considered for formulary addition; however, this process could also be prompted by the approval of a new drug to market, a scheduled class review, a response to an action by the FDA, or newly published efficacy or safety data about a medication. Selection of formulary medications should be made on the basis of safety, efficacy, and cost-effectiveness, with considerations for the potential for medication errors and error reduction.[11,13,23] The request process also requires mechanisms for effective communication to educate all personnel involved in the medication use process.

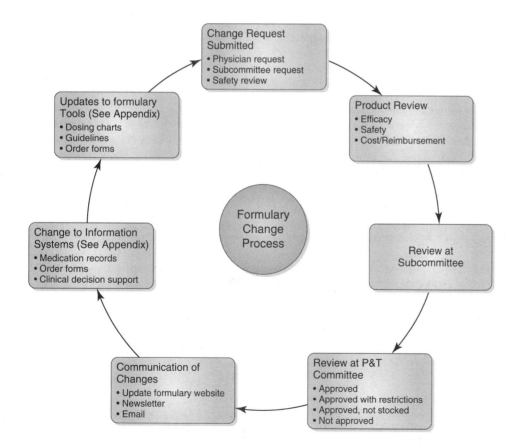

**FIGURE 18-6** Formulary system review process.

| CASE STUDY 18-1 | Tbo-filgrastim (Granix™) Request Process |

**Background**

You are a clinical pharmacy specialist in oncology working for a large cancer hospital. During rounds one morning, a physician colleague tells you about a new version of filgrastim, called tbo-filgrastim (Granix). Although this new drug was approved via the normal pathway for biologic drugs, it is widely regarded as the first biosimilar medication to be marketed in the United States. Much like the concept of generic medications, these biosimilars aim to provide comparable efficacy to the originator product at a discounted price. After further discussion, the physician tells you that he would like to start using tbo-filgrastim in some of his patients and wants to know how he can order this product.

**Question**

What next steps should you tell the physician to take?

**Answer**

If the physician would like to replace filgrastim with this new product, he should submit a formal request to add tbo-filgrastim to the formulary. These requests are typically submitted via a request form containing the name, dosage form, strength, and intended use of the medication; details regarding its clinical evidence (e.g., literature citations); and any other special considerations (e.g., financial reimbursement requirements). The requestor should also disclose any potential conflicts of interest that are pertinent to the medication being requested. **Appendix 18-A** provides an example of a request change form.

## PRODUCT REVIEW

Members of the P&T Committee should be provided with thorough, accurate, nonbiased, and current reviews, often in the form of a formulary monograph, for the medication undergoing formulary consideration.[11,12] Various review types are acceptable based on Committee preference and the nature of the request: full drug monograph, therapeutic class review, or expedited review. Full formulary monographs are the most common type of evaluation and are appropriate for most medication reviews.

Regardless of the mechanism initiating the formulary change process (e.g., new drug approval, provider request), a full drug monograph should normally be prepared for the P&T Committee's review and evaluation. Although the final document should be tailored to the needs of the specific formulary and institution, the typical components of a formulary monograph are included in **Figure 18-7**. A detailed description of the components of a formulary monograph is provided in **Appendix 18-B**. The P&T Committee is charged with the task of reviewing the literature provided in the monograph and making decisions on the appropriateness for the organization's patient population based on the safety, efficacy, and cost-effectiveness of the medication.

In addition to formulary monographs, reviews of entire therapeutic classes should be performed regularly to ensure that formulary medications are of appropriate efficacy, safety, and costs compared with other therapeutic alternatives. Class reviews should include all commercially available products in the therapeutic class, regardless of formulary status.

Because this review allows for class comparisons of safety, efficacy, and pharmacoeconomic data, it is reasonable to expect decisions regarding formulary addition, as well as formulary deletion of more costly therapeutically similar products. This ultimately leads to the refinement of formulary-selected medications within a therapeutic class.

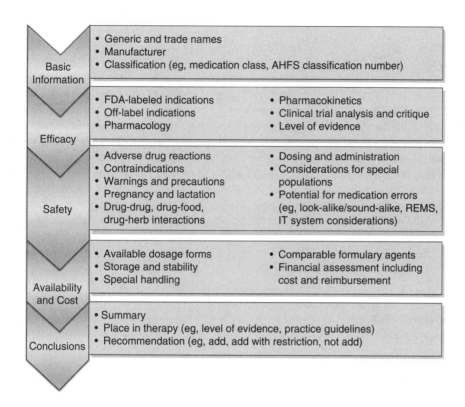

**FIGURE 18-7**  Components of a product review for formulary consideration.

---

### Background

The attending physician has submitted a formal request to the Pharmacy and Therapeutics Committee asking for tbo-filgrastim to be added to the formulary. After discussing the request with the chair of the Committee, you are asked to create and present a formulary monograph at the next meeting.

### Question

What are the components of a formulary monograph and the type of information that should be discussed in each section?

### Answer

The components, length, and overall detail of a formulary monograph may vary depending on the institution and type of medication being reviewed. Nevertheless, most monographs contain the same basic components that are used to evaluate the efficacy, safety, and cost of therapy. Appendix 18-B provides an example of the typical components of a formulary monograph and a description of the contents. While preparing the monograph, it is important to consider what medication use policies, guidelines, charts, or other documents would be affected by a potential change. **Appendix 18-C** provides a checklist example of this type of review.

Periodically, previous formulary decisions should be reviewed by the P&T Committee to determine the current relevance of the prior decision. For example, when new safety or efficacy data become available or significant changes to the cost of the medication occur, an abbreviated reevaluation is warranted. Additionally, if the FDA approves a new dosage form or strength of a medication currently on the formulary, the P&T Committee may decide to conduct an abbreviated review because the safety and efficacy of the medication have been reviewed previously. Additionally, newly published efficacy and/or safety data or action by the FDA (e.g., Boxed Warning, newly approved indication) could prompt an abbreviated review for an individual formulary medication. This type of review may also be an appropriate choice for consideration of newly marketed medications. Novel medications with no therapeutic alternatives may undergo an abbreviated review to ensure availability for specific patient populations (e.g., HIV medications, cancer treatments); the P&T Committee may also choose to impose a waiting period (e.g., 1 year) before reviewing a therapeutically similar medication. This waiting period would allow for the collection of postmarketing safety data.

Following the product review, it is the responsibility of the P&T Committee to make decisions regarding each medication under consideration. The P&T Committee may vote to add the medication to the formulary for widespread use throughout the organization without restrictions. It may also vote to add a medication but assign restrictions or guidelines for use. Finally, the P&T Committee may vote to not add the medication to the formulary for various reasons, including therapeutic duplication, unacceptable risk for medication errors, economic concerns, or lack of supporting safety or efficacy data over currently available medications.

When considering formulary additions, discussion regarding deletions of certain products from the formulary may be warranted. Low utilization of a formulary medication, newly identified safety concerns, superior efficacy and/or safety data with a newly approved medication, and market discontinuation are viable reasons a medication may require deletion. These action items may be the responsibility of a specific subcommittee.

Although many organizations use internal resources to prepare product reviews, there are commercially available resources (e.g., the Formulary Monograph Service), or information can be made available through group purchasing organizations. Academy of Managed Care Pharmacy (AMCP) formulary dossiers are an additional resource used by healthcare plans as well as healthcare systems.

## APPLICATION OF LITERATURE EVALUATION SKILLS

Several key concepts are important for a thorough understanding of formulary evaluation and management. Clinical and anecdotal experience can be misleading when making decisions about entire patient populations; therefore, evaluation of clinical trial data is an important component of formulary decision making. Sources of evidence include a variety of strengths and types, ranging from meta-analyses and randomized controlled clinical trials to case reports. Consensus statements from professional organizations and expert opinions can also be useful in preparing a product review in the absence of or in addition to stronger sources of evidence. The goal of a formulary review is to base the decision on evidence-based practice. Various resources for evidence-based practice are presented in **Table 18-1**.[24] Essential Evidence Plus defines *evidence-based practice* as "making a conscientious effort to base clinical decisions on research that is most likely to be free from bias, and using interventions most likely to improve how long or well patients live."[24]

| TABLE 18-1 | Resources for Evidence-Based Practice |
|---|---|
| **Resource** | **Availability** |
| *Evidence Rating Scales* | |
| **Centre for Evidence-Based Medicine, Oxford (1a-5)** | www.cebm.net/?o=1025 |
| **SORT: Strength-of-Recommendation Taxonomy (A, B, C)** | *American Family Physician.* 2004;69(3):548-556<br>www.aafp.org/afp/2004/0201/p548.html |
| **GRADE: Grading of Recommendations Assessment, Development and Evaluation (A, B, C, D)** | www.gradeworkinggroup.org |
| **Various practice guidelines rating scales** | Essential Evidence Plus: www.essentialevidenceplus.com/product/ebm_loe.cfm |
| *Online Products or Other Resources* | |
| **The Cochrane Library** | www.thecochranelibrary.com/view/0/index.html |
| **National Guideline Clearinghouse** | www.guideline.gov |
| **Agency for Healthcare Research and Quality** | www.ahrq.gov |
| **EBM Guidelines** | onlinelibrary.wiley.com/book/10.1002/0470057203 |
| **Centre for Evidence-Based Medicine** | www.cebm.net |
| **Essential Evidence Plus** | www.essentialevidenceplus.com |
| *The Philosophy of Evidence-Based Medicine* | J. H. Howick (Wiley-Blackwell, 2011) |
| *How to Read a Paper* | T. Greenhalgh (Wiley-Blackwell, 2014) |
| *Evidence-Based Decisions and Economics: Health Care, Social Welfare, Education, and Criminal Justice* | I. Shemilt, ed. (Wiley-Blackwell, 2010) |

Data from Evidence-Based Practice Overview. Essential Evidence Plus. 2013. http://www.essentialevidenceplus.com/product/ebm_overview.cfm. Accessed July 24, 2014.

When preparing a formulary review, it may be helpful to determine the level of evidence to summarize the strength of evidence for the literature evaluation. Level-of-evidence scales are commonplace in published guidelines; however, not all clinical scenarios have guidelines available for review. Therefore, some organizations elect to use general published evidence ratings scales and modify them to meet their needs.

## Pharmacoeconomic Evaluation

Careful economic assessment is necessary when evaluating medications for formulary addition; thus, a description of these analyses is warranted in this context. The pharmacoeconomic analysis should incorporate all costs and consequences relevant to the addition.[25] This analysis can be as simple as just a review of costs compared with therapeutic equivalents. Depending on the organization, the cost will be dependent on several factors, including, but not limited to, the following: wholesale acquisition cost, group purchasing agreements, manufacturer-specific contracts, and 340B outpatient pricing. Reimbursement should also be considered, because it may affect any potential cost savings. The cost and reimbursement figures should then be applied to actual or projected utilization to determine the annualized impact on the budget. Some organizations, especially PBMs, will complete more in-depth reviews. A brief description of the types of pharmacoeconomic analyses and their role in the formulary decision process follows.

Cost-minimization analyses are appropriate when new medications are considered to be therapeutically equivalent; therefore, they are typically included in a

| CASE STUDY 18-3 | Tbo-filgrastim (Granix™) Evaluation |
| --- | --- |

## Background

Upon reviewing the literature for tbo-filgrastim, you come across several observational studies and randomized controlled trials (RCTs). You decide to follow the principles of evidenced-based medicine and review only those studies with the strongest level of evidence.

## Question

Based on the studies listed in **Table 18-2**, choose three articles that would be most appropriate to include in your formal clinical trial review. Why did you choose these articles? What is the level of evidence?

## Answer

Based on the search results listed in Table 18-2, it would be most appropriate to include studies 1, 4, and 5. These studies are all prospective RCTs. Interventional studies, such as RCTs, generally provide the highest quality of evidence because they can better establish cause-and-effect relationships compared with observational designs. They are also less susceptible to bias and confounders due to their randomized treatment assignment. Studies 1, 4, and 5 also have a greater sample size compared with the other studies listed in Table 18-2. Generally, studies with a larger sample can detect smaller differences between treatments and can provide better insight about the total population at risk. The observational studies 2, 3, and 6 should still be reviewed, as they may add additional information pertinent to the overall discussion and recommendation.

    Level of evidence can be determined by different mechanisms. Table 18-1 provides examples of evidence rating scales. **Appendix 18-D** provides an example of a level of evidence rating system. Using Appendix 18-D, the level of evidence is listed in **Table 18-3**.

| TABLE 18-2 | Literature Search Results for Tbo-filgrastim | | |
| --- | --- | --- | --- |
| **Study** | **Design** | **Population** | **Intervention** |
| Study 1 | P, R, MC, PC, AC | 348 patients with breast cancer requiring chemotherapy | Tbo-filgrastim (n = 140) vs. filgrastim (n = 136) or placebo (n = 72) |
| Study 2 | Obs | 14 patients requiring collection of PBSC for autologous transplantation after induction | Tbo-filgrastim with plerixafor before apheresis |
| Study 3 | Obs | 58 patients requiring PBSC transplantation | Tbo-filgrastim (n = 32) vs. lenograstim (n = 26) |
| Study 4 | P, R, MC, AC | 92 with non-Hodgkins lymphoma requiring chemotherapy | Tbo-filgrastim (n = 63) vs. filgrastim (n = 29) |
| Study 5 | P, R, MC, AC | 240 patients with small cell/non–small cell lung cancer requiring chemotherapy | Tbo-filgrastim (n = 160) vs. filgrastim (n = 80) |
| Study 6 | Obs | 22 patients undergoing allogenic stem cell transplant | Tbo-filgrastim (n = 11) versus "reference" GCSF agent (n = 11) |

AC = active controlled; GCSF = granulocyte colony stimulating factor; MC = multicenter; Obs = observational study; P = prospective; PBSC = peripheral blood stem cells; PC = placebo controlled; R = randomized.

| TABLE 18-3 | Level of Evidence Ratings | | |
| --- | --- | --- | --- |
| **Study** | **Level of Evidence** | **Study** | **Level of Evidence** |
| Study 1 | 1B | Study 4 | 1B |
| Study 2 | 1C | Study 5 | 1B |
| Study 3 | 1C | Study 6 | 1C |

| CASE STUDY 18-4 | Tbo-filgrastim (Granix™) Evaluation |
|---|---|

## Background

After reviewing the efficacy and safety of tbo-filgrastim, you now wish to determine the financial feasibility of using this medication. The hospital in this example uses filgrastim in both the inpatient and outpatient settings. The supply chain manager reports that the hospital has a group purchasing agreement for tbo-filgrastim and qualifies for 340B outpatient pricing. The group purchasing agreement states that a 70% institution market share will provide a 7% rebate, with an additional 3% rebate if the purchasing group maintains a 45% market share.

## Question

What are some of the factors/costs you would want to know in order to perform an economic analysis?

## Answer

There are many factors to consider in regard to cost and reimbursement, including, but not limited to, the following: inpatient and outpatient cost, contract pricing, purchasing incentives, reimbursement, and real or projected utilization. Depending on the organization, costs can be determined by the following:

- Wholesale acquisition costs (WAC), average sales price (ASP), average wholesale price (AWP), 340B price
- Group purchasing agreements
- Manufacturer-specific contracts

Purchasing agreements and other contracts typically have market-share requirements for the single agent or bundled with other products. Additionally, it is important to review differences in these costs from inpatient to outpatient and compare them with other available products. When considering an addition or switch in formulary products, the costs should be applied to real or projected utilization to determine what estimated annualized increases or savings may be realized. Lastly, there should be an evaluation of the reimbursement in the outpatient setting.

This hospital reviewed the costs, purchasing agreements, and Amgen-specific contracts for filgrastim. **Table 18-4** shows that acquisition cost is similar for inpatient use; however, the cost is more favorable for filgrastim in the outpatient setting.

A review of previous-year utilization shows 550 doses outpatient and 1,488 doses inpatient (73% market share). If all use is changed to tbo-filgrastim, this hospital would realize approximately $6,000 in annual savings. If only inpatient use is changed to tbo-filgrastim, the hospital would realize up to $30,000 in annual savings. Assuming similar usage, there may be concern that the market-share requirements may not always be achieved, which would minimize those cost-savings projections.

| TABLE 18-4 | Acquisition Cost Information | | |
|---|---|---|---|
| **Medication** | **Available Strength(s)** | **Inpatient Cost per Unit ($)** | **Outpatient Cost per Unit ($)** |
| Tbo-filgrastim (Granix™) | 300 micrograms, PFS | 230 | 180 |
| | 480 micrograms, PFS | 355 | 278 |
| Filgrastim (Neupogen®) | 300 micrograms, PFS | 243 | 142 |
| | 480 micrograms, PFS | 385 | 227 |
| | 300 micrograms/mL, 1 mL SDV | 230 | 120 |
| | 480 micrograms/mL, 1 mL SDV | 363 | 189 |

PFS = prefilled syringe, SDV = single-dose vial.

| TABLE 18-5 | Tbo-filgrastim Reimbursement Information |
|---|---|
| Supplied | 300- and 480-microgram, single-use, prefilled syringe<br>NDC: 63459-910-11 and 63459-912-11, respectively<br>Charge code: *Not available at the time of this review*<br>HCPCS code: J1446<br>Billing unit: 5 micrograms = 1 billing unit (BU) |
| Diagnosis and administration code | *ICD-9 Code*: 288.0, neutropenia, with 780.61 for any associated fever<br>*Administration (CPT) Code*: 96372, subcutaneous or intramuscular injection |
| Cost | See Table 18C-4 |
| Inpatient Use | Cost will come out of the DRG assigned to the admission. |
| Outpatient Use | • Medicare: FDA-approved indications only<br>     300 microgram<br>     480 microgram<br>  Medicare Part B allowable charge (WAC + 6%)<br>     $243.90<br>     $390.32<br>  Medicare pays 80%<br>     $195.12<br>     $312.26<br>  Patient secondary insurance pays 20%<br>     $48.78<br>     $78.06<br>• Medicaid: No additional reimbursement for drug if given in a hospital-based clinic.<br>• Private payers: Prior authorization required.<br>• *Recommended to fill as an outpatient prescription if the patient has coverage and have the patient self-administer.* |
| Special considerations | Has not been added to the state local coverage determination (LCD) for colony-stimulating factors at the time of this review. |
| Reimbursement assistance programs | • Teva CORE: 1-888-587-3263<br>• Patient assistance program<br>• No copayment support listed |

**Table 18-5** shows the reimbursement evaluation. Reimbursement for inpatient use will always be part of the payments made based on the diagnosis-related group (DRG) assigned at admission. Therefore, costs for the drug may or may not be covered during that admission. Outpatient reimbursement is based on the patient's payer. Most payers follow the reimbursement guidelines provided by the Centers for Medicare and Medicaid Services (CMS). Medicare will provide reimbursement based on the FDA-approved indications unless otherwise stated by the state's local coverage determination (LCD). If covered, reimbursement is based on the ASP or WAC, with Medicare paying 80%. Based on the outpatient acquisition costs in Table 18-5, the payments by Medicare would provide up to $30 in revenue per dose. Additional revenue may be realized if the patient has a secondary payer or covers the 20% not covered by Medicare. Off-label use would not be covered by Medicare and would require prior authorization by private payers. Medicaid coverage is determined by each state, so reimbursement for medications administered in a hospital-based clinic may or may not be covered. Therefore, any cost savings would need to be weighed against the potential for revenue loss.

formulary review. This analysis accounts for the cost of the medication, as well as non-medication-related costs (e.g., administration costs, monitoring, length of hospital stay). Cost-benefit analyses measure inputs and outcomes in monetary terms and are applied to clinical scenarios. Cost-benefit analyses are favored for their ability to measure clinical outcomes (e.g., avoidance of death, reduction in blood pressure) and assign a monetary value on those outcomes. However, the limitation with this type of analysis is the questionable meaningfulness of the result due to assumptions of perceived value. Cost-effectiveness analyses assess the incremental difference in investment required to produce an incremental difference in clinical outcome and are complex in nature. This is the most common type of pharmacoeconomic analysis found in the pharmacy literature; however, it is not often used for formulary decision making due to its complexity. Cost-utility analyses allow for the relation of therapeutic outcomes to pharmaceutical costs or services and patient preferences. Cost-utility analyses measure costs per unit of utility, defined as the amount of satisfaction gained from the medication or service.

Pharmacoeconomic analyses published in the literature can also be a valuable resource when making formulary decisions. Careful attention should be paid to the assumptions in the economic model to ensure the results are applicable to the organization. Rigorous pharmacoeconomic procedures may not be possible for all formulary product reviews; however, a basic financial evaluation should be included at a minimum.

## STRATEGIES FOR FORMULARY MANAGEMENT

A variety of strategies are used to manage individual formularies, whether managed care preferred drug lists or organizational formularies. Several of those strategies are described below and summarized in **Figure 18-8**.

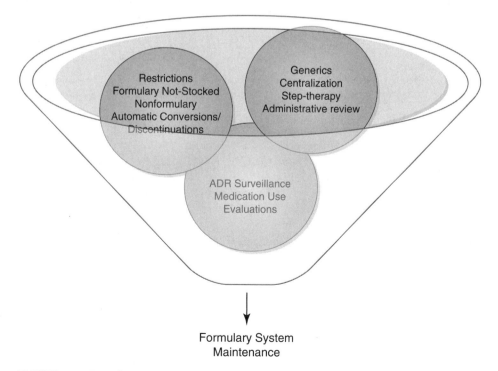

**FIGURE 18-8** Formulary management and maintenance strategies.

One important reason for the adoption of drug formularies is their cost-saving potential. Given this concern, generic drug utilization is an important strategy for management.[11] Most organizations and PBMs allow and encourage the use of generic equivalents (e.g., AB-rated drug products) in order to provide optimal patient care in the most cost-effective manner.

Adding a medication to the formulary with use restricted by approved criteria is also a common management strategy. The purpose of restricting a medication is to ensure patient safety and appropriate utilization. Medications may be restricted by physician specialty, whereby the P&T Committee believes a higher degree of expertise is needed to appropriately prescribe a medication. Medications may also be restricted to a specific patient population, clinical indication or criteria, or patient care area. Restriction classifications may vary among organizations and should reflect the needs and characteristics of the specific organization.

Unique product designations have also been used to help manage formulary use. Traditionally, medications have been classified into one of three formulary categories: on formulary without restriction, on formulary with restriction, and nonformulary. Recently, however, the use of a newer formulary designation—known as formulary not stocked—has become more prevalent among hospitals. This new category permits a medication to be added to the formulary without the need to keep it stocked in the pharmacy. Doing so allows hospitals to retain the advantages of a formulary medication (e.g., safe integration into computer software, better purchasing power), while also avoiding the costly inventory burden (e.g., risk of wasting expensive, unused medications). This designation is often applied to high-cost, low-use medications; to medications with limited therapeutic use requiring special expertise; or to medications associated with a high risk of serious toxicity. This category may be more beneficial in the outpatient setting where there is the luxury of time to order products for patient care needs. For the inpatient setting, this designation may not be appropriate as the clinical situation may be more urgent, which would not allow for procurement time. Therefore, some large organizations (i.e., those that have more than one pharmacy location) prefer to centralize predetermined quantities of rarely used, high-cost medications (e.g., designated antivenins, antidotes, factors) sufficient to last through emergency situations.

Another common management strategy is the use of automatic conversions and discontinuations.[11,26] These strategies allow for use of preferred agents over nonformulary drugs or help to limit the use of medications. **Therapeutic alternatives** differ from generic equivalents in that they are drug products with different chemical structures, but are of the same pharmacologic and/or therapeutic class. These medications can usually be expected to have similar therapeutic effects and safety profiles when administered to patients in equivalent doses and regimens. Legally, therapeutic alternatives cannot be interchanged for one another without notification and authorization of the prescriber. Therefore, the development of therapeutic interchange protocols can be instrumental in streamlining medication use in selected classes. This strategy allows for the exchange of one product for another according to previously approved guidelines by the organization.

For example, if the preferred proton pump inhibitor of an organization is pantoprazole, then a protocol may be developed for the conversion of all other proton pump inhibitors to pantoprazole based on previously established and approved written guidelines or protocols within a formulary system. This strategy provides pharmacists with the authorization to exchange formulary alternatives in place of a nonformulary or nonpreferred medication without having to contact the prescriber. It is important to consider that the prescriber should retain the authority to opt out of the interchange if an appropriate justification is provided (e.g., allergy or therapeutic failure to preferred product). One limitation of the substitutions is the inconsistency of reconciling the medication at discharge to ensure the patient is restarted on the therapy that he was stabilized on at home prior to admission. Therefore, it is important to ensure that the organization has a well-established medication reconciliation process. Many computerized provider order entry (CPOE) systems allow for presentation of this substitution information at the point of prescribing and also present this substitution to the provider at discharge.

Another type of automatic conversion would be to establish intravenous (IV)–to–oral (PO) protocols. Intravenous products are typically more expensive, can be difficult to administer, and may a pose greater risk to a patient compared with an oral formulation; therefore, it is prudent to limit their use to patients who cannot take anything by mouth. IV-to-PO conversion protocols allow the substitution of the oral formulation based on specific predefined conditions for specific agents and appropriate doses. Similar to therapeutic conversions, these protocols allow the pharmacist to make the substitution without contacting the prescriber. However, it is important to consider factors, other than the patient's PO status, when developing inclusion and exclusion criteria for the conversion.

In addition, automatic order discontinuations can be used to control medication use and help to promote cost-effective and safe medication management. The use of an electronic health record promotes the use of these where necessary, because it allows for the order to discontinue automatically. The duration of the order may be based on the potential increased adverse effects after a certain number of days of treatment. For example, the Boxed Warning for ketorolac indicates that it should be reserved for short-term (i.e., less than 5 days) management of moderate-to-severe pain. Therefore, some organizations have placed an automatic stop on the order at 48 hours to allow for reassessment of the patient. If continued therapy is warranted, it may be ordered again; however, the full duration should not exceed 5 days. There are also clinical scenarios where it would be unsafe to allow an order based on a specific concomitant order or when certain lab values are present. In these scenarios, an organization may elect to establish a hard stop so that the order cannot be processed until the unsafe combination is resolved. For example, the CPOE system would not allow the provider to enter an order for IV ethanol when a patient has an active order for metronidazole.

Step-therapy measures are useful when a therapeutic treatment plan is administered in a stepwise approach. For example, it is often appropriate to begin therapy for gastroesophageal reflux disease (GERD) with an $H_2$-receptor antagonist, such as famotidine, before progressing to therapy with a proton pump inhibitor. Similarly, many formularies require a failure, documented allergy, or adverse reaction to an angiotensin-converting enzyme inhibitor (e.g., lisinopril) before allowing the use of an angiotensin II receptor antagonist (e.g., losartan).

Lastly, administrative review, also known as second-level review, has been described with high-cost medications and serves to ensure appropriate use of the medication and increase awareness of the cost among prescribers. This review considers not only the cost of a medication but also the anticipation of reimbursement. The individual or team conducting the review is often part of P&T leadership (e.g., director of pharmacy, committee chair) and/or medical staff leadership (e.g., chief medical officer). The ordering provider may be asked to present the case, and the reviewing party will either approve the use or refer the case to another committee for further information and follow-up (e.g., ethics consultation service, palliative care committee, ad-hoc peer review team). Although this process is important to ensure fiscally responsible use of medications, it may be prohibitive to patient care in urgent or emergent situations.

# STRATEGIES FOR FORMULARY SYSTEM MAINTENANCE

## NONFORMULARY USE

An important consideration in formulary maintenance is the realization that medications not included on the formulary may be necessary for individual patients. Although the intent of the formulary process is to select the most appropriate medications for the majority of patients covered by the formulary, the need for nonformulary medications will arise. Organizations should have a provision in place that allows for procurement and dispensing of a nonformulary product if the use is justified. Nonformulary use may be appropriate if an individual has tried and failed formulary alternatives or has an allergy or intolerance to the formulary agents. Furthermore, patients with a rare diagnosis or condition may require treatment with a nonformulary medication for which there is no formulary alternative.

Nonformulary use should be monitored and reported to the P&T Committee. This evaluation allows the Committee to monitor trends in nonformulary prescribing. For inappropriate prescribing habits, educational measures (e.g., academic detailing) can be employed to encourage prescribing of formulary alternatives. However, tracking nonformulary prescribing identifies medications that should undergo formulary review due to frequent use.

## ROLE OF ADVERSE DRUG REACTION AND MEDICATION ERROR SURVEILLANCE AND REPORTING PROGRAMS

The estimated incidence and projected costs attributed to medication misadventures underscore the necessity for effective surveillance programs, primarily due to the impact of these events on patient safety. The 2000 publication by the Institute of Medicine, *To Err is Human: Building a Safer Health System*, revealed the significance of both medication errors and adverse drug reactions (ADRs) in the lay and medical literature.[27] The report shed light on the common occurrence of medication errors and ADRs in every health system. Identification of a medication misadventure is critical for improvement in patient safety and optimal formulary management.

Surveillance programs are instrumental in raising awareness of the prevalence of ADRs and the resultant harm. Such programs are necessary due to limited clinical experience with medications and limitations in ADR detection in clinical trials. Surveillance programs help to optimize patient safety and improve patient outcomes by identifying trends in institutions. Results from surveillance programs should be reviewed by the P&T Committee regularly to implement appropriate changes to the formulary.

With regard to medication errors, it is important to consider that, while no harm is incurred with some medication errors, all events should be reported because there is a potential for a patient, a visitor, or an employee to incur harm due to the conditions of the environment. These types of errors are referred to as *near misses* and are instrumental in improving processes within a formulary system.

From a formulary perspective, safeguarding the use of medications can be achieved through careful product selection. Reducing the number of medications and dosage forms on the formulary, standardizing the available concentrations and volumes of intravenous medications, and removing high-alert medications (e.g., concentrated electrolytes) from clinical areas serve to reduce the potential for errors to occur.

| CASE STUDY 18-5 | Tbo-filgrastim (Granix™) Formulary Recommendation |
|---|---|

## Background

You have now finished compiling the formulary monograph for tbo-filgrastim and are ready to make your recommendation. Based on your review of the literature, you have determined that tbo-filgrastim is efficacious for its labeled indication to reduce the length of severe neutropenia in patients with nonmyeloid malignancies being treated with chemotherapy. However, data for nonlabeled indications (e.g., use in bone marrow transplant, use in pediatrics) are lacking compared with its innovator product, filgrastim. Overall, adverse reactions are comparable with filgrastim, although slightly more bone pain was seen in the clinical trials with tbo-filgrastim. Based on the financial evaluation, you have determined that there is some cost savings with the inpatient use of tbo-filgrastim; however, the limited anticipated use in the outpatient setting minimizes the cost savings. Additionally, with the uncertainty with outpatient reimbursement, there may be some revenue lost. Lastly, some providers are hesitant to transition treatment for certain patients to tbo-filgrastim because the FDA has not approved extended labeling.

## Question

Given this scenario, how would you summarize the review for formulary addition? Would you add it to the formulary? Would you place any restrictions on its use?

## Answer

Although this medication is not officially classified as a biosimilar product by the FDA, it has been utilized for several years in Europe as such. For a medication to be classified as a biosimilar product by the FDA, several steps must be completed to demonstrate similarity to the reference drug. These include demonstrating similarities in chemical structure, toxicity, pharmacokinetic and pharmacodynamic properties, immunogenicity, and clinical safety and effectiveness. Even though similarities have been demonstrated with tbo-filgrastim, to date, no product has been approved as a biosimilar in the United States. With no precedent being set, it is difficult to determine if the FDA would indeed grant biosimilar status to this medication if the manufacturer were to apply. The FDA is less specific and states that similarity among indications will be taken on a case-by-case basis. Although it is fairly clear that this medication could be efficacious for the FDA-approved indication, data for nonlabeled indications are lacking. The demonstrated similarities between tbo-filgrastim and filgrastim might suggest that any differences would be minimal. Additionally, this medication is included in the National Comprehensive Cancer Network (NCCN) guidelines regarding myeloid growth factors next to filgrastim for the prophylaxis and treatment of febrile neutropenia.

One potential benefit with the use of an agent such as tbo-filgrastim over the current formulary product is cost savings. Based on the financial evaluation, a complete switch from filgrastim to tbo-filgrastim would account for annual cost savings of about $6,000. On the other hand, a switch only to use in the inpatient setting would account for a cost savings of approximately $30,000. Another factor to consider is the impact of reimbursement with use in the outpatient setting. Currently reimbursement, especially for nonlabeled indications, is questionable.

With this information, a full formulary switch to tbo-filgrastim is likely to be efficacious and safe in patients. However, for nonlabeled indications, this belief is based on the extrapolation of data from patients with no disease or other conditions. A full switch may also incur a cost savings, but not to a large enough degree to overcome a potential for large operational changes; questions regarding nonlabeled use; and questionable reimbursement over a more established drug. Therefore, it is recommended that tbo-filgrastim *not be added* to the formulary at this time.

After discussion with the Hematology/Oncology subcommittee, it was determined that there should not be any use of tbo-filgrastim until there are more data for nonlabeled uses and/or the cost differences for outpatient use changes. Therefore, the P&T Committee voted to add tbo-filgrastim to the "nonformulary restricted" list, meaning that nonformulary use is not allowed under any circumstance. Clinical and financial data will be re-reviewed in 6 months.

Finally, formulary decisions should consider the potential for medication errors. As discussed previously, the formulary review process requires the need for potential medication errors to be identified. This should entail a careful evaluation of the product packaging; storage conditions; look-alike, sound-alike nature of the medication name; and commercially available concentrations and products.

## MEDICATION USE POLICY DEVELOPMENT

As mentioned previously, the formulary system incorporates more than the list of medications available for use within the organization. The formulary system has evolved to include development of policies on the use of medications and medication use processes, as well as multidisciplinary plans of best clinical practice. Medication use policy can be summarized as using best practices for the safe and effective delivery of medication therapy. This is achieved through effective formulary management with oversight by the P&T Committee. It allows organizations to not only comply with various regulatory and statutory requirements, but also encourages a culture of safety and efficiency. It includes strategies to modify prescribing behaviors, including medication guidelines, prescribing tools, clinical pathways (also known as critical paths, care maps, or patient pathways), evidence-based order sets, and collaborative drug therapy management agreements.[28]

# CONTINUOUS QUALITY IMPROVEMENT

## MEDICATION USE EVALUATIONS

Quality assessment and improvement is a function of ongoing process evaluation and assessment. In order to evaluate quality, it must be adequately defined. Organizations rely on several governing and accrediting bodies to provide appropriate definitions of quality. The Joint Commission (www.jointcommission.org), the Centers for Medicare and Medicaid Services (CMS) (www.cms.gov), the National Committee for Quality Assurance (www.ncqa.org), the Agency for Healthcare Research and Quality (www.ahrq.gov), and the Institute for Safe Medication Practices (www.ismp.org) each provide standards, guidelines, and recommendations for ensuring quality in patient care. These resources are used to strengthen the medication use process and enhance the quality of patient care.

Medication use evaluations (MUEs) are a quality improvement measure that examine aspects of the medication use process from prescribing to monitoring (see **Figure 18-9**).[11,29] Organizations conduct MUEs to evaluate the medication use process

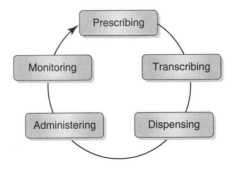

**FIGURE 18-9** Medication use cycle.

with the goal of optimizing patient outcomes. An MUE may be applied to an individual medication (e.g., propofol use in the neurosurgical intensive care unit); therapeutic class (e.g., thiazolidinedione use and the presence of weight gain, edema, or congestive heart failure); a disease state or condition (e.g., assessment of potentially inappropriate medications according to the Beers criteria in patients who are at least 65 years of age); a specific clinical event (e.g., concomitant administration of proton pump inhibitors and clopidogrel in patients admitted with myocardial infarction); a medication use process (e.g., time to initiation of patient-controlled analgesia pumps); or a specific outcome (e.g., adherence to formulary restriction guidelines for prescribing of ezetimibe).

MUEs are a systematic way to monitor, evaluate, and improve medication use throughout a system or organization. They are an important aspect of formulary management and may be a tool to measure the effectiveness of an intervention, such as the evaluation of a newly added formulary medication.

# SPECIAL CONSIDERATIONS

## OFF-LABEL USE

**Off-label use** refers to the use of a medication outside of the labeled indications, route, dose, or specified patient population and is a common practice in institutions.[11,22,30] Although the ultimate responsibility for off-label prescribing rests with the prescriber, the formulary review should include evaluation of efficacy and safety data for off-label prescribing if it is part of the initial request.

## INVESTIGATIONAL DRUG USE

Many practitioners in academic and nonacademic organizations are involved with clinical investigation of medications, which may include prescription and nonprescription products. Although investigational use of a medication may occur regardless of formulary status, members of the P&T Committee should be aware of the investigational use of a medication within the organization. Similar considerations for the safe use of medications within the institution apply in these circumstances.

## PROCUREMENT CHALLENGES

Drug shortages create significant difficulty and challenges for healthcare professionals.[31,32] In many cases, an appropriate therapeutic alternative exists and, while concerns about the therapeutic alternative are alleviated, the logistical impact remains. For example, temporary alternatives to formulary medications, such as a conversion to phenytoin in the event of the fosphenytoin shortage, requires changes to information systems (e.g., preprogrammed infusion pumps and order forms) and widespread education efforts for prescribers, pharmacists, and nurses.

During drug shortages, the role of the P&T Committee is important and serves to set organizational priorities. Processes should be in place within organizations to involve key personnel for handling such challenges. Unlike routine formulary changes, drug shortages are abrupt and require a swift response. Therefore, the following should be considered in the event of a shortage: designating appropriate alternatives; identifying strategies for managing the remaining stock, including the establishment of use restrictions; and implementing evidence-based review procedures. Routine and thorough communication with staff and patients is imperative when managing shortages.

Market withdrawals and drug recalls present another challenge to inventory management and procurement personnel. Recalls occur when a product is defective or potentially harmful. Recalls are initiated by the manufacturer directly, by an FDA request, or by an FDA order. They are classified by severity (i.e., Class I, II, or III), with Class I being the most severe.[33] Organizations should have adequate strategies in place to identify affected products in order to remove the items from stock.[34]

# EFFECTIVE COMMUNICATION

Clear and consistent communication is one of the most important aspects of patient safety in health care. The P&T Committee should ensure that there are established mechanisms to communicate with healthcare professionals, patients, and payers about changes within the formulary system.[11,35,36] The goal should be to provide effective communication, provide transparent formulary management, and convey all implemented drug policies. Additionally, academic detailing should be provided by pharmacy staff to meet the needs of the professional staff in regard to the use of medications within the organization.

A published formulary is a valuable communication tool. Historically, this was available as a hard copy reference; however, there are many ways to host a formulary in an electronic format. Many organizations use a website to host the formulary through a specific vendor. **Table 18-6** lists a number of different vendors.[37-44] Such sites provide

| **TABLE 18-6**    Formulary Hosting Resources | | |
|---|---|---|
| **Formulary Hosting Resource** | **Company** | **Type of Resource** |
| **Amplifi®** | Wolters Kluwer Health–Pharmacy OneSource® | Formulary hosting—health systems |
| **Epocrates** | | Formulary hosting—health systems and commercial payers |
| **FormChecker** | Elsevier–Gold Standard | Formulary hosting—health systems |
| **FormWeb** | Formulary Productions | Formulary hosting—health systems |
| **Formulary Advisor®** | Truven Health Analytics | Formulary hosting—health systems |
| **Lexicomp® FORMULINK** | Wolters Kluwer Health–Lexicomp® | Formulary hosting—health systems |
| **RxFlex** | Adaptive Rx–Pharmacy Benefit Solutions | Formulary hosting—commercial payers |
| **Zynchros™ Commercial Plan Pro™ Medicare Part D Pro™** | SXC Health Solutions | Formulary hosting—commercial payers |

*Data* from Amplifi®. Wolters Kluwer Health – Pharmacy OneSource®. http://www.pharmacyonesource.com/applications/amplifi/. Accessed July 24, 2014; Epocrates® Formulary Hosting. Epocrates® – An AthenaHealth Company. http://www.epocrates.com/formulary-hosting. Accessed July 24, 2014; FormChecker. Elsevier Gold Standard. http://www.goldstandard.com/product/pricing-analysis-cost-control/form-checker/. Accessed July 24, 2014; FormWeb. Formulary Productions. http://formweb.com/. Accessed July 24, 2014; Micromedex 2.0 – Formulary Advisor®. Truven Health Analytics. http://www.truvenhealth.com/your_healthcare_focus/hospital_patient_care_decisions/medication_management.aspx. Accessed July 24, 2014; Lexicomp® FORMULINK. Lexicomp®. http://www.lexi.com/institutions/products/formulary/. Accessed July 24, 2014; RxFlex – Formulary Management Simplified. AdaptiveRx – Pharmacy Benefit Solutions. http://www.adaptiverx.com/rxflex.jsp. Accessed July 24, 2014; Zynchros Services. http://www.zynchros.com/services/. Accessed July 24, 2014.

a list of medications available on the formulary and may also help drive compliance with TJC medication management guidelines; create cost savings; promote patient safety (e.g., links to Boxed Warnings and FDA warnings); increase staff productivity (e.g., links to other point-of-care resources); and centralize all the P&T Committee-approved guidelines, dosing charts, protocols, and order forms.

Other mechanisms of communication include newsletters, continuing education programs, blogs, and e-mails. A P&T Committee newsletter can provide not only the action items of the Committee, but also articles relative to medication use, reports from medication use evaluations, links to FDA safety alerts, and updates on drug shortages, to name a few.

# SUMMARY

Formulary management is a complicated practice and requires a keen understanding of the multiple components of the process. Regardless of the setting (e.g., health system, managed care organization), ensuring safe, effective, and cost-effective use of medications are underlying principles of a formulary. Furthermore, formulary management is a dynamic process, which requires a multidisciplinary approach involving the medical, pharmacy, nursing, and ancillary staff. Strategies discussed in this chapter should be implemented to ensure safe and effective medication use within organizations.

# REFERENCES

1.  Summary of NDA approvals & receipts, 1938 to present. U.S. Food and Drug Administration, Centers from Drug Evaluation and Research website. http://www.fda.gov/AboutFDA/WhatWeDo/History/ProductRegulation/SummaryofNDAApprovalsReceipts1938tothepresent/default.htm. Accessed July 24, 2014.
2.  2012 novel new drugs summary: January 2013. U.S. Food and Drug Administration, Centers from Drug Evaluation and Research website. http://www.fda.gov/downloads/Drugs/DevelopmentApprovalProcess/DrugInnovation/UCM337830.pdf. Accessed July 24, 2014.
3.  ANDA (Generic) drug approvals. U.S. Food and Drug Administration, Centers from Drug Evaluation and Research website. http://www.fda.gov/Drugs/DevelopmentApprovalProcess/HowDrugsareDevelopedandApproved/DrugandBiologicApprovalReports/ANDAGenericDrugApprovals/default.htm. Accessed July 24, 2014.
4.  Kaitin KI, DiMasi JA. Pharmaceutical innovation in the 21st century: new drug approvals in the first decade, 2000-2009. *Clin Pharmacol Ther.* 2011;89(2):183-188.
5.  Mullard A. 2011 FDA drug approvals. *Nat Rev Drug Discov.* 2012;11(2):91-94.
6.  Edwards R. In struggle to cut expenses, hospitals eye the pharmacy. H&HN: Hospitals & Health Networks®. 2011. http://www.hhnmag.com/hhnmag/jsp/articledisplay.jsp?dcrpath=HHNMAG/Article/data/11NOV2011/1111HHN_FEA_pharmacy&domain=HHNMAG. Accessed July 24, 2014.
7.  Anagnostis E, Wordell C, Guharoy R, Beckett R, Price V. A national survey on hospital formulary management processes. *J Pharm Pract.* 2011;24(4):409-416.
8.  Hoffman JM, Li E, Doloresco F, et al. Projecting future drug expenditures in United States non-federal hospitals and clinics—2013. *Am J Health Sys Pharm.* 2013;70(6):525-539.
9.  Academy of Managed Care Pharmacy. Formulary management; 2009. http://amcp.org/WorkArea/DownloadAsset.aspx?id=9298. Accessed July 24, 2014.
10. Scroccaro G. Formulary management. *Pharmacotherapy.* 2000;20(10 Pt 2):317S-321S.
11. Tyler LS, Cole SW, May JR, et al; ASHP Expert Panel on Formulary Management. ASHP guidelines on the pharmacy and therapeutics committee and the formulary system. *Am J Health Syst Pharm.* 2008;65(13):1272-1283.

12. Trice S, Devine J, Mistry H, Moore E, Linton A. Formulary management in the Department of Defense. *J Manag Care Pharm*. 2009;15(2):133-146.

13. Boucher BA. Formulary decisions: then and now. *Pharmacotherapy*. 2010;30(6 Pt 2):35S-41S.

14. Nair KV, Wolfe P, Valuck RJ, McCollum MM, Ganther JM, Lewis SJ. Effects of a 3-tier pharmacy benefit design on the prescription purchasing behavior of individuals with chronic disease. *J Manag Care Pharm*. 2003;9(2):123-133.

15. Hieber KA. Is your pharmacy benefit designed for your employees or the big drug companies? Pharmacy Benefit Design Considerations. PBM Plus Inc. 2008 http://www.pbmplus.com/docs/pharmacy_benefit_design.pdf. Accessed July 24, 2014.

16. Cowen DL. The Edinburgh Pharmacopoeia. *Med Hist*. 1957;1(4):340-351.

17. Balu S, O'Connor P, Vogenberg FR. Contemporary issues affecting P&T Committees, Part 1: the evolution. *P&T*. 2004;29(11):709-711.

18. American Society of Hospital Pharmacists. Minimum standard for pharmacies in hospitals. *Am J Hosp Pharm*. 1958;15:992-994.

19. American Medical Association. AMA policy on drug formularies and therapeutic interchange in inpatient and ambulatory patient care settings. *Am J Hosp Pharm*. 1994;51(14):1808-1810.

20. Chase KA. Medication management. In: Holdford DA, Brown TR, eds. *Introduction to Hospital and Health-System Pharmacy Practice*. Bethesda, MD: American Society of Health-System Pharmacists; 2010:59-80.

21. Pedersen CA, Schneider PJ, Scheckelhoff DJ. ASHP national survey of pharmacy practice in hospital settings: prescribing and transcribing—2004. *Am J Health Syst Pharm*. 2005;62(4):378-390.

22. Durán-García E, Santos-Ramos B, Puigventos-Latorre F, Ortega A. Literature review on the structure and operation of Pharmacy and Therapeutics Committees. *Int J Clin Pharm*. 2011;33(3):475-483.

23. Schiff GD, Galanter WL, Duhig J, et al. A prescription for improving drug formulary decision making. *PLoS Med*. 2012;9(5):1-7.

24. Evidence-based practice overview. Essential Evidence Plus website. http://www.essentialevidenceplus.com/product/ebm_overview.cfm. Published 2013. Accessed July 24, 2014.

25. Lipsy RJ. Institutional formularies: the relevance of pharmacoeconomic analysis to formulary decisions. *Pharmacoeconomics*. 1992;1(4):265-281.

26. Gray T, Bertch K, Galt K, et al. Guidelines for therapeutic interchange—2004. *Pharmacotherapy*. 2005;25(11):1666-1680.

27. Kohn LT, Corrigan JM, Donaldson MS, eds. *To Err Is Human: Building a Safer Health System*. Washington, DC: National Academies Press; 2000.

28. Vermeulin LC, Rough SS, Thielke TS, et al. Strategic approach for improving the medication-use process in health systems: the high performance pharmacy practice framework. *Am J Health-Syst Pharm*. 2007;64(16):1699-1710.

29. American Society of Health-System Pharmacists. ASHP guidelines on medication-use evaluation. *Am J Health-Syst Pharm*. 1996;53(16):1953-1955.

30. Vargas-Rivas JE, Sabater-Hernández D, Calleja-Hernández MA, Faus MJ, Martínez-Martínez F. Role of the hospital pharmacy and therapeutics committee in detecting and regulating off-label drug use. *Int J Clin Pharm*. 2011;33(5):719-721; author reply 722-723.

31. Fox ER, Birt A, James KB, Kokko H, Salverson S, Soflin DL. ASHP guidelines on managing drug product shortages in hospitals and health systems. *Am J Health Syst Pharm*. 2009;66(15):1399-1406.

32. Jensen V, Kimzey LM, Goldberger MJ. FDA's role in responding to drug shortages. *Am J Health Syst Pharm*. 2002;59(15):1423-1425.

33. Drug recalls. U.S. Food and Drug Administration, Centers from Drug Evaluation and Research website. http://www.fda.gov/Drugs/Drugsafety/DrugRecalls/default.htm. Accessed July 24, 2014.

34. Generali JA. Managing medication recalls effectively. *Hosp Pharm*. 2011;46(1):5-6.

35. Abarano T, Cecere D. A multi-hospital formulary and drug information website. *Pharmacy Purchasing Products*. 2012;9(2):44.

36. Reddan JG, Seehan AH, Eskew J, Elmes G. Integration of a medication management infrastructure in a large, multihospital system. *Am J Health Syst Pharm*. 2004;61(23):2557-2561.

37. Amplifi®. Wolters Kluwer Health—Pharmacy OneSource®. http://www.pharmacyonesource.com/applications/amplifi/. Accessed July 24, 2014.

38. Epocrates® Formulary Hosting. Epocrates®—An AthenaHealth Company. http://www.epocrates.com/formulary-hosting. Accessed July 24, 2014.

39. FormChecker. Elsevier Gold Standard. http://www.goldstandard.com/product/pricing-analysis-cost-control/form-checker/. Accessed July 24, 2014.

40. FormWeb. Formulary Productions. http://formweb.com. Accessed July 24, 2014.

41. Micromedex 2.0—Formulary Advisor®. Truven Health Analytics. http://www.truvenhealth.com/your_healthcare_focus/hospital_patient_care_decisions/medication_management.aspx. Accessed July 24, 2014.

42. Lexicomp® FORMULINK. Lexicomp®. http://www.lexi.com/institutions/products/formulary/. Accessed July 24, 2014.

43. RxFlex—Formulary Management Simplified. AdaptiveRx—Pharmacy Benefit Solutions. http://www.adaptiverx.com/rxflex.jsp. Accessed July 24, 2014.

44. Zynchros Services. http://www.zynchros.com/services/. Accessed July 24, 2014.

APPENDIX

# 18-A

# EXAMPLE OF A REQUEST TO CHANGE THE FORMULARY

# INSTRUCTIONS

The Pharmacy and Therapeutics Committee makes formulary decisions based on published data from controlled clinical trials. The Committee considers the efficacy, safety, approved indication(s), tolerability, and cost/reimbursement of a medication when determining its formulary status.

Please fill out this form completely. This form consists of three parts: part A—request to add to the formulary or make a change in restriction; part B—request for deletion from the formulary; and part C—conflict of interest statement. **You must be an attending-level physician or an attending-level dentist to initiate a change to the formulary.** In addition, the appropriate department chair or division chief must countersign this form. To submit the form, click the submit button on the electronic PDF or send the completed form to the Drug Information Center.

> **Drug Information Center**
> Department of Pharmacy Services
> Telephone: XXX-XXXX; Facsimile: XXX-XXXX
> Email: XX@CCC.EDU
> *Formulary and Drug Information Resources Link*

## Part A: For Additions to the Formulary or Changes in Restriction

Generic name:

Trade name:

Manufacturer:

Dosage form(s) and strength(s) requested for addition:

Is a change in restriction required:          Yes
If so, what is the requested change?

Why is this medication superior to or significantly better than current formulary agents?

Improved Safety Profile       Improved Efficacy            More Convenient Dosing Regimen

Less Prone to Med Errors      Additional Indications       More Cost Effective

Based on the above information, please provide the literature citations to support formulary addition or change in restriction.

What indications do you intend to use this medication to prevent or treat?

Please provide any additional information you think pertinent to assist the Pharmacy and Therapeutics Committee in evaluating this agent for formulary addition or change in restriction in the space provided below.

Will this medication require any specialized financial reimbursement requirements (e.g., preapproval from the insurer, obtained from a specialty pharmacy)?

          Yes                 No                Unknown

What medications(s) may be deleted from the formulary?

Were you involved in the clinical trials for this medication?       Yes        No

Did a pharmaceutical representative prompt this request?       Yes        No

---

## Part B: For Deletions from the Formulary

Generic name:

Trade name:

Manufacturer:

Dosage form(s) and strength(s) requested for deletion:

Please provide justification for the deletion of this product from the formulary:

**Part C: Disclosure**

**Note:** This information is shared with the Pharmacy and Therapeutics Committee members and is considered when evaluating your request. A potential conflict of interest does not preclude a person from requesting a medication for formulary addition or a change in restriction. The Committee appreciates that many members of the Medical Staff have relationships with pharmaceutical companies, and that physicians with an area of expertise often receive research grants or other support from industry. The Committee considers it important to disclose these relationships to eliminate any concerns regarding potential conflicts of interest. Please provide the following information to the best of your knowledge:

Companies involved in the development, production, and distribution of the requested medication:

Companies with pharmaceutical products that may be major competitors with the requested medication:

Do you, or an immediate member of your family, have a proprietary interest in any of these companies listed?                     Yes                     No

    If yes, which companies?

    Please check all that apply:
        Own stock in one of the above companies (excluding mutual funds)
        Serve on the Board of Directors for one of these companies
        Expect to receive (or currently receive) royalties from one of these companies
        Other: _____

Have you received any financial support in the last 12 months from the companies listed?                     Yes                     No

    If yes, which companies?

    Please check all that apply:
        Received more than $5,000 in research funding
        Received support for presenting continuing education or professional education programs supported by the company (defined as more than 1 lecture for the same company in a 12-month period)
        Received an educational grant of more than $5,000
        Received more than $500 in travel support, personal gifts, compensation, or rewards in the past 12 months
        Other: _____

**Requester:**

Name: _____ Department: _____

Contact information: _____ (phone) _____
(e-mail) _____

Department Chair/Division Chief/Service Line Medical Director: _____

Contact information: _____ (phone) _____
(Email) _____

Date Form Completed:
___/___/___

---

**Drug Information Services Use Only**

Date Request Received: ___/___/___ Upcoming Letter Sent ___/___/___
Outcome Letter Sent ___/___/___

# FORMULARY MONOGRAPH
# TEMPLATE

**Generic Name (Trade Name):**
**Manufacturer:**
**AHFS Classification:**

| |
|---|
| **Recommendations:** |
| • Provide recommendation for formulary addition (i.e., add, add with restriction, no add). <br> • Provide reasons for the recommendation and other comments as needed. |
| **Subcommittee Recommendation:** |
| • If this medication is to be presented at a subcommittee meeting, then that group's recommendation will be recorded here. |

**Executive Summary:** Provide a summary of the formulary review (see example).

**Indication:** Only FDA-approved indications will be reviewed unless a specific off-label indication was requested by the attending physician. Regardless of request, the first paragraph of this section should include FDA-approved indications only and, if an off-label indication was requested, then the second paragraph will discuss this information.

**Pharmacology:** This section will describe in general the pharmacology and any pharmacodynamic principles for the medication or medication class.

**Pharmacokinetics:** This section will review the general pharmacokinetics, including absorption, distribution, metabolism, and excretion.

**Selected Clinical Trials:** This section will review, at a minimum, two relevant clinical trials that demonstrate the efficacy and safety of the medication compared with placebo and/or an active comparator(s). The *Grading of Evidence Worksheet* will provide an evidence rating for each trial and will be included at the end of each article review with an explanation for the specific rating.

Example: *This clinical trial was rated 1A because of its randomized, double-blind, placebo-controlled design. It shows that clevidipine is a safe and effective treatment for blood pressure following cardiac surgery, but its significance is questionable due to its placebo-controlled nature.*

**Adverse Reactions:** This section summarizes the most common adverse reactions associated with the medication. Additionally, severe but rare reactions will be presented.

**Pregnancy and Lactation:** This section will review any issues related to use during pregnancy and/or lactation.

**Contraindications:** This section will contain all labeled contraindications.

**Warnings/Precautions:** This section will contain any pertinent warnings and precautions from the labeling or the FDA.

**Drug Interactions:** This section will describe any documented or theoretical drug–drug, drug–herb, drug–disease, drug–alcohol, and/or drug–lab interactions.

**Potential for Medication Errors:** This section will describe any documented or potential medication errors based on look-alike, sound-alike potentials and/or packaging details.

**Monitoring Parameters:** This section will list any specific monitoring parameters.

**Dosage and Administration:** This section will contain specific dosing and administration information to include, but not limited to, the following: initial dose, any specific dose titration schedule, maximum dose, special dosing based on age or end-organ function, specific administration techniques (e.g., IV push, continuous infusion), and stability/compatibility.

**Dosage Forms Available:** This section will list the available dosage forms and any specific storage or handling requirements.

**Smart Pump Infusions:** If applicable, minimum and maximum concentrations, rate, and/or doses will be specified. These will be added to the smart pump drug infusion library. *(IV medications only)*

**Reconstitution and Filtration Requirements:** This section will contain information on reconstitution, dilution, and any filtration requirements for injectable medications. *(Injectable medications only)*

**Storage/Handling Requirements:** This section will contain information on stability of the medication at controlled room temperature, under refrigeration, and when frozen.

**Sample Status:** All oral medications, excluding chemotherapy, are available for sampling in the outpatient clinics. If there are potential safety concerns, sampling may be denied for a specific medication.

**Risk Evaluation Mitigation Strategy (REMS) Requirement:** This section will list any REMS requirements that are mandated for a medication by the Food and Drug Administration (FDA).

**Cost Comparison/Reimbursement:** The acquisition cost of the medication will be compared with formulary agents with similar indications or mechanisms of action. If possible, the potential utilization and annualized cost should be determined. Additionally, reimbursement criteria and allowable charges should be discussed.

**Discussion:** The discussion will summarize the details for the monograph, which will lead to the recommendation. Summarize efficacy, safety, other advantages/disadvantages (e.g., pharmacokinetics, drug–drug interactions), place in therapy based on published guidelines, and cost in this section.

**Recommendation:** The recommendation can be to add, add with specific restrictions (e.g., service line, patient population, indication, area), or not add the medication to the formulary.

**References:** Use the National Library of Medicine guidance document, *Citing Medicine* (www.nlm.nih.gov/citingmedicine).

All information MUST be verified and validated in at least two sources unless original data.

Examples of appropriate references include the following:

- Package insert
- Micromedex®, AHFS Drug Information, etc. (pull original literature when cited)
- Review articles
- Guidelines

# EXAMPLE OF A FORMULARY ACTIVITY CHECKLIST

*The following checks should be made during drug information review and changes made according to decisions of the Pharmacy and Therapeutics Committee.*

| Drug—Generic Name (Brand Name) | Form(s) | | Strength(s) |
|---|---|---|---|
| | Yes | No | Responsible/Comments |
| Online formulary changes<br>• Formulary medication list<br>• Updates to other pages | | | |
| Restricted Medication List | | | |
| Bed Placement Infusion Chart | | | |
| Adult Continuous Infusion Chart | | | |
| Pediatric Continuous Infusion Chart | | | |
| NICU Continuous Infusion Chart | | | |
| Electrolyte Guidelines—Adult and Pediatric | | | |
| IV Push Guidelines—Adult and Pediatric | | | |
| Drug Refrigeration Chart | | | |
| Filtration Chart | | | |
| Chemotherapy Reconstitution Guidelines | | | |
| General Reconstitution Guidelines | | | |
| Insulin Products Comparison Chart | | | |
| Opioid Analgesia Comparison Chart | | | |
| Food–Drug Interaction Chart | | | |
| Food–Drug Interaction Patient Brochure | | | |
| Natural Products Interaction Chart | | | |
| Natural Products Interaction Patient Brochure | | | |
| IV-to-PO Conversion Chart | | | |
| Chemotherapy/ Hazardous Medication List | | | |
| Smart Pump Libraries | | | |
| Provide monograph/change details to the following:<br>• Informatics team (Pharmacy/Orders)<br>• Pharmacy Operations Committee<br>• Order Forms Committee | | | |
| Order Forms | | | |
| Outpatient Reimbursement Plan | | | |

# EXAMPLE OF GRADING LEVELS OF EVIDENCE WORKSHEET

The grid should be completed for each study reviewed. For each question, indicate if it is yes (Y), no (N), or unknown (U). Total the number of yes responses to assign the Grading Evidence as follows: 0–4 = C (Poor); 5–7 = B (Fair); 8–10 = A (Good).

| Questions | Study 1 | Study 2 | Study 3 | Study 4 | Study 5 | Study 6 | Study 7 | Study 8 |
|---|---|---|---|---|---|---|---|---|
| Are the patients similar to general practice? | | | | | | | | |
| Was the study controlled? | | | | | | | | |
| Were the subjects randomly assigned? | | | | | | | | |
| Were steps taken to conceal the treatment assignment? | | | | | | | | |
| Were patients and study personnel "blinded"? | | | | | | | | |
| Were all patients properly accounted for:<br>• Was follow-up complete?<br>• Was there intent-to-treat analysis? | | | | | | | | |
| Were the intervention and control groups similar? | | | | | | | | |
| Are the results clinically as well as statistically significant? | | | | | | | | |
| In a negative trial, was the power adequate? | | | | | | | | |
| Were there NO other factors that may have affected study outcomes? | | | | | | | | |
| Level of Benefit<br>Is the benefit > risk? (if Y = 1; if N = 2) | | | | | | | | |
| Total number of yes (Y) responses | | | | | | | | |
| **Grade of Evidence**[*] | | | | | | | | |

| References | |
|---|---|
| Study 1 | |
| Study 2 | |
| Study 3 | |
| Study 4 | |
| Study 5 | |
| Study 6 | |
| Study 7 | |
| Study 8 | |

# ACADEMIC DETAILING AND INDUSTRY RELATIONSHIPS

Michael Gabay, PharmD, JD, BCPS
Yvette Grando Holman, RPh, PharmD, BCPS

## CHAPTER OBJECTIVES

▸ Describe academic detailing.

▸ List the key principles involved in effective academic detailing.

▸ Summarize the steps in establishing an academic detailing program.

▸ Summarize the guidelines that define pharmacist–pharmaceutical industry relationships.

▸ Define the limitations of pharmaceutical industry–sponsored education.

# CHAPTER OUTLINE

# KEY TERMS

# INTRODUCTION

**Academic detailing** may be defined as "noncommercial, evidence-based direct outreach to clinicians" that aids prescribers regarding appropriate clinical decision making based on the best available efficacy, safety, and cost-effectiveness data.[1,2] This innovative approach usually involves a one-on-one interaction between a prescriber and another health professional (i.e., pharmacist, nurse, physician) specifically trained in effectively communicating the most recent evidence-based data regarding medications or other interventions.[3] Academic detailing is the brainchild of Dr. Jerry Avorn, Professor of Medicine at Harvard Medical School and Chief of the Division of Pharmacoepidemiology and Pharmacoeconomics at Brigham and Women's Hospital. Dr. Avorn knew that prescribers often lack sufficient time to remain current on the comparative effectiveness, safety, and costs of various treatments. In addition, he recognized the success of pharmaceutical sales representatives, and their concise, effective methods of providing drug information, in driving prescribing patterns. Academic detailing basically merges the "interactive, one-on-one communication approach of industry detailers with the evidence-based noncommercial information of academia."[3] The goals of academic detailing are to improve clinician decision making, positively impact patient outcomes, and reduce costs. Academic detailing programs have been established internationally in countries such as Australia, the United Kingdom, Canada, and the Netherlands. They have also been established in a number of U.S. states, including New Hampshire, Vermont, Pennsylvania, Massachusetts, Maine, New York, and South Carolina. In addition, integrated health systems (e.g., Kaiser) have developed and implemented their own academic detailing services.

Avorn and colleagues found academic detailing to be a successful approach to improving drug therapy decisions as far back as 1983.[4] In their initial study, three drug categories with less than optimal prescribing patterns were targeted: propoxyphene, cerebral and peripheral vasodilators, and cephalexin. Physicians included in the study were randomized to one of three groups: a print-only group that received educational materials regarding the targeted medications, a face-to-face group that received not only the printed materials but also an in-person educational intervention by a trained clinical pharmacist, or a control group that received no interventions. Results revealed that the face-to-face group reduced prescribing of the target medications by 14% compared to controls ($p = 0.0001$). In addition, the face-to-face intervention resulted in an average decrease in prescribing costs of $105 per physician for the three drug groups ($p = 0.002$ vs. the control group).

# ACADEMIC DETAILING

Academic detailing programs may be utilized to counteract a variety of negative prescribing patterns, including administration of medications with low benefit/risk ratios when safer alternatives are available; prescribing of ineffective or marginally effective therapies for treatable conditions; polypharmacy in vulnerable populations; use of expensive medications when effective, less costly medications are available; and under-utilization of evidence-based therapies for major disease states. In 1990, Soumerai and Avorn published a special communication that summarized important principles of academic detailing in order to improve clinical decision making.[5] These principles include defining specific problems and objectives, conducting market research, establishing credibility, targeting high-potential prescribers, involving opinion leaders, using two-sided communication, promoting active learner involvement, incorporating repetition and reinforcement, providing brief graphic print materials, offering practical alternatives, and selecting and training of academic detailers. **Table 19-1** provides a brief overview of each of these important principles. The majority of these principles have been found to be effective in adult education and patient compliance research.[5] Academic detailing programs should incorporate these principles to some degree in order to be successful.

## ESTABLISHING AN ACADEMIC DETAILING PROGRAM

Beyond application of the core principles of academic detailing, other issues involving program components, delivery, administration, and financing need to be considered when establishing an academic detailing service. When initially developing clinical materials for an academic detailing service, it is of vital importance to choose a topic that is of genuine interest to prescribers and not simply a cost-cutting measure.[6] Oftentimes, clinical topics that pose a conundrum for prescribers are similarly an issue for payers, so identifying an appropriate topic should not be too difficult. Examples of clinical modules that have been implemented by various state academic detailing programs include appropriate pain management following the safety concerns involving cyclooxygenase-2 (COX-2) inhibitors and appropriate therapy for heartburn. Following topic selection, a complete and extensive search of the biomedical literature should be performed. The results of this search should be compiled into a summary report. The information within this report should be further distilled into engaging educational materials that contain brief key messages rooted in the evidence. Educational materials should be developed for both prescribers and patients (i.e., prescribers may share developed materials with their patients in order to enhance the one-on-one detailing between the educator and the prescriber). One of the challenges with academic detailing programs is keeping educational materials up-to-date. Programs should develop a process for keeping materials current.

Although Soumerai and Avorn[5] state that targeting high-potential prescribers is one of the principles of academic detailing, other sources state that program delivery should be generally available instead of targeted to specific prescribers.[6] Targeted prescribers may view academic detailing programs as an intrusion into their clinical practice and not as an educational endeavor. In addition, program delivery should be voluntary, not mandatory. A voluntary approach fits well with the educational, one-on-one nature of most academic detailing programs. The initial detailing visit should be devoted to establishing the credibility of the program and answering general questions from the prescriber regarding the purposes of academic detailing. The importance of establishing credibility and trust in the one-on-one relationship between the prescriber and the

**TABLE 19-1    Principles of Academic Detailing**

| Principle | Comments |
|---|---|
| Define specific problems and objectives | • Key first step.<br>• Define areas to be addressed and behaviors to be encouraged or discouraged. |
| Conduct market research | • Understand the motivation behind a prescriber's use of a specific therapy.<br>• Motivational factors can be determined by conducting focus groups and prescriber surveys and ongoing communication between educators and prescribers.<br>• Research aids in identifying key nonclinical and clinical motivational factors regarding prescribing patterns.<br>• May need to conduct multiple focus groups or surveys of various representative samples of target prescribers in order to develop an effective detailing message. |
| Establish credibility | • Credibility is an essential component of effective academic detailing.<br>• Credibility can be established through use of unbiased organizational identities and respected educators. |
| Target high-potential prescribers | • Identify and target prescribers where academic detailing may have the most impact on negative prescribing patterns.<br>• Potentially provide feedback to individual prescribers to demonstrate prescribing patterns outside the norm. |
| Involve opinion leaders | • Identify and enlist "educationally influential" prescribers within the targeted population; these individuals can exponentially aid in the success of the academic detailing program. |
| Use two-sided communication | • Present both sides of an issue.<br>• Acknowledge disadvantages of the medication being promoted by the academic detailing program.<br>• Do not completely discount the positive attributes of an alternative intervention. |
| Promote active learner involvement | • Engage in two-way communication in order to improve behavior change.<br>• Do not overquestion the prescriber; this may lead to the prescriber feeling that his or her time is being wasted or that the detailer is being manipulative. |
| Incorporate repetition and reinforcement | • Concentrate on a small number of important messages during detailing.<br>• Provide feedback of improved behavior with reinforcement. |
| Provide brief graphic print materials | • Illustrated materials that emphasize key clinical recommendations are useful adjuncts to the one-on-one interaction. |
| Offer practical alternatives | • Offer the prescriber an alternate effective pharmacologic or nonpharmacologic therapy.<br>• Consider the practicality and availability of alternatives. |
| Select and train academic detailers | • Doctoral-level clinical pharmacists may be effective academic detailers and require a minimal amount of training.<br>• Training topics should include clinical issues, communication and persuasion skills, and recommendations regarding the target drug and alternatives. |

Data from Soumerai SB, Avorn J. Principles of educational outreach (academic detailing) to improve clinical decision making. *JAMA.* 1990;263(4):549-556.

detailer cannot be overstated. Delivery of educational materials may also be leveraged through the use of existing channels in states or organizations. Academic detailing programs should examine ways to collaborate with these organizations while steering clear of any potential conflicts of interest.

Administration of an academic detailing program is another area that requires time and effort. Identifying detailers with an appropriate clinical background willing to effectively interact with prescribers can be difficult. In addition, salaries for these individuals must be competitive in order to attract necessary expertise. Generally, academic detailers work "in the field" and are managed remotely.[6] A system for reporting time, managing prescriber visits, and handling other administrative support issues must be identified and implemented. Some programs provide continuing medical education (CME) to physicians who participate in academic detailing. Obtaining and maintaining CME accreditation can be a laborious process in itself. In addition, detailing programs should develop a mechanism for evaluating materials, encounters, and changes in prescribing patterns. Evaluations can be used to improve upon the program as well as justify funding.

Financing for academic detailing programs may be accomplished via several different mechanisms.[6] Some states (i.e., Maine and Vermont) impose, or have proposed imposing, fees on manufacturers and labelers of prescription medications in order to fund academic detailing programs. Similarly, the District of Columbia has funded its detailing service through licensing fees that industry detailers pay in order to conduct business within the District. Other potential partial or full funding mechanisms include foundation and federal grants, pharmaceutical industry settlement funds, Medicaid match funding, or consortium funding.

## ACADEMIC DETAILING PROGRAMS ON THE STATE AND FEDERAL LEVELS

Academic detailing initiatives at the state level continue to expand. A summary of selected state-level programs is presented in **Table 19-2**.[2,7] Many of these programs are partnerships between state health agencies and universities. Some contract with the Independent Drug Information Service (IDIS; www.rxfacts.org) for clinical support. The IDIS is a team of physicians and researchers at Harvard Medical School that completes ongoing searches of the biomedical literature and condenses drug information from these searches into concise, clinically relevant summaries for physicians and patients. These summaries can then be used for academic detailing programs. The number of academic detailers within each state program varies; however, all are healthcare professionals, primarily nurses, physicians, and pharmacists. The overall budget for these programs varies significantly from state to state, as does the mechanism by which the programs are financed.

At the federal level, the U.S. House of Representatives and Senate introduced legislation titled the Independent Drug Education and Outreach Act (IDEA) in 2009. The goal of IDEA is to affect prescribing patterns by sending trained pharmacists, nurses, and other healthcare professionals into prescribers' officers to provide them with independent, evidence-based information on the full spectrum of treatment options available for various disease states.[8] This goal is to be achieved by federally funded grants and/or contracts through the Agency for Healthcare Research and Quality (AHRQ) to train and deploy healthcare professionals and to develop educational materials that show the relative safety, effectiveness, and cost of prescription drugs for the same indication, including generic and over-the-counter alternatives. To be awarded an IDEA-related contract or grant, applicants may not receive financial support from any pharmaceutical

**TABLE 19-2**   Academic Detailing Programs at the State Level

| State (Program Start Date) | Program Description |
| --- | --- |
| Maine (2009) | • Legislation was passed in 2007 mandating that the Department of Health and Human Services establish an academic detailing program in Maine.<br>• Clinical topics offered include atypical antipsychotics, chronic pain management, atrial fibrillation, hypertension, antiplatelet therapy, type 2 diabetes, and obesity.<br>• Two academic detailers (physician assistant and physician).<br>• Offers CME.<br>• 2009 budget: $150,000. |
| Massachusetts (2009) | • Program is directed by the Department of Public Health in conjunction with Commonwealth Medicine.<br>• Contracts with the Independent Drug Information Service for clinical support.<br>• Two academic detailers (nurse and physician).<br>• Initial clinical topic: type 2 diabetes.<br>• 2008 budget: $200,000. |
| New York (2008) | • Program directed by the Department of Health in conjunction with the State University of New York and the University of Massachusetts Medical School.<br>• Contract with the Independent Drug Information Service for clinical support.<br>• Clinical topics include RSV bronchiolitis, hypertension, diabetes, and hepatitis C.<br>• 20 academic detailers (pharmacists).<br>• Offers CME.<br>• Supported by general funds offset by savings. |
| Oregon (2009) | • Rural Oregon Academic Detailing (ROAD) project.<br>• Partnership between the Oregon State University College of Pharmacy and the Oregon Rural Practice-based Research Network at Oregon Health and Science University.<br>• Focus on Medicaid providers in rural Oregon.<br>• Clinical topics focused in the area of mental health.<br>• Three academic detailers (pharmacists).<br>• Funded by a grant from the Pew Prescription Project and the Oregon Department of Human Services. |
| Pennsylvania (2005) | • The Pharmaceutical Assistance Contract for the Elderly (PACE) program in Pennsylvania contracts with the Independent Drug Information Service for clinical support.<br>• Clinical topics include pain management, upper GI symptom treatment, anticoagulants, lipid-lowering therapies, and blood pressure treatment.<br>• 11 academic detailers (nurses and pharmacists).<br>• Budget: $1 million annually financed through lottery funds. |
| South Carolina (2007) | • Collaborative effort between the South Carolina College of Pharmacy and the Department of Health and Human Services (Medicaid).<br>• Officially known as the South Carolina Offering Prescribing Excellence (SCORxE) program.<br>• Clinical topics include atypical antipsychotics in children, asthma and ADHD therapy in children, smoking cessation, and mental health topics.<br>• Program staff of eight (pharmacists and administrative support).<br>• Budget: Approximately $1 million annually. |
| Vermont (1999) | • Offered by the University of Vermont's Office of Primary Care with funding from various sources, including the State of Vermont.<br>• Topics include approaches for discontinuing medications, management of ADHD, migraine therapy, and treatment of chronic low back pain.<br>• Six academic detailers (physicians and pharmacists).<br>• Offers CME.<br>• 2007 budget: $200,000. |

Data from The Hilltop Institute. Academic detailing: a review of the literature and states' approaches. http://www.hilltopinstitute.org/publications/AcademicDetailing-ReviewOfTheLiteratureAndStates%27Approaches-December2009.pdf. Accessed July 24, 2014; Academic detailing: an interview with Jerry Avorn, MD. AARP Rx Watchdog Report. http://assets.aarp.org/www.aarp.org_/cs/health/206907rxwatchdog_dec_09.pdf. Accessed July 24, 2014.

manufacturer whose medication is part of the program. In 2009, the IDEA Act did not move beyond initial committee review in both houses of Congress.

## ADDITIONAL RESOURCES

The following are academic detailing resources beyond state-specific program sites:

- *National Resource Center for Academic Detailing (NaRCAD)*. NaRCAD is supported by a grant from AHRQ. The program is housed in the Division of Pharmacoepidemiology and Pharmacoeconomics in the Department of Medicine at Brigham and Women's Hospital and Harvard Medical School. NaRCAD provides organizations with support and guidance in establishing new academic detailing programs, as well as evaluating and improving existing ones.
- *Independent Drug Information Service (IDIS)*. This service provides summaries of clinical topics for healthcare providers, medication information for patients, and summaries of new clinical research findings. These resources can be utilized in academic detailing programs. The IDIS is run by the Alosa Foundation.

# INDUSTRY RELATIONSHIPS

Pharmacists cannot execute their jobs without the pharmaceutical industry as it exists today. Before the days of mass manufacturing, pharmacists were more like chemists, who had their "laboratories" inside the apothecaries where powders and liquids were mixed and formulated into physician-requested recipes. Robust data did not exist to support these concoctions. Sometimes these compounds made people sicker than they were prior to taking these medications. As manufacturing processes modernized, the pharmaceutical companies gained technology to mass-produce tablets, capsules, liquids, suppositories, and troches, so that this compounding became less and less a part of a pharmacist's job responsibility. Instead, the pharmacist was able to purchase products ready to be administered, transforming the job to more of a dispensary rather than a mixing chemist.

As technology moved forward, intravenous medications for hospitalized patients were added to the manufacturing process. This was an important step in the evolution of pharmacy, because sterility issues related to making an intravenous medication was of the utmost importance to the health and welfare of the patient. This was not to be taken lightly. It further allowed for an expansion of pharmacy services, which we take for granted today. Imagine how a hospital pharmacy might function if manufactured intravenous medications were not available.

## THE CURRENT PHARMACEUTICAL INDUSTRY MARKET

Needless to say, today's pharmacists could not do their jobs without the pharmaceutical industry, and the industry could not do its job without pharmacists to educate, prepare, and dispense its products. The relationship is symbiotic. The pharmaceutical industry is a for-profit business, with shareholders to which it must report. The industry creates products that help people feel better and live longer. This is no small task. The industry invests a huge amount of money into research and development. Current estimates indicate that it takes $1 billion to bring a drug to market,[9] with a limited patent time to recoup this investment before the patent expires, allowing a generic manufacturer to produce the same molecular entity. Compared to other industries, the pharmaceutical industry reinvests a higher percentage of its profits into research and development. Approximately 12% of a company's profit is put back into research and development, compared to an average of 4% by all other industries.[10] Another challenge for pharmaceutical scientists involves the time in which a patent is filed. When a company finds a chemical entity in the laboratory that has any chance of possibly becoming a drug for use in humans, a patent must be filed very early in the development process. Even though a drug is still in laboratory and clinical development, the patent lifespan starts ticking. It may take 7-10 years to actually develop the chemical entity into a safe and efficacious drug for humans. It also requires the approval of the Food and Drug Administration (FDA). All this while, the pharmaceutical company has less and less time to recoup its investment before the patent expires at 17 years. It is estimated that of every 5,000 compounds synthesized, one will come to market as a drug. Only 30% of those drugs that do make it to market will recoup their research and development costs.

In addition, market factors make it even more difficult for companies to recoup their investment. Until the 1980s, it was typical for a patient to visit his physician when ill and receive a prescription, which was filled at the patient's neighborhood pharmacy. The patient would likely pay cash for a name-brand prescription; generic drugs were not widely available. If fortunate enough to have a prescription drug plan, the patient would keep the pharmacy receipt and submit it on a paper form to his insurance plan once he arrived home. A few weeks later, a check would arrive in the mail at the patient's home to reimburse a portion of the drug bill. Today, a multitude of external market factors affect this process. Many patients covered by prescription insurance plans belong to a group plan that follows a **formulary**, which is a list of products that are acceptable for use based on efficacy, safety, and cost. If the drug is *on-formulary*, a copay is rendered at the pharmacy after the pharmacist electronically bills the insurance company. The formulary may have multiple levels, so that some drugs are *preferred*, or first tier, and others are on a second or third tier. The patient pays more for a higher tiered drug. The drug may not be on the insurance company's formulary at all, a status called **nonformulary**, in which case a patient may be asked to pay the full cash price for the drug. This is often an expensive endeavor. If there is more than one product available in a specific therapeutic area, then the likelihood of the insurance plan influencing the prescriber to one product is high. This is even more apparent when a class of drugs has a mix of generic and branded drugs available, with the insurance company keeping generic formulations as a first tier and branded products in higher tiers to control costs, regardless of improvements in drug factors that may be had with newer, branded products.

Hospital pharmacies work in a similar way. Hospitals, too, use formularies to control inventory and costs. Instead of tiers, hospitals will usually designate products as on-formulary or nonformulary. This means a provider either has access to the product, or not, for inpatients. Patients often are discharged from the hospital on new drug regimens that they will take as outpatients. To maintain continuity of care, it is preferable for patients to maintain taking the same product that was started in the inpatient setting. Therefore, hospital formularies will influence outpatient prescription writing habits. Because hospitals focus on using cost-effective drugs as formulary agents, which are often generic drugs, a patient will often leave the hospital on a generic drug regimen.

Both insurance companies and hospitals use a **pharmacy and therapeutics committee** (P&T committee) to determine whether a product will be available for general use. P&T committees usually appoint a physician chairperson, with members including physicians from multiple specialties, pharmacists, nurses, and administrators. P&T committee membership is confidential to outsiders, as are its meeting agenda items. P&T committee meetings are usually scheduled monthly. Some will employ the aid of subcommittees to work with specialized agents, such as an oncology or infectious disease subcommittee, which will report back to the parent committee with recommendations for focused drug classes. Pharmaceutical companies have broadened their efforts to educate in recent years in light of the impact of nonprescribers who are members of P&T committees who choose which products are available on plans and in hospitals. This process of formulary or nonformulary status in both outpatient and inpatient settings results in intense competition for market share by pharmaceutical companies.

Why is all of this important? It drives the pharmaceutical industry, a for-profit industry with shareholder stakes, on where sales can be made. The pharmaceutical industry is motivated to get its products on insurance formularies at a low tier so that prescribers can readily write prescriptions for these products, and patients will have a low copay. Similarly, the industry is motivated to get its products approved on hospital formularies so that physicians can prescribe the drug for inpatients, who eventually become outpatients, and may be on a particular product chronically.

In contrast, healthcare insurance companies and hospitals are under intense pressure to keep costs as low as possible. This often means substituting older generic drugs in place of potentially better (but more expensive) branded drugs. Therein lies the conflict.

## GOVERNANCE OF PHARMACEUTICAL INDUSTRY RELATIONSHIPS

The pharmaceutical industry is self-regulated by the Pharmaceutical Research and Manufacturers of America (PhRMA). The organization has defined the guidelines by which industry representatives may interact with healthcare practitioners as they relate to marketing practices. This Code on Interactions with Healthcare Professionals[11] was developed in 2009 and is optional for companies to choose to follow. Member companies are listed in the document. The code is intended to define how manufacturers can inform healthcare professionals about the benefits and risks of products to achieve appropriate patient use, to provide guidance on communicating scientific and educational information, and to define interactions with research and consultation services. The intent is that pharmaceutical marketing practices will follow all legal requirements and set a high ethical standard. Representatives of companies who are committed to this code have pledged that their marketing practices will be accurate and not misleading; that claims about a product will be communicated only if substantiated; that both risks and benefits will be presented; and that FDA legal requirements are met. Company representatives are allowed to provide occasional modest meals in-office for healthcare professionals. Recreational events as part of product promotion are not allowed. Promotional activities must not be associated with any CME, but can be supported via a third-party vendor. Manufacturers may hire medical experts for consultation purposes and also for speaker programs intended to be promotional in nature. These speaker programs are strictly for on-label drug messaging only, and are separate from CME programs. Companies that employ consultants or speakers are encouraged to cap yearly earnings for these healthcare practitioners. The code encourages these practitioners to disclose their financial relationships with manufacturers so as to avoid the appearance (real or perceived) of bias. Implementation of this code in 2009 initiated the elimination of company-sponsored pens, notepads, and other "reminders" bearing a company logo. The pharmaceutical industry in the United States also has governmental approval to market prescription drugs directly to patients, a practice not seen anywhere else in the world. This direct-to-consumer advertising can be in print form, such as magazines, or via television or social media.

Hospitals may also have individual policies on working with industry representatives. The American Society of Health-System Pharmacists (ASHP) in 1992 defined guidelines for pharmacists indicating the sole consideration for pharmacists must be toward patient care.[12] Guidelines for beneficial interactions with vendors of the pharmaceutical industry are defined, such that policies and procedures are shared, registration while on hospital property occurs, and contact information is recorded. Vendors should have appointments established before coming into the hospital, and the representative should display a name badge. It may be the hospital's policy that only formulary-approved drugs may be discussed while doing business inside the hospital. Vendors should never go into patient-care areas without explicit permission and must abide by all confidentiality expectations. Some hospitals may allow vendors to exhibit. Drug samples are generally not accepted in the inpatient setting. The pharmaceutical industry may provide funding for educational programming or work with healthcare providers as consultants, advisors, or in the capacity of clinical research.[13] A code of ethics for pharmacists was published in 1996 by ASHP and has been adapted by all facets of the profession.[14] It is intended to guide pharmacists on the moral and ethical obligations and virtues in relationships with patients, healthcare professionals, and society. Article IV addresses professional relationships, stating "A pharmacist acts with honesty and integrity." A pharmacist must act with conviction of conscience, avoid discriminatory practices, and ensure that the patient is at the center of each decision.

Additionally, in 2008, the American College of Clinical Pharmacy (ACCP) released its position statement on guidelines for ethical interactions between pharmacists and members of industry.[15] It was expanded from its original version to include the pharmaceutical industry as well as medical device companies, wholesalers, and computer manufacturers. The intent of this document was to recognize federal and organizational guidelines for industry that address real and perceived ethical conflicts with members of the healthcare team. These relationships can be mutually beneficial; however, pharmacists must be diligent to ensure that these interactions are appropriate and do not lead to a negative impact on patients. The welfare of the patient is the pharmacist's primary concern. A pharmacist must act with honesty and integrity in all professional relationships. Pharmacists should not accept gifts from industry that may influence their objectivity, real or perceived. Appropriate gifts are defined as being nominal in value (defined as less than $100 and having an educational nature, such as a textbook or anatomical model, slides, patient informational guides, or drug monographs). Inappropriate gifts include cash payments, social events, entertainment, personal gifts, sporting events, travel or registration to symposiums, or direct payment for meeting attendance. Any compensation related to a drug purchase is unacceptable. Pharmacists who have a real or perceived conflict of interest must disclose this information. When involved in formulary or drug purchasing decisions, pharmacists must not make choices based on established relationships. Examples of these relationships include employment, acting as a consultant, receiving an honorarium, stock ownership or options (excluding diversified mutual funds), expert testimony, grants, patents, royalties, or any other financial relationships. It should be noted that PhRMA, ASHP, and ACCP guidelines are not intended to limit the legitimate exchange of prudent scientific information.

Sometimes established relationships may come into conflict, such as when there is a decision relating to formulary inclusion. In this case, it is advised that pharmacists should disclose these relationships with companies to achieve transparency. Greater scrutiny and transparency are necessary to ensure appropriate ongoing relationships between pharmacists and their patients. However, healthcare organizations and associations have not done an adequate job of identifying and managing conflicts of interest. A 2008 survey of medical schools indicates that 38% had written a conflict of interest policy, 37% were developing one, and 25% had not developed any guideline.[16] Pharmacy schools must address this issue, and students must be provided education on proper interactions with the pharmaceutical industry. To address this, the University of Wisconsin School of Public Health has developed a lecture dedicated to this topic that was added to the curriculum of second-year medical students.[17] The Oregon Society of Health-System Pharmacists has addressed the topic at a statewide meeting to introduce policies set forth by ASHP and PhRMA in an open format to better understand how pharmacists and pharmaceutical industry members can work together within regulatory guidance and for the best outcome of patients.

In 2013, the Centers for Medicare and Medicaid Services (CMS) enacted the Physician Payments Sunshine Act as part of the Affordable Care Act.[18] The law requires manufacturers of drugs, biologics, and devices to report transfers of value to physicians and teaching hospitals on a public website. Manufacturers must report instances where physicians receive more than $10 per event or more than $100 per year. Exceptions include drug samples, honoraria for accredited CME, and gifts that benefit patients. An annual report will be released by each manufacturer listing the name of the physician recipient and the amount of money transferred. The intent is to allow patients access to this information for making decisions about their own health care. In effect, the law will put pressure on physicians to decide if public disclosure of industry relationships is warranted. The Sunshine Act is in accordance with other conflict of interest disclosure requirements, such as those imposed by ASHP and ACCP; however, pharmacists at this time are exempt from the industry reporting requirements of the act.

Ultimately, pharmacists should avoid situations where conflicts are established and decisions must be made regarding formulary choices. Guidelines that dictate behavior from both pharmacists and from industry state that grants, scholarships, subsidies, support, consulting contracts, and educational or practice-related items should not be provided or offered to a healthcare professional in exchange for prescribing products or for a commitment to continue prescribing products. Research and development and education must be differentiated from industry sales and marketing. Disclosure and transparency must be fully declared, and the health and welfare of the patient must always come first.

---

**CASE STUDY 19-1     P&T Committee Conflict?**

Kaye is a clinical pharmacist manager who sits on her hospital's P&T committee and holds a leadership position as P&T secretary. Her husband works as a pharmaceutical sales representative for AzmaTech, a manufacturer of inhalers. The company's new drug, Dilator®, has recently been approved by the FDA for the treatment of patients with asthma. A physician with privileges in the hospital has approached the committee about adding Dilator® to the formulary. It is Kaye's responsibility to research the benefits, risks, cost-effectiveness, and comparative information on Dilator® versus other inhalers already on formulary at the hospital to determine if the committee should add the new drug to the formulary.

## Questions

1. What potential for bias exists for Kaye?
2. Should Kaye be responsible for the research on Dilator® required by the committee for review?
3. Does Kaye need to disclose any conflict of interests?
4. Should Kaye be involved with the formulary decision?

## STRUCTURE OF THE PHARMACEUTICAL INDUSTRY

There are approximately 7,000 pharmacists working in the pharmaceutical industry, which accounts for approximately 2.7% of all pharmacists. Pharmacists employed in industry work in many areas, including drug discovery, manufacturing, marketing, medical information, product development or management, quality assurance, sales, regulatory, health outcomes research, legal, safety, information technology, training and development, and scientific communications.[19]

For pharmacists who are customers of the pharmaceutical industry, the most common relationship encountered is meeting with the account representative working in sales, or a medical liaison. In 2004 (before PhRMA guidelines were enacted), the U.S. pharmaceutical industry spent an estimated $57.5 billion on marketing, with $12-$18 billion specifically targeting practicing physicians and residents.[20] This represents approximately $8,000-$13,000 spent on each physician every year.[17]

Generally, the sales team reports up through a sales hierarchy within the company, whereas a medical liaison will report up through a research and development (R&D) hierarchy. Company structure tends to keep sales separate from R&D. A company's sales arm will most commonly employ individuals who have sales, marketing, or business backgrounds; however, this person could come from a medical background, such as nursing or pharmacy. Sales teams are highly trained on their particular product and competitors and meet directly with physicians and other healthcare providers to influence prescribing habits. A representative employed in sales may not, under any circumstances, communicate information contradictory to a product's package insert. In contrast, the medical liaison is usually a PharmD, PhD, or MD. Individuals employed as medical liaisons hold a scientific degree with the intention of being able to communicate information in select cases that may be off-label from a product's package insert. Both of these types of industry representatives work in field territories with local hospitals, physicians, and other healthcare professional customers. Their goal is to achieve formulary acceptance of drug products, which results in a purchase for the company.

## PHARMACEUTICAL BUYING CONTRACTS

When drugs are added to a hospital formulary, a company may offer a buying contract. Contracts can be based on market share or volume. They may be offered to individual hospitals or to groups of hospitals. A contract based on market share would offer discounted prices for the hospital if a certain market share is maintained. For example, if a new inhaler is added to the formulary, the hospital may attempt to keep it available to practitioners so that it is utilized 80% of the time compared to other inhalers in the same therapeutic class. By maintaining an 80% market share, the pharmaceutical company will allow the hospital to purchase the inhaler at the lowest contract price. If the hospital allows too many of the competitive inhalers to be used, the company reserves the right to charge more for the new inhaler since the contract was not met. These contracts can be complicated and may tie unrelated products into a buying contract. This contracting technique is known as *bundling*. Using our inhaler example, a company may ask for 80% market share for the best price on the inhaler and then offer another 5% savings if a certain percentage of other products it also markets (e.g., its vaccine and its antibiotic) also hit their contract targets. Other contracts can be volume based. In this setting, the more a drug is purchased by the hospital, the lower resulting unit price. Ultimately, patients' illnesses dictate what drugs are purchased, so hospitals may be penalized if not enough patients present with the illness the contracted drug is meant to treat. Contracts may also be offered to group purchasing organizations (GPOs) so that loosely related hospitals may collaborate on purchases. If the group of hospitals meets company-mandated targets, discounts are offered. It can become very difficult to manage these contracts based on patient populations, physician preferences, and coordination challenges. It is the responsibility of company representatives to present these contracts to the director of pharmacy or purchasing coordinator within a hospital.

## PHARMACEUTICAL INDUSTRY PROVISION OF EDUCATION

Educational efforts by pharmaceutical companies are defined by PhRMA. The traditional way for industry representatives to disseminate their company's information is via face-to-face meetings. This includes both sales representatives and medical science liaisons. Representatives will arrange for an appointment with a healthcare professional. Representatives are allowed to utilize sales brochures produced by their companies. These documents go through extensive scrutiny before approval for sales teams. They are developed by a marketing team, reviewed by corporate attorneys, and ultimately must be in sync with PhRMA guidelines and the FDA's governance on pharmaceutical marketing practices. This means that claims about a product must be substantiated with sound clinical data, and the messages must be consistent with FDA-approved labeling. These one-on-one meetings can be an effective means to discuss new products or updates in product labeling. It is important to note that every contact made between an industry representative and a healthcare provider dictates that the representative will provide a balanced discussion of the product to include both benefits and risks. A package insert must be left behind at each discussion. Contents of the discussion may only include FDA-approved labeling of the drug. If questions arise from the healthcare professional that a sales representative cannot answer, the inquiry must be forwarded to a scientific colleague, such as a medical science liaison or a drug information specialist employed by the company.

An effective tool for pharmacists to utilize when meeting with sales representatives, using the acronym PEACEFUL, has been proposed:[21]

P = Patient's profile best suited for the new drug
E = Efficacy of the drug compared with placebo and gold standard
A = Availability on hospital or health plan formularies
C = Cost
E = Ease of use/convenience
F = Formulations, such as tablet, capsule, syrup, injections
U = Unwanted adverse effects (minor and major)
L = Lay educational material (video, pamphlet)

Pharmacists can ensure that they are collecting unbiased data when the PEACEFUL tool is utilized during a meeting with a drug representative. The information captured in this format will provide the pharmacist a meaningful collection of data that can then be used to determine the best patient profile for a particular drug therapy.

Group presentations are another format for education. Representatives are allowed under PhRMA guidelines to provide a modest meal for educational purposes. Inside the hospital, this may mean in-servicing departments on a newly approved formulary drug, utilizing information that is FDA approved and included in a package insert. Speaker programs may occur outside the hospital in a dinner setting with a company-paid speaker educating healthcare practitioners on the merits of a product. It should be noted that these promotional programs require speakers to disseminate only information that is FDA approved. Unless an audience member asks an unsolicited off-label question, the speaker must remain on task with the slide presentation provided by the pharmaceutical company. It is not standard for these programs to present comparative data between products. It is also important to note that these speakers are hired by the company to present the company's data. Again, as a pharmacist, it is important to assess any potential or real conflict of interest when accepting a meal under the pretenses of a promotional message.

Unrestricted continuing education sponsored by industry is no longer allowed. However, some companies may provide unrestricted grants to hospitals or foundations that may then use this funding to provide education to healthcare practitioners without the input of industry representatives. This type of funding may go toward hospital grand rounds presentations or other educational formats.

## Opportunities to Partner with the Pharmaceutical Industry to Improve Patient Care

Once a drug has gained formulary acceptance within a hospital, it opens opportunities for the representative to provide education of healthcare practitioners. Generally, a representative can then ethically promote the drug product in a manner consistent with hospital policy and PhRMA guidelines. This may include in-services for target healthcare professionals, such as nurses, physicians, pharmacists, respiratory therapists, microbiologists, or discharge planners, depending on the product. Healthcare practitioner targets for education are ultimately determined by the company's marketing team and will depend upon the type of drug promoted and who will influence its use. A potential successful partnership may include the industry representative teaming with a clinical pharmacist for these in-services. The benefits of this partnership are many. Representatives are obliged to speak only on the information contained in the product package insert; pharmacists can supplement important clinical information during in-services to fill in gaps. Pharmacists can also convey the approved pharmacy and therapeutics intent of the product, such as a specific patient population that would particularly benefit from the product or limitations of usage of the product in certain patients.

Representatives and pharmacists can also successfully partner to help a hospital meet quality core measures when products meet these indications. For instance, teaming with a vaccine manufacturer to educate nurses about the importance of administering a pneumococcal vaccine to all patients older than 65 years will help to improve compliance with this national core measure. Another quality measure, the prevention of 30-day readmissions of patients who leave the hospital on anticoagulants, can be attained by working with representatives to help educate nurses and pharmacists on counseling patients on these drugs. Patients with chronic obstructive pulmonary disease or asthma can avoid emergency readmissions with proper inhaler technique, which can be helped by educational efforts for discharge counseling or practice with placebo inhalers obtained from the manufacturer. The goal of meeting these important core measures can be a partnership with industry representatives to improve hospital scorecards and ultimately patient care. The benefits of these working relationships can be exceptional.

Another area for partnership is in the growing use of risk evaluation and mitigation strategies (REMS). REMS were developed by the FDA in 2007 as a response to the increasing number of drug withdrawals from the marketplace due to safety concerns. REMS are designed to manage a known or potential serious risk associated with a drug by using postmarketing surveillance data. REMS are not standardized throughout the pharmaceutical industry, which can be problematic for pharmacists and physicians to ensure full compliance with each REMS program within a hospital. Components of REMS may include patient guides, patient package inserts, or communication plans for healthcare providers. Education can be direct from a medical science liaison or web based for providers. It may include requirements for special training or certification for prescribing or dispensing, dispensing only under certain circumstances, special monitoring, or the use of patient registries. The need for REMS is determined by the FDA at the time of drug approval. To meet the differing requirements of each REMS, it is prudent that healthcare providers understand the regulations for each product. To do so, working directly with pharmaceutical company representatives can increase the likelihood of succeeding with the REMS requirements and thus providing optimal care for the patient. REMS programs should be communicated to hospital P&T committees and medication safety committees. Educational efforts should also include health-system administration, risk management, nursing leadership, and medical staff within a hospital.[22]

# SUMMARY

Academic detailing is an innovative approach to communicating the most recent evidence-based data regarding medications or other interventions from one health professional to another in order to better patient outcomes, improve clinical decision making, and reduce costs. This form of one-on-one communication is derived from the historically successful interactions between pharmaceutical sales representatives and prescribers. The relationship between pharmacists and pharmaceutical industry remains symbiotic yet continues to evolve, particularly with the more recent introduction of codes and statements discussing ethical interactions between pharmacists and industry members. Opportunities to partner with pharmaceutical industry to improve patient care are numerous and include educational efforts, implementation of REMS programs, and aid in achieving quality core measures.

# REFERENCES

1. Fischer MA, Avorn J. Academic detailing can play a key role in assessing and implementing comparative effectiveness research findings. *Health Aff (Millwood)*. 2012;31(10):2206-2212.
2. The Hilltop Institute. Academic detailing: a review of the literature and states' approaches. http://www.hilltopinstitute.org/publications/AcademicDetailing-ReviewOfTheLiteratureAndStates%27Approaches-December2009.pdf. Accessed July 24, 2014.
3. National Resource Center for Academic Detailing. http://www.narcad.org. Accessed July 24, 2014.
4. Avorn J, Soumerai SB. Improving drug-therapy decisions through educational outreach. *N Engl J Med*. 1983;308(24):1457-1463.
5. Soumerai SB. Avorn J. Principles of educational outreach (academic detailing) to improve clinical decision making. *JAMA*. 1990;263(4):549-556.
6. Prescription Policy Choices. A template for establishing and administering prescriber support and education programs: a collaborative, service-based approach for achieving maximum impact. http://www.policychoices.org/documents/ADPITemplate91708.pdf. Accessed July 24, 2014.
7. Academic detailing: an interview with Jerry Avorn, MD. AARP Rx Watchdog Report. http://assets.aarp.org/www.aarp.org_/cs/health/206907rxwatchdog_dec_09.pdf. Accessed July 24, 2014.
8. Gabay M. Academic detailing and the IDEA Act. *Hosp Pharm*. 2010;45(11):839-840.
9. Pharmaceutical and Research Manufacturers of America. Pharmaceutical marketing in perspective: its value and role as one of many factors informing prescribing. http://www.phrma.org/sites/default/files/pdf/phrma_marketing_brochure_influences_on_prescribing_final.pdf. Accessed July 24, 2014.

10. Pharmaceutical industry: by the numbers. Texas Trial Lawyers website. http://www.ttla.com /index.cfm?pg=bynumbersdrugs. July 24, 2014.

11. Pharmaceutical and Research Manufacturers of America. Code on Interactions with Healthcare Professionals: ethical interactions with healthcare professionals are critical to our mission. http:// www.phrma.org/code-on-interactions-with-healthcare-professionals. Accessed July 24, 2014.

12. American Society of Hospital Pharmacists. ASHP guidelines on pharmacists' relationships with industry. *Am J Hosp Pharm*. 1992;49(1):154.

13. American Society of Hospital Pharmacists. ASHP guidelines for pharmacists on the activities of vendors' representatives in organized health care systems. *Am J Hosp Pharm*. 1994;51(4):520-521.

14. American Society of Hospital Pharmacists. Code of ethics for pharmacists. *Am J Health-Syst Pharm*. 1996;53:1805.

15. Pharmacists and industry: guidelines for ethical interactions. American College of Clinical Pharmacy position statement. *Pharmacotherapy*. 2008;28(3):410-420.

16. Ehringhaus SH, Weissman JS, Sears JL, et al. Responses of medical schools to institutional conflicts of interest. *JAMA*. 2008;299(6):665-671.

17. Soyk C, Pfefferkorn B, McBride P, et al. Medical student exposure to and attitudes about pharmaceutical companies. *WMJ*. 2010(109)3:142-148.

18. *Remington: The Science and Practice of Pharmacy*. 21st ed. Philadelphia, PA: Lippincott Williams & Wilkins, 2005.

19. Centers for Medicare and Medicaid Services. Medicare, Medicaid, Children's Health Insurance Programs: transparency reports and reporting of physician ownership or investment interests. *Fed Regist*. 2013;78:9457-9528.

20. Gagnon MA, Lexchin J. The cost of pushing pills: a new estimate of pharmaceutical promotion expenditures in the United States. *PLoS Med*. 2008;5:e1.

21. Reynolds B. Visits from pharmaceutical reps can be "PEACEFUL." *Pharmacy Today*. 2007(2):24.

22. Shane R. Risk evaluation and mitigation strategies: impact on patients, healthcare providers, and health systems. *Am J Health-Syst Pharm*. 2009;66:S6-S12.

# MEDICAL WRITING AND PEER REVIEW

Heather J. Ipema, PharmD, BCPS
Maria G. Tanzi, PharmD

## CHAPTER OBJECTIVES

▸ Describe medical writing and tips to becoming a successful writer.

▸ Explain the various parts of a manuscript and key information that belongs in each section.

▸ Explain various ethical issues that impact medical writing.

▸ Describe factors that authors might consider when choosing a journal for article submission.

▸ Describe the process and requirements for articles submitted to biomedical journals.

▸ Explain the purpose and importance of article peer review.

▸ Describe the process of article peer review.

▸ Describe ethical standards of the article peer review process.

## CHAPTER OUTLINE

## KEY TERMS

# INTRODUCTION

The ability to write clearly and effectively is a key skill needed by healthcare professionals to perform numerous aspects of their jobs. Some have even stated that writing is the action catalyst in health care.[1] From physician offices to pharmacists to third-party insurers, writing is the primary means of recording activities and, in most cases, is the mandatory form of communication. The push toward electronic patient medical records will only further enhance the need for healthcare professionals to know how to write clearly and accurately.

Medical writing is an essential skill for pharmacists to master, as many of the activities pharmacists are involved in require a writing component.[1] For example, daily tasks such as updating patient records, interacting with insurers, and answering drug information questions usually involve writing. Beyond these daily tasks, pharmacy-related projects such as in-service presentations, newsletters, formulary monographs, clinical algorithms, adverse drug reaction reports, continuing education programs, patient educational materials, and manuscripts must all be written. Pharmacy students are also faced with the task of writing numerous documents such as progress notes, discharge summaries, and teaching materials.

Documents authored by pharmacists and other healthcare professionals can be classified into four categories: patient care, clinical reports, research publications, and administrative documents.[1] Patient care documents encompass reports such as a patient consult note, a progress note, or a pharmacist care plan. Clinical reports are those that are generally generated for the healthcare institution and include items such as a clinical algorithm or guideline, a drug utilization review or evaluation, or a formulary review. Medical writing focusing on research can include the generation of a book chapter or review, a grant proposal or review, or a poster or **manuscript** for publication. The administrative type of medical writing can encompass such items as a letter of recommendation for a fellow colleague or student, a memorandum, a performance evaluation, a utility analysis report, or a variance report. Therefore, mastering the skills needed to write a wide range of documents allows healthcare professionals to effectively do their jobs. This chapter will focus on the recommended steps when writing a research paper, with an emphasis on the various sections of scientific manuscripts and the submission and peer review process.

# WRITING A RESEARCH PAPER: TIPS FOR SUCCESS

In an article written by R. Grant Steen, the author discusses the key qualities a medical author should strive to be, including original, honest, innovative, organized, careful, clear, modest, fair-minded, frank, persistent, rigorous, and realistic.[2] Organization is essential, because many medical documents have specific formats that must be followed. For example, scientific papers submitted for publication are generally required to follow the **International Committee of Medical Journal Editors (ICMJE) Uniform Requirements for Manuscript Submission**;[3] a detailed review of these requirements will be covered in a subsequent section of this chapter.

When deciding to write a paper, following certain steps may help ease the process. The decision to write a paper is the first step, as making a conscious commitment to start and complete a paper is essential.[4] In addition, healthcare professionals who are on the academic track must write papers for publication to advance via promotion and tenure. Once the decision is made, conferring with a mentor and reviewing the available literature is the next logical step. A mentor can give the writer his or her honest opinion about the topic selected and how to design the paper to be unique and informative and contribute something of value to the current literature pool. When conducting a literature search, it is important to be as thorough as possible to ensure that nothing of importance is missed. All articles that relate to the topic should be pulled and reviewed, and literature searches should be at least 2 months current to the time the paper will be submitted.

Creation of a timetable is another key step, because dividing a larger task into smaller steps with anticipated completion dates will make the writing project more manageable.[4] An example timetable for writing a manuscript has been proposed by Kliewer and is summarized in **Table 20-1**.[4]

| **TABLE 20-1** Example Timetable for Developing a Manuscript |
| --- |
| **Session 1**: Take notes on the literature, outline selected papers, and set provisional dates for completion. |
| **Session 2**: Devise an outline and title for the manuscript. |
| **Session 3**: Create a rough, initial draft. |
| **Sessions 4 and 5**: Create second and third drafts. |
| **Session 6**: Prepare tables and graphs and give the paper to coauthors. |
| **Session 7**: Incorporate suggestions from coauthors. |
| **Session 8**: Prepare all figures and the abstract. |
| **Session 9**: Proof all changes and extensively review the final product. |
| **Session 10**: Send out the paper. |

Modified from Kliewer MA. Writing it up: a step-by-step guide to publication for beginning investigators. *AJR Am J Roentgenol.* 2005;185(3):591-596.

**CASE STUDY 20-1**    **Determining the Need for a Publication**

A pharmacy student has an idea for a review article and presents her idea to her faculty mentor during a routine advising session. Upon questioning the student, the faculty mentor realizes that the student has not conducted a literature search on the proposed topic. How should the faculty mentor now advise the student?

The faculty mentor should educate the student that a thorough literature search needs to be conducted to determine if the review article will be informative and contribute something of value to the current literature pool. The student and faculty mentor should determine if other similar review articles have been published and, if so, how the proposed review may be different from articles already in the public domain.

When developing an **outline**, main headings should be created to serve as a template for subsequent section development. Filling in the outline with notes and phrases, rather than complete sentences, is recommended, as this will allow the writer to more easily insert the notes taken from the literature or other sources.[4] Once the outline is complete, the initial draft should be created as freely and extemporaneously as possible, always keeping in mind that subsequent drafts will be needed. In a book written by Deborah St James, the author summarizes seven steps to successful writing, with one being **freewrite**.[5] The author notes that the best way to get ideas on paper is to just start writing whatever comes to mind for approximately 10 minutes, because this is a good way to get the creative side of the brain working and additional ideas flowing. For the initial rough draft, the focus should not be on grammar, punctuation, organization, and spelling, because subsequent drafts can focus on editing for clarity and correctness.

As noted, the revision process should focus on unity and coherence.[5] Subsequent drafts should be assessed for unity by determining if all the sentences in each paragraph contribute to the development of the paragraph's central idea. Coherence should be assessed by determining if there is a relationship between each sentence and each paragraph and whether the content is clear to the reader. Transition words or phrases are helpful in working toward coherence and connecting ideas. Once the draft has been revised, proofreading is one of the final key steps in ensuring that the best possible written piece has been created. Asking someone else to read over the work is a good idea, because it may be difficult to find errors after working on the same content for some time. Another trick to catching errors is to read the written work out loud, listening for mistakes that might have been overlooked.

## PARTS OF A MANUSCRIPT

Although medical writing can take on many forms, development and submission of a manuscript is the main focus of this chapter. Understanding ICMJE's requirements for manuscript submission and what should be contained in each section of a scientific manuscript will aid the writer tremendously during the manuscript development process. In addition, being familiar with the **CONsolidated Standards of Reporting Trials (CONSORT) Statement** will help those who are writing papers about **randomized controlled trials**.[6] This chapter gives only a brief overview of the key components of a scientific manuscript, and readers are encouraged to review the information on both ICMJE's website (www.icmje.org) and the CONSORT website (www.consort-statement.org) for more details.[3,6]

# Title

The title of the article is the first thing people will read when determining if they want to read the full paper. Titles should be concise and informative.[3] The title should contain some key bits of information, such as the study design (e.g., randomized, double-blind trial), but the title should generally not be indicative of the results of the trial. Authors should include all information in the title that will make electronic retrieval both sensitive and specific. It is recommended that a few titles be written, with selection of the best title once the contents of the paper have been fully developed.[7]

# Introduction

The introduction section should generally be brief and include elements such as the objective or purpose of the paper, key background information and prior literature, and the hypothesis of the study (if applicable).[8] When discussing background information, the nature of the problem and its significance should be stressed.[3] The introduction section should make it clear to the reader why the paper is needed.[4] In addition, only directly pertinent references should be cited, and no data or conclusions from the current work should be included in this section. It has been noted that this section should be used as the lead-in to persuade readers to keep reading.[8] The introduction for reports of **original research** may be written before the research is performed as part of an **institutional review board** application or grant proposal.

# Methods

The methods section of a scientific paper contains a multitude of information, such as study design, selection and description of participants, interventions, outcomes, and statistical analyses. When describing the methods, it should be written in a way so that an outsider can reproduce the results.[3] If writing a review paper, the search strategy should be clearly defined in the methods section. Key questions that should be answered in the methods section are presented in **Table 20-2**.[8] The methods section of an original research report is often written before research begins to ensure that all individuals involved in the study are aware of the approved protocol and procedures.

Per ICMJE, **inclusion** and **exclusion criteria** of study participants must be clearly established, in addition to the reasons certain groups were selected or actively excluded.[3] In addition, if drugs or chemicals were used, all identifying information, such as generic name(s), doses(s), and route(s) of administration, should be included. For the statistical analyses, the specific computer software that was used to analyze the results should also be included. Clinical outcomes and surrogate markers should also be clearly defined in the methods section, with reference to key trials that have established their relevance.[9] Documentation of protection of research subjects is another essential component that must be included in this section. Approval from a local ethics committee should be described to ensure that patient rights were protected.

| TABLE 20-2   Key Questions That Should Be Answered in the Methods Section |
| --- |
| Who or what was examined? |
| What was done (in detail)? |
| Were there controls? |
| How was bias avoided and objectivity maintained? |
| What statistical methods were used? |

Data from Griscom NT. Your research: how to get it on paper and in print. *Pediatr Radiol*. 1999;29(2):81-86.

## RESULTS

The results section is often referred to as the most important part of the paper or the core of the paper.[7,9] This section is for data presentation only; it should not include any comments, discussions, or inferences about the data.[10] Numerous authors note that this section should be as clear and to the point as possible.[7-9] ICMJE recommends that results be presented in a logical sequence as text, tables, and figures.[3] If data are summarized in tables or figures, the same information should not be presented in great detail in the text. The text should be written in such a way that it summarizes the results and refers to the tables and figures for more detail.[10]

When describing the results, all patients enrolled in the study should be accounted for, and use of a CONSORT flow diagram is the preferred method to show the flow of participants throughout a randomized controlled trial.[6] In addition, results for the outcomes specified in the methods section should be reported. Numeric results should be given not only as derivatives, such as percentages, but also as absolute numbers to show the reader how the derivatives were calculated.[3] The statistical methods used to analyze the data should also be clearly specified.

When generating illustrations for the paper, an article by Fraser notes that writers need to ask themselves, "Is it really helpful or necessary?"[10] Fraser developed some general rules that should be followed when creating illustrations, and these rules are summarized in **Table 20-3**.[10]

## DISCUSSION

The discussion section is generally divided into three main parts: the explanation of the current work, arguments and comparisons with other work, and the implications of the current work.[10] For experimental studies, it is useful to begin the discussion by briefly summarizing the main findings, then exploring possible mechanisms or explanations for these findings, comparing and contrasting the results with other relevant studies, stating the limitations of the study, and exploring the implications of the findings for future research and for clinical practice.[3]

When discussing the current results, the meaning of the results should be clearly stated, along with possible biases and flaws, and other comments about the validity of the data.[10] When comparing the current work with those of others, it should be compared against recent reports and present knowledge and understanding of the subject matter. This section of the discussion will contain the most references to published work. The final section should review implications for current knowledge, discuss aspects that remain open to question, and give specific suggestions for future work.

## ABSTRACT AND KEYWORDS

Most journals have clear instructions on what they want in the **abstract**. The abstract is generally structured and usually is restricted by a specific word count. Most abstracts will

| **TABLE 20-3**  General Rules for Creating Figures in a Manuscript |
|---|
| Do not overcrowd the figure. |
| Do not extrapolate beyond the data points. |
| Present time or any other independent variable on the horizontal axis and the dependent variable on the vertical axis. |
| Do not suppress the zero. |

Data from Fraser HS. Writing a scientific paper. *West Indian Med J.* 1995;44(4):111-114.

contain a brief introduction, the purpose of the study, a brief summary of the methods, the most important results, and a statement of conclusion.[10] ICMJE also notes that the funding source should be cited in the abstract.[3]

## REFERENCES

This section is one of the easiest to complete and can be done quickly if a few items are kept in mind. References should be numbered consecutively based upon use in the text and formatted according to the journal's style. This style can vary and may follow the Uniform Requirements, the *American Medical Association Manual of Style*, the *Chicago Manual of Style*, or the *Publication Manual of the American Psychological Association*.[3,11-13] Authors should cite original work as much as possible and avoid citing review articles or other works that summarize original papers.[3] Other tips from ICMJE on appropriate references to be used in the paper include avoid citing abstracts, other unpublished works, and personal communications.

# ETHICAL ISSUES IN MEDICAL WRITING

Authors have numerous duties and responsibilities to ensure that their work meets certain publication ethics. The work should be as transparent as possible, with the author reporting all sources of funding, any potential conflicts of interest, and only including coauthors who actually participated in the development of the paper.[14] If others were involved in helping analyze the data or other aspects of the research, these individuals should be recognized in the acknowledgments section. Medical **ghostwriting** is a process in which a pharmaceutical company drafts favorable scientific articles and sends them to academic researchers to sign on as authors.[15] This process is usually done with the help of medical education and communication companies and is considered a serious breach of medical ethics and a violation of most major medical journals' policies.

According to the ICMJE, an author is one who takes responsibility for at least one component of the work, is able to identify who is responsible for other components, and is confident in his or her coauthors' ability and integrity.[3] **Authorship** credit should only be given to those who fulfill all three of the following requirements: (1) substantial contributions to conception and design, acquisition of data, or analysis and interpretation of data; (2) drafting the article or revising it critically for important intellectual content; and (3) final approval of the version to be published.

The integrity of the work will also be assessed, and can only be maintained with works that do not contain false data, fabricated data, manipulated images, or plagiarized statements.[14] If data are considered to be false or fabricated, editors may ask to review the raw data to ensure that the results are real. **Plagiarism** is another serious problem and is defined as an intentional or unintentional copying of the words of another person.[16] It can be further broken down into *direct plagiarism*, which is a direct copy of text; *mosaic plagiarism*, which is the borrowing of ideas and opinions; and *self-plagiarism*, which is reusing one's own work without citations. To minimize the occurrence of plagiarism, the author should cite all the original sources used and use direct quotes when the exact words of other authors are used.

Another issue that is considered to be author misconduct is duplicate submission or duplicate publication.[17] This is the process in which a manuscript is submitted to two journals simultaneously or the work has already been published by one journal and now the authors submit a minimally revised version to another journal. Once the work has been submitted to a journal and accepted, it should not be submitted to an alternate journal for publication.

# MANUSCRIPT SUBMISSION

Preparation of manuscript content is only the beginning of the manuscript submission process. Authors must also decide which journal is most appropriate for the manuscript and follow that journal's submission requirements. The following sections describe these next steps in more detail.

## SELECTING A JOURNAL

Journal selection can occur at several points during the manuscript preparation process. Some authors decide where to submit their manuscript before it is written, which can prevent future revision required to conform to the journal's formatting requirements. Other authors may prefer to prepare the manuscript first so that the final depth and scope of the project is known before choosing the best journal.

### Journal Characteristics

With both approaches to the timing of journal selection, similar factors must be considered prior to making a final decision. **Table 20–4** describes important journal characteristics that some authors may consider.[18] Information about these characteristics can be found on the journal's website or printed in a current issue of the journal. Some journals also provide explicit assistance to authors considering their journal, such as the *British Medical Journal (BMJ)* web page titled "Is the BMJ the right journal for my research article?"[19] Less

| TABLE 20-4 | Characteristics of Medical Journals of Importance to Authors |
|---|---|
| Journal Characteristic | Questions to Ask |
| Audience | Who typically reads the journal (e.g., physicians, pharmacists, non-healthcare professionals)? What type of reader would be most interested in the manuscript (e.g., clinicians, researchers, academic practitioners)? How technical is the manuscript language? Will target readers be able to understand the language? How large is the journal's circulation audience? What countries are represented in the audience? |
| Purpose/scope | Does the journal focus more on basic or clinical research? |
| Types of articles published | What type of article is the manuscript (e.g., original research report, review article, case report)? Does the journal publish this type of article? Does the manuscript meet the journal's requirements for this type of article? |
| Reputation | How prestigious is the journal compared to similar journals? What is the journal's impact factor (or other journal ranking metric)? Is the journal indexed in a searchable database (e.g., MEDLINE, Embase)? Do articles in the journal undergo peer review? |
| Timeliness | How timely are the manuscript's findings or conclusions? What is the typical delay between manuscript submission and publication? |
| Access | Is the journal available electronically? Is the desired target audience more likely to read in-print or electronic articles? Does the journal have open access, or does it require a subscription? |

Data from Chipperfield L, Citrome L, Clark J, et al. Authors' submission toolkit: a practical guide to getting your research published. *Curr Med Res Opin*. 2010;26(8):1967-1982.

**CASE STUDY 20-2**    **Choosing a Journal for Publication**

A hospital pharmacist has authored a manuscript describing the process and outcomes associated with implementing a new clinical protocol at his institution. After researching journals for manuscript submission, the pharmacist has a list of three potential journals. Which journal should the pharmacist consider submitting to first?

- Journal A: National audience of various healthcare providers in a variety of practice settings; publishes mostly landmark multicenter clinical trials; offers early publication online.
- Journal B: Audience is a mix of hospital and community pharmacists; articles are not peer reviewed; pharmacist knows a member of the editorial staff.
- Journal C: Audience is hospital pharmacists, technicians, and administrators; accepts manuscripts describing protocol implementation; pharmacist has been rejected from this journal before.

Although the pharmacist has previously submitted manuscripts that were rejected by journal C, the journal's audience and scope make it the best match for his current manuscript. Journal B could be a second choice if the manuscript is not accepted to journal C but may be a less desirable option due to the lack of peer review. Journal A is a prestigious journal, but it is probably unlikely that journal A would publish a manuscript that relates to the clinical experience of a single institution.

experienced authors may find it helpful to solicit journal recommendations from more seasoned colleagues.

Prior to actually submitting the manuscript, it may be prudent to conduct a presubmission inquiry with the journal editors.[18] By inquiring about a topic before manuscript preparation/submission, authors may be able to save unnecessary time and effort submitting to a journal that is not suitable for the manuscript or not interested in the topic. **Presubmission inquiries** may be particularly useful for time-sensitive manuscripts or other unusual circumstances that require special editorial attention. Many pharmacy (e.g., *American Journal of Health-System Pharmacy*) and nonpharmacy journals (e.g., *New England Journal of Medicine*) have formal processes for prospective authors to submit manuscript ideas to the journal's editorial staff for feedback.[18,20,21] Other journals usually allow authors to inquire about potential manuscript topics by emailing the editors.[18]

## Impact Factor

Several metrics that compare journal influence and prestige have been developed. The most well-established metric is called the **impact factor**. Impact factors are calculated yearly for more than 11,000 journals and are published in the subscription-only Thomson Reuters Journal Citation Reports.[22] The calculation involves the number of times during the report year that articles published in the journal during the prior 2 years were cited divided by the number of citable articles published in the prior 2 years.[23] Citable articles include original research reports and review articles.[22] A high impact factor suggests that the journal publishes important articles that inform subsequent research, and is therefore a more prestigious journal than those with lower impact factors.

Authors should be aware that comparison of journal impact factors is only appropriate within individual disciplines.[24,25] For example, the *New England Journal of Medicine* had a 2013 impact factor of 54.420, whereas the leading cardiology journal (*Journal of the American College of Cardiology*) had an impact factor of 15.343 due to inherent differences in its audience and scope compared to the *New England Journal of Medicine*.[22] The 2013 impact factors for some popular pharmacy journals are provided in **Table 20-5**.

**TABLE 20-5**  The 2013 Impact Factors of Selected Pharmacy Journals

| Journal Name | 2013 Impact Factor |
| --- | --- |
| Annals of Pharmacotherapy | 2.923 |
| Journal of Managed Care Pharmacy | 2.682 |
| American Journal of Health-System Pharmacy | 2.205 |
| Pharmacotherapy | 2.204 |
| Journal of the American Pharmacists Association | 0.929 |

Data from Journal Citation Reports. ISI Web of Knowledge website.

Use of the journal impact factor as a measure of a journal's importance has been criticized for various reasons. Some authors feel that the calculation itself is biased because some journals are excluded from the database (including those published in languages other than English), only citations of citable articles are considered, and self-citation is not assessed.[22,26] It has also been noted that journals with a large number of review articles often have higher impact factors because review articles tend to be heavily cited.[26,27] The 2-year citation window may not be long enough for disciplines that typically see a peak in article citations after a longer period of time.[24] Also, there has been an unfortunate trend of using impact factors to evaluate author quality in areas such as academic promotion and tenure and awarding of research funds rather than journal quality.[24,28]

### Other Journal-Ranking Metrics

Due to the limitations and criticism of the journal impact factor, several other metrics for evaluating journal quality and importance have been developed.[24,27,28] The **Eigenfactor Metrics** is probably the best-known alternative metric because it is reported along with the impact factor in the Journal Citation Reports.[22] The Eigenfactor Metrics considers the number of times during the report year that articles published in the journal during the prior 5 years were cited, omits self-citations, ranks journals according to importance during the citation process (similar to the way Google ranks websites), can be used to compare journals across disciplines, and is freely available online.[29,30]

### Final Journal Choice

Authors generally want to publish in the most reputable journal possible, but the most prestigious journals are also the most competitive because they receive a large number of manuscript submissions. For example, the *BMJ* currently accepts only 7% of submitted manuscripts, and the *Journal of the American Medical Association* (*JAMA*) has an acceptance rate of only 9%.[19,31] In comparison, the more specialized, and therefore lower impact, *American Journal of Health-System Pharmacy* accepts 36% of submitted manuscripts.[32] Overall, authors usually have the best chance of publishing if they choose a journal whose audience and purpose are most compatible with the manuscript rather than focusing solely on journal reputation.[18] If the manuscript has been written by numerous authors, all authors should agree with the final journal choice.

## MANUSCRIPT SUBMISSION PROCESS AND REQUIREMENTS

A vital action before final manuscript preparation and submission is review of the chosen journal's **instructions for authors**.[18] These instructions are available on the journal's website and may also be published yearly in the journal itself. Important issues such as

| **TABLE 20-6**   Types of Articles Published in Medical Journals | |
| --- | --- |
| **Common Article Types** | **Less Common Article Types** |
| Original research report | Short report of original research |
| Case report | Clinical practice guideline |
| Review article | Meta-analysis |
| Letter to the editor | Clinical/problem-solving case |
| Editorial | Special report |

article types, formatting, and other submission requirements are explained in detail in the instructions for authors. Although checking the instructions may be intuitive, numerous journal editors have noted that manuscript characteristics such as "not following manuscript preparation instructions" and "submitting a manuscript in a format that does not match what the journal publishes" are leading reasons for manuscript rejection.[33,34]

## Article Types

Most journals only publish certain types of articles. Examples of common article types in medical journals are provided in **Table 20-6**. Original research reports and other articles with clinical research results may have formatting requirements but may not have limits on their word count, number of tables/figures, or number of references. In contrast, space limitations of in-print journals may require the journal to cap the length of more summative (review) articles or require submission of letters to the editor within a short time period in order to decrease the number of letters published. All of these requirements are clearly stated in the author instructions.

## Manuscript Formatting

Failure to adhere to instructions for formatting may prevent editors from seriously considering manuscripts that might otherwise be considered high quality.[18] Formatting requirements differ among journals. Potential manuscript elements with specific requirements may include font choice, text spacing, margins, reference formats, table/figure titles or structure, information required on the cover page, and number of electronic files that can be submitted for each manuscript. The journal's style may mimic the Uniform Requirements, may follow other common manuscript styles (e.g., *AMA Manual of Style*, *Publication Manual of the American Psychological Association*, *Chicago Manual of Style*, National Library of Medicine referencing), or may be unique to the journal.[3,11-13,35]

In addition to basic formatting, many journals require that manuscripts adhere to their preferred organizational structure. A common organization scheme is introduction, methods, results, and discussion (IMRAD) for original research reports. This type of common structure allows the reader to efficiently find information of interest in the published article.[34,36] Following the IMRAD format, some journals may also require the use of structured abstracts with defined headings.

## Other Requirements for Manuscript Submission

Most journals require submission of additional information or materials before a manuscript can be fully considered for publication.[18] A title page should be included with the manuscript. All journals have preferences regarding the information required on the title page (e.g., manuscript title, author names and affiliations, keywords, word count).

Journals that employ a double–blind peer review process may require a title page without author names. It is also common for authors to submit a cover letter with the manuscript. There are no standard elements for manuscript cover letters, but authors may choose to comment on why the manuscript would be an important addition to the literature, why it would be of interest to the journal's readership, and whether the manuscript has been previously published or submitted for publication elsewhere. Other disclosures that may be required by the journal (e.g., conflicts of interest, transfer of copyright from the authors to the journal upon publication, contributions of each author) can be included in the cover letter. Alternatively, the journal may have forms to formally document disclosures and other ethical/legal matters.

### Manuscript Checklists

A desire among medical journal editors to increase transparency, accountability, and quality of research reports has led to the development of numerous manuscript checklists. **Manuscript checklists** aim to standardize the type of information included in published study reports, and medical journals are increasingly recommending or requiring their use.[37] Most elements of these checklists involve the manuscript content; therefore, authors should consult the relevant checklist at the beginning of the writing process in case they decide to submit to a journal that requires the checklist as part of manuscript submission.

The most common manuscript checklist is the CONSORT checklist for randomized, controlled trials; checklists for other types of articles can be found in **Table 20-7**.[6,37-45] Examples of elements recommended for inclusion in a report of a randomized controlled trial are completely defined prespecified primary and secondary endpoints; an explanation of how the sample size was determined; descriptions of randomization and blinding methods used; and the number of participants randomized to treatment, received treatment, and included in the final analysis.[6] When considered together, these recommended

| **TABLE 20-7** Selected Manuscript Checklists | |
|---|---|
| **Checklist** | **Article Type** |
| CHERRIES | Internet surveys |
| CONSORT | Randomized, controlled trials |
| GNOSIS | Phase I and II studies |
| MOOSE | Meta-analysis of observational studies in epidemiology |
| PRISMA (formerly QUORUM) | Meta-analyses, systematic reviews |
| SQUIRE | Quality improvement projects |
| STROBE | Observational studies in epidemiology |
| TREND | Nonrandomized intervention trials |

Data from CONSORT: Transparent Reporting of Trials website. http://www.consort-statement.org. Accessed July 22, 2014; Larson EL, Cortazal M. Publication guidelines need widespread adoption. *J Clin Epidemiol.* 2012;65(3):239-246; Vollmer WM. Responsibilities of authorship. *Chest.* 2007;132(6):2042-2045; Eysenbach G. Improving the quality of web surveys: the checklist for reporting results of Internet e-surveys (CHERRIES). *J Med Internet Res.* 2004;6(3):e34; Chang SM, Reynolds SL, Butowski N, et al. GNOSIS: guidelines for neuro-oncology: standards for investigational studies-reporting of phase 1 and phase 2 clinical trials. *Neuro Oncol.* 2005;7(4):425-434; Stroup DF, Berlin JA, Morton SC, et al; Meta-analysis Of Observational Studies in Epidemiology (MOOSE) group. Meta-analysis of observational studies in epidemiology: a proposal for reporting. *JAMA.* 2000;283(25):2008-2012; PRISMA: Transparent Reporting of Systematic Reviews and Meta-Analyses website. http://www.prisma-statement.org. Accessed July 22, 2014; SQUIRE: Standards for Quality Improvement Reporting Excellence website. http://squire-statement.org. Accessed July 22, 2014; STROBE statement website. http://www.strobe-statement.org. Accessed July 22, 2014; Transparent Reporting of Evaluations with Nonrandomized Designs (TREND). Centers for Disease Control and Prevention website. http://www.cdc.gov/trendstatement/. Accessed July 22, 2014.

elements comprise the minimum information needed to provide readers with a clear description of the study methods, statistical analysis, results, and potential importance of the study findings.

### Overall Manuscript Submission Process

Contemporary manuscript submission is usually done online, but some journals may accept hard-copy submissions from authors without electronic access. Completely submitted manuscripts (including ancillary materials) may undergo an initial review by a member of the editorial staff to assess suitability for the journal and adherence to submission requirements.[11,46] The initial review process may also involve an assessment of the manuscript's scope and overall quality to eliminate papers with a very low chance of publication.[11,46,47] Manuscripts meeting initial review criteria go through the peer review process, which will be discussed in more detail later in this chapter. Upon acceptance, the manuscript goes through a final editorial review for clarity, accuracy, and style.[11] The author may be contacted at this point to provide clarification on unclear wording and ensure that the editorial changes made were appropriate. Authors also review the final manuscript layout (called *galleys* or *proofs*) for completeness and accuracy. Publication of the final article occurs in the next available issue with an opening for the article type, although timely articles or those that may have a high impact on clinical practice may be published sooner or released online prior to publication in print.

As previously stated, manuscript rejection is common.[47] Authors can appeal the journal's decision or choose to resubmit the manuscript to a different journal. Appeals are not accepted by all journals, and authors choosing to appeal the original journal's decision should be aware that appeals are typically a low priority for journal editors and responses may be delayed.[11,18] Consideration of the feedback and specific comments from the peer reviewers or editors can help guide the authors' decision to try another journal.[18,47] If major methodological flaws were identified, it may be unlikely that any other journals would accept the manuscript. However, if the rejection was based on overall suitability for the journal's scope and readership, a more compatible journal may have a high interest in the manuscript. Publication may be more likely if the manuscript is revised according to reviewer suggestions, because similar feedback is likely to be received from reviewers of the second journal. In highly specialized fields where individuals are likely to serve as peer reviewers for numerous journals, responding to prior feedback may be critical.

# PEER REVIEW PROCESS

Manuscript peer review has been commonly used by biomedical journals since the 1940s.[11,48] Although final decisions regarding the fate of manuscripts submitted for publication remain with journal editors, feedback from peer reviewers can help editorial decision making.

## PURPOSE OF ARTICLE PEER REVIEW

A universal definition of article peer review does not exist.[48] In essence, article **peer review** involves peer experts in the author's field providing feedback and recommendations on submitted manuscripts to the author and journal editors. Although authors may not always welcome criticism of their written work, the purpose of the peer reviewer's comments is to provide constructive suggestions to improve the manuscript and increase its chance of publication.[11] The two major areas that peer review should address are the manuscript's overall importance and quality. *Importance* considers whether the published article would increase knowledge or directly assist practicing clinicians or researchers. Assessment of article *quality* considers the research question, conclusion, and description of the study methods and data analysis. Both criteria can be considered independent of study outcomes, which implies that well-conducted studies with negative results should be considered for publication in an equal manner as those with positive results.

Despite numerous studies of the peer review process and several International Congresses on Peer Review in Biomedical Publication, questions remain regarding whether peer review effectively increases the quality of published articles.[48] A 2007 Cochrane review on this topic concluded that evidence is insufficient to support the idea that peer review results in higher quality literature.[49] Similarly, a systemic review published in *JAMA* in 2002 determined that so little evidence regarding the effect of peer review exists that it should be considered an untested process.[50]

## Reviewer Selection

Although some journals allow authors to identify individuals who could serve as reviewers or those that the author prefers do not review the manuscript, selection of peer reviewers is at the discretion of the journal editors.[11,47] Many journals maintain a list of reviewers, their areas of interest, and quality or timeliness of their prior reviews.[11] Other individuals who may be invited to review are known experts in the field or authors of prior publications on the same topic. Clinicians who desire to review for a specific journal can express their interest by contacting the journal editors.[48] Little has been published regarding reviewer demographics, but one report from 1993 concluded that the most effective reviewers for the studied journal (*Journal of General Internal Medicine*) were "young, from strong academic institutions, [and] well known to the editors."[51] Peer review is usually conducted on a volunteer basis, with individual motivations to review, including development of literature evaluation skills, early access to new information, or giving back to colleagues and editors.[48] Multiple (two to five) peer reviewers evaluate each manuscript, and editors may also consult a statistical reviewer if the peer reviewers are unable to adequately evaluate the statistical methods.[11]

## Review Process

Numerous publications provide guidance and advice to peer reviewers.[48,52-56] In addition, most journals provide reviewers with instructions for completing the review that contain general information on the desired scope and tone of the review. Reviewers are expected to read the entire manuscript, including any supplementary material, and provide a critique and specific suggestions for improvement to the authors. Examples of potential manuscript aspects for which reviewers can provide feedback are provided in **Table 20-8**.[48,52,53] Notably, peer reviewers rarely comment on grammatical issues because these are addressed by the editors.[11] A literature search is usually required to confirm whether similar articles have been previously published and to ensure that the author cited all relevant articles. Overall, comments to the author should be direct, specific, actionable, and aimed at increasing the manuscript's quality.

In addition to author feedback, reviewers often provide comments and recommendations directly to the editors. These comments to the editor are generally not shared with the authors. Feedback to editors should include comments on the overall importance and quality of the manuscript and provide a recommendation regarding

**TABLE 20-8** Potential Manuscript Aspects for Peer Review Feedback to Authors

| Manuscript Aspect | Potential Content of Feedback to Authors |
|---|---|
| Title | Adequately summarizes and describes the article? |
| Keywords | Appropriate? Any to include or omit? |
| Abstract | Completely summarizes the article? Same conclusion as the body? Appropriately structured (if applicable)? |
| Introduction | Clearly explains objective? Is objective interesting, relevant, and novel? Focused on overall objective? Enough information presented to meet objective? |
| Study design and methods | Clearly and completely described? Appropriate patients included? Appropriate number of patients included? Statistics adequately described? |
| Results | Are both safety and efficacy discussed? Should either be emphasized more or less? Results summarized clearly? All relevant results provided? |
| Tables and figures | Clear? Needed? Appropriately labeled? Information duplicated in tables and text? Could some info be converted from text to a table/figure? |
| Conclusions | Supported by data presented? Clearly stated? Appropriate limitations identified? |
| References | All relevant references included? |
| Length and layout | Length appropriate for article type? Headings appropriate/needed? Overall organization clear? Does the content flow? |

Data from Sylvia LM, Herbel JL. Manuscript peer review—a guide for health care professionals. *Pharmacotherapy*. 2001;21(4):395-404; Brand RA. Reviewing for clinical orthopaedics and related research. *Clin Orthop Relat Res.* 2012;470(9):2622-2625; and Paice E. How to write a peer review. *Hosp Med.* 2001;62(3):172-175.

the manuscript's acceptance. Any concern regarding a breach of author ethics (e.g., plagiarism, data fabrication, duplicate publication) should be brought to the editor's attention. Most journals have a defined set of potential actions, which may include accept as-is, accept with revision, revise and rereview, and reject. Reviewers may also be able to recommend that the manuscript be resubmitted as a different type of article, such as a letter to the editor. Comments to both authors and editors, along with the reviewer's recommendation, are usually submitted online. Depending on the journal, reviews are due within 10–30 days of the manuscript being sent for peer review. Following receipt of all peer reviews for the manuscript, the editor communicates the journal's final decision to the authors. Manuscripts are rarely accepted as-is and requests for revision are common.

Authors whose manuscripts require revision receive comments from all of the reviewers and the editor, along with a deadline for resubmission. Resubmission usually requires the edited manuscript and a point-by-point response that details the action taken on each reviewer comment or suggestion. This level of detail is especially important for suggestions not incorporated into the manuscript so the reviewers know why their recommendations were not accepted. The edited manuscript and response are sent to the same reviewers for re-review, and the reviewers subsequently provide similar feedback on the revised version to the authors and editors. Several revisions may be needed before the editor arrives at a final decision on manuscript acceptance or rejection.

| CASE STUDY 20-3 | Peer Review Process |
| --- | --- |

Three months after article submission, an author receives the comments and suggestions provided by the journal's peer reviewers. Communication from the journal editor indicates that the article will not be accepted unless the changes are made. The author is surprised by the number of comments, and notices that the reviewers have requested a few major organizational changes, along with many minor grammatical changes. What should the author do next?

The author currently has several options. If she makes all the changes suggested by the peer reviewers, the article is likely to be accepted. However, this may take a substantial amount of time, especially because some of the changes require restructuring of the entire article. Alternatively, the author can make only some of the suggested changes (such as the easier, minor changes), but the article will probably not be accepted unless the major issues are addressed. The author could also submit the article as-is to another journal, but this may not be a productive option because it is likely that reviewers of the second journal would request similar major changes as those requested by the first journal. The author's action will likely be based on a combination of factors, including whether she currently has the time to make the requested changes, her confidence that making the requested changes will lead to article acceptance, and her overall motivation to publish the article.

## PEER REVIEWER ETHICS

Peer review has been criticized because it is a highly subjective process with the potential for bias.[11] For example, competition for research funding or other recognition may tempt reviewers to use information in unpublished manuscripts for their own benefit or provide unfavorable reviews to their competitors.[53,55] Conversely, reviewers may be more likely to provide favorable reviews for manuscripts written by individuals with whom they have professional relationships or other affiliations. Potential bias in the peer review process has prompted many authors to articulate standards for ethical reviewer behavior. These best practices for ethical peer review include disclosure of potential **conflicts of interest** before agreeing to conduct the review and maintenance of confidentiality.[54,55] Reviewers may be able to perform unbiased reviews even when potential conflicts of interest exist, but the editor should decide whether the review would be appropriate in these situations. All submitted manuscripts should be regarded as privileged and confidential, and manuscript content should not be shared with others or used for the reviewer's personal gain. Unfortunately, adherence to these standards depends on the professionalism and integrity of the individual reviewer because journal editors do not have reliable mechanisms for enforcing ethical peer review behavior.

### Blinding in Peer Review

Journals differ in their approach to **blinding** as a way to decrease bias during article peer review.[11] Authors are nearly always blinded to reviewer identity, which may permit reviewers to provide more honest, frank feedback than they would otherwise. Reviewers, on the other hand, may or may not be aware of the authors' identity. Unblinded reviewers may be biased toward author identity, credentials, or institutional affiliations, which could hinder the provision of objective reviews. However, blinded reviewers may not be able to tailor their feedback appropriately to the author's training and expertise. Numerous studies investigating the effect of reviewer blinding on the quality of reviews have been conducted, with no clear consensus.[57-63] Interestingly, a recent effort to increase transparency of the review process has led to some journals requiring that reviewers agree to have their identified, signed reviews posted on the journal website as an accompaniment to the published article.[64] Although the desire to increase transparency is noble, there is some concern that journals with fully unblinded peer review may have more difficulty recruiting reviewers.[60,61]

## SUMMARY

Healthcare professionals, including pharmacists, must frequently communicate in writing. Medical writing can be made easier by approaching the project in an organized and systematic manner and performing several revisions of the completed work to assess for clarity, brevity, and completeness. When writing for medical journals, careful attention to formatting requirements from the journal and national or international organizations may increase the potential for favorable peer review and successful publication.

## REFERENCES

1. Assa-Eley MT, Ward CT, Hobson EH. Communication: an overview. In: Nemire RE, Kier KL, eds. *Pharmacy Student Survival Guide*. 2nd ed. New York, NY: McGraw Hill; 2009. http://www.accesspharmacy.com.proxy.cc.uic.edu/content.aspx?aid=5256398. Accessed July 22, 2014.
2. Steen RG. Writing for publication in a medical journal. *Indian J Endocrinol Metab*. 2012;16(6):899-903.
3. Uniform Requirements for Manuscripts Submitted to Biomedical Journals. International Committee of Medical Journal Editors website. http://www.icmje.org. Accessed July 22, 2014.
4. Kliewer MA. Writing it up: a step-by-step guide to publication for beginning investigators. *AJR Am J Roentgenol*. 2005;185(3):591-596.
5. St James D. *Writing and Speaking for Excellence: A Brief Guide for the Medical Professional*. Sudbury, MA: Jones & Bartlett Publishers; 1998.
6. CONSORT: Transparent Reporting of Trials website. http://www.consort-statement.org. Accessed July 22, 2014.
7. Biswas J. Practical suggestions in the writing of a research paper. *Indian J Ophthalmol*. 1998;46(4):247-250.
8. Griscom NT. Your research: how to get it on paper and in print. *Pediatr Radiol*. 1999;29(2):81-86.
9. Alexandrov AV. How to write a research paper. *Cerebrovasc Dis*. 2004;18(2):135-138.
10. Fraser HS. Writing a scientific paper. *West Indian Med J*. 1995;44(4):111-114.
11. AMA Manual of Style Committee. *AMA Manual of Style: A Guide for Authors and Editors*. 10th ed. New York, NY: Oxford University Press; 2007.
12. *The Chicago Manual of Style*. 15th ed. Chicago, IL: University of Chicago Press; 2003.
13. American Psychological Association. *Publication Manual of the American Psychological Association*. 6th ed. Washington, DC: Author; 2010.
14. Morton NS. Publication ethics. *Paediatr Anaesth*. 2009;19(10):1011-1013.
15. Anekwe TD. Profits and plagiarism: the case of medical ghostwriting. *Bioethics*. 2010;24(6):267-272.
16. Masic I. Ethical aspects and dilemmas of preparing, writing and publishing of the scientific papers in the biomedical journals. *Acta Inform Med*. 2012;20(3):141-148.
17. Brice J, Bligh J. Author misconduct: not just the editors' responsibility. *Medical Education*. 2004;39:83-89.
18. Chipperfield L, Citrome L, Clark J, et al. Authors' submission toolkit: a practical guide to getting your research published. *Curr Med Res Opin*. 2010;26(8):1967-1982.
19. Is the BMJ the right journal for my research article? British Medical Journal website. http://www.bmj.com/about-bmj/resources-authors/forms-policies-and-checklists/bmj-right-journal-my-research-article. Accessed July 22, 2014.
20. For Authors and Reviewers. The American Journal of Health-System Pharmacy website. http://www.ajhp.org/site/misc/ifora.xhtml. Accessed January 13, 2015.
21. Presubmission Inquiries. The New England Journal of Medicine website. https://cdf.nejm.org/misc/authors/PresubmissionInquiries.aspx. Accessed July 22, 2014.
22. Journal Citation Reports. ISI Web of Knowledge website. http://admin-apps.webofknowledge.com.proxy.cc.uic.edu/JCR/help/h_info.htm#information. Accessed December 4, 2014.
23. The Thomson Reuters Impact Factor. Thomson Reuters website. http://thomsonreuters.com/products_services/science/free/essays/impact_factor/. Accessed March 5, 2013.

24. Haeffner-Cavaillon N, Graillot-Gak C. The use of bibliometric indicators to help peer-review assessment. *Arch Immunol Ther Exp (Warsz)*. 2009;57(1):33-38.
25. Mathur VP, Sharma A. Impact factor and other standardized measures of journal citation: a perspective. *Indian J Dent Res*. 2009;20(1):81-85.
26. Makeham JM, Pilowsky PM. Journal impact factors and research submission pressures. *ANZ J Surg*. 2003;73(3):93-94.
27. Bernstein J, Gray CF. Content factor: a measure of a journal's contribution to knowledge. *PLoS One*. 2012;7(7):e41554.
28. Bornmann L, Marx W, Gasparyan AY, Kitas GD. Diversity, value and limitations of the journal impact factor and alternative metrics. *Rheumatol Int*. 2012;32(7):1861-1867.
29. Bergstrom CT, West JD. Assessing citations with the Eigenfactor Metrics. *Neurology*. 2008;71(23):1850-1851.
30. Eigenfactor Metrics website. http://eigenfactor.org. Accessed July 22, 2014.
31. About JAMA. JAMA: The Journal of the American Medical Association website. http://jama.jamanetwork.com/public/About.aspx. Accessed July 22, 2014.
32. Hasegawa GR. Publication of residency projects: another perspective. *Am J Health Syst Pharm*. 2012;69(1):77-78.
33. Pierson DJ. The top 10 reasons why manuscripts are not accepted for publication. *Respir Care*. 2004;49(10):1246-1252.
34. Audisio RA, Stahel RA, Aapro MS, Costa A, Pandey M, Pavlidis N. Successful publishing: how to get your paper accepted. *Surg Oncol*. 2009;18(4):350-356.
35. Wendling D, ed. *Citing Medicine: The NLM Style Guide for Authors, Editors, and Publishers*. 2nd ed. Bethesda, MD: National Library of Medicine; 2007. http://www.ncbi.nlm.nih.gov/books/NBK7256/?redirect-on-error=__HOME__&amp=&depth=2. Accessed July 22, 2014.
36. Dimitroulis G. Getting published in peer-reviewed journals. *Int J Oral Maxillofac Surg*. 2011;40(12):1342-1345.
37. Larson EL, Cortazal M. Publication guidelines need widespread adoption. *J Clin Epidemiol*. 2012;65(3):239-246.
38. Vollmer WM. Responsibilities of authorship. *Chest*. 2007;132(6):2042-2045.
39. Eysenbach G. Improving the quality of web surveys: the checklist for reporting results of internet e-surveys (CHERRIES). *J Med Internet Res*. 2004;6(3):e34.
40. Chang SM, Reynolds SL, Butowski N, et al. GNOSIS: guidelines for neuro-oncology: standards for investigational studies-reporting of phase 1 and phase 2 clinical trials. *Neuro Oncol*. 2005;7(4):425-434.
41. Stroup DF, Berlin JA, Morton SC, et al; Meta-analysis Of Observational Studies in Epidemiology (MOOSE) group. Meta-analysis of observational studies in epidemiology: a proposal for reporting. *JAMA*. 2000;283(25):2008-2012.
42. PRISMA: Transparent Reporting of Systematic Reviews and Meta-Analyses website. http://www.prisma-statement.org. Accessed July 22, 2014.
43. SQUIRE: Standards for Quality Improvement Reporting Excellence website. http://squire-statement.org. Accessed July 22, 2014.
44. STROBE statement website. http://www.strobe-statement.org. Accessed July 22, 2014.
45. Transparent Reporting of Evaluations with Nonrandomized Designs (TREND). Centers for Disease Control and Prevention website. http://www.cdc.gov/trendstatement. Accessed July 22, 2014.
46. Publication Process. New England Journal of Medicine website. http://www.nejm.org/page/media-center/publication-process. Accessed July 22, 2014.
47. Woolley KL, Barron JP. Handling manuscript rejection: insights from evidence and experience. *Chest*. 2009;135(2):573-577.
48. Sylvia LM, Herbel JL. Manuscript peer review—a guide for health care professionals. *Pharmacotherapy*. 2001;21(4):395-404.
49. Jefferson T, Rudin M, Brodney Folse S, Davidoff F. Editorial peer review for improving the quality of reports of biomedical studies. *Cochrane Database Syst Rev*. 2007;(2):MR000016.
50. Jefferson T, Alderson P, Wager E, Davidoff F. Effects of editorial peer review: a systematic review. *JAMA*. 2002;287(21):2784-2786.
51. Evans AT, McNutt RA, Fletcher SW, Fletcher RH. The characteristics of peer reviewers who produce good-quality reviews. *J Gen Intern Med*. 1993;8(8):422-428.
52. Brand RA. Reviewing for clinical orthopaedics and related research. *Clin Orthop Relat Res*. 2012;470(9):2622-2625.
53. Paice E. How to write a peer review. *Hosp Med*. 2001;62(3):172-175.
54. Levine AM, Heckman JD, Hensinger RN. The art and science of reviewing manuscripts for orthopaedic journals: part I. Defining the review. *Instr Course Lect*. 2004;53:679-688.

55. Christenbery TL. Manuscript peer review: a guide for advanced practice nurses. *J Am Acad Nurse Pract*. 2011;23(1):15-22.

56. Araújo CG. Peer review: a constantly-evolving scientific process. *Arq Bras Cardiol*. 2012;98(2):e32-e35.

57. McNutt RA, Evans AT, Fletcher RH, Fletcher SW. The effects of blinding on the quality of peer review: a randomized trial. *JAMA*. 1990;263(10):1371-1376.

58. van Rooyen S, Godlee F, Evans S, Smith R, Black N. Effect of blinding and unmasking on the quality of peer review: a randomized trial. *JAMA*. 1998;280(3):234-237.

59. Godlee F, Gale CR, Martyn CN. Effect on the quality of peer review of blinding reviewers and asking them to sign their reports: a randomized controlled trial. *JAMA*. 1998;280(3):237-240.

60. van Rooyen S, Godlee F, Evans S, Black N, Smith R. Effect of open peer review on quality of reviews and on reviewers' recommendations: a randomised trial. *BMJ*. 1999;318(7175):23-27.

61. van Rooyen S, Delamothe T, Evans SJ. Effect on peer review of telling reviewers that their signed reviews might be posted on the web: randomised controlled trial. *BMJ*. 2010;341:c5729.

62. Alam M, Kim NA, Havey J, et al. Blinded vs. unblinded peer review of manuscripts submitted to a dermatology journal: a randomized multi-rater study. *Br J Dermatol*. 2011;165(3):563-567.

63. Fisher M, Friedman SB, Strauss B. The effects of blinding on acceptance of research papers by peer review. *JAMA*. 1994;272(2):143-146.

64. Linder S, Schliwa M, Werner S, Gebauer D. Transparent peer review—an appreciation of the reviewers' contribution to a published article. *Eur J Cell Biol*. 2010;89(11):779.

# INFORMATICS AND CLINICAL DECISION SUPPORT

Christine D. Sommer, PharmD, MA

## CHAPTER OBJECTIVES

- ▸ Define *informatics*.
- ▸ Provide a brief history of informatics.
- ▸ Describe events that led to an increase in health IT adoption.
- ▸ Define *meaningful use*.
- ▸ Define common clinical screenings available through clinical decision support.

## CHAPTER OUTLINE

## KEY TERMS

Biomedical informatics

Clinical decision support

Clinical informatics

Computerized provider order entry

Electronic health record

Health Information Technology for
   Economic and Clinical Health Act

Meaningful use

# INTRODUCTION

Informatics is one of the fastest growing areas of healthcare, and the majority of pharmacists will interact with the field of informatics in some way over the course of their career. Informatics can be broken down into two broad categories: basic research, which constitutes the field of biomedical informatics, and applied research and practice, which constitutes the fields of translational bioinformatics, clinical research informatics, clinical informatics, consumer health informatics, and public health informatics.

The American Medical Informatics Association (AMIA) defines **biomedical informatics** (formerly called *medical informatics*) as "the interdisciplinary field that studies and pursues the effective uses of biomedical data, information, and knowledge for scientific inquiry, problem solving and decision making, motivated by efforts to improve human health." This discipline incorporates both technology and social/behavioral sciences into the development, study, and application of theories, methods, and processes through basic research efforts. These efforts are mostly undertaken within academia, research institutes, and corporate research labs. The research undertaken by the biomedical informatics community benefits the users of its practical implementation.[1]

The practical implementation of this research constitutes the field of health informatics, which includes both population informatics and clinical informatics. **Clinical informatics** is defined by AMIA as "the application of biomedical informatics methods and techniques, including information technology, to deliver healthcare services." While many pharmacists may think of clinical informatics as merely their pharmacy computer system or perhaps the electronic health record system, it is really much broader than that. Clinical informatics forms an umbrella over the subdivisions of informatics that focuses on the use of technology within the various healthcare divisions: medical informatics, nursing informatics, pharmacy informatics, etc. Many aspects of care fall within its realm, including the design, implementation, and adoption of image systems, clinical documentation, computerized provider order entry (CPOE), pharmacy computer systems, and **clinical decision support** (CDS), including medication decision support (MDS), found within these systems.[1]

# HISTORY OF INFORMATICS

The history of informatics is obviously strongly tied to the history of the development of the computer. The first digital computers were developed in the 1940s and by the 1950s were beginning to enter the marketplace. Early computers were mainframe systems in which computer resources were "time shared." The MEDINET project at General Electric is considered the earliest attempt at developing a hospital information system in the United States using this technology. Programs at Massachusetts General Hospital in Boston, Massachusetts; Latter Day Saints Hospital in Salt Lake City, Utah; Kaiser Permanente in Oakland, California; and Stanford University in Stanford, California, followed. The development of the microcomputer and advances in networking capabilities led to another approach in healthcare computing—the use of individual computers in specialty areas (such as pharmacy, lab, admitting) that relied on a central shared database. In the 1980s, the modern personal computer was introduced. Hundreds of vendors began developing applications for use in health care. Within pharmacy, the first widespread use of computers outside a health-system pharmacy was for patient profiling and online adjudication of claims. Gradually, medication decision support was incorporated through the screening for potential drug–drug interactions and allergic reactions. In the late 1990s, the widespread development of high-speed networks and applications allowed more facilities to adopt clinical information systems.[2-4]

For students working within major medical centers, the presence of a hospital **electronic health record** (EHR), system may seem the norm; however, that is still far from the case. As of 2012, only 44.5% of acute care nonfederal hospitals had at least a "basic" EHR system with clinician notes in place; however, that represents a fourfold increase over the 9.4% adoption level in 2008.[5] Why the dramatic increase? Perhaps the two biggest drivers of the explosion in the adoption of health information systems were the identification of an epidemic and a global recession.

In 1999, the Institute of Medicine (IOM) released a landmark report that shook the healthcare community: *To Err Is Human: Building a Safer Health System*. According to extrapolation of two previously published studies on the rate of medical errors in Colorado, New York, and Utah hospitals, between 45,000 and 98,000 Americans die each year from medical errors. Medical errors were defined as either the failure of a medical plan to be completed as intended or the use of a wrong plan to treat a patient. To put these numbers into perspective, each year medical errors kill more Americans than motor vehicle accidents, breast cancer, or AIDS—in fact the number of deaths is equivalent to a fully loaded jumbo jet crashing every day.[6]

But errors do not just result in death. There are financial impacts as well. Errors cost the U.S. healthcare system between $8.5 billion and $14.5 billion annually.[6] More and more large purchasers of health care, such as the federal government, insurance companies, and employers, are attempting to limit reimbursement for medical errors,[7,8] which will shift these costs to the systems that provide care. There are also nonmonetary costs, both to patients, who develop a distrust of the healthcare system and who may be burdened with the physical and psychological ramifications of a medical error, and to society, which suffers from decreased productivity and health as a whole.[6] Finally, the healthcare worker is often referred to as the "second victim" of a medical error. Healthcare workers involved in medical errors often develop dysfunctional behaviors and may face financial and legal issues after a medical error.[9]

Less than 10 years after the epidemic of medical errors was identified, the Great Recession began. December 2007 marked the beginning of a global economic decline that began with the U.S. subprime mortgage crisis and subsequent financial crisis. In response to this crisis, the American Recovery and Reinvestment Act of 2009 (ARRA) was passed. ARRA increased spending in the areas of energy, health, and infrastructure; provided federal tax incentives; and increased safety net provisions, such as expansion of unemployment and welfare. ARRA included the **Health Information Technology for Economic and Clinical Health Act** (HITECH).[10] The goal of HITECH is to improve health care through the meaningful use of technology by ensuring that clinicians have access to complete and accurate information and encouraging patient involvement through access to their medical information. HITECH provides $25.9 billion for the adoption and use of interoperable health information technology. The act provides incentive payments from Medicaid and Medicare for the meaningful adoption of certified EHRs. Beginning in 2015, hospitals and doctors will face Medicare penalties for not using EHRs.[10]

## MEANINGFUL USE

A key aspect of HITECH is the **meaningful use** requirement. Funded EHRs must use technology to improve care coordination, reduce health disparities, engage patients and caregivers, improve population and public health, and ensure privacy and security. Meaningful use criteria and requirements are being rolled out in three stages (**Table 21-1**). Stage 1 included requirements for **computerized provider order entry** (CPOE) for medications; drug–drug and drug–allergy interaction checking; demographic information (language, sex, race, ethnicity, date of birth, smoking status); vital signs; problem and medication lists; allergy profiling; clinical decision support; electronic prescribing; and system security. Stage 2 added requirements for CPOE for laboratory and radiology, an electronic medication administration record, and the adoption of three of the following six objectives: capability of electronic submission of syndromic surveillance data to public health agencies; electronic notes within patient records; electronic copies of imaging results and reports; recording of patient family health history as structured data; capability of reporting of cancer rates to state registries; and the capability to report other specific cases to specialized registries. Stage 3 requirements are currently being proposed and are scheduled to become effective in 2016.[11]

What does this mean for health care? For hospitals, it means more choices and assistance with the financial burden of purchasing and installing a system. Because systems will be required to communicate with each other, hospitals will no longer need to choose

| TABLE 21-1    Focus of Meaningful Use Criteria | | |
|---|---|---|
| **Stage 1: Data Capture and Sharing (2011–2012)** | **Stage 2: Advanced Clinical Processes (2014)** | **Stage 3: Improved Outcomes (2016)** |
| Electronically capturing health information in a standardized format | More rigorous health information exchange (HIE) | Improving quality, safety, and efficiency, leading to improved health outcomes |
| Using that information to track key clinical conditions | Increased requirements for e-prescribing and incorporating lab results | Decision support for national high-priority conditions |
| Communicating that information for care coordination processes | Electronic transmission of patient care summaries across multiple settings | Patient access to self-management tools |
| Initiating the reporting of clinical quality measures and public health information | More patient-controlled data | Access to comprehensive patient data through patient-centered HIE |
| Using information to engage patients and their families in their care | | Improving population health |

Reproduced from How to Attain Meaningful Use. HealthIT.gov website. http://www.healthit.gov/providers-professionals/how-attain-meaningful-use. Accessed March 27, 2014.

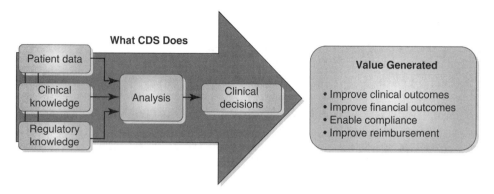

**FIGURE 21-1** How CDS/MDS improves care.

Courtesy of First Databank, Inc.

between an integrated system (one system from a single vendor that is used system wide) that may not completely meet the needs of every department and a "best of breed" option that requires labor-intense programming in order for the various systems (such as admitting, lab, pharmacy, etc.) to pass data between each other. As of March 2014, there were more than 3,700 products certified to meet 2011 meaningful use requirements in either the ambulatory care or inpatient environments, with 1,929 of these being complete EHR systems. As of this same time, there were 984 products already certified to meet 2014 meaningful use requirements, with 198 of these being complete EHR systems. More than 1,200 different vendors supply these systems, providing lots of choice in the marketplace.[12]

For clinicians, it means increased e-prescribing, more access to patient data, and more patient-specific alerting. It also means that almost all pharmacists will interact with the field of informatics through the use of either a pharmacy computer system or EHR. CDS and MDS data are designed to improve patient care by providing integrated, real-time data to the clinician within their workflow (**Figure 21-1**). In other words, the computer generates an alert to the clinician based upon the drug being ordered and patient-specific data within the EHR, without the clinician needing to stop to consult a tertiary reference. Numerous studies have shown that CDS has the ability to reduce errors.[13-15] CPOE backed by CDS allows orders to be screened for allergies, inappropriate dosages, contraindications, and drug interactions at the time the order is written and at the same time eliminates readability issues of handwritten orders. It can also provide prompts to prevent errors of omission, such as forgetting to order labs or other monitoring parameters. Although there are hundreds of system vendors, the market for CDS data is more consolidated, with most systems selecting from a handful of CDS vendors. With the use of these systems comes a responsibility of being an informed user (**Table 21-2**).

| TABLE 21-2    Responsibilities of Clinical Decision Support End-Users |
|---|
| Know the name of your system vendor. |
| Know the name of your data provider. |
| Understand what alerts are on, off, and/or filtered. |
| Understand editorial policies of activated modules. |
| Know how often your system is updated. |
| Know the procedure for questioning data within the system. |
| Stay current on system changes. |
| Avoid workarounds—ask for improvements instead. |
| Be familiar with downtime procedures. |
| Remember, it is decision *support*; it should not replace professional judgment. |

# CLINICAL DECISION SUPPORT AND MEDICATION DECISION SUPPORT DATA

CDS and MDS data are gathered from various sources, such as labeling, guidelines, and the primary medical literature. Each data vendor has its own editorial policies that govern the data provided in its products. These policies guide not only what is included and excluded in its databases, but how the data are described (**Figure 21-2**). Data provided include both product data and clinical data. Product data include attributes such as the National Drug Code (NDC), trade name, ingredients, strength, dosage form, quantity, manufacturer, and price. Clinical data may include allergy alerts, compatibility issues, contraindications, dosing, drug–drug interactions, drug–food interactions, indications, and patient education materials. Updates are provided to customers at various frequencies, such as weekly or monthly. In others, the system vendor is the actual customer of the data vendor and updates are provided to the vendor, who then processes them for local use. In other cases, institutions or health systems may be direct customers of the data vendor and receive their updates directly. In either case, the data are only as current as the last update supplied by the data vendor and applied to the system by either the system vendor or the institution.

Despite the fact that there are fewer data vendors compared to system vendors, no two vendor systems will be identical because of the many ways that vendor data can be implemented. It is important to distinguish between the data that are provided by the vendor and the implementation by the system vendor. The two most widely implemented CDS tools are those mandated by Stage 1 of meaningful use: drug allergy screening and drug–drug interaction screening.

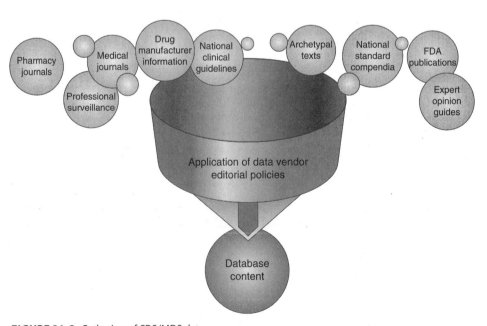

**FIGURE 21-2** Gathering of CDS/MDS data.

Courtesy of First Databank, Inc.

Most vendors provide two levels of allergy alerts: direct allergy (e.g., the use of ampicillin in a patient allergic to penicillin) and potential cross-sensitivities (e.g., the use of cephalexin in a patient allergic to penicillin). One issue with screening for allergens is that it is very dependent on what, if anything, is profiled in the patient's EHR. The EHR can only screen against profiled allergies. Many "allergies" that are documented are frequently intolerances (e.g., nausea with codeine) and not true immune system-generated responses. This can result in false alerts for related ingredients that the patient may tolerate. Many also provide screening against inactive ingredients to which patients may be allergic, such as dyes in tablets. This presents another issue—if a product is profiled instead of an active ingredient, many systems will assume that the patient is also allergic to the inactive ingredients within the product.

Drug–drug interaction data are also widely implemented. Some systems may use a comprehensive database of drug–drug interactions, whereas others use a subset of clinically significant drug–drug interactions. Databases differ not only in their content, but their classification as well. Each vendor has its own proprietary system for categorizing drug–drug interactions. Drug–drug interaction data are frequently cited as a source of alert fatigue for EHR users. Studies have shown that drug–drug interaction alerts are frequently overridden.[16,17] Although these numbers may be artificially high because most studies assume that all overridden alerts are ignored, when in fact a user may override the alert and then order appropriate labs to monitor the interaction, there is room for improvement.[18] Currently, most drug–drug interaction alerts are triggered solely by the presence of two drugs. As EHRs advance, there will be additional opportunities to fine-tune alerts by incorporating additional patient-specific data. For example, if the recommended action to manage a potential drug–drug interaction is to monitor the patient's serum potassium and there is already an order for a daily basic metabolic profile (BMP), which includes a serum potassium level, the alert could be suppressed. In the meantime, EHR systems typically allow institutions to filter interactions differently for different types of clinicians (e.g., physicians may see only the most clinically significant, whereas pharmacists see additional alerts) and allow some customization of the interaction data. Some sites may be unwilling to assume the increased liability and maintenance requirements of customization.

## OPPORTUNITIES FOR PHARMACISTS

For interested pharmacists, the expansion of informatics means increased job opportunities in almost every aspect of the field (**Figure 21-3**). System and data vendors require experienced clinicians to assist in designing and maintaining their products. Health systems and larger pharmacy chains hire pharmacy informatics personnel to assist with training, maintenance of formularies, creation of order sets, and applying updates. Students and pharmacists interested in the field can find out more information from the various associations that focus on informatics (**Table 21-3**).

## SUMMARY

Informatics is one of the most rapidly expanding healthcare areas. There are two broad categories of informatics—basic research (i.e., biomedical informatics) and applied research and practice. Clinical informatics, one of the applied research and practice fields, is defined as the application of biomedical informatics methods and techniques, including information technology, to deliver healthcare services.

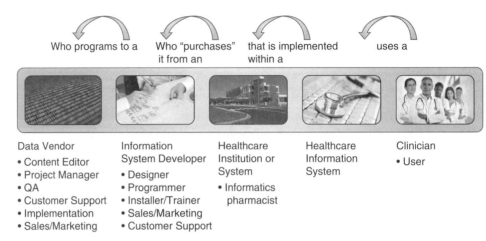

Who programs to a    Who "purchases"    that is implemented    uses a
                     it from an         within a

Data Vendor
• Content Editor
• Project Manager
• QA
• Customer Support
• Implementation
• Sales/Marketing

Information
System Developer
• Designer
• Programmer
• Installer/Trainer
• Sales/Marketing
• Customer Support

Healthcare
Institution or
System
• Informatics
  pharmacist

Healthcare
Information
System

Clinician
• User

**FIGURE 21-3**  Career options in informatics.

Courtesy of First Databank, Inc. Photos (L to R): © Johan Swanepoel/Shutterstock, © iStockphoto/Thinkstock, © Konstantin L/Shutterstock, © Ioana Davies (Drutu)/Shutterstock, © holbox/Shutterstock.

The development of the informatics field has been closely associated with the progression of computer technology. Initial hospital information systems in the United States were mainframe systems in which computer resources were "time-shared." As technology progressed, computer systems were used for patient profiling, claims adjudication, and drug–drug interaction or allergic reaction screening. Today, more hospitals and health systems have some form of an EHR and there is an increase in electronic prescribing, clinical and medication decision support data, and patient-specific alerts.

With the expansion of healthcare-related informatics, there are increased job opportunities for pharmacists. These include assisting in designing and maintaining products for system and data vendors, maintaining formularies, creating order sets, and applying updates for health systems and large pharmacy chains.

| TABLE 21-3    Associations Focusing on Informatics | | | |
|---|---|---|---|
| **Association** | **Acronym** | **Website** | **Representation** |
| American Medical Informatics Association | AMIA | www.amia.org | Represents biomedical and health informatics professionals. |
| American Society of Health-System Pharmacists | ASHP Section of Pharmacy Informatics and Technology | www.ashp.org | Represents pharmacists working in pharmacy informatics. |
| Healthcare Information and Management Systems Society | HIMSS | www.himss.org | Represents clinicians, corporations, and nonprofit associations interested in health IT. |
| Pharmacy Health Information Collaborative | Pharmacy HIT | www.pharmacyhit.org | Represents the interests of pharmacy in health IT matters. |

| CASE STUDY 21-1 | How Are Olanzapine and Cholestyramine Chemically Related? |
|---|---|

You are an inpatient pharmacist at a hospital utilizing an electronic health record (EHR) system. In this setting, prescribers enter orders electronically into the medical record. Orders are then verified by a pharmacist before being delivered/administered to the patient. You are a pharmacist verifying medication orders in the hospital inpatient pharmacy. While verifying an order, you receive the following alert. Why are you receiving this alert and what should you do?

WARNING: ALLERGY CONTRAINDICATION

Zyprexa Zydis® is contraindicated based upon documented allergy to Questran®.

This alert is being triggered because the patient's allergy profile contains a brand name product. Because Zyprexa Zydis® tablets and Questran® suspension both contain aspartame, an allergy alert is triggered.

What you should do is investigate which of the two clinical possibilities is true:

1. *The alert is a false positive.* In this instance, the patient is really only allergic to cholestyramine, not aspartame. Allergies are frequently entered by nonclinician personnel, who often enter the allergy exactly as stated by the patient or may pick a "representative" of the allergy, such as a common brand name. The EHR system was either programmed to assume or was told by the individual who entered the allergy that the patient was allergic to all ingredients, both active and inactive, in the product.
2. *The alert is valid.* Many excipients can cause allergic reactions in patients, including aspartame.

Before dispensing the product, you should attempt to verify what the patient's true allergy is, and its manifestation, by questioning the patient, if the patient is alert and oriented. Patients with true allergic reactions to excipients will usually know they are allergic to the excipient, such as aspartame, or be allergic to many different things, all of which may have aspartame in them.

If the patient is not alert or oriented, you can attempt to determine if the patient has already received aspartame in another product, either on their home medication list, during a previous admission, or in this admission, without an allergic reaction.

If you cannot determine whether the patient is truly allergic to aspartame, substituting another medication may be the safest course of action. If the medication cannot be substituted, or is urgently needed, advise nursing to closely observe the patient for signs and symptoms of an allergic reaction.

If you are able to verify the patient's true allergy, update the patient's allergy profile accordingly.

| CASE STUDY 21-2 | Why Do Interactions Differ Across Town? |
|---|---|

You have decided to work some extra shifts at a hospital across town. You thought it would be easy to adjust because they have the same EHR system as the hospital at which you work full time. One Saturday you realize that some interactions you remember seeing as alerts at your facility do not generate alerts at your relief site. You have also realized that some interactions that are generated at both sites have different severity classifications. Why aren't you seeing the same interactions at each facility?

The differences may be the result of several possibilities, such as timing issues, customization, different data providers, and a problem with one of the systems.

One reason for these differences could be that the "missing" interaction was recently added by the data vendor, who also updated the severity classifications on some interactions. The "differences" come from the fact that one hospital has not yet loaded the update into the system. Data vendors typically provide updates to clinical data on a weekly or monthly basis. In some cases, the data update is provided to the vendor, who either installs it remotely into its systems or redistributes it to its customers. In other cases, the EHR owner (hospital or health system) contracts directly with the data vendor and receives the updates directly from the data vendor. It is then up to the EHR owner to actually install the updates.

Another reason may be customization. One or both facilities may have customized the data they receive from their data vendor. No two hospitals will have the same mix of patients and providers. For example, a rural community hospital will have a much different mix of patients and providers than an urban teaching hospital or a pediatric hospital. As new tools are developed to help facilities customize data (a capability requirement of meaningful use), it is growing more and more common for them to do so. One or both facilities may have customized the data to better fit their facility.

Differences in data providers may also be the reason. Although the hospitals use the same EHR vendor, they may subscribe to different data providers. Several EHR vendors program to more than one data provider. The EHR purchaser can then select which data vendor's product to purchase for use within its system. Each of the data providers has its own editorial policies about what is and is not included and how to classify drug–drug interactions.

Lastly, although a remote possibility, it could be that there is a problem with how one facility's system has been implemented.

Be a responsible end-user. Ask about the differences you are seeing.

# REFERENCES

1.  Glossary of Acronyms and Terms Commonly Used in Informatics. AMIA website. http://www.amia.org/glossary. Accessed July 22, 2014.
2.  Hardy C. Pharmacy information systems. In: Dumitru D. *The Pharmacy Informatics Primer.* Bethesda, MD: American Society of Health-Systems Pharmacists; 2009:65-76.
3.  Rose E, Jones MA. Clinical decision support. In: Dumitru D. *The Pharmacy Informatics Primer.* Bethesda, MD: American Society of Health-Systems Pharmacists; 2009:35-64.
4.  Shortliffe ER, Blois MS. The computer meets medicine and biology: emergence of a discipline. In: Shortliffe ER, Perreault LE. *Medical Informatics Computer Applications in Health Care and Biomedicine.* 2nd ed. New York, NY: Springer; 2001:3-40.
5.  Charles D, King J, Patel V, Furukawa MF. Adoption of electronic health record systems among U.S. non-federal acute care hospitals: 2008–2012. ONC Data Brief, no 9. Washington, DC: Office of the National Coordinator for Health Information Technology; March 2013.
6.  Kohn LT, Corrigan JM, Donaldson MS. *To Err Is Human: Building a Safer Health System.* Washington, DC: National Academies Press; 2000:1-4.
7.  Carlson, L. Quality care lowers costs along with medical errors. *Employee Benefit News.* 2004;18(12):52-55.
8.  Shepherd L. Bad medicine: feds, insurers refusing to pay for medical errors. *Employee Benefit News.* 2007;21(14):53-54.
9.  Wu A. Medical error: the second victim. The doctor who makes the mistake needs help too. *BMJ (Clinical Research Ed.).* 2000;320(7237):726-727.
10. HITECH Act. HealthIT.gov website. http://www.healthit.gov/policy-researchers-implementers/hitech-act-0. Accessed March 27, 2014.
11. How to Attain Meaningful Use. HealthIT.gov website. http://www.healthit.gov/providers-professionals/how-attain-meaningful-use. Accessed March 27, 2014.
12. CHPL Product Information Database. http://oncchpl.force.com/ehrcert. Accessed March 27, 2014.
13. Armada ER, Villamañán E, López-de-Sá E, et al. Computerized physician order entry in the cardiac intensive care unit: effects on prescription errors and workflow conditions. *J Crit Care.* 2014;29(2):188-193.
14. Kaushal R, Shojania KG, Bates DW. Effects of computerized physician order entry and clinical decision support systems on medication safety: a systematic review. *Arch Intern Med.* 2003;163(12):1409-1416.
15. Milani RV, Oleck SA, Lavie CJ. Medication errors in patients with severe chronic kidney disease and acute coronary syndrome: the impact of computer-assisted decision support. *Mayo Clin Proc.* 2011;86(12):1161-1164.
16. Shah NR, Seger AC, Seger DL, et al. Improving acceptance of computerized prescribing alerts in ambulatory care. *J Am Med Inform Assoc.* 2006;13(1):5-11.
17. Taylor LK, Tamblyn R. Reasons for physician non-adherence to electronic drug alerts. *Stud Health Technol Inform.* 2004;107(Pt 2):1101-1105.
18. Nanji KC, Slight SP, Seger DL, et al. Overrides of medication-related clinical decision support alerts in outpatients. *J Am Med Inform Assoc.* 2014;21(3):487-491.

## CHAPTER 22

# BASIC PRINCIPLES OF PHARMACOECONOMICS

Jennifer C. Samp, PharmD, MS
Yash J. Jalundhwala, MS
Alexandra Perez, PharmD, MS
Simon Pickard, PhD

## CHAPTER OBJECTIVES

▸ Describe the importance of economic evaluations in health care and pharmacy.

▸ Describe the basic types of economic evaluations.

▸ Introduce terminology commonly used in pharmacoeconomic studies.

▸ Identify the relevant types of costs and outcomes included in economic evaluations.

▸ Discuss the different perspectives of an evaluation and the costs and outcomes relevant to each perspective.

▸ Discuss the interpretation of the results of economic evaluations.

▸ Describe the role of decision analysis and identify the different parts of a decision tree.

▸ Describe the role and types of sensitivity analyses.

▸ Discuss preference-based measurement of health and its relevance to economic evaluations.

▸ Discuss the relevance of comparative effectiveness research to pharmacoeconomics.

▸ Discuss economic evaluations of clinical pharmacy services.

▸ Understand the key components of an economic evaluation and be able to critically evaluate the literature on this topic to inform healthcare decisions.

▸ Identify guidelines for conducting and interpreting pharmacoeconomic studies and their use in health technology assessment.

## CHAPTER OUTLINE

## KEY TERMS

Cost–benefit analysis
Cost-effectiveness analysis
Cost-of-illness studies
Cost-minimization analysis
Cost–utility analysis
Decision analysis
Direct costs

Economic analysis
Incremental costs
Indirect costs
Intangible costs
Marginal costs
Opportunity cost
Sunk costs

## INTRODUCTION

In the United States and around the world, healthcare expenditures have risen dramatically over the past several decades. In the 1960s, healthcare expenditures made up 5.1% of the U.S. gross domestic product (GDP); today, healthcare expenditures account for 17.9% of GDP and total nearly $2.7 trillion. Increased spending on pharmaceuticals has accompanied the rise in overall healthcare expenditures. Roughly 10% of current healthcare spending is on pharmaceuticals, totaling approximately $263 billion in 2011.[1]

Concerns over escalating healthcare costs have preoccupied decision makers in many countries, and jurisdictions that wished to incorporate costs and outcomes into their decision-making processes were early adopters of economic evaluations of healthcare programs in order to improve allocative efficiency. This is particularly relevant to pharmaceuticals, as the decision to reimburse for new drug therapies can be costly, and the value for money needs to be informed by evidence. Application of the framework used in economic evaluations of healthcare interventions in the context of pharmaceuticals gave rise to the field of pharmacoeconomics. Pharmacoeconomics has emerged as an area of study that attracts experts from a variety of fields, including economists, decision scientists, engineers, pharmacists, health services researchers, physicians, and others, resulting in a rich multidisciplinary field. The purpose of this chapter is to introduce the concepts and terminology that form the foundations of pharmacoeconomics, provide an overview of the main components of economic evaluations, and discuss areas of application that are relevant to pharmacists.

# ECONOMIC EVALUATIONS

Several types of evaluation are central to medical decision making, particularly with respect to drugs: Is it safe? Can it work (e.g., is it efficacious)? Does it work in actual practice (e.g., is it effective)? And, can I afford it? The latter question is a key issue for the patient from an individual perspective, and a key issue from a system perspective, when some or all of the cost is borne by a payer that is not the patient, such as a government program or insurance company. Economic evaluations help us make choices using a structured approach to decision making by identifying and comparing relevant costs and/or outcomes associated with two or more competing alternatives (e.g., a new drug compared to the existing standard of care).

## COMPONENTS OF ECONOMIC EVALUATIONS

**Economic analysis** has been defined as "a comparative analysis of alternative courses of action in terms of both their costs and consequences."[2] Costs and consequences must be determined in order to perform an economic evaluation, where the differences in costs (inputs) and the difference in consequences (outputs) of two or more competing alternatives are compared.

### Outcomes

Outcomes are also often referred to as the outputs, benefits, consequences, or effects of a healthcare intervention. Outcomes are the results of the intervention. According to the ECHO framework,[3] outcomes can be placed into three major categories: economic, clinical, and humanistic. Economic outcomes include differences in future costs associated with each alternative (pharmaceutical product or service), expressed in monetary units. Clinical outcomes are direct medical consequences associated with the intervention, program, or service. These can be expressed in natural units; examples include changes in blood pressure, hemoglobin A1c values, or hospitalization rates. Humanistic outcomes are patient- or health-related quality of life (HRQoL), patient satisfaction, and other consequences felt by the patient or patient's family. A specific type of outcome unit, the quality-adjusted life year (QALY), is derived from a particular type of HRQoL known as a utility or preference-based measure. This will be discussed in greater detail later in the chapter.

Economic, clinical, and humanistic outcomes can be thought of as a Venn diagram with three overlapping circles (**Figure 22-1**). Outcomes may fall under one of these categories or under two or three. For example, if an antidepressant therapy causes an increase in symptom-free days, the outcome of increased symptom-free days may be considered both a clinical outcome and a humanistic outcome. Depression severity is measured by markers of days with depression, and this makes it a clinical outcome. Additionally, symptom-free days make the patient feel better and more productive. When the patient "feeling better" is quantified, this can be seen as a humanistic outcome. It is important to consider all relevant outcomes from the ECHO framework in an economic evaluation. In the case of pharmacoeconomic evaluation, we would note that this

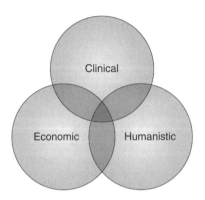

**FIGURE 22-1** ECHO framework.

framework for considering costs as economic outcomes is not ideal, because costs are deemed inputs and are separated from the health outcomes, consequences, or effects— that is, outputs—of an economic evaluation, because difference in costs constitutes the numerator and difference in consequences the denominator.

## Costs

Costs include the resources utilized in implementing the intervention.[2] When conducting economic evaluations, it is important to include the costs associated with the interventions of interest. The costs that are included will depend on the perspective, the patient population, and the question of interest.

Costs are often categorized as direct, indirect, or intangible. **Direct costs** are directly tied to a product or service and involve an exchange of money. These are generally the easiest costs to obtain because they are often documented in medical records or insurance claims databases. In healthcare evaluations, direct costs are either medical or nonmedical. Medical costs are any health-system cost. Nonmedical costs are costs that are associated with a medical service but not a direct part of the service. An example of nonmedical costs would include the transportation costs to and from a doctor's office.

Costs often involve money, but they can also involve other things, such as time and productivity loss. These are referred to as **indirect costs**. Because there is no direct exchange of money with indirect costs, these may be harder to measure. Person time is important because there is a monetary value associated with an individual's time. There are a few different ways to place a value on a person's time. The human capital approach is one common way to value person time. In this approach, people are viewed as productive resources, and time is valued by the potential earnings that could have been made during that time. For example, if a person is sick with the flu for 3 days, the human capital approach would have valued the loss of productivity as the wages that would have been made during those 3 days. The human capital approach is an acceptable approach to value individuals' time because it is intuitively easy to understand and it is relatively easy to implement (i.e., use a wage rate to put a dollar value on time). However, this approach also has a few disadvantages. First, the human capital approach makes it difficult to value those who do not report an income, such as homemakers, children, volunteers, and retirees. As a result, the human capital approach is subject to the biases that are a result of discrimination in the labor force. The human capital method also assumes that patients are not paid during sick time. This is often not the case for salaried employees, who may have a certain number of sick days available without pay reduction.

The willingness to pay method is another way to value person time. In this approach, individuals are asked to state a maximum monetary value that they would pay for a given outcome or outcome avoided. For example, a study may find that individuals will pay $30, on average, for a flu shot in order to avoid the having the flu later. This value would represent the willingness to pay to avoid the flu. The disadvantage of this approach is that situations are hypothetical. Therefore, willingness to pay estimates may actually overestimate indirect costs.[2,4,5]

The final type of cost that has been historically discussed is **intangible costs**; these consequences are difficult to measure, such as pain and suffering. They are no longer separately considered in economic evaluations because they are not strictly intangible and can be measured and valued using utility and willingness to pay approaches.[2]

In addition to direct, indirect, and intangible costs, there are a few other commonly used cost terms in pharmacoeconomics that are important to understand. It is important to remember that there are costs to any decision that is made. This is because the resources could have been used elsewhere. The benefit that is forgone from the next best alternative is called the **opportunity cost**. Costs included in an economic evaluation should only include current and future costs; this is because costs from the past are already incurred and will not be recovered, from an economic point of view. Costs that have occurred in the past are known as **sunk costs**. Marginal costs and incremental costs are other important cost terminologies. These terms are sometimes mistakenly used interchangeably because both refer to the additional costs. **Marginal costs**, more specifically, are the additional costs from producing one additional unit. Marginal costs are used to determine if it is cost-effective to produce additional units. Suppose a clinical pharmacy service sees 10 patients per day. The marginal cost is the additional cost required to serve the 11th patient. The fixed costs of the clinical pharmacy service would not be included in the marginal cost, because fixed costs remain the same regardless of the number of patients seen. Variable costs, such as the cost of additional patient forms, lab work, and additional pharmacist's time, may be included in marginal cost of the 11th patient. **Incremental costs** are a broader type of additional cost. Incremental costs are the additional (total) costs of implementing one option compared to that of an alternative intervention. An example is if a hospital were deciding between two drugs to place on the formulary: (1) antihypertensive drug A and (2) antihypertensive drug B. Drug A is more costly but has a greater effect. Therefore, the additional (total) cost that would be incurred if drug A were on formulary compared to drug B is called the incremental cost. In economic evaluations, the incremental cost is compared to the additional benefit gained to determine if the added costs are worth the additional effect (or benefit) realized.

## Discounting

Because people prefer having money and health in the present, rather than in the future, future values of these may be discounted. Discounting enables a higher value to be placed on present costs and a lower value to be placed on future costs. It is typical to consider discounting for economic evaluations that span a length of time greater than 1 year. Although discounting is typically applied to costs, there is debate over the extent to which outcomes should be discounted.[2,5] Note that the discount rate is not the same as the interest rate. An interest rate is a percentage of principle that is charged by a lender to a borrower for use of certain assets.

A discount factor can be calculated from the following equation:

$$\text{Discount factor} = 1 \div (1 + r)^t$$

where $r$ is the discount rate and $t$ is the number of years the cost is incurred.

The discount rate used in economic evaluations may also vary. Guidelines suggest a range of rates; a discount rate of 3–5% is commonly used, but other discount rates can be applied depending on other factors, including the current interest rate. The higher the discount rate, the more valuable money is considered in the present in comparison to the future. Discounting does not reduce the benefit in the future; rather, it gives higher value to benefits in the present in comparison to those realized in the future.[6,7]

## Perspective

Determining the viewpoint, or perspective, of the analysis will assist in determining which types of costs and outcomes should be included in a specific evaluation. The most common perspectives include the patient, payer, health system, and society.[2,8]

An analysis from the patient perspective incorporates costs incurred by the patient. Examples of direct costs include out-of-pocket medical costs, insurance deductibles, and insurance premiums. Indirect costs to the patient are also important to consider in analyses from the patient's perspective. Patient time or losses in productivity are indirect patient costs. Direct nonmedical patient costs can also include transportation costs to the health system or child care costs while the patient is seeking medical treatment.

The payer perspective is the perspective that is taken when looking at the costs and outcomes from the viewpoint of the primary payer of the health care. The payer may be the insurance company, the employer, or the government. The government may be considered the primary payer in countries where there is a national healthcare system or, in the United States, Medicare and Medicaid. The costs considered in the payer perspective are usually direct medical costs needed to make the intervention of interest. For insurance companies, this would include the costs that are paid by the insurance company for medical services, exclusive of the patient's contribution. Sometimes, the perspective of the employer is used; this can comprise insurance premiums, paid by the employer. Indirect costs such as lost work days or losses to productivity may also be considered in analyses from the employer's perspective.

Economic evaluations from the viewpoint of the health system (i.e., hospital, physician groups, etc.) are performed from the provider perspective. These evaluations should include the actual direct costs of providing medical care that arise from the intervention of interest. Indirect costs are generally not included with this perspective. A comprehensive evaluation from the provider perspective would collect the costs of medical treatment of a patient, including laboratory tests, procedures, hospitalizations, emergency room visits, prescriptions, healthcare professional salaries, and overhead costs. However, actual costs of providing care to patients can be difficult to estimate because true costs are often not known. Instead, health–system charge data (or insurance claims) are often used to estimate costs from the provider perspective. Charge data is the dollar amount that is billed to the insurance company or payer following services. Use of charge data has limitations because it may not reflect the dollar amount that is actually reimbursed to the provider for the service.

An analysis from the societal perspective is the broadest perspective and evaluates the net costs and consequences inclusive of all relevant perspectives. The end result is meant to demonstrate the overall cost and benefit to society. Costs should include all direct costs, indirect costs, and intangible costs, if possible. Outcomes should include those seen in both the short and long term. Other perspectives that take a narrower view may not include all of these components; however, if we think of society as the payer, all costs and outcomes, whether incurred immediately or later on, will ultimately be realized by the society. Therefore, when determining the best option among a set of choices with the societal perspective, one needs to consider all possible costs and outcomes. For example, treating patients for diabetes with drug A may appear more costly in the short term. If drug A reduces hospitalizations, emergency room visits, morbidity, and mortality in the long term, then it will likely have reduced costs in the long term. Narrower perspectives, such as those of the payer or provider, may fail to account for this because the benefits are not realized immediately. Countries with national health systems tend to favor the societal perspective in economic evaluations because society is the ultimate end payer.

## TYPES OF ECONOMIC EVALUATIONS

As previously noted, economic evaluations are "the comparative [analyses] of alternative courses of action in terms of both their costs and consequences."[2] Economic evaluations can be classified into partial and full economic evaluations. Partial economic evaluations include studies that consider costs and/or outcomes but do not compare interventions and/or link the costs to the outcome. Partial economic evaluations include (1) cost analyses, (2) cost–outcome description, (3) cost description, (4) outcome description, and (5) cost-of-illness studies. Full economic evaluations compare both cost and outcomes of two or more alternative options. The four main types of full economic evaluations include (1) cost-minimization analysis (CMA), (2) cost-effectiveness analysis (CEA), (3) cost–utility analysis (CUA), and (4) cost–benefit analysis (CBA). We will look at some of these types of evaluation in detail in the following sections.

### Partial Economic Evaluations

#### Cost-of-Illness Studies

Cost-of-illness (COI) studies are partial economic evaluations, but they are widely used to inform decision making. **Cost-of-illness studies** seek to provide insight into the economic burden of a disease state.[9] The intended use is to help understand appropriate resource allocation to prevent, treat, or manage a disease state. COI studies are conducted using the prevalence approach or the incidence approach. The prevalence approach is more commonly used, and it captures the total cost of the disease in a year, among all individuals at any stage of the disease. The incidence approach estimates the lifetime costs of the disease for patients who are newly diagnosed in the given year. All types of costs (direct, indirect, and intangible) are included in a COI study. COI studies may be used by pharmaceutical companies, government bodies, and insurance companies to inform policy, pricing, and budget allocation decisions.[10,11] An example of this type of evaluation is the annual economic estimate of diabetes presented by the American Diabetes Association. In 2012, the cost of diabetes for the U.S. population was estimated to be $245 billion.[12] When using the results from these studies, care must be taken to understand the methodology used for estimating the costs and types of costs included. Differences in methodologies can result in a large variation of estimates.[9,13,14]

### Full Economic Evaluations

#### Cost-Minimization Analyses

**Cost-minimization analysis** (CMA) is the simplest type of full pharmacoeconomic evaluation, because the consequences of competing alternatives are assumed to be similar or inconsequential. Consequently, classification of CMA as a full evaluation has been questioned. CMAs are often used in the comparison of acquisition costs; thus, they are not widely seen in published studies. There are also concerns around the uncertainty of the costs measured in the evaluation.[15,16] Some of the most popular comparisons where

CMAs are used are to compare generic (or brand name) drugs with the same drug moiety,[17,18] drug classes used to treat a condition,[19] diagnostic approaches,[20] different routes of administration of the same drug,[21] or the same drug given in different settings (e.g., home IV infusion versus hospital, inpatient versus outpatient).[22] It is important to consider the perspective when calculating costs. Costs from a hospital system's perspective may not be necessary in a CMA from a payer's perspective. Clinical outcomes may be assumed to be equal based on empirical evidence or scientific opinion. Only the final costs of the alternatives are compared. The alternative that has the lowest cost is the favorable choice.

## Cost-Effectiveness Analyses

**Cost-effectiveness analysis** (CEA) is an economic evaluation that compares alternative interventions by measuring both costs and outcomes (in natural units of clinical effect). Because the interventions are compared by the natural unit of effect, often the comparison can be made only for interventions for the same condition. Examples of possible units of effect are mm Hg reduction in blood pressure,[23] number of symptom-free days,[24,25] number of cases detected/prevented,[26] and the number of lives saved.[27] Units of natural disease can include both intermediate and primary outcomes as well as efficacy and effectiveness outcomes.[28] Costs are measured depending on the perspective of the analyses. Both costs and consequences are discounted, as relevant.[29]

In analyzing the costs and effects of various options, a systematic process is followed. First, the options are ranked by increasing cost. The least costly option is always preceded by the option of "no intervention" or "no treatment." "No intervention" is associated with zero costs and zero effects and is included to provide a baseline of "not doing anything at all." Each option is then compared to the prior option. An option is considered first-order dominated, and thus eliminated, if it has higher costs and lower units of effect compared to another possible option. The final result of a CEA is expressed in terms of the ratio of incremental costs and incremental effects when comparing two alternatives. This yields a cost per unit of effect called the *incremental cost-effectiveness ratio* (ICER) (Case Study 22-1). The ICER will aid in understanding the cost per unit increase of the natural health effect. Because there is increasing willingness to pay, organizations will be more likely to pay higher costs per unit of effect.[30-32] CEA studies help us understand the value of the money spent.

## Cost–Utility Analyses

A **cost–utility analysis** (CUA) is a type of full pharmacoeconomic evaluation that compares two or more alternatives based on their costs and outcomes, where outcomes are measured in units of quality-adjusted life years (QALYs) or disability-adjusted life-years (DALYs).[33] QALYs are specific utility-based units that form the outcome in the denominator of a CUA. Due to its similarities with CEA studies (they differ only in the type of outcome measured), many people consider CUAs to be a specific type of CEA. QALYs are calculated from time spent in a given health state and the quality of life associated with that health state; the quality or utility of that health state is obtained from a utility measure. Utilities are measured on a scale of 0 to 1, with 1 representing the best imaginable health state and 0 representing dead, although some measures allow for states worse than dead (i.e., negative values). CUAs are different from CEAs in that comparisons can be made across different diseases or programs. This is possible because utilities are measured on a common scale and, therefore, can be compared in different disease states.[34-36] Similar to CEAs, results are expressed as an incremental ratio of costs to a ratio of effects (i.e., QALYs), called an *incremental cost–utility ratio* (ICUR) (Case Study 22-2). Measurement of utilities will be discussed in greater detail in the section on health-related quality of life later in this chapter.

| CASE STUDY 22-1 | Calculate the Incremental Cost-Effectiveness Ratio |
|---|---|

A hospital administrator is deciding which of three diabetes drugs to place on formulary: drug A, drug B, or drug C. Drug A costs $50 per year, and 10% of patients reach controlled HbA1c values. Drug B costs $70 per year, and 10% of patients reach controlled HbA1c values. Drug C costs $200 per year, and 15% of patients reach controlled HbA1c values. The incremental cost-effectiveness ratio (ICER) will tell us the added cost of the percentage increase in patients with controlled HbA1c.

**Step 1.** Starting with no treatment, the options are placed in order of increasing costs.

| Option | Cost | Effect (% with Improvement in HbA1c) | ICER |
|---|---|---|---|
| No treatment | $0 | 0 | |
| Drug A | $50 | 10 | |
| Drug B | $70 | 10 | |
| Drug C | $200 | 15 | |

**Step 2.** Delete any options with higher costs and a same or lower effect than a comparator treatment, because they are not rational options. These are referred to as first-order dominated options. In this example, drug B is a dominated option because it has a higher cost and the same effect as drug A.

| Option | Cost | Effect (% with Controlled HbA1c) | ICER |
|---|---|---|---|
| No treatment | $0 | 0 | |
| Drug A | $50 | 10 | |
| ~~Drug B~~ | ~~$70~~ | ~~10~~ | |
| Drug C | $200 | 15 | |

**Step 3.** Calculate the ICER for each drug compared to the previous option by dividing the difference in costs by the difference in effect. In this example, the ICER of drug A is calculated by comparing drug A to no treatment. The ICER of drug C is calculated by comparing drug C to drug A.

| Option | Cost | Effect (% with Controlled HbA1c) | ICER |
|---|---|---|---|
| No treatment | $0 | 0 | |
| Drug A | $50 | 10 | ($50 − $0) ÷ (10 − 0) = $5 |
| Drug C | $200 | 15 | ($200 − $50) ÷ (15 − 10) = $30 |

This example shows that drug A has an ICER of $5 per percentage increase in patients with controlled HbA1c compared to no treatment. Drug C has an ICER of $30 per percentage increase in patients with controlled HbA1c.

We can see that drug A and drug C are in order of increasing incremental cost-effectiveness ratios, with drug A's ICER being lower than that of drug C. This is appropriate, and no further calculations are needed. The decision maker should now choose between placing drug A or drug C on formulary. This decision will be driven by the price that the hospital is willing to pay per unit of effect. A hospital's budget will likely drive its willingness to pay.

In Case Study 22-2, we will show a scenario where one option has a higher ICER than a subsequent option.

Incremental cost-effectiveness (or utility) ratios can also be displayed graphically on a plane with the costs on the *y*-axis and the benefits on the *x*-axis. **Figure 22-2** graphically displays the costs and effects for drugs A, B, C, and D from Case Study 22-2. The slopes of the lines that connect the options represent the ICERs. In an ideal situation, all slopes in Figure 22-2 would increase in magnitude. However, drug B is a first-order-dominated option because it is above and to the left of drug A with a negative slope. Therefore, this option should be eliminated. With the remaining options, drug A has the lowest cost

**CASE STUDY 22-2**    **Calculate Incremental Cost–Utility Ratios**

The government wants to determine the incremental cost–utility ratio (ICUR) of several chemotherapy options for breast cancer. Drug A costs $100,000 and extends patients' lives by an average of 4 years at a constant utility of 0.75. Drug B costs $150,000 and extends life by 2.5 years with a utility of 0.8. Drug C costs $200,000 and extends life by 5 years with utility also at 0.8. Drug D costs $300,000 and restores individuals to perfect health (utility = 1.0). Life is extended by 6 years. Eliminate dominated treatment options and identify the cost-effective options.

**Step 1**. Calculate the QALYs for each treatment option.

| Option | Utility | Years of Life | QALYs Gained |
|---|---|---|---|
| Drug A | 0.75 | 4 | $0.75 \times 4 = 3$ |
| Drug B | 0.8 | 2.5 | $0.8 \times 2.5 = 2$ |
| Drug C | 0.8 | 5 | $0.8 \times 5 = 4$ |
| Drug D | 1 | 6 | $1.0 \times 6 = 6$ |

**Step 2**. Starting with no treatment, put the options in order of increasing costs in a table format. The QALY value that was calculated serves as the effect. For no treatment, assume zero effect.

| Option | Cost | Effect (QALYs Gained) | ICUR |
|---|---|---|---|
| No treatment | $0 | 0 | |
| Drug A | $100,000 | 3 | |
| Drug B | $150,000 | 2 | |
| Drug C | $200,000 | 4 | |
| Drug D | $300,000 | 6 | |

**Step 3**. Delete any first-order-dominated options. In this example, drug B is a dominated option because it has a higher cost and lower effect than drug A.

| Option | Cost | Effect (QALY) | ICUR |
|---|---|---|---|
| No treatment | $0 | 0 | |
| Drug A | $100,000 | 3 | |
| ~~Drug B~~ | ~~$150,000~~ | ~~2~~ | |
| Drug C | $200,000 | 4 | |
| Drug D | $300,000 | 6 | |

**Step 4**. Redraw the table without the dominated option (drug B). Calculate the ICUR for each drug compared to the previous option by dividing the difference in costs by the difference in effect.

| Option | Cost | Effect (QALY) | ICUR |
|---|---|---|---|
| No treatment | $0 | 0 | |
| Drug A | $100,000 | 3 | $(\$100,000 - 0) \div (3 - 0) = \$33,333$ per QALY gained |
| Drug C | $200,000 | 4 | $(\$200,000 - \$100,000) \div (4 - 3) = \$100,000$ per QALY gained |
| Drug D | $300,000 | 6 | $(\$300,000 - \$200,000) \div (6 - 4) = \$50,000$ per QALY gained |

**Step 5**. Examine the ICUR results. A treatment option is second-order dominated if it has a higher ICUR compared to the subsequent treatment. In this example, drug C has a higher ICUR ($100,000) than drug D ($50,000). Therefore, drug C is second-order dominated, and it should be removed from the analysis. Recalculate the ICURs for drug A and drug D after drug C has been removed.

| Option | Cost | Effect (QALY) | ICUR |
|---|---|---|---|
| No treatment | $0 | 0 | |
| Drug A | $100,000 | 3 | ($100,000 – 0) ÷ (3 – 0) = $33,333 per QALY gained |
| Drug D | $300,000 | 6 | ($300,000 – $100,000) ÷ (6 – 3) = $66,000 per QALY gained |

This example shows that drug A has an ICUR of $33,333 per QALY gained. Drug D has an ICUR of $66,000 per QALY gained.

with the smallest effect. Moving from drug A to the next option, it is preferable to have a smaller slope (i.e., ICER). The line from drug A to drug C has a higher slope than drug A to drug D. Drug C is, therefore, a second-order-dominated therapy with a higher cost per unit of effectiveness. Drug C can thus be eliminated.

## Cost–Benefit Analyses

A **cost–benefit analysis** (CBA) is the final type of economic evaluation that will be discussed. In CBAs, both the costs and the outcomes are measured in monetary units. Health benefits such as years of life gained, reductions in cholesterol, or disability days avoided are translated into a monetary value. Translating clinical benefits into a monetary value can be difficult; however, this approach allows comparison of alternatives with different units of outcomes because the outcomes are converted to a common unit (i.e., dollars). These outcomes are compared to the costs of implementing the intervention of interest. The ratio of the costs of the option is divided by the outcomes of the program, in monetary units.[37-40]

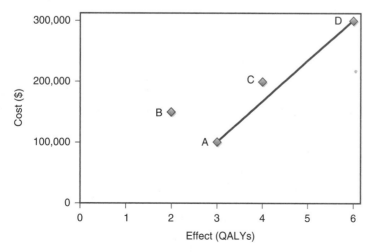

**FIGURE 22-2** Incremental cost and benefit for drugs A, B, C, and D.

CBA is often used when deciding where to spend monetary resources in order to achieve the greatest impact. Suppose that one hospital administrator believes money should be used to implement a smoking cessation program. Another hospital administrator wants to use the same money to start a diabetes education program. Each option has different clinical and humanistic outcomes. In a CBA, outcomes (i.e., benefits) are monetized so that the cost–benefit ratios can be directly compared. This allows the comparison of two different programs with different units of benefits. Some of the examples where CBA has been used include evaluation of vaccinations programs,[41,42] health screening programs,[43,44] programs aimed at preventing or controlling a condition,[45] comparing drugs and/or non-drug treatment options (e.g., diet, exercise, surgery) for a condition,[46-48] drug-dependence treatment services,[49] diagnostic tests,[50,51] and educational/counseling efforts.[52,53]

### Net Benefit Calculation

As discussed earlier, benefits, in addition to costs, can be discounted in economic evaluations. Similar to costs, it is preferential to have benefits in the present rather than in the future. Therefore, future healthcare benefits are often discounted to reflect this preference. The *net benefit calculation* (also referred to as the *net cost calculation*) is used to determine the present value of costs and benefits in the future for one intervention. For example, suppose that a pharmacy is considering implementing a diabetes outreach program for the next 10 years. The program will cost \$5,000 to start up the first year, and it will cost \$2,000 every year thereafter to maintain. The pharmacy projects that the diabetes program will not have any monetary benefits the first year. It will have \$1,000 in benefits the second year, \$2,000 in benefits the third year, and \$3,000 each year thereafter. The pharmacy wants to know if the monetary benefits will outweigh the costs of the diabetes outreach program. Because benefits and costs occur over time, it is necessary to account for the discounted value of costs and benefits. In order to do this, the discount rate can be used to bring all future costs and benefits to the present value. This can be accomplished with the following net benefit calculation:

$$\sum_{t=0}^{n}\left(\frac{B^t}{(1+r)^t}\right) - \sum_{t=0}^{n}\left(\frac{C^t}{(1+r)^t}\right)$$

The equation represents the difference between the sum of the discounted benefits and the sum of the discounted cost from time 0 through time $n$. When this calculation is positive, the net benefits are greater than the net costs, and the program should be implemented. When choosing between implementing one of several programs, all of which have positive net benefits, the choice should be made toward the program with the highest net benefit.

### Budget Impact Analysis

*Budget impact analysis* (BIA) is specific form of economic evaluation that quantifies the financial impact of adopting a new program or intervention on the provider's expenditure and budget.[54] Adoption of the new program will change the resource utilization; this may cause differences in the expenditure for the target group. Because the primary purpose of BIA is to capture this impact on the budget from a payer's or provider's perspective, the analyses generally look at these implications in the short term (i.e., 1-3 years), assuming the population characteristics. The use of BIAs by healthcare decision makers is increasing.[55]

### Interpreting Results of an Economic Evaluation

The previous discussion provided an overview of the most common methods in conducting a full economic evaluation, where costs and outcomes are both considered.

| Cost-Effectiveness | New intervention has lower cost. | New intervention has equal cost. | New intervention has higher cost. |
|---|---|---|---|
| **New intervention has lower effectiveness.** | How much effectiveness is given up for the reduced cost? Examine the ICER. | Choose standard option. | Choose standard option. |
| **New intervention has equal effectiveness.** | Choose new intervention. | Arbitrary. | Choose standard option. |
| **New intervention has higher effectiveness.** | Choose new intervention. | Choose new intervention. | How much more does the new intervention cost per additional unit of effectiveness? Examine the ICER. |

**TABLE 22-1    Interpreting the Results of an Economic Evaluation When Compared to Standard (Current) Treatment**

Data from Rascati KL. *Essentials of Pharmacoeconomics.* Philadelphia, PA: Lippincott Williams & Wilkins: 2009.

When costs and outcomes are combined in economic evaluations, one of nine scenarios can be obtained. **Table 22–1** demonstrates these nine possible scenarios when a new intervention is compared to an alternative (or status quo).

When a program has a higher cost and a lower effect than a comparator, this is known as the *dominated option*. A dominated program would never be selected. Similarly, a new program with a lower cost but high benefit in comparison to the alternative should be adopted. This is called the *dominant option*. To determine whether to implement a new program with a higher cost and a higher benefit, look at the ICER. The ICER is the difference in costs of the options divided by the difference in effects. Pending budget availability, the new program should be implemented if the added cost is worth the additional benefit. Otherwise, a new program would be selected if it is less costly and equally efficacious or incurs the same costs but is more effective. In opposite scenarios, the new program would be rejected. When looking at equal costs and effectiveness, different factors should be taken into consideration when making allocation decisions.

**Figure 22–3** graphically displays the plane of costs and benefits. An economic evaluation is most useful when there are other options with a higher cost but improved

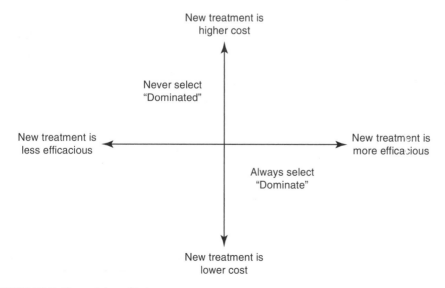

**FIGURE 22-3** The cost–benefit plan.

effect or options with a lower cost and decreased effect. The goal of the evaluation is to determine if the increased cost (or decreased cost) is worth the change in effect. In cases of cost-effectiveness studies, the points plotted to the right of the threshold line are considered to be cost-effective.[56]

# DECISION ANALYSIS

**Decision analysis** is a systematic way to compare alternative choices in instances of uncertainty. Different values for outcomes and costs are synthesized from multiple sources.[57] Decision analysis is a helpful tool to aid in pharmacoeconomic analyses comparing two or more alternatives in complex scenarios. A complex scenario is that in which several events must be considered; when choosing between two drugs we usually consider effectiveness, side effects, and complications. Decision analysis allows for the incorporation of all these factors.

Decision analyses typically use models that include different elements of the alternative choices, chance of occurrence of the events, and final outcomes of the alternatives. The inputs for the probability of outcomes and costs information are gathered from best available information and can include a variety of sources, including clinical trials, observational studies, survey research, literature reviews, expert panels, and internal resources. These values can then be used to calculate a weighted cost and outcome for each alternative that incorporates the likelihood of these events. When the weighted costs and outcomes are compared, this yields an expected value for each option given the information available and the uncertainty around this information. The option with the lowest cost per unit of outcome is the preferred option.

Decision analyses aid the decision maker in clearly outlining the possible choices, the consequences of the choices, areas of uncertainty, and the expected value of the choices, where the value is described in cost per desired outcome. Decision analyses have been used to aid decisions in both healthcare and non-healthcare settings. The outcome used in a specific decision analysis will vary depending on the type of economic analyses being undertaken.[33,58,59]

When conducting decision analyses, decision trees help to graphically display the logical sequence of possible outcomes and events for scenarios over a short-term time period. When decision trees are created, a conventional format is generally followed. Branches of the tree represent different pathways and are displayed with lines. Nodes are points between the branches that represent divergence of a branch. A square denotes a decision node for two or more possible choices. The decision node is placed at the leftmost part of the tree. The resulting options and events are placed in order of occurrence, with the options placed immediately following the decision node and the chance events in order thereafter. The pathway of specific events occurring is based on the probability of each event occurring. A circle denotes a chance node. All events diverging from a specific chance node must have probabilities that sum to 100% or 1.0, and they must be mutually exclusive. It is best practice to limit the number of chance events occurring from a single chance node to two.[58] For example, if a patient takes drug A, there is a certain probability ($n$) that the patient will experience an adverse event. The chance that the patient does not experience the adverse event will equal $100\% - n\%$. The event pathway ends with a terminal node represented with a triangle-shaped node. Typically, decision analyses can be created using computer software such as Microsoft Excel, TreeAge, and Crystal Ball, among others. The formatting generally remains the

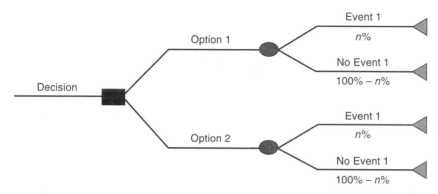

**FIGURE 22-4**  General decision tree structure.

same across all decision analysis software. **Figure 22-4** is an example of a graphically displayed decision tree.

After decision trees are graphically displayed, the calculation of the final expected values for each option is very simple. For each pathway, the probabilities of each event occurring are multiplied together. This will yield a probability for the occurrence of that specific pathway of events. This number is then multiplied by the total cost events of that pathway. Likewise, a "folding back" method can be implemented. Starting from the right–hand side, the probability of each event is multiplied by the cost of that event. This is done for each event in the pathway, and the numbers are added together. Once each event pathway is calculated in either manner, the value for each pathway is summed together. This yields the expected value for the decision. Many patients are flowing through the pathways of events, and the expected value is the average cost of a person in the specific decision. The option with the lowest expected values is the preferred option.

Decision trees are often used to model acute conditions; in instances where a longer time period is needed (i.e., chronic conditions) and health states may change, Markov modeling can be done. Markov analyses allow for a more accurate representation of complex scenarios in chronic conditions where the patients may move back and forth in the health states.[60-62]

**CASE STUDY 22-3** | **Using a Decision Tree to Guide Pharmecoeconomic Considerations for Formulary Management**

A formulary committee is deciding between two antibiotic medications to put on the hospital formulary: drug A and drug B. The pharmacist on the committee decides to use a decision tree to determine the expected value for each drug. Drug A costs $5. Of those who use drug A, 90% will be cured (treatment success) and 15% will experience an injection site reaction. Drug B costs $10. Among those who use drug B, 95% will be cured and 5% will experience an injection site reaction. Treatment failures cost approximately $1,000, and injection site reactions cost approximately $50 to treat.

**Step 1**. Draw out the design of the decision tree. Squares are used to denote decision nodes. In this case, the decision is between drug A and drug B. Circles are used to denote chance events. In this example, chance events are the chance that patients are cured and the chance that patients experience an injection site reaction. Triangles denote the completion of the pathway of events or the end of the tree branch.

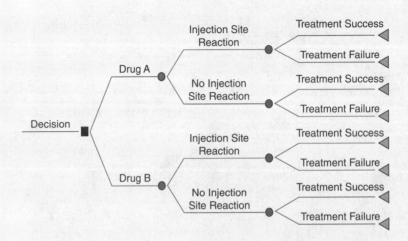

**Step 2**. Determine the expected value for drug A and drug B by calculating the costs and probabilities of each pathway and then calculating the expected value for all pathways.

| Pathways for Drug A | | | | | | |
|---|---|---|---|---|---|---|
| Pathway | Event | Event Costs | Pathway Costs | Event Probabilities | Pathway Probabilities | Expected Value of Pathway |
| Pathway 1 | Drug A | $5 | $55 (5 + 50 + 0) | N/A | 0.135 (0.15 × 0.90) | $7.425 ($55 × 0.135) |
| | Injection site reaction | $50 | | 0.15 | | |
| | Success | $0 | | 0.90 | | |
| Pathway 2 | Drug A | $5 | $1,055 (5 + 50 + 1,000) | N/A | 0.015 (0.15 × 0.10) | $15.825 ($1,055 × 0.015) |
| | Injection site reaction | $50 | | 0.15 | | |
| | Failure | $1,000 | | 0.10 | | |
| Pathway 3 | Drug A | $5 | $5 (5 + 0 + 0) | N/A | 0.765 (0.85 × 0.90) | $3.825 ($5 × 0.765) |
| | No injection site reaction | $0 | | 0.85 | | |
| | Success | $0 | | 0.90 | | |
| Pathway 4 | Drug A | $5 | $1,005 (5 + 0 + 1,000) | N/A | 0.085 (0.85 × 0.10) | $85.425 ($1,005 × 0.085) |
| | No injection site reaction | $0 | | 0.85 | | |
| | Failure | $1,000 | | 0.10 | | |

**Expected Value of Drug A: $7.425 + $15.825 + $3.825 + $85.425 = $112.50**

| Pathways for Drug B | | | | | | |
|---|---|---|---|---|---|---|
| **Pathway** | **Event** | **Event Costs** | **Pathway Costs** | **Event Probabilities** | **Pathway Probabilities** | **Expected Value of Pathway** |
| Pathway 1 | Drug B | $10 | $60 (10 + 50 + 0) | N/A | 0.0475 (0.05 × 0.95) | $2.85 |
| | Injection site reaction | $50 | | 0.05 | | |
| | Success | $0 | | 0.95 | | |
| Pathway 2 | Drug B | $10 | $1,060 (10 + 50 + 1,000) | N/A | 0.0025 (0.05 × 0.05) | $2.65 |
| | Injection site reaction | $50 | | 0.05 | | |
| | Failure | $1,000 | | 0.05 | | |
| Pathway 3 | Drug B | $10 | $10 (10 + 0 + 0) | N/A | 0.9025 (0.95 × 0.95) | $9.025 |
| | No injection site reaction | $0 | | 0.95 | | |
| | Success | $0 | | 0.95 | | |
| Pathway 4 | Drug B | $10 | $1,010 (10 + 0 + 1,000) | N/A | 0.0475 (0.95 × 0.05) | $47.975 |
| | No injection site reaction | $0 | | 0.95 | | |
| | Failure | $1,000 | | 0.05 | | |

Expected Value of Drug B: $2.85 + $2.65 + $9.025 + $47.975 = $62.50

Based on this decision analysis, in which only costs are being considered for the final decision, drug B has a lower expected value than drug A. Therefore, even though drug B has a higher drug cost, the analysis suggests that the formulary committee should put drug B on formulary because the overall medical costs of patients on drug B is lower than for patients on drug A.

## SENSITIVITY ANALYSES

Sensitivity analyses are another decision analysis tool that can help to address the uncertainty of the model inputs by allowing variation in the inputs around a certain range of values. In sensitivity analyses, the values of some or all parameters can be varied around upper- and lower-bound values that are thought to be inclusive of the true value. The upper and lower bounds can be determined from comparison of values to other references. Varying the values of certain parameters will show whether the inputs have a large effect on the expected value of each option. If the expected values change, then the option with the lowest cost per unit of effect may also change. If the expected values of the options do not significantly change and the preferred option does not change, then there is more confidence in the model result. This would mean that the model is robust to variations in the parameters, and the overall decision would remain the same. When the expected values of the alternatives change significantly when the parameters are varied, the final estimate is less robust, and there may be less confidence in which is the preferred option.[57]

When the value of one model parameter is changed at a time, it is called a one-way sensitivity analysis. Two-way sensitivity analyses involve changing two parameters simultaneously. Monte Carlo simulation is a type of sensitivity analysis that is based on probability. Unlike the one-way or two-way sensitivity analyses, the parameters in Monte Carlo simulations are defined by a distribution (e.g., beta, gamma, log normal). In multiple iterations of rerunning the model, inputs based on the defined probability distributions are used. The end result is an estimated outcome based on the average input values from the distribution.[63,64]

Because decision trees are tools to conduct economic evaluations, they follow many of the same rules as other pharmacoeconomic analyses. For example, the perspective for the decision analysis will determine the relevant costs and outcomes for inclusion. All relevant options should be compared. Because alternative options are compared against each other, omitting a relevant option would change the results and lead to biased conclusions. More information on modeling best practices can be found in the ISPOR-SMDM Modeling Good Research Practice Guidelines.[57]

# HEALTH-RELATED QUALITY OF LIFE

Health-related quality of life (HRQoL) was mentioned during the discussions of humanistic outcomes and cost–utility analyses; it is a growing field in pharmacoeconomics and deserves further discussion here. HRQoL is a subset of quality of life that is multidimensional in nature; it includes physical, mental, and social functioning, as well as overall well-being.[65,66]

Instruments used to measure HRQoL are part of a wider set of tools referred to as *patient-reported outcomes* (PROs). PROs include other outcomes that patients self-report, such as symptom-free days and patient satisfaction. The use of HRQoL in determining allocation of resources in a healthcare system and its association with other humanistic outcomes highlights its use in decision making. HRQoL may be an important endpoint in the assessment of medications used in palliative care[67] and chronic conditions where medications can provide symptom relief and improve quality of life, but not necessarily survival time, such as asthma, depression, cancer, and rheumatoid arthritis.

Broadly, a patient's HRQoL can be measured using condition-specific or general health measures. Condition-specific HRQoL instruments are designed for use in specific diseases (e.g., asthma), populations (e.g., older adults), or health problems (e.g., pain) and may assess functional issues (e.g., sexual functioning) that are generally associated with the particular disease state. For this reason, these measures have the advantage of being able to capture small changes that may not be captured otherwise in a more general instrument. Some examples of disease-specific HRQoL instruments include the LupusQol for lupus,[68] the Functional Assessment of Cancer Therapy (FACT) for cancer,[69] and Asthma Quality of Life (AQoL) for asthma.[70]

Generic measures of HRQoL, on the other hand, are intended to measure common core dimensions of HRQoL without regard to a particular disease/condition. An advantage of these instruments is that health states can be compared across diseases.[65,71] Generic instruments measure general domains of health and may not capture smaller changes in health that are specific to a particular disease state. Broadly, these measures can be categorized as health status measures (health profile) and preference-based measures.

Health profiles provide a variety of scores, one for each domain, and typically do not provide an overall summary score. Perhaps the best-known example is the Medical Outcome Trust Short Form-36 items (SF-36).[72] The SF-36 is a profile measure that consists of eight domains; it also produces two aggregate scores: a physical component score (PCS) and a mental component score (MCS). U.S. population norm–based scores for PCS and MCS are available and can serve as a basis for interpretation of scores and burden of disease.[73]

In contrast, preference-based measures are designed to provide a single summary score. As noted previously, these measures generate utility scores for health states described by multiattribute health state classifier systems that are subsequently used in the calculation of QALYs.

For instance, the health state classifier system of the EQ-5D (3L), one of the most widely used preference-based measures, consists of five one-item dimensions, each describing three levels of functioning (e.g., no problems, some problems, extreme problems).[74]

EQ-5D has many country-specific preference sets (see www.euroqol.org), including value sets based upon the general population of the United States[75] and the United Kingdom (UK).[76] Recently, a five-level version of EQ-5D has also been developed.[77] Other preference-based measures include the Quality of Well-Being (QWB),[78] the Health Utilities Index (HUI-2 and HUI-3),[79,80] and the SF-6D, which was derived from the SF-36 and has six levels of severity across six domains of health.[81]

Due to the importance of cost–utility analysis to inform reimbursement decisions related to new drug treatments, there is a demand for measures that can generate utilities. For this reason, a utility approach has been applied to new and existing disease-specific measures, as well as studies that have mapped items from existing measures onto the EQ-5D and SF-6D in order to generate utility scores.[82-85] A diverse list of disease-specific and generic instruments for measuring quality of life and health-related quality of life is available from the PROQOLID database.

The most widely used HRQoL instruments have a broad array of studies to support their use for many applications, and the evidence base can help to make an informed choice when selecting an appropriate measure. There are a number of important considerations when selecting a measure: the basis for the measure, validity, reliability, responsiveness, interpretability, burden, availability of alternative forms, and cultural/language adaptations.[86] Psychometric studies focus on the properties of reliability and validity of the instrument. Reliability is the ability of an instrument to generate consistent scores over time when the value of the state is held constant. Validity is the ability of an instrument to measure the construct it is intended to measure. Responsiveness, which is a type of construct validity (longitudinal), refers to the ability of an instrument to capture changes over time when meaningful change occurs. Responsiveness and sensitivity are sometimes employed synonymously, but sensitivity specifically refers to the ability to capture change, regardless of whether meaningful change has occurred.[87] Burden is relevant both in terms of the length and complexity of the illness from the patient's perspective and also to the administrative burden. Manuals and websites are available to assist with scoring and interpretation, as well as for translation and cultural adaptations for measures such as the SF-36 and EQ-5D, which have gained wide acceptance internationally as generic measures of HRQoL.[71]

Perhaps the single most significant development in PROs and health measurement in recent years has been the Patient Reported Outcomes Measurement Information System (PROMIS), a system of measures that has been developed based on item-response theory. Initiated in 2004, PROMIS is an ongoing program funded by the National Institutes of Health (NIH). PROMIS consists of banks of items from many existing measures of health. It utilizes computer adaptive testing (CAT) to precisely calibrate the level of health for a given dimension of health, selecting items informed by the previous responses of the individual to provide a precise estimate of health using a minimal number of uninformative items. The aim is to develop a generic measure of HRQoL that is precise and feasible to be implemented in clinical practice across multiple settings and conditions. Although originally intended to be a measure of health status, there is interest in generating a preference-based score from PROMIS items.[88,89]

An increasing use of HRQoL to aid economic evaluations has resulted in a surge in its use in clinical trials and real-world clinical settings.[90,91] The recent note by the U.S. Food and Drug Administration (FDA) most appropriately sums up the increasing attention to HRQoL: "The use of PRO instruments is part of a general movement toward the idea that the patient, properly queried, is the best source of information about how he or she feels."[92] Guidelines for reporting patient-reported outcomes in randomized trials are available via the CONSORT-PRO extension.[114]

This is further prompted by the collective desire to incorporate a patient's perspective in measuring the outcome and/or quality of pharmaceuticals and healthcare services. This view is endorsed by the recent efforts of the Patient Centered Outcomes Research Institute (PCORI)[93] and the UK Department of Health.[94] In addition to evaluating the effectiveness of health services and pharmaceuticals, the measurement of HRQoL in population health studies can also guide health policy making.[95,96] The International Society for Quality of Life Research (ISOQOL) has developed guidelines to help implement PRO assessment in clinical practice.[115]

# COMPARATIVE EFFECTIVENESS RESEARCH

Comparative effectiveness research (CER) has recently emerged as a paradigm that has clear implications and relevance to the field of pharmacoeconomics and outcomes research. CER emphasizes the need to understand the effectiveness of medications as used in actual practice. CER emerged from the recognition that randomized controlled trials (RCTs) are conducted under ideal and controlled settings that differ from the real world, thereby providing only limited information to inform clinical practice. One of the limitations of RCTs is the selection criteria for patient populations; this is typically intended to minimize heterogeneity among patients so that a difference between the treatment and comparator can be detected. RCTs also tend to achieve high medication compliance rates, because there is usually rigorous patient monitoring. Therefore, RCTs are designed to assess the internal validity and determine if a drug "can work." This helps in determining the *efficacy* of the drug. However, this may not necessarily hold true when a drug becomes widely available and is used in a much broader patient population. In real-world settings, patients have suboptimal medication adherence, comorbidities, and polypharmacy issues, and often discontinue medication. Drug use in a real-world setting assesses the external validity to determine if the drug "does work." This is referred to as *effectiveness*. Different types of CER studies can include the following: randomized head-to-head trials in real-world settings (e.g., ALLHAT), prospective observational studies (e.g., Women's Health Initiative), retrospective studies using insurance/claims databases, medical chart reviews, systematic reviews of literature, meta-analyses, and mixed-treatment comparisons. Real-world studies that estimate the safety and effectiveness of drugs can be used as inputs for costs and outcomes in pharmacoeconomic models. One of the main challenges of CER studies is that treatment comparisons based on secondary data sources are subject to threats to internal validity, particularly confounding by indication, due to lack of randomization. Interest in CER has driven the development of increasingly sophisticated statistical methods that attempt to mitigate the limitations of real-world data, such as using propensity scores and other pharmacoepidemiological methods, as well as interest in prospective study designs that attempt to capture real-world practices using pragmatic clinical trials.

# ECONOMIC EVALUATION OF CLINICAL PHARMACY SERVICES

The evolution of clinical pharmacy services has advanced pharmacists' involvement in providing pharmaceutical care as part of multidisciplinary healthcare teams. Costs are incurred when clinical pharmacy services are offered, and as a result, economic evaluations of clinical pharmacy services are often performed to determine if the additional cost is worth the benefits of the service. The procedure for conducting a pharmacoeconomic evaluation is the same for clinical pharmacy services and drugs. Over the last few years, improved study designs and more robust results from economic evaluations of clinical pharmacy services have helped in justifying the economic viability of these services and making a case for reimbursement of services.[97-101]

# EVALUATING THE PHARMACOECONOMIC LITERATURE

As with all other types of research, the quality of economic evaluations can vary widely. Additionally, the generalizability of study results must carefully consider the patient population, which may not be comparable to other populations.[102,103] Although there are many types of economic evaluations, each should include some of the same key elements. The following checklist outlines key elements to look for when reviewing an economic evaluation:

1. As in any other study, economic evaluations should begin with a clear objective and research question.[104] In full economic evaluations, this objective usually involves assessing the costs and outcomes of two or more healthcare options.
2. The type of study (i.e., CEA, CUA, or CBA) should be examined to determine if the study design is appropriate to address the research question.
3. The comparisons included in the study should be comprehensive and reflective of all possible comparators. For example, if we are interested in the cost-effectiveness of a new second-line therapy for patients with colon cancer, all available second-line therapies for that target patient population should be included. If a study fails to include a relevant option, the results should be interpreted with this potential bias in mind.
4. Similar to other types of studies, economic evaluations may be limited to a patient population with specific socioeconomic and clinical characteristics. This is important to note in determining if the results for the decision can be generalized to the entire population. This is known as *external validity*. The narrower the study population, the more external validity is compromised, because the results may not be comparable to what would occur in other populations.
5. The values of the inputs should be reflective of true values or the best available estimates. The included inputs should also be appropriate and comprehensive given the research question and study design. The perspective of the study will guide which inputs (i.e. costs and outcomes) are relevant for the research question of interest. For example, studies taking a societal perspective should, ideally, include all direct, indirect, and intangible costs that could be incurred. A study under the payer's perspective will include costs sustained by the payer; therefore, intangible costs (e.g., pain and suffering) and indirect costs (e.g.,

lost productivity) are generally not included in a health-system perspective study. Conversely, the indirect costs of lost productivity may be important for studies with an employer perspective. As this chapter has demonstrated, each economic evaluation is unique, and the compilation of study inputs is often specific to the particular research question. When the inputs are appropriately selected, it is more likely that the study results are reflective of the true results. This is known as *internal validity*. It is also important to note that some studies may claim to take a particular perspective while the examination of the inputs may show otherwise. This further demonstrates why the inputs and their values should be assessed for appropriateness when reviewing economic evaluations.

6. All economic evaluations should clearly state all assumptions. Results can then be interpreted with these assumptions and the corresponding limitations in mind.

7. Decision analysis modeling studies should be transparent and include the decision tree (model) structure.[105]

8. Study conclusions should align with the data and study results.

9. If incorporated, sensitivity analyses should be clearly explained and results stated.

10. The source of funding should be clearly stated and the authors' conflict of interests disclosed. Reviewers may wish to consider who sponsored the research, as this may introduce bias that is not otherwise discussed.

Many other details should be assessed when reviewing an economic evaluation. Although only the key ones have been highlighted in this section, more extensive guidelines have been developed on this issue. The International Society for Pharmacoeconomics and Outcomes Research (ISPOR) has published several sets of guidelines for various pharmacoeconomic topics. In particular, the ISPOR-AMCP-NPC Task Force has developed a questionnaire that can assist in decision making based on evaluating pharmacoeconomic modeling studies.[106] These may be found at www.ispor.org. Nonetheless, the basic principles just described can be applied to assess any economic evaluation, whether it is a cost evaluation of drug therapies, a cost–benefit analysis of healthcare programs, or an assessment of pharmaceutical services.

## FUTURE CHALLENGES

A major challenge to the field of healthcare economics and pharmacoeconomics is that value can be defined using a variety of approaches; this ultimately requires judgment and assumptions that can affect the outcome of an evaluation.[104] In spite of having clear strengths in aiding evidence-based decisions, policies at national levels have not uniformly advocated for the use of pharmacoeconomic data in healthcare decision making, in part, because it must be recognized that no pharmacoeconomic study is without limitations and assumptions. Additionally, particular care must be taken in cases where economic evaluations are (mis)used for rationing of health care.[107] Lack of robust methodology and data input may also cause bias in some estimates. The potential for bias may further limit their use in healthcare decision making,[108] as there are concerns about a possible publication bias in the pharmacoeconomic literature. Published studies may be more likely to report favorable results, particularly studies funded by the industry or those not reporting/using rigorous methodology.[109] These concerns may be allayed by recent efforts like the CHEERS guidelines, which attempt to standardize reporting of pharmacoeconomic studies.[104] A need for robust and parsimonious national guidelines on the reporting of HRQoL and pharmacoeconomic data remains. In the United States, in particular, the acceptance of CEAs by decision makers has been slow. Lack of transparency, absence of a U.S. agency dedicated to pharmacoeconomic research, inadequate inputs, and reluctance of accepting industry-funded research could be some of the possible reasons for a slow uptake. Although many guidelines are available, there is lack of a uniform standard to assess cost-effectiveness. In CUA studies, the threshold of willingness to pay used to measure if a drug is worthwhile is not uniform across patient groups and conditions. Some researchers believe that the reason may also be more political, with a desire to not use CEA studies for rationing of health care. PCORI specifically discourages the use of cost/QALY as a decision-making metric. The Patient Protection and Affordable Care Act explicitly prohibits the use of cost–utility analysis, specifically QALY, in directing recommendations about healthcare technologies, treatment, and services. In addition, a certain amount of antipathy to the cost-effectiveness information exists because it may expose uncomfortable choices about the costs of treatments and their benefits.[110,111]

In spite of these challenges, pharmacoeconomic studies are unlikely to diminish in their relevance. Although the direct use of cost-effectiveness information may not be seen in the United States in the near future, its indirect use to aid decision making is only likely to grow.[112,113] Hospital systems in the United States continue to use pharmacoeconomic data in making formulary decisions. The Department of Defense (DoD) Pharmacoeconomic Center (PEC) conducts clinical and cost-effectiveness evaluations to support the DoD pharmacy and therapeutics (P&T) committee that maintains the Military Health System (MHS) formularies. The Academy of Managed Care Pharmacy's (AMCP) format for drug dossier formulary submissions includes a section on economics, in addition to safety and efficacy information. Health plans and payers are increasingly seeking budget impact models to understand the budgetary impact of adding drugs to their formulary. These are special cases of CEAs and may include an option to vary the costs per person/month. (See the ISPOR best practice guidelines for budget impact analysis.[54,55]) A positive global trend in the increasing number of pharmacy education programs offering some level of formal training in pharmacoeconomics highlights the importance of these studies in making evidence-based decisions.[116,117]

# ACKNOWLEDGMENTS

The authors would like to acknowledge Kibum Kim and Iulia D. Ursan for their input and review of this chapter.

# SUMMARY

Although decision makers have traditionally relied on information from clinical trials and other efficacy studies, economic evaluations are increasingly recognized as an important tool to aid in healthcare decision making. Pharmacy and therapeutics committee members may consider economic evaluations when deciding whether to put a drug on a hospital formulary. Managed care companies often use economic information in deciding what tier to place a new drug. Guidelines committees can use economic information for deciding a drug's place in therapy relative to other compounds. And, finally, pharmacists and other healthcare providers may use economic evaluations to inform patients of the benefits of a therapy relative to the costs in the context of other options.

This chapter has discussed the growing importance of the evaluation of healthcare services, products, and interventions. As costs for health care rise, it is necessary to be able to demonstrate the value of increased expenditure. This justification can be shown through comparison of costs and benefits in economic evaluations. Understanding these concepts will aid in assessing economic evaluation studies to determine their usefulness for ascertaining value and resource allocation.

# REFERENCES

1. Center for Disease Control and Prevention. Health Expenditures, United States 2012–Table 113. http://www.cdc.gov/nchs/data/hus/hus12.pdf#113. Accessed July 28, 2014.
2. Drummond MF, Sculpher MJ, Torrance GW, O'Brien BJ, Stoddart GL. *Methods for the Economic Evaluation of Health Care Programmes.* 3rd ed. New York, NY: Oxford University Press; 2005.
3. Kozma CM, Reeder CE, Schulz RM. Economic, clinical, and humanistic outcomes: a planning model for pharmacoeconomic research. *Clin Ther.* 1993;15(6):1121-1132; discussion 1120.
4. Koopmanschap MA, Rutten FF. A practical guide for calculating indirect costs of disease. *Pharmacoeconomics.* 1996;10(5):460-466.
5. Gold MR, Siegel JE, Russell LB, Weinstein MC, eds. *Cost-effectiveness in Health and Medicine.* New York, NY: Oxford University Press; 1996.
6. Krahn M, Gafni A. Discounting in the economic evaluation of health care interventions. *Med Care.* 1993;31(5):403-418.
7. Smith DH, Gravelle H. The practice of discounting in economic evaluations of healthcare interventions. *Int J Technol Assess Health Care.* 2001;17(2):236-243.
8. Byford S, Raftery J. Perspectives in economic evaluation. *BMJ.* 1998;316(7143):1529-1530.
9. Drummond MF. Cost-of-illness studies: a major headache? *Pharmacoeconomics.* 1992;2(1):1-4.
10. Johnson JA, Bootman JL. Drug-related morbidity and mortality. A cost-of-illness model. *Arch Intern Med.* 1995;155(18):1949-1956.
11. Rice DP. Cost of illness studies: what is good about them? *Inj Prev.* 2000;6(3):177-179.
12. American Diabetes Association. Economic costs of diabetes in the U.S. in 2012. *Diabetes Care.* 2012;36(4):1033-1046.
13. Koopmanschap MA. Cost-of-illness studies. Useful for health policy? *Pharmacoeconomics.* 1998;14(2):143-148.
14. Bloom BS, Bruno DJ, Maman DY, Jayadevappa R. Usefulness of US cost-of-illness studies in healthcare decision making. *Pharmacoeconomics.* 2001;19(2):207-213.
15. Briggs AH, O'Brien BJ. The death of cost-minimization analysis? *Health Econ.* 2001;10(2):179-184.
16. Newby D, Hill S. Use of pharmacoeconomics in prescribing research. Part 2: cost-minimization analysis—when are two therapies equal? *J Clin Pharm Ther.* 2003;28(2):145-150.
17. Duerden MG, Hughes DA. Generic and therapeutic substitutions in the UK: are they a good thing? *Br J Clin Pharmacol.* 2010;70(3):335-341.
18. Ramesh L. Economic evaluation of antibiotic prescriptions: a cost minimization analysis. *J App Pharm Sci.* 2013;3(6).
19. Hilleman DE, Mohiuddin SM, Lucas BD Jr, Stading JA, Stoysich AM, Ryschon K. Cost-minimization analysis of initial antihypertensive therapy in patients with mild-to-moderate essential diastolic hypertension. *Clin Ther.* 1994;16(1):88-102; discussion 187.
20. Harewood GC, Wiersema MJ, Edell ES, Liebow M. Cost-minimization analysis of alternative diagnostic approaches in a modeled patient with non-small cell lung cancer and subcarinal lymphadenopathy. *Mayo Clin Proc.* 2002;77(2):155-164.
21. Martello JL, Pummer TL, Krenzelok EP. Cost minimization analysis comparing enteral N-acetylcysteine to intravenous acetylcysteine in the management of acute acetaminophen toxicity. *Clin Toxicol (Phila).* 2010;48(1):79-83.
22. Farmer KC, Schwartz WJ 3rd, Rayburn WF, Turnbull G. A cost-minimization analysis of intracervical prostaglandin E2 for cervical ripening in an outpatient versus inpatient setting. *Clin Ther.* 1996;18(4):747-756; discussion 702.
23. Logan AG, Milne BJ, Achber C, Campbell WP, Haynes RB. Cost-effectiveness of a worksite hypertension treatment program. *Hypertension.* 1981;3(2):211-218.
24. Lave JR, Frank RG, Schulberg HC, Kamlet MS. Cost-effectiveness of treatments for major depression in primary care practice. *Arch Gen Psychiatry.* 1998;55(7):645-651.

25. Oba Y, Salzman GA. Cost-effectiveness analysis of omalizumab in adults and adolescents with moderate-to-severe allergic asthma. *J Allergy Clin Immunol.* 2004;114(2):265-269.

26. Dasgupta K, Schwartzman K, Marchand R, Tennenbaum TN, Brassard P, Menzies D. Comparison of cost-effectiveness of tuberculosis screening of close contacts and foreign-born populations. *Am J Respir Crit Care Med.* 2000;162(6):2079-2086.

27. Sonnenberg A, Delco F, Inadomi JM. Cost-effectiveness of colonoscopy in screening for colorectal cancer. *Ann Intern Med.* 2000;133(8):573-584.

28. Rascati KL. *Essentials of Pharmacoeconomics.* Philadelphia, PA: Lippincott Williams & Wilkins; 2009.

29. Lazaro A. Theoretical arguments for the discounting of health consequences: where do we go from here? *Pharmacoeconomics.* 2002;20(14):943-961.

30. Weinstein MC, Stason WB. Foundations of cost-effectiveness analysis for health and medical practices. *N Engl J Med.* 1977;296(13):716-721.

31. Weinstein MC, Siegel JE, Gold MR, Kamlet MS, Russell LB. Recommendations of the Panel on Cost-effectiveness in Health and Medicine. *JAMA.* 1996;276(15):1253-1258.

32. Siegel JE, Weinstein MC, Russell LB, Gold MR. Recommendations for reporting cost-effectiveness analyses. Panel on Cost-Effectiveness in Health and Medicine. *JAMA.* 1996;276(16):1339-1341.

33. Berger M, Bingefors K, Hedblom E, Pashos C, Torrance G. *Healthcare Cost, Quality and Outcomes: ISPOR Book of Terms.* Lawrenceville, NJ: ISPOR; 2003.

34. Robinson R. Cost-utility analysis. *BMJ.* 1993;307(6908):859-862.

35. Robinson R. Economic evaluation and health care. What does it mean? *BMJ.* 1993;307(6905):670-673.

36. Coons SJ, Kaplan RM. Cost-utility analysis. In: Bootman JL, Townsend RJ, McGhan WF, eds. *Principles of pharmacoeconomics.* Cincinnati, OH: Wharvey Whitney Books; 1996:102-126.

37. Pauker SG, Kassirer JP. Therapeutic decision making: a cost-benefit analysis. *N Engl J Med.* 1975;293(5):229-234.

38. Johannesson M, Jonsson B. Economic evaluation in health care: is there a role for cost-benefit analysis? *Health Policy.* 1991;17(1):1-23.

39. Robinson R. Cost-benefit analysis. *BMJ.* 1993;307(6909):924-926.

40. Johannesson M, Weinstein MC. Designing and conducting cost-benefit analyses. In: Spilker B, ed. *Quality of Life and Pharmacoeconomics in Clinical Trials.* Philadelphia, PA: Lippincott Williams & Wilkins; 1995:1085-1092.

41. Bridges CB, Thompson WW, Meltzer MI, et al. Effectiveness and cost-benefit of influenza vaccination of healthy working adults: a randomized controlled trial. *JAMA.* 2000;284(13):1655-1663.

42. Nichol KL. Cost-benefit analysis of a strategy to vaccinate healthy working adults against influenza. *Arch Intern Med.* 2001;161(5):749-759.

43. Mohle-Boetani JC, Miller B, Halpern M, et al. School-based screening for tuberculosis infection. A cost-benefit analysis. *JAMA.* 1995;274(8):613-619.

44. Lappalainen M, Sintonen H, Koskiniemi M, et al. Cost-benefit analysis of screening for toxoplasmosis during pregnancy. *Scand J Infect Dis.* 1995;27(3):265-272.

45. Chaix C, Durand-Zaleski I, Alberti C, Brun-Buisson C. Control of endemic methicillin-resistant Staphylococcus aureus: a cost-benefit analysis in an intensive care unit. *JAMA.* 1999;282(18):1745-1751.

46. Johannesson M, Fagerberg B. A health-economic comparison of diet and drug treatment in obese men with mild hypertension. *J Hypertens.* 1992;10(9):1063-1070.

47. Carrasco G, Molina R, Costa J, Soler JM, Cabre L. Propofol vs midazolam in short-, medium-, and long-term sedation of critically ill patients. A cost-benefit analysis. *Chest.* 1993;103(2):557-564.

48. Le Pen C, Levy E, Ravily V, Beuzen JN, Meurgey F. The cost of treatment dropout in depression. A cost-benefit analysis of fluoxetine vs. tricyclics. *J Affect Disord.* 1994;31(1):1-18.

49. Cartwright WS. Cost-benefit analysis of drug treatment services: review of the literature. *J Ment Health Policy Econ.* 2000;3(1):11-26.

50. Sonnenberg A. Cost-benefit analysis of testing for Helicobacter pylori in dyspeptic subjects. *Am J Gastroenterol.* 1996;91(9):1773-1777.

51. Lubell Y, Reyburn H, Mbakilwa H, et al. The impact of response to the results of diagnostic tests for malaria: cost-benefit analysis. *BMJ.* 2008;336(7637):202-205.

52. Avorn J, Soumerai SB. Improving drug-therapy decisions through educational outreach. A randomized controlled trial of academically based "detailing." *N Engl J Med.* 1983;308(24):1457-1463.

53. Rutz W, Carlsson P, von Knorring L, Walinder J. Cost-benefit analysis of an educational program for general practitioners by the Swedish Committee for the Prevention and Treatment of Depression. *Acta Psychiatr Scand.* 1992;85(6):457-464.

54. Sullivan SD, Mauskopf JA, Augustovski F, et al. Budget impact analysis-principles of good practice: report of the ISPOR 2012 Budget Impact Analysis Good Practice II Task Force. *Value Health*. 2014;17(1):5-14.

55. Mauskopf JA, Sullivan SD, Annemans L, et al. Principles of good practice for budget impact analysis: report of the ISPOR Task Force on good research practices—budget impact analysis. *Value Health*. 2007;10(5):336-347.

56. Black WC. The CE plane: a graphic representation of cost-effectiveness. *Med Decis Making*. 1990;10(3):212-214.

57. Weinstein MC, O'Brien B, Hornberger J, et al. Principles of good practice for decision analytic modeling in health-care evaluation: report of the ISPOR Task Force on Good Research Practices—Modeling Studies. *Value Health*. 2003;6(1):9-17.

58. Detsky AS, Naglie G, Krahn MD, Naimark D, Redelmeier DA. Primer on medical decision analysis: part 1—getting started. *Med Decis Making*. 1997;17(2):123-125.

59. Rascati KL. Decision analysis techniques: practical aspects of using personal computers for decision analytic modeling. *Drug Benefit Trends*. 1998:33-36.

60. Briggs AH, Sculpher M. An introduction to Markov modelling for economic evaluation. *Pharmacoeconomics*. 1998;13(4):397-409.

61. Naimark D, Krahn MD, Naglie G, Redelmeier DA, Detsky AS. Primer on medical decision analysis: part 5—working with Markov processes. *Med Decis Making*. 1997;17(2):152-159.

62. Sonnenberg FA, Beck JR. Markov models in medical decision making: a practical guide. *Med Decis Making*. 1993;13(4):322-338.

63. Briggs AH, Gray AM. Handling uncertainty in economic evaluations of healthcare interventions. *BMJ*. 1999;319(7210):635-638.

64. Briggs AH, Claxton K, Schulpher MJ. *Decision Modelling for Health Economic Evaluation*. New York, NY: Oxford University Press; 2006.

65. Guyatt GH, Feeny DH, Patrick DL. Measuring health-related quality of life. *Ann Intern Med*. 1993;118(8):622-629.

66. Patrick DL, Erickson P. *Health Status and Health Policy: Quality of Life in Health Care Evaluation and Resource Allocation*. New York, NY: Oxford University Press; 1993.

67. Badia X, Herdman M. The importance of health-related quality-of-life data in determining the value of drug therapy. *Clin Ther*. 2001;23(1):168-175.

68. Jolly M, Pickard AS, Wilke C, et al. Lupus-specific health outcome measure for US patients: the LupusQoL-US version. *Ann Rheum Dis*. 2010;69(1):29-33.

69. Cella DF, Tulsky DS, Gray G, et al. The Functional Assessment of Cancer Therapy scale: development and validation of the general measure. *J Clin Oncol*. 1993;11(3):570-579.

70. Juniper EF, Guyatt GH, Cox FM, Ferrie PJ, King DR. Development and validation of the Mini Asthma Quality of Life Questionnaire. *Eur Respir J*. 1999;14(1):32-38.

71. Coons SJ, Rao S, Keininger DL, Hays RD. A comparative review of generic quality-of-life instruments. *Pharmacoeconomics*. 2000;17(1):13-35.

72. Ware JE Jr, Sherbourne CD. The MOS 36-item short-form health survey (SF-36). I. Conceptual framework and item selection. *Med Care*. 1992;30(6):473-483.

73. Ware JE, Kosinski M, Bjorner JB, Turner-Bowker DM, Gandek B, Maruish ME. *User's manual for the SF-36v2 Health Survey*. 2nd ed. Lincoln, RI: Quality Metric Inc; 2007.

74. Rabin R, de Charro F. EQ-5D: a measure of health status from the EuroQol Group. *Ann Med*. 2001;33(5):337-343.

75. Shaw JW, Johnson JA, Coons SJ. US valuation of the EQ-5D health states: development and testing of the D1 valuation model. *Med Care*. 2005;43(3):203-220.

76. Dolan P. Modeling valuations for EuroQol health states. *Med Care*. 1997;35(11):1095-1108.

77. Herdman M, Gudex C, Lloyd A, et al. Development and preliminary testing of the new five-level version of EQ-5D (EQ-5D-5L). *Qual Life Res*. 2011;20(10):1727-1736.

78. Kaplan RM, Anderson JP, Ganiats TG. The Quality of Well-Being Scale: rationale for a single quality of life index. In: Walker SR, Rosser R, eds. *Quality of Life Assessment: Key Issues in the 1990s*. London: Kluwer Academic; 1993:65-94.

79. Feeny D, Furlong W, Boyle M, Torrance GW. Multi-attribute health status classification systems. Health Utilities Index. *Pharmacoeconomics*. 1995;7(6):490-502.

80. Feeny D, Furlong W, Torrance GW, et al. Multiattribute and single-attribute utility functions for the health utilities index mark 3 system. *Med Care*. 2002;40(2):113-128.

81. Brazier JE, Roberts J, Deverill M. The estimation of a preference-based measure of health from the SF-36. *J Health Econ*. 2002;21(2):271-292.

82. Xie F, Pullenayegum EM, Li SC, Hopkins R, Thumboo J, Lo NN. Use of a disease-specific instrument in economic evaluations: mapping WOMAC onto the EQ-5D utility index. *Value Health.* 2010;13(8):873-878.

83. Brazier JE, Yang Y, Tsuchiya A, Rowen DL. A review of studies mapping (or cross walking) non-preference based measures of health to generic preference-based measures. *Eur J Health Econ.* 2010;11(2):215-225.

84. Lin FJ, Longworth L, Pickard AS. Evaluation of content on EQ-5D as compared to disease-specific utility measures. *Qual Life Res.* 2013;22(4):853-874.

85. Kontodimopoulos N, Aletras VH, Paliouras D, Niakas D. Mapping the cancer-specific EORTC QLQ-C30 to the preference-based EQ-5D, SF-6D, and 15D instruments. *Value Health.* 2009;12(8):1151-1157.

86. Aaronson N, Alonso J, Burnam A, et al. Assessing health status and quality-of-life instruments: attributes and review criteria. *Qual Life Res.* 2002;11(3):193-205.

87. Liang MH. Longitudinal construct validity: establishment of clinical meaning in patient evaluative instruments. *Med Care.* 2000;38(9 Suppl):II84-90.

88. Cella D, Yount S, Rothrock N, et al. The Patient-Reported Outcomes Measurement Information System (PROMIS): progress of an NIH Roadmap cooperative group during its first two years. *Med Care.* 2007;45(5 Suppl 1):S3-S11.

89. Revicki DA, Kawata AK, Harnam N, Chen WH, Hays RD, Cella D. Predicting EuroQol (EQ-5D) scores from the patient-reported outcomes measurement information system (PROMIS) global items and domain item banks in a United States sample. *Qual Life Res.* 2009;18(6):783-791.

90. Acquadro C, Berzon R, Dubois D, et al. Incorporating the patient's perspective into drug development and communication: an ad hoc task force report of the Patient-Reported Outcomes (PRO) Harmonization Group meeting at the Food and Drug Administration, February 16, 2001. *Value Health.* 2003;6(5):522-531.

91. Willke RJ, Burke LB, Erickson P. Measuring treatment impact: a review of patient-reported outcomes and other efficacy endpoints in approved product labels. *Control Clin Trials.* 2004;25(6):535-552.

92. Bren L. The importance of patient-reported outcomes ... it's all about the patients. *FDA Consum.* 2006;40(6):26-32.

93. Butt Z, Reeve B. Enhancing the patient's voice: standards in design and selection of patient-reported outcomes measures (PROMS) for use in patient-centered outcomes research: methodology committee report. Submitted to the Patient Centeredness Workgroup, PCORI Methodology Committee; March 30, 2012.

94. Devlin N, Appleby J. *Getting the Most out of PROMS.* London: The Kings Fund, Office of Health Economics; 2010.

95. Burstrom K, Johannesson M, Diderichsen F. Swedish population health-related quality of life results using the EQ-5D. *Qual Life Res.* 2001;10(7):621-635.

96. Hennessy CH, Moriarty DG, Zack MM, Scherr PA, Brackbill R. Measuring health-related quality of life for public health surveillance. *Public Health Rep.* 1994;109(5):665-672.

97. Schumock GT, Meek PD, Ploetz PA, Vermeulen LC. Economic evaluations of clinical pharmacy services—1988-1995. The Publications Committee of the American College of Clinical Pharmacy. *Pharmacotherapy.* 1996;16(6):1188-1208.

98. Schumock GT, Butler MG, Meek PD, Vermeulen LC, Arondekar BV, Bauman JL. Evidence of the economic benefit of clinical pharmacy services: 1996-2000. *Pharmacotherapy.* 2003;23(1):113-132.

99. Perez A, Doloresco F, Hoffman JM, et al. ACCP: economic evaluations of clinical pharmacy services: 2001-2005. *Pharmacotherapy.* 2009;29(1):128.

100. Chisholm-Burns MA, Graff Zivin JS, Lee JK, et al. Economic effects of pharmacists on health outcomes in the United States: a systematic review. *Am J Health Syst Pharm.* 2010;67(19):1624-1634.

101. Touchette DR, Doloresco F, Suda KJ, et al. Economic evaluations of clinical pharmacy services: 2006-2010. *Pharmacotherapy.* 2014;34(8):771-793.

102. Mason J. The generalisability of pharmacoeconomic studies. *Pharmacoeconomics.* 1997;11(6):503-514.

103. Mason JM, Mason AR. The generalisability of pharmacoeconomic studies: issues and challenges ahead. *Pharmacoeconomics.* 2006;24(10):937-945.

104. Husereau D, Drummond M, Petrou S, et al. Consolidated Health Economic Evaluation Reporting Standards (CHEERS) statement. *Value Health.* 2013;16(2):e1-e5.

105. Eddy DM, Hollingworth W, Caro JJ, Tsevat J, McDonald KM, Wong JB. Model transparency and validation: a report of the ISPOR-SMDM Modeling Good Research Practices Task Force-7. *Med Decis Making.* 2012;32(5):733-743.

106. Caro JJ, Eddy DM, Kan H, et al. Questionnaire to assess relevance and credibility of modeling studies for informing health care decision making: an ISPOR-AMCP-NPC Good Practice Task Force report. *Value Health*. 2014;17(2):174-182.

107. Shaw JW. Lack of support for cost-utility analysis in the health care reform law: a case of ignorance or political posturing? *Clin Ther*. 2010;32(6):1091-1092.

108. Drummond MF. The future of pharmacoeconomics: bridging science and practice. *Clin Ther*. 1996;18(5):969-978; discussion 968.

109. Bell CM, Urbach DR, Ray JG, et al. Bias in published cost effectiveness studies: systematic review. *BMJ*. 2006;332(7543):699-703.

110. Neumann PJ, Weinstein MC. Legislating against use of cost-effectiveness information. *N Engl J Med*. 2010;363(16):1495-1497.

111. Neumann PJ. What next for QALYs? *JAMA*. 2011;305(17):1806-1807.

112. Luce BR. What will it take to make cost-effectiveness analysis acceptable in the United States? *Med Care*. 2005;43(7 Suppl):44-48.

113. Neumann PJ, Sullivan SD. Economic evaluation in the US: what is the missing link? *Pharmacoeconomics*. 2006;24(11):1163-1168.

114. Calvert M, Blazeby J, Altman DG, Revicki DA, Moher D, Brundage MD. Reporting of patient-reported outcomes in randomized trials: the CONSORT PRO extension. *JAMA*. 2013;309(8):814-822.

115. Snyder CF, Aaronson NK, Choucair AK, et al. Implementing patient-reported outcomes assessment in clinical practice: a review of the options and considerations. *Qual Life Res*. 2012;21(8):1305-1314.

116. Nwokeji ED, Rascati KL. Pharmacoeconomic education in colleges of pharmacy outside of the United States. *Am J Pharm Educ*. 2005;69:348-355.

117. Reddy M, Rascati K, Wahawisan J, Rascati M. Pharmacoeconomic education in US colleges and schools of pharmacy: an update. *Am J Pharm Educ*. 2008;72(3):51.

# GLOSSARY

**A posteriori** Determined afterward; literally, "from the one behind."

**A priori** Determined beforehand; literally, "from the one before."

**Absolute risk difference** The difference in risk of an outcome between groups that is calculated using subtraction (i.e., experimental event rate minus control event rate).

**Absolute risk reduction** Absolute change in risk between the control and treatment groups; the risk of the event in the control group minus the risk of the event in the treatment group; expressed as a percentage.

**Abstract** A brief summary of the main points of an article.

**Academia** The environment concerned with the pursuit of research, scholarship, and education.

**Academic detailing** Noncommercial, evidence-based direct outreach to clinicians that aids prescribers regarding appropriate clinical decision making based on the best available efficacy, safety, and cost-effectiveness data.

**Accessible population** The portion of a larger population that is available to a researcher and from which sample subjects will be selected for inclusion in a clinical study.

**Accuracy** The relative proximity of a measurement to the real value.

**Active control** An intervention that has an effect on outcomes (rather than no effect, as with placebo) and is compared to an investigational intervention.

**Active treatment group** The group in a clinical study in which subjects will receive the intervention under investigation; also referred to as the *study group*.

**Adherence bias** Another term for compliance bias.

**Admission rate bias** A type of selection bias in which the rates of exposed and unexposed individuals enrolled in a study systematically differ from the rates of exposed and unexposed individuals not enrolled in the study as a result of the setting in which the subjects are selected; also referred to as *Berkson bias* or *Berkson's paradox*.

**Adverse drug event** An injury resulting from medical care involving medication use.

**Adverse drug reaction** A nonpreventable adverse drug event that occurs when a medication is used in the recommended manner and results in an undesired response.

**AGREE Instrument** An acronym that stands for Appraisal of Guidelines Research and Evaluation. This is an instrument that can be used by policy makers, guideline developers, healthcare professionals, and educators to assist in the evaluation of clinical practice guidelines.

**Alpha (α)** The significance level or threshold for "accepting" the null hypothesis; this value is commonly set at 0.05.

**Alternative hypothesis** The hypothesis that is accepted when the null hypothesis is rejected; normally, that there is a true difference between comparator groups that is not due to random chance, but rather some characteristic of the groups themselves.

**Analysis of covariance** A statistical test used to compare continuous outcomes in more than two groups when controlling for confounding variables.

**Analysis of variance** A statistical test used to compare continuous outcomes in more than two groups.

**Analytical study** A study that tests hypotheses to determine associations between a characteristic or exposure and a disease or outcome.

**Assay sensitivity** The ability of a clinical trial to distinguish an effective treatment from an ineffective treatment.

**Attention bias** A type of information bias that can occur when subjects change their behavior because they know that their actions are being observed; also referred to as *observation bias*.

**Authorship** The process of making substantial contributions to scientific research and manuscript preparation that qualify individuals to be listed as authors of the manuscript.

**Automated dispensing cabinet** Computerized drug storage and distribution systems that allow medications to be stored securely in patient care areas.

**Background information** Additional data that further clarifies the drug information question that is being asked.

**Bar diagram** A method of data presentation where the discrete variables are placed on the $x$-axis and the count or frequency on the $y$-axis.

**Baseline characteristics** The significant attributes of subjects in each clinical study group at the time of subject enrollment.

**Benchmarks** Something that can be used as a way to judge the quality or level of other, similar things.

483

**Berkson bias** Another term for *admission rate bias*.

**Berkson's paradox** Another term for *admission rate bias*.

**Best practice** Commercial or professional procedures that are accepted or prescribed as being correct or most effective.

**Beta (β)** In hypothesis testing, the probability of committing a type II error.

**Bias** In clinical research, an identifiable and sometimes quantifiable circumstance that is systematically, or nonrandomly, introduced consciously or unconsciously by actions or decisions made by persons connected to the research and that leads to an error in the interpretation of study results.

**Biomedical informatics** The interdisciplinary field that studies and pursues the effective uses of biomedical data, information, and knowledge for scientific inquiry, problem solving, and decision making; motivated by efforts to improve human health.

**Blinding** In clinical research, the process of ensuring that certain participants in a clinical study, such as subjects, investigators, and/or data analysts, are unaware of subject group assignment. May also refer to a way to decrease bias during peer review.

**Blocked randomization** A randomization technique that ensures approximately equal numbers of subjects in all groups throughout the duration of the enrollment period.

**Boolean operators** Allow searching with multiple terms by creating relationships between those terms within a search; Boolean operator AND returns articles containing both search terms. The operator OR returns articles with one or more of the search terms. The operator NOT returns articles that do not contain the search term.

**Box plot** A method of data presentation where the continuous variable is represented on the $y$-axis and the time or measurement point is on the $x$-axis. The box extends from the 25th to the 75th percentiles and the median is denoted by a line drawn in the middle.

**Case-control study** A retrospective observational study used to identify etiologies of a disease by comparing exposures/characteristics in cases versus controls.

**Case report (case series)** Provides a detailed description of a patient's or patients' disease; may include signs, symptoms, diagnosis, treatment, and outcomes. Commonly provides information on rare or novel scenarios in medicine.

**Categorization** The act of classifying a drug information request into a specific question type.

**Chance** In clinical research, an unidentifiable circumstance that is randomly introduced into a clinical study and that causes an error in the interpretation of the results of the study.

**Chi-square** A statistical test used to evaluate nominal data.

**Clinical decision support** The use of electronic medical knowledge in combination with electronic patient data to support decision making about patients.

**Clinical informatics** The application of biomedical informatics methods and techniques, including information technology, to deliver healthcare services.

**Clinical practice guidelines** Statements developed through a systematic process, including review of current evidence and recommendations, to optimize patient care.

**Clinical research** Original investigations in living subjects that are intended to provide insight into an aspect of biology, health, or medical care in the same types of subjects as the investigation is conducted.

**Clinical significance** The ability to establish whether a result is meaningful enough to be able to incorporate a change in patient care.

**Clinically significant difference** The minimum magnitude of difference between the effects of different interventions that would cause a meaningful change in practice.

**Closed formulary** Limited availability of medications for use within an organization based on safety, efficacy, and cost-effectiveness.

**Cluster randomization** A two-step randomization technique that involves formation of groups (i.e., clusters) of subjects and then randomly assigning all subjects in each cluster to a study or control group in order to keep the specific clusters of individuals together throughout the study.

**Cluster sampling** A two-stage probability sampling technique in which members of the accessible population are divided into logical heterogeneous groups (i.e., clusters) based on a characteristic of convenience, such as location; randomly selecting clusters; and then randomly selecting samples from the clusters.

**Cochrane Database of Systematic Reviews** A database that provides rigorous systematic reviews of the primary literature.

**Coefficient of determination** Value that indicates how much of the variance in one variable can be explained or accounted for by one or more other variables. It is the square of the correlation coefficient and is represented by $r^2$ when one dependent and one independent variable are used. When more than two variables are used, the coefficient is represented by $R^2$.

**Cohort study** Researchers follow a group of people (a cohort), some of whom have the exposure of interest and some of whom do not.

**Collaborative practice drug therapy management agreements** Agreements between a pharmacist and a physician allowing a pharmacist to manage or initiate drug therapy under the supervision of the physician. What the pharmacist may do is regulated by individual state boards of pharmacy.

**Combined outcome** A clinical study outcome consisting of multiple individual dependent variables that should be similar with regard to cause and impact; also referred to as a *composite outcome*.

**Comparative effectiveness research** Research that compares benefits and harms of different therapies.

**Compliance bias** A type of information bias that occurs when more subjects in one group systematically fail to properly follow study protocols than subjects in another group do because of inconvenience of or intolerance to their assigned intervention or when equal amounts of noncompliance between groups exists, but the noncompliance affects the outcomes of one group more than it affects the outcomes of another. Also referred to as *adherence bias*.

**Composite outcome** A clinical study outcome consisting of multiple individual dependent variables that should be similar with regard to cause and impact. Also referred to as a *combined outcome*.

**Computerized provider order entry** The ordering of medications, procedures, tests, etc., for a patient by a provider inputting information into a computer system.

**Concordance** The degree of agreement that exists when different individuals use the same instrument to make a measurement. Also referred to as *inter-rater reliability*.

**Conditions for Coverage** Health and safety standards that healthcare organizations must meet in order to begin and continue participating in the Medicare and Medicaid programs.

**Conditions of Participation** Health and safety standards that healthcare organizations must meet in order to begin and continue participating in the Medicare and Medicaid programs.

**Confidence interval** A range of values that is likely to contain the true parameter value.

**Confidence interval bounds** The greatest and least probable effects of an intervention, as quantified by a confidence interval.

**Conflict of interest** Any relationship or affiliation that may hinder objective, unbiased participation in the scientific research or publishing process.

**Confounders** Extraneous factors that correlate with both the dependent and independent variables.

**CONsolidated Standards of Reporting Trials (CONSORT) Statement** An evidence-based, minimum set of recommendations for reporting of randomized controlled trials.

**Constancy assumption** The expectation that the effect of an intervention will be the same in a current clinical trial as it was in historical clinical trials.

**Contamination bias** Another term for *migration bias*.

**Content expert** A person who attends the journal club who provides depth, expertise, and perspective on the subject matter discussed at the journal club; provides insight into implications for practice.

**Continuing professional development** The lifelong process of active participation in learning activities that assists individuals in developing and maintaining continuing competence, enhancing their professional practice, and supporting achievement of their goals.

**Control** In clinical research, the intervention, condition, or lack thereof to which the study intervention or condition is being compared.

**Control group** The group in a clinical study in which subjects will receive the active comparator intervention, inactive placebo, or no intervention, or in which the condition of interest does not exist.

**Convenience sampling** A nonprobability sampling technique in which subjects are chosen based on availability to investigators.

**Correlation** Used to determine to what degree two variables change together or *covary*.

**Correlation coefficient** A measure indicating the strength and direction of a relationship between two variables that is represented by *r*. Also known as *Pearson's correlation coefficient* or *Pearson's product-moment correlation coefficient*.

**Cost–benefit analysis** An economic evaluation where both costs and outcomes are measured in monetary units.

**Cost-effectiveness analysis** An economic evaluation that compares alternative interventions by measuring both costs and outcomes.

**Cost-of-illness studies** Partial economic evaluations that are aimed at providing insight into the economic burden of a disease state.

**Cost-minimization analysis** An analysis where the health outcomes can be considered to be equivalent between treatment alternatives and therefore the interest is only on which of the alternatives has the lower cost.

**Cost–utility analysis** An economic evaluation that compares two or more alternatives based on their costs and outcomes, where outcomes are measures in units of quality-adjusted life years or disability-adjusted life years.

**Covariance** A measure of the joint variance of two or more variables.

**Covariates** Variables that are measured and accounted for in the statistical analysis in addition to the primary variables as factors that may affect the outcome.

**Critical appraisal** The process of systematically evaluating a clinical trial or research for value and relevance.

**Crossover study** Clinical study in which each subject is exposed to each intervention or exposure in a sequential manner and in which each subject's outcome data are directly compared to one another, thus allowing each subject to serve as his or her own control.

**Cross-sectional study** A study used to characterize a population at one moment in time and to determine prevalence of a characteristic or outcome.

**Cumulative Index of Nursing and Allied Health Literature (CINAHL)** A database that contains bibliographic information from journals specific to nursing and allied health professionals, such as respiratory therapists, physical therapists, occupational therapists, and pharmacists.

**Data and safety monitoring board** A committee that is independent of a study's investigators and whose purpose is to periodically assess the risks versus benefits of continuing a clinical study. Also referred to as a *data monitoring committee*.

**Data dredging** The process of analyzing large volumes of data from clinical research to identify patterns that may or may not accurately reflect the larger population. Also referred to as *data mining*.

**Data mining** The process of analyzing large volumes of data from clinical research to identify patterns that may or may not accurately reflect the larger population. Also referred to as *data dredging*.

**Data monitoring committee** A committee that is independent of a study's investigators and whose purpose is to periodically assess the risks versus benefits of continuing a clinical study. Also referred to as a *data and safety monitoring board.*

**Database of Abstracts of Reviews of Effects (DARE)** A database that provides summaries of systematic reviews and meta-analyses published in the literature.

**Decision analysis** A systematic way to compare alternative choices in instances of uncertainty.

**Demographics** Professional and/or contact information of the requestor.

**Dependent variable** In clinical research, the condition that is expected might be altered by the independent variable.

**Descriptive study** A study that provides a description (often frequency and/or pattern) of a disease or outcome in a population.

**Detection bias** A type of selection bias that can occur when the methods of screening for the condition of interest differ between the control group and the experimental group.

**Dichotomous variable** Variables with only two possible outcomes.

**Direct costs** Costs that are directly tied to a product or service and involve an exchange of money.

**Direct outcome** An outcome that is an important and meaningful event or aspect of an individual's condition and that represents a significant temporary or permanent change to that individual's life.

**Disproportional allocation** The process of intentionally assigning more subjects to one group than to another in a predefined ratio.

**Double-blind trial** An interventional study design in which both investigators and subjects are unaware of group assignments.

**Double-dummy** A blinding technique that is used to match differing dosage forms, providing a placebo in each group that matches the intervention in the other group(s).

**Drug information** A clinical practice that involves the efficient retrieval, evaluation, and communication of medication information in order to assist in care decisions, develop evidence-based recommendations, and improve patient outcomes.

**Drug information residency** A residency program designed to effectively train pharmacists as organizational leaders in the development of safe and effective medication use policies and/or processes and in the expert analysis of medication-related information.

**Drug information specialist** A specially trained individual who has the clinical knowledge and skills that allow for the provision of clear, concise, and accurate recommendations regarding drug use.

**Dummy** A placebo that is intended to resemble or simulate an active intervention.

**Economic analysis** A comparative analysis of alternative courses of action in terms of both their costs and their consequences.

**Effect size** The magnitude of difference observed between groups for an outcome in a clinical study; often symbolized by the Greek uppercase letter delta ($\Delta$).

**Effectiveness** A measure of how well an intervention works for a condition outside the boundaries of clinical research, taking into account such factors as its efficacy, safety, and accessibility.

**Efficacy** The degree to which a therapy produces a desired outcome under ideal study conditions.

**Efficacy outcome** Any clinical study outcome that examines whether the intervention of interest has a desired effect on the condition of interest.

**Eigenfactor Metrics** A newer measure for comparing quality and significance among journals.

**Electronic health record** A digital health record that can be accessed by multiple users.

**Endpoint** In clinical research, the result of a studied hypothesis. Also referred to as an *outcome.*

**Entry time bias** A subtype of detection bias that can occur when subject entry times significantly differ between groups. Also referred to as *starting time bias.*

**Equivalency study** A clinical study that endeavors to determine if two interventions are not meaningfully different from one another with regard to an outcome of interest.

**Error** In clinical research, a deviation between the truth about a phenomenon in a population and what is observed in a clinical study about that phenomenon that is significant enough in magnitude to result in a false conclusion being drawn.

**Ethical review board** A committee that is independent of a study's investigators and whose purpose is to review protocols for studies conducted in human subjects. Also referred to as an *institutional review board* or *independent research ethics committee.*

**Evidence-based clinical practice guidelines** Those clinical practice guidelines based on evidence supported by results from clinical trials.

**Evidence-based medicine** The conscientious, explicit, and judicious use of current best evidence in making clinical decisions about the care of individual patients. The practice of evidence-based medicine means integrating individual clinical experience with the best available external clinical evidence from systematic research.

**Exclusion criteria** A defined set of specific characteristics that will preclude a potential subject from study participation or that could lead to involuntary study withdrawal.

**Experimental study** Trial in which researchers assign subjects a therapy or treatment and measure the desired effect. Such trials contain at least two groups in which members of one group receive active therapy and members of the other group may receive the standard of care or placebo.

**Exposure suspicion bias** A type of information bias that can occur when subjects in one group are systematically exposed to diagnostic procedures or investigations that subjects in another group are not as a result of the researchers' knowledge or beliefs about the group to which individual subjects have been assigned.

**External validity** The extent to which the results apply to the population of interest; sometimes referred to as *generalizability.*

**Failure modes and effects analysis** A method to proactively assess risk associated with introduction of a new process, medication, or device into a system.

**False negative** In hypothesis testing, an error in which no meaningful difference between groups is observed for an outcome when a meaningful difference actually does or would exist in the population; that is, failing to reject the null hypothesis when we should have rejected it. Also referred to as a *type II error*.

**False positive** In hypothesis testing, an error in which a meaningful difference between groups is observed for an outcome when that difference actually does not or would not exist in the population; that is, rejecting the null hypothesis when we should have failed to reject it. Also referred to as a *type I error*.

**Fisher's exact test** A statistical test used to evaluate nominal data; used either when the total sample size is less than 20 or if the expected number of observations for any one of the cells would be less than 5.

**5 Million Lives Campaign** A campaign started by the Institute for Healthcare Improvement to reduce morbidity and mortality in health care, including adverse drug events and surgical complications.

**Fixed-effects meta-analysis** A less conservative meta-analytic method that assumes there is one true effect size of a treatment present in all studies analyzed and that any variation is due to random chance.

**Formulary** A list of medications that are deemed appropriate for use by an organization.

**Formulary system** Ongoing process by which changes are made to the formulary.

**Freewrite (freewriting)** An approach to writing in which the author simply puts his or her ideas on paper without using an outline or other organizational tools.

**Ghostwriting** The unethical process of manuscript preparation and submission by individuals who are paid employees of the research sponsor and are not listed as authors of the manuscript.

**Gold standard** An instrument or method for taking a measurement that is considered to be the best available at a given time and under a given set of conditions.

**GRADE** An acronym that stands for Grading of Recommendations, Assessment, Development, and Evaluation. It is a working group whose goal is to create a standardized process to rate the quality of literature and determine the appropriate level of evidence of a recommendation.

***h* index** A surrogate value for the cumulative impact and relevance of an individual researcher's published work; taking into account the number of his or her publications and the number of times those publications have been cited in other works.

**Hawthorne effect** a type of bias in which patients respond to therapy (either control or treatment) because they are being studied.

**Hazard ratio** Chance of an event occurring in the treatment arm divided by the chance of the event occurring in the control arm; the risk of occurrence of the hazard is expressed as a rate or number of events per unit time; written as a decimal.

**Head-to-head trial** A type of interventional study design in which two or more active interventions are directly compared to each other with the ultimate goal of establishing comparative effectiveness, efficacy, or safety.

**Health Information Technology for Economic and Clinical Health Act** Part of the American Recovery and Reinvestment Act of 2009 that provides funding to promote and expand the use of interoperable health information technology.

**Hierarchy of evidence** A ordered representation of primary literature with the meta-analysis at the top and expert opinion at the bottom.

**High-alert medication** A medication that is not necessarily associated with a higher rate of adverse events, but is associated with an increased risk of significant patient harm when used in error.

**High-benefit medications** Medications that must be used properly within a defined time window that can positively affect patient outcomes.

**Histogram** A method of data presentation where the $x$-axis provides the measurement range of the variable of interest (divided into equal units or class intervals) and the $y$-axis represents the frequency or relative frequency. Histograms are sometimes used to visualize whether a dataset is a bell-shaped distribution or it is skewed.

**Identical placebo** An inactive intervention that is designed to be identical to the study intervention in all regards except that it does not contain an active ingredient or is otherwise purposefully ineffectual. Also referred to as a *matched placebo*.

**Impact factor** The average number of times each article appearing in a journal during a given period of time was cited during a subsequent period of time; used as a surrogate value for the importance that the scientific community places on articles published in a journal.

**Improvement maps** A free, interactive, web-based tool from the Institute for Healthcare Improvement designed to bring together the best knowledge available on the key process improvements that lead to exceptional patient care. The Improvement Map aims to help make care safer, smooth patient care transitions, lead improvement efforts effectively, reduce costs, and increase quality.

**Incidence** The number of new cases of a disease, condition, or event that occur in a specific time frame in the individuals who are at risk for developing the new disease, condition, or event.

**Incidence rate** A representation of the incidence that accounts for the specific time frame in the actual incidence. These include measures such as patient-years or person-days.

**Incident reports** Voluntary reporting of safety concerns or events by healthcare providers, patients, or caregivers.

**Inclusion criteria** Criteria that are used to choose individuals for participation in clinical research studies.

**Incremental costs** The additional (total) costs of implementing one option compared to that of an alternative intervention.

**Independent data** Data in a parallel study, where individuals are assigned to only one group and remain in that group.

**Independent research ethics committee** A committee that is independent of a study's investigators and whose purpose is to review protocols for studies conducted in human subjects. Also referred to as an *institutional review board* or *ethical review board*.

**Independent variable** In clinical research, the intervention, exposure, condition, or contributing factor that is under investigation and that is expected to possibly have an effect on the dependent variable.

**Indirect costs** Costs, such as time and productivity loss, that involve no direct exchange of money and therefore may be harder to measure.

**Inferential statistics** Statistics used to make generalizations about a population based on the response illustrated by a sample of the population.

**Information bias** Any type of bias that causes a systematic error in the measurement, analysis, interpretation, or reporting of data in a clinical study.

**Informed consent** The process by which a potential study subject is presented with information about a clinical study and willingly volunteers to participate in that study.

**Institutional review board** A committee that is independent of a study's investigators and whose purpose is to review protocols for studies conducted in human subjects. Also referred to as an *independent research ethics committee* or *ethical review board*.

**Instructions for authors** Rules for manuscript preparation and submission that are specific to individual journals.

**Instrument** A piece of equipment, calculation, algorithm, survey, or other device for measuring a phenomenon.

**Intangible costs** Costs such as pain and suffering.

**Intention-to-treat analysis** A method of analyzing data from all patients in the group to which they were initially assigned, regardless of whether they completed the trial or violated protocol. Individual trials may define the intention-to-treat population differently.

**Internal validity** The degree to which the results of a study can be believed based on how the study was planned and conducted.

**International Committee of Medical Journal Editors (ICMJE) Uniform Requirements for Manuscript Submission** International standards for the information that should be contained in a scientific manuscript upon submission for publication.

**Interquartile range** The values between the 25th and 75th percentiles of a dataset.

**Inter-rater reliability** The degree of agreement that exists when different individuals use the same instrument to make a measurement. Also referred to as *concordance*.

**Interval data** A type of quantitative data where the difference between each unit of a measurement scale is equal, but there is no absolute zero.

**Intervention** In medicine or clinical research, any act on the part of a healthcare professional or researcher that is intended to alter the course of a patient's or subject's condition; an intervention could be a test, a drug, a procedure, surgery, counseling, etc. Also referred to as a *maneuver*.

**Interventional study** A clinical investigation in which the researcher alters the normal course of events. Also referred to as an *experimental study*.

**Journal club coordinator** Designated person who provides oversight, structure, and consistency for each journal club session;

may be one role or may be divided into two roles. This can be an educator/faculty member, preceptor, or practitioner.

**Kruskal–Wallis** A statistical test used to compare more than two groups of independent, ordinal, or non-normally distributed data.

**Maneuver** In medicine or clinical research, any act on the part of a healthcare professional or researcher that is intended to alter the course of a patient's or subject's condition; a maneuver could be a test, a drug, a procedure, surgery, counseling, etc. Also referred to as an *intervention*.

**Mann–Whitney U** A statistical test used when there are two independent samples to compare the distribution of ranked results between the groups.

**Manuscript** A complete article that is not yet published.

**Manuscript checklist** Published lists of minimum requirements for preparing a specific type of article.

**Marginal costs** The additional costs from producing one additional unit.

**Matched placebo** An inactive intervention that is designed to be identical to the study intervention in all regards except that it does not contain an active ingredient or is otherwise purposefully ineffectual. Also referred to as *identical placebo*.

**Matched study** A clinical study in which each subject is assigned to a single group and his or her outcome data are directly compared with those of a similar subject in another group.

**McNemar** A statistical test used for nominal data that are paired.

**Mean** Value obtained by summing the values associated with each individual data point and then dividing by the total number of data points.

**Meaningful use** Using certified electronic health record technology to improve the quality, safety, and efficacy of health care while reducing disparities, engaging patients and family, improving care coordination and population and public health, and maintaining privacy and security of patient health information.

**Meaningfulness** In clinical research, the significance of an outcome to subjects in a clinical study and individuals in the represented population.

**Measurement** The act of assigning a value to an observation.

**Median** The value of the data point that is in the middle, or 50th percentile, of the dataset distribution.

**Medical surveillance bias** A type of selection bias that can occur in retrospective studies when the inclusion of subjects is limited to those who have received a certain nonroutine screening or diagnostic test.

**Medication error** Any error, through an act of commission or omission, occurring in any step of the medication use process.

**Medication guideline** A subset of written policies that provide guidance for clinicians in selecting and monitoring appropriate therapy. A clinical directive where patient-specific factors and the clinical situation may warrant an occasional deviation from usual practice.

**Medication management standards** A list of standards required by The Joint Commission that guide pharmacists in developing a medication management strategy featuring all stages of medication use, including selection, storage, ordering, dispensing, administration, and monitoring.

**Medication safety** Freedom from accidental injury during the course of medication use; this term encompasses activities to avoid, prevent, or correct adverse drug events that may occur due to medication use.

**Medication use evaluation** A performance improvement method focused on the evaluation and improvement of medication-use processes to optimize patient outcomes.

**Medication use policy** Defines or clarifies an operational or clinical standard of medication use.

**Medication use process** Prescribing, transcribing, dispensing, administering, and monitoring medications.

**MEDLINE** A secondary resource database that contains 19 million biomedical journal abstracts and citations from around the world.

**Membership bias** A type of selection bias that can occur when subjects in one group have a higher prevalence of a characteristic that may alter their outcomes than subjects in another group have, and that characteristic is systematically tied to another characteristic upon which group assignments are based.

**MeSH** an acronym for Medical Subject Headings, which is the U.S. National Library of Medicine's controlled vocabulary (i.e., thesaurus); this vocabulary gives uniformity and consistency to the indexing and cataloging of biomedical literature.

**Meta-analysis** A systematic review with quantitative pooling of data in order to produce a summary result that is a weighted average of the existing data.

**Metrics** Standards of measurement.

**Migration** The circumstance in which a subject assigned to a group associated with a specific course transitions to a course that is more associated with a different group, even if that group does not exist in the study, but is still counted as if he or she were following the course associated with his or her original group.

**Migration bias** A type of information bias that can occur when subjects unintentionally start following a protocol that is more similar to a group to which they are not assigned than to the group to which they are assigned, but whose outcome data are not missing and are treated as still belonging to their assigned group. Also referred to as *contamination bias*.

**Mimicry bias** A subtype of unmasking bias in which the inciting condition presents similarly to the condition of interest.

**Missing data bias** A type of information bias that can occur when data that are absent are omitted, assumed, imputed, or otherwise treated.

**Mode** The most frequently occurring value in a dataset.

**Modified intention-to-treat analysis** A data analysis procedure in which data from all subjects who were enrolled in a clinical study and who continued to a prespecified point early in the study are used, even if some of the subjects' data must be assumed because they are missing.

**Negative predictive value** The proportion of all negative measurements made by an instrument that are true negatives, which yields the probability that a negative measurement represents a

negative case. Calculated by dividing the number of true negatives by the total number of true and false negatives.

**Negative study** A study that does not demonstrate what the researchers intended to demonstrate.

**Neyman bias** Another term for *prevalence-incidence bias*.

**95%-95% confidence interval approach** A method used to determine a noninferiority margin by considering the entire effect of the active control versus placebo as well as the largest loss of effect that an investigational drug may have in order to be considered noninferior.

**Nominal data** A type of qualitative data where the categories are unrelated and no scale or direction is implied.

**Noncontemporaneous control bias** A subtype of detection bias that can occur when historical control subjects are used.

**Nonformulary** Term for a medication that is not approved for inclusion on the formulary.

**Nonformulary medication** Medication not approved for inclusion on the formulary.

**Noninferior** An intervention that is not worse than a comparator by a predefined amount of difference. In exchange for allowing an intervention to be slightly worse than a comparator, some benefit of the intervention or the trial design is gained.

**Noninferiority margin** The furthest extent of loss of effect that an investigational drug may have versus an active control in order to be considered noninferior.

**Noninferiority study** A clinical study that endeavors to determine if one intervention is not meaningfully worse than another intervention, the latter of which was previously established as efficacious with regard to an outcome of interest.

**Nonparametric tests** Statistical tests used to evaluate ordinal and nominal data and data that are not normally distributed.

**Nonprobability sampling** Any sampling method that is accomplished in a systematic, nonrandom manner. Also referred to as *nonrandom sampling*.

**Nonrandom sampling** Any sampling method that is accomplished in a systematic, nonrandom manner. Also referred to as *nonprobability sampling*.

**Nonresponse bias** Participation bias, usually in the context of survey research.

**Normal distribution** A distribution that has the appearance of a bell-shaped curve; both sides of the curve are symmetric about the middle of the curve.

**Null hypothesis** The hypothesis that there is no true difference between comparator groups and that any difference discovered is due to random chance.

**Number needed to harm** The number of patients who need to be treated for a specified period of time to see one patient harmed.

**Number needed to treat** The number of patients who need to be treated to prevent one event; reciprocal of the absolute risk reduction expressed as a decimal proportion; usually rounded to a whole number.

**Objective measurement** In medicine and clinical research, an assignment of a value to a phenomenon that involves a relatively low amount of human interpretation.

**Observation bias** Another term for *attention bias*.

**Observational study** A clinical study in which the researcher only witnesses events and describes their circumstances, but does not intervene in any way. Observational studies may be either retrospective or prospective.

**Odds ratio** The odds of having the outcome in the exposed group divided by the odds of having the outcome in the control group.

**Off-label use** Use of a medication outside the FDA-approved indication(s), route, dose, or specified patient population.

**One-sided superiority study** A clinical study that only allows for determination of favor of one intervention relative to the other, but not the reverse. Also referred to as a *one-tailed superiority study*.

**One-tailed superiority study** A clinical study that only allows for determination of favor of one intervention relative to the other, but not the reverse. Also referred to as a *one-sided superiority study*.

**Open formulary** Unrestricted list of medications available for use within an organization.

**Open label trial** An interventional study design in which all participants, including investigators, subjects, and data analysts, are aware of group assignments.

**Opportunity cost** The benefit that is foregone from the next best alternative.

**Order set** A standard list of medical and medication orders for practitioners that are commonly used for specific conditions and procedures, but may be modified for individual patients. They typically contain specific elements to support quality care and regulatory requirements.

**Ordinal data** A type of qualitative data where a scale or direction is associated with the categories.

**Original research** Interventional or observational research studies that seek to generate new scientific information.

**Outcome** In clinical research, the result of a studied hypothesis. Also referred to as an *endpoint*.

**Outline** An organizational tool used when writing that serves as a blueprint for the major points and flow of a writing project.

**Paired data** Individual subject differences are measured as in pretest-posttest and crossover study designs where an individual's data are in both groups.

**Paired *t*-test** Test that measures whether means from a within-subjects test group vary over two test conditions.

**Parallel study** A clinical study in which each subject is assigned to a single group and his or her outcome data are pooled with others in the same group for the purposes of analysis.

**Parametric tests** Statistical tests used to evaluate continuous data that are normally distributed.

**Participation bias** A type of selection bias that can occur when the subjects who are willing to participate in a study have different characteristics than those who are unwilling to participate in the study, and those characteristics have an impact on an outcome of interest.

**PDCA cycle** A continuous cycle of improving quality through the plan-do-check-act approach.

**Peer review** A structured process whereby persons who have similar competence to the authors of a work of literature and knowledge in the work's subject matter evaluate submitted manuscripts and supply feedback to the authors before the work is published.

**Per-protocol analysis** A method of analyzing data only from patients who adhered to the trial protocol; individual trials may define the per-protocol population differently.

**Person approach** Response to human error that involves considering the individual most directly involved in the error to be at fault for causing the error.

**Pharmacy and therapeutics committee** A multidisciplinary group, including physicians and pharmacists, that oversees the formulary process and medication management in a health system or organization.

**PICO** An acronym that stands for patient (or problem), intervention, comparison (or control), and outcome, which are the four parts to a well-built question.

**Pie charts** A method of data presentation where each discrete variable is visualized as a slice of the "pie." The size of each slice is determined by the proportion of each relative to the total of the pie.

**Placebo** A type of intervention that does not possess any pharmaceutical activity or that simulates a medical intervention, but that does not itself have any recognizable effect. A placebo may or may not be designed to resemble an intervention under investigation.

**Placebo-controlled trial** A type of interventional study design that uses a placebo in place of an active intervention in one group and that is intended to establish whether an active intervention is efficacious for a given condition.

**Placebo effect** The phenomenon that exists when subjects who are receiving an inactive or ineffectual intervention exhibit changes in the course of a condition of interest, despite the lack of a true intervention; a potential example of attention bias.

**Plagiarism** Using the ideas, words, or data of another individual without properly acknowledging that individual, implying that the ideas, words, or data are your own.

**POEM** An acronym that stands for patient-oriented evidence that matters. POEMs answer a single question, providing the best review of evidence, taking into account not only safety and efficacy of a therapy, but also patient-specific parameters, such as quality of life, activities of daily living, cost-effectiveness, and long-term outcomes.

**Policy** A written statement that provides guidance on the position and values of an organization. It can be considered a directive that must always be followed.

**Polychotomous variable** Variables with more than two possible outcomes.

**Population** An entire group of individuals having some defined characteristic of interest in common.

**Position statement** A written statement released by an organization that explains or justifies their stance on an issue.

**Positive predictive value** The proportion of all positive measurements made by an instrument that are true positives, which yields the probability that a positive measurement represents a positive case; calculated by dividing the number of true positives by the total number of true and false positives.

**Positive study** A study that demonstrates what the researchers intended to demonstrate.

**Post-hoc analysis** An evaluation of a previously undesignated hypothesis using the data already collected from a clinical study.

**Pragmatic trials** Measure effectiveness or the benefit of interventions under real-world conditions; may be referred to as *naturalistic randomized control trials*.

**Precision** The relative proximity to one another of multiple measurements of an actually identical characteristic or value.

**Presubmission inquiry** The process of contacting a journal prior to manuscript submission to inquire about the suitability of a manuscript topic.

**Prevalence** All of the cases (new and existing) or events in the population in a given time frame.

**Prevalence-incidence bias** A type of selection bias that can occur in studies in which cases that are mild and self-resolving and those that are rapidly fatal are not captured, resulting in a systematic failure to include these cases. Also referred to as *Neyman bias*.

**Primary literature** Written accounts of original thought or discovery directly derived from firsthand observation or research.

**Primary outcome** The main hypothesis under investigation in a clinical study. Also referred to as the *study objective*.

**Probability distribution** A visual representation of the probability that an event will or will not occur.

**Probability sampling** Any sampling technique that allows each member of the accessible population an equal chance of being selected for the actual study sample.

**Probability value** The value provided as a result from inferential statistical tests that represents the probability that the result was due to chance. Also known as *p*-value.

**Procedure selection bias** A type of selection bias that most commonly occurs when individual subjects are decidedly assigned to groups based on clinical judgment instead of being randomly assigned.

**Prospective cohort study** A study that follows a population from the present to the future, measuring characteristics periodically over time to determine possible risk and/or protective factors for a disease or outcome.

**Prospective study** A clinical study orientation that uses events that occur and data that are collected after the initiation of the study; prospective studies may be observational or interventional.

**Publication bias** A type of information bias that can occur as a result of the propensity against researchers submitting articles to biomedical journals describing negative studies for publication and the propensity for biomedical journal publishers to pass over such articles that are submitted in favor of publishing positive studies.

**Purposive sampling** A nonprobability sampling technique in which subjects are nonrandomly chosen to achieve a predefined study population.

**Qualitative variable** Used to describe data that can be classified into categories that are discrete.

**Quality improvement** Systematic and continuous actions that lead to measurable improvement in healthcare services and the health status of targeted patient groups.

**Quantitative variable** An outcome that is represented by a number. Also referred to as a *continuous variable*.

**Quota sampling** A type of purposive sampling accomplished by choosing participants based on a fixed quota, which can be either proportional, resulting in equal numbers of subjects between groups, or disproportional, in which one group will have more participants than the other in a fixed ratio, and in which the formation of groups and selection of subjects are based on predefined criteria and characteristics.

**Random allocation** A subject allocation process that ensures that all subjects have the same chance of being assigned to a study or control group in an unpredictable manner. Also referred to as *randomization*.

**Random effects meta-analysis** A more conservative meta-analytic method that allows for the true effect size of a treatment to vary between studies analyzed and allows for the influence of variation due to random chance.

**Random sampling** The most basic form of probability sampling in which each member of the accessible population is available for selection to be included in the study sample with equal chances of selection.

**Randomization** A subject allocation process that ensures that all subjects have the same chance of being assigned to a study or control group in an unpredictable manner. Also referred to as *random allocation*.

**Randomized controlled trial** A prospective study that randomizes patients to an intervention or control group to determine efficacy and safety of an intervention within a specific population; commonly considered the gold standard for clinical trials.

**Ratio data** A type of quantitative data where there is an absolute zero.

**Recall bias** A type of information bias that can occur when subjects are asked to remember events from the past.

**Receive** The interactive process of accepting a drug information question from a requestor.

**Record** Documenting the drug information process for quality assurance purposes.

**Refereeing** The process of conducting peer review.

**Reference bias** A type of information bias that can occur when a published article cites only references that do not accurately represent the entire body of knowledge on the topic.

**Reference point** The point of no difference between treatments in statistical comparisons. In absolute comparisons, the reference point is 0; in relative comparisons, it is 1.

**Regression** Used to predict the value of one variable (response or outcome variable) based on the value of one or more other variables (predictor or explanatory variables).

**Regression coefficient** A coefficient used in a regression model that represents the amount of change in one variable ($y$) for each unit change in a second variable ($x$). May be referred to as a regression constant in a regression model and is analogous to the slope of a straight line. Represented by $b_1$ or $\beta_1$ for samples and populations, respectively.

**Regression model** An equation that allows for the prediction of the value of one variable based the value of one or more other variables. For linear regression, the model is $Y = \beta_0 + \beta_1 X + \cdots + \beta_k X_k$. For logistic regression, the model is $Y = 1 \div [1 + e^{-(\beta_0 + \beta_1 X + \cdots + \beta_k X_k)}]$.

**Relative risk** The risk of an event occurring in the exposed group compared to the control group. Also known as the *risk ratio*.

**Relative risk reduction** One minus the relative risk; expressed as a percentage.

**Repeatability** The degree of agreement that exists when the same individual uses an instrument to make multiple measurements of the same value under the same conditions. Also referred to as *test-retest reliability*.

**Repeated measures ANOVA** A statistical test used when an outcome is studied in the same individual but under different conditions or multiple time periods.

**Requestor** An individual who requires assistance to answer a drug information question.

**Research** Reviewing appropriate drug information and medical resources to inform the final drug information response.

**Respond** Communicating a formal recommendation directly to the requestor.

**Response bias** A type of information bias that can occur when subjects respond to questions in a way that they believe the researcher wishes them to answer, rather than in a truthful way.

**Retrospective cohort study** A study that looks at data on characteristics and outcomes that have already been collected on a population in order to determine possible risk and/or protective factors for a disease or outcome.

**Retrospective power** The actual power of a statistical test as calculated by using the actual sample size and data values that were collected in a study, as opposed to the sample size and data values that were predicted; useful when a null hypothesis has not been rejected.

**Retrospective study** A clinical study orientation that uses events that occurred and data that were collected before the initiation of the study.

**Rhetorical bias** A type of information bias that can occur when authors of scientific literature use language and innuendo to lead the reader to a conclusion that is not supported by evidence.

**Root cause analysis** A method to identify active and latent failures that contributed to an error once an error or near miss is identified.

**Safety analysis** An evaluation of the risks associated with an intervention in a clinical study.

**Sample** A relatively small group that is chosen from a larger population and that is assumed to be a fair representation of that population.

**Sample size** The number and distribution of subjects used in a clinical study, which affects the study's statistical power.

**Sample size bias** A type of information bias that occurs because too few or too many subjects than are appropriate are included in the study.

**Sampling** The process of identifying a sample.

**Scale degradation bias** A type of information bias that can occur when data are not analyzed in the most specific and precise manner possible.

**Scatterplot** A graphical representation of the relationship between two variables; the value of one variable is graphed against the value of a second variable.

**Secondary outcome** A hypothesis under investigation in a clinical study that is important enough to alter the design of the study, but that is not the main hypothesis under investigation.

**Secondary resources** Resources that index or abstract the primary literature and are used to locate pertinent primary literature.

**Selection bias** Any type of bias that causes a systematic difference between the probability of choosing or assigning one individual from the target population and the probability of choosing or assigning another individual from the same population.

**Sensitivity** The ability of a test to indicate the presence of disease when the patient has the disease; a measure of "true positives."

**Simple random sampling** A probability sampling technique that is accomplished by enumerating all possible selections from the accessible population and choosing numbers at random to obtain a sample.

**Simple randomization** A randomization technique in which subjects are assigned to groups with a known and equal probability.

**Single-blind trial** An interventional study design in which only one group of participants, either the investigators or subjects, is unaware of group assignment.

**Skewed distribution** A distribution that is not symmetric about the middle of the curve.

**Specificity** The ability of a test to correctly recognize those without a disease; a measure of "true negatives."

**Standard of care** The interventions that should be made by a clinician in the course of caring for an individual with a specific condition or circumstance.

**Standard deviation** A measure of dispersion around the mean for interval or ratio-level data that are normally or near-normally distributed; expressed mathematically as the square root of the variance.

**Standard error of the mean** The theoretical mean of all the potential samples from a given population.

**Standards of practice** In health care, practice standards serve as guideposts for a profession and as a way of communicating to peers, patients, policy makers, other professionals, and the public the roles and responsibilities of members of the profession. Practice standards also provide a benchmark for evaluating the quality of services and patient care.

**Standardized regression coefficient** A regression coefficient that has been rescaled, or standardized, to allow for direct comparison of the contributions of each variable to the regression model. Standardization is based on standard deviation units.

**Starting time bias** A subtype of detection bias that can occur when subject entry times significantly differ between groups. Also referred to as *entry time bias*.

**Statistical power** The probability of a statistical test to detect a statistically significant difference when one truly exists; usually calculated with predicted data when planning a clinical study to determine the sample size required; may also be calculated retrospectively with actual observed data when a null hypothesis has not been rejected.

**Statistical significance** The circumstance of having a relatively low probability of having committed a type I error; conventionally, when the calculated *p*-value is equal to or less than the prespecified and accepted alpha value.

**Statistically significant difference** A difference between groups that cannot be attributed to chance alone, but rather to a specific cause (e.g., treatment, patient characteristics, etc.). It is generally present when a null hypothesis is rejected.

**Stratified random sampling** A probability sampling technique in which all members of the accessible population are divided into homogenous groups by specified characteristics (e.g., gender or race) and then randomly selecting individuals from the divided groups, allowing for the characteristic to be fairly represented and even distributed.

**Stratified randomization** A randomization technique that attempts to balance groups with regard to one or more specific characteristics.

**Student's *t*-test** A statistical test used to evaluate two independent groups with continuous data.

**Study group** The group in a clinical study in which subjects will receive the intervention under investigation. Also referred to as the *active treatment group*.

**Study hypothesis** The proposed circumstance in a clinical study in which the independent variable does affect the dependent variable. Also referred to as the *alternative hypothesis*.

**Study objective** The main hypothesis under investigation in a clinical study. Also referred to as the *primary outcome*.

**Study orientation** The position in time of an investigation relative to when the data for the investigation are collected; study orientation may be retrospective, prospective, or instantaneous.

**Study population** The individual subjects actually included in a clinical study.

**Subgroup analysis** An evaluation of the certain results of a clinical study in a subset of subjects who share a specific characteristic.

**Subject allocation** The process of assigning enrolled subjects into study groups, which may be random or nonrandom.

**Subjectivity** The amount of interpretation required in taking a measurement, which directly affects the precision of the instrument or method used to take the measurement.

**Sunk costs** Costs that have occurred in the past.

**Superiority study** A clinical study that endeavors to determine if an intervention is better than no intervention or another intervention with regard to an outcome of interest; superiority studies may be one or two sided.

**Superiority testing** Statistical testing that aims to detect whether an intervention is better than a comparator.

**Surrogate outcome** An outcome that, although less meaningful than a direct outcome, is more convenient to measure than the direct outcome and is a suitable substitute for the direct outcome because it has been shown to predict or be otherwise associated with the direct outcome.

**Systematic review** Identification, evaluation, and synthesis of existing evidence on a particular topic in order to provide increased power and precision of the efficacy and safety of an intervention.

**Systematic sampling** A probability sampling technique in which the sample is chosen by using a preidentified sampling interval and a randomly selected starting point.

**Systems approach** Response to human error that considers errors to be the result of a culmination of many system weaknesses or failures.

**Target population** A smaller portion of a larger population that is identified by investigators in which to test a clinical question.

**Temporal truth** The state of reality as it exists in a population at a single instant in time, which clinical research endeavors to identify and quantify.

**Tertiary literature** General or specialized information gathered from primary and secondary literature. Examples include textbooks, reference books and databases, monographs, and review articles.

**Tertiary outcome** A hypothesis under investigation in a clinical study that is exploratory in nature and that is generally not important enough to significantly alter the design of the study.

**Test–retest reliability** The degree of agreement that exists when the same individual uses an instrument to make multiple measurements of the same value under the same conditions. Also referred to as *repeatability*.

**Therapeutic alternative** Drug products with different chemical structures but of the same pharmacologic and/or therapeutic class.

**Tracer methodology** An evaluation method in which surveyors select a patient, resident, or client and use that individual's record as a roadmap to move through an organization to assess and evaluate the organization's compliance with selected standards and the organization's systems of providing care and services.

**Triple-blind trial** An interventional study design in which all participants, including investigators, subjects, and data analysts, are unaware of group assignments.

**True negative** An accurate measurement in which a nonexisting condition is identified as being absent.

**True positive** An accurate measurement in which an existing condition is identified as being present.

**Two-sided superiority study** A clinical study that allows for determination of favor of either of two interventions relative to the other. Also referred to as a *two-tailed superiority study*.

**Two-tailed superiority study** A clinical study that allows for determination of favor of either of two interventions relative to the other. Also referred to as a *two-sided superiority study*.

**Type I error** Erroneously rejecting the null hypothesis; a false positive result.

**Type II error** Falsely accepting a null hypothesis; a false negative result.

**Type III error** An error in which a meaningful difference between groups is observed for an outcome when the opposite difference actually does or would exist in the population.

**Ultimate question** The true drug information question to which the pharmacist will respond.

**Unblinding** The circumstance in which a study participant, such as an investigator, subject, or data analyst, who was intended to be held unaware of a subject's group assignment, intentionally or unintentionally becomes aware of the group to which a subject was assigned.

**Unmasking bias** A type of information bias that can occur when an inciting condition that is unrelated to a condition of interest creates a situation in which the condition of interest is more likely to be discovered.

**Validation** The process by which the precision and accuracy of an instrument are determined.

**Variance** A measure of the spread of data, based on the distance of an individual data point from its mean.

**Virtual journal club** A self-directed approach to a journal club in which participants with common interests in different locations can discuss published research in real time, and have asynchronous discussions, within an electronic environment format.

**Volunteer effect** The propensity for systematic differences to exist between individuals more open to participating in research and those less willing to participate in research.

**Wilcoxon rank sum** A statistical test, used when there are two independent samples, that compares the distribution of ranked results between the groups.

**Wilcoxon signed rank** A statistical test, used when paired ordinal or non-normally distributed continuous data are being compared.

**Withdrawal bias** A subtype of missing data bias that occurs as the result of a disproportionate number of subjects between groups or high numbers of subjects in all groups discontinuing their participation in a study.

**$y$-intercept** A constant in a regression model that represents the theoretical value of $y$ and when $x = 0$; represented by $b_0$ or $\beta_0$ for samples and populations, respectively.

# INDEX

**Note:** Page numbers followed by *b, f,* and *t* indicate material in boxes, figures, and tables respectively.